Sports Injury
Prevention &
Rehabilitation

Sports Injury
Prevention &
Rehabilitation

Eric Shamus, PhD, PT, CSCS

Sports Medicine Track Coordinator
Masters of Medical Science
Assistant Professor of Physical Therapy
Nova Southeastern University
Fort Lauderdale, Florida

Jennifer Shamus, PhD, MSPT, CSCS

HealthSouth Foot and Ankle, and Running Instructor
HealthSouth Orthopedic Clinical Specialist
Site Coordinator
HealthSouth Sports Medicine and Rehabilitation Center
Fort Lauderdale, Florida

McGraw-Hill

MEDICAL PUBLISHING DIVISION

New York Chicago San Francisco Lisbon London Madrid Mexico City
Milan New Delhi San Juan Seoul Singapore Sydney Toronto

McGraw-Hill

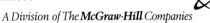

A Division of The McGraw·Hill Companies

Sports Injury Prevention and Rehabilitation

1234567890 DOCDOC 0987654321

ISBN: 0-07-135475-1

This book was set in Aster by Pine Tree, Inc.
The editors were Martin J. Wonsewicz, Stephen Zollo, Susan R. Noujaim, and Peter J. Boyle.
The production supervisor was Clara B. Stanley.
The cover designer was Elizabeth Schmitz; the interior designer was Robert Freese.
The index was prepared by Patricia Perrier.
R. R. Donnelley & Sons was printer and binder.

This book is printed on acid-free paper.

Cataloging-in-publication data is on file for this book at the Library of Congress.

*This book is dedicated to
OUR PARENTS
for their love, support,
and guidance.*

Contents

Contributors

Clive E. Brewster, MS, PT
Area Manager and Coordinator
HealthSouth Sports Medicine and
Rehabilitation Center
Los Angeles, California
Chapter 2

William W. Briner, MD
Family Practice
Lutheran General Hospital
Park Ridge, Illinois
Chapter 4

George J. Davies, MEd, PT, SCS, ATC,
CSCS
Professor, Physical Therapy
Graduate Physical Therapy Program
University of Wisconsin-La Crosse
Director of Clinical and Research Services
Gunderson Lutheran Sports Medicine
La Crosse, Wisconsin
Chapter 15

David M. Drexler, DO
Family Practice
Lutheran General Hospital
Park Ridge, Illinois
Chapter 4

Chris Durall, MS, PT, ATC, CSCS
Sports Physical Therapy Resident
Gunderson Lutheran Sports Medicine
Graduate Faculty
University of Wisconsin-La Crosse
Onalaska, Wisconsin
Chapter 15

Dennis Fater, PhD, PT, CSCS
Associate Professor, Physical Therapy
Graduate Physical Therapy Program
University of Wisconsin
La Crosse, Wisconsin
Staff Physical Therapy
Gunderson Lutheran Sports Medicine
Onalaska, Wisconsin
Chapter 15

Bill Foran, MS, CSCS
Strength and Conditioning Coach
Miami Heat
Miami, Florida
Chapter 13

John P. Frappier, MS
Medical Advisory Board
US Association of Independent
Gymnastics Clubs
Physical Therapy Faculty
University of North Dakota
School of Medicine
President, Acceleration Products
Fargo, North Dakota
Chapter 1

Suzanne Gasse, PT, ATC, CSCS
Area Administrator
HealthSouth Sports Medicine and
Rehabilitation Center
Fort Lauderdale, Florida
Chapter 14

Paul R. Geisler, MA, ATC/L
Instructor and Program Director
Sports Medicine and Athletic Training
Department of Health and Kinesiology
Georgia Southern University
Statesboro, Georgia
Founder and Owner, KineticGolf
Program
Chapter 7

Brian R. Hoke, PT, SCS
Adjunct Faculty
Old Dominion University
Norfolk, Virginia
Touro College
Bay Shore, New York
Physical Therapist, Sports Clinical
Specialist
Atlantic Physical Therapy, PC
Virginia Beach, Virginia
Chapter 9

Jane Jarosz-Hlis, PT, CSCS
Site Coordinator
HealthSouth Sports Medicine and
Rehabilitation Center
USPTA Certified Teaching Professional
Plantation, Florida
Chapter 3

William Kelleher, PhD
Associate Professor
Center for Psychological Studies
Director, Community Clinic for Older
Adults
Coordinator, Clinical Health Psychology
Concentration for the PhD and PsyD
Nova Southeastern University
Fort Lauderdale, Florida
Chapter 13

Susan Lefever-Button, MA, PT, ATC
President
San Juan Physical Therapy
Friday Harbor, Washington
Chapter 16

Moira N. McPherson, PhD
Associate Professor
School of Kinesiology
Lakehead University
Thunder Bay, Ontario, Canada
Chapter 11

Karen J. Mohr, PT, SCS
Research Director
Kerlan-Jobe Orthopedic Clinic
Los Angeles, California
Chapter 2

William J. Montelpare, PhD
Associate Professor
School of Kinesiology
Lakehead University
Thunder Bay, Ontario, Canada
Chapter 11

Megan Neyer, PhD LPC, NCC
Director
Total Performance Systems
Decatur, Georgia
Director of Sports Psychology Services,
United States Diving
1980 Olympian 3 Meter and 10 Meter
1982 World Champion
15 Time US National Champion, 8 Time
NCAA Champion
Chapter 6

Neil Purves, MSc
Research Associate
School of Kinesiology
Lakehead University
Thunder Bay, Ontario, Canada
Chapter 11

Jonathan C. Reeser, MD, PhD
Department of Physical Medicine
Marshfield Clinic
Marshfield, Wisconsin
Chapter 4

Eric Shamus, PhD, PT, CSCS
Sports Medicine Track Coordinator
Masters of Medical Science
Assistant Professor of Physical Therapy
Nova Southeastern University
Fort Lauderdale, Florida
Chapter 13

Jennifer Shamus, PhD, PT, CSCS
HealthSouth Foot and Ankle, and
Running Instructor
HealthSouth Orthopedic Clinical
Specialist
Site Coordinator
HealthSouth Sports Medicine and
Rehabilitation Center
Fort Lauderdale, Florida
Preface

Charles Shapiro, MEd, PT
Assistant Professor of Physical Therapy
Nova Southeastern University
Fort Lauderdale, Florida
Chapter 5

Kirsten Snellenburg, MPT, LMT
1990–1996 International Olympic Coach,
US Windsurfing Team
1989–1993 US Sailing Team
St. Petersburg, Florida
Chapter 8

J. Richard Steadman, MD
Executive Director
Steadman-Hawkins Sports Medicine
Foundation
Vail, Colorado
Physician, United States Olympic Ski
Team
Chapter 10

Stephen C. Swanson, MS
Biomechanist
Institute for Sport Science and Medicine
The Orthopedic Specialty Hospital
Chair, Technology Sciences
Sixth IOC World Congress on Sports
Science and Medicine
Research Director
Acceleration Products
Salt Lake City, Utah
Chapter 1

Michael R. Torry, PhD
Director, Biomechanics Research
Laboratory
Steadman-Hawkins Sports Medicine
Foundation
Vail, Colorado
Chapter 10

Brian J. Tovin, MMSc, PT, SCS, ATC,
FAAOMPT
Clinic Director
The Sports Rehabilitation Center at
Georgia Tech
Director of Rehabilitation
Georgia Sports Medicine
Atlanta, Georgia
Head Athletic Trainer for Aquatics Sports,
1996 Olympic Games
Former Staff Trainer, United States
Diving Team
Chapter 6

Ryan P. Vermillion, BEd, PT, ATC
Director of Rehabilitation
Associate Athletic Trainer
Washington Redskins, Ltd
Chapter 12

Preface

Most healthcare practitioners at some point in their careers have been asked to evaluate an injured athlete. Understanding the sport in which an athlete participates contributes greatly to accurate diagnosis and treatment of injury. This was the inspiration for the book *Sports Injury Prevention and Rehabilitation*. It is the purpose of this book to familiarize healthcare practitioners with the biomechanics of several popular sports and how they relate to the prevention and rehabilitation of common injuries.

Each chapter covers one sport and is written by one or more experts on that sport. The authors describe the biomechanics of the basic skills performed. Then the components of injury prevention are discussed. These include recommendations for warm-up, stretching, and strengthening programs. In season and out of season periodization concepts are also reviewed. Common intrinsic and extrinsic risk factors are explained with the assumption that injury prevention is the first step in decreasing the incidence and severity of injury.

Despite the best designed athletic programs, injuries will occur. The injuries most frequently sustained are described in each chapter. Rehabilitation tips are offered, including how to protect an injured area and decrease inflammation, how to restore range of motion, and how to increase strength and proprioception. Sport-specific drills and specific criteria for a safe return to the sport are included as well.

Sports Injury Prevention and Rehabilitation will lend insight to any healthcare provider who comes in contact with an athlete, whether recreational or professional or somewhere in-between. This book will provide the tools necessary for providing the most efficient and effective training programs and rehabilitation. This book will also bring the team of qualified coaches, athletic trainers, orthopedic surgeons, and physical therapists to the top of their game.

—Jennifer Shamus

Acknowledgements

We would like to thank and acknowledge all of the individuals who contributed to this book. Without their expertise and dedication, this book would not have been possible.

Special thanks to Steve Zollo and the McGraw-Hill staff for their never ending help and encouragement.

And we cannot forget to thank the many athletes that challenged and inspired us and encouraged us to share this knowledge with others.

CHAPTER 1

Biomechanics: An Interdisciplinary Tool

Stephen C. Swanson

John P. Frappier

Introduction and Historical Perspective

Human movement has long fascinated scientists, clinicians, philosophers, and artists. Some of the greatest minds in history have expressed an interest in describing and understanding human motion. The famous Greek philosopher Aristotle (384–322 B.C.), the Roman physician Galen (131–201 A.D.), the brilliant Leonardo da Vinci (1452–1519), and Italian scientist Giovanni Borelli (1608–1679) all provided detailed and insightful descriptions of human movement and functional anatomy.[3] Although these descriptions were purely qualitative, the astute observations and attention to detail were similar in many ways to modern biomechanics. The similarities lie in the fact that their descriptions were rooted in a desire to better understand the human body as a whole, either from a biologic perspective or from an artist's need to better represent human movement in paintings and sculpture. In either case, human movement analysis was used as a tool to provide better understanding of the questions at hand.

The dawn of modern biomechanics coincided with the development of measurement tools that allowed the analyses to become quantitative. The advent of the motion picture camera allowed scientists and photographers to investigate details of human motion that go beyond the capacity of the naked eye. In addition, innovative techniques for recording ground reaction forces and displacements, as well as more precise time measurements, facilitated some of the first studies that could be classified as biomechanics or even exercise science. Nobel prize winner A. V. Hill, a physiologist who many consider to be the "father" of modern exercise science, integrated physiologic and mechanical measures to provide valuable insight into the mechanics of muscle contraction, energy expenditure, and the efficiency of distance running and to create the first description of the velocity curve in sprinting.[13,18] Wallace Fenn, one of Hill's students in physiology, used similar instrumentation to pioneer calculation of the work done by the body against gravity as well as an estimation of the work done by individual segments.[10,11] Herbert Elftman, a biologist, conducted the first true "biomechanics" study using mechanical principles to estimate the contribution of muscles during the motion sequences recorded by Fenn.[7–9] The preceding works again demonstrate that biomechanics can best be described as an interdisciplinary tool used by physiologists, engineers, biologists, and artists.

The advancement and widespread use of high-speed film in the 1960s and early 1970s facilitated publication of biomechanical research studies related to sports. Refinement in instrumentation techniques using newly available microelectronics devices resulted in improved measurements of force, acceleration, muscle activity, and physiologic parameters. For the first time, detailed descriptions of the movements, forces, and metabolic characteristics of athletes during different activities were made available to clinicians and researchers. Thus the fields of sports medicine and sport science began to grow and assemble a body of literature and associated professional societies. College curricula for students in physical therapy, coaching, medicine, physiology, and exercise science started to include classes in biomechanics and kinesiology. The study of human movement became an integral part of the preparation of professionals in many areas.

Over the last 25 to 30 years, the proliferation of sports medicine and sport science literature related to human movement has been phenomenal. For the sports medicine professional, modern biomechanics research can be especially helpful in understanding injury mechanisms, prescription of rehabilitation programs, performance enhancement, and improved athletic equipment. However, the level of detail in many biomechanics research studies may be beyond the needs of the clinician. Thus the clinician has the daunting task of sorting through the immense amount of

research literature generated each year and deciding what is relevant for improving the level of care given to a patient or athlete following an injury. Hopefully, this text will be helpful in providing both an overview of the detailed biomechanics associated with a broad range of sports and suggested techniques for effective rehabilitation.

Kinesiology or Biomechanics?

Among movement scientists and clinicians, there is often disagreement over the use of the terms *kinesiology* and *biomechanics*. The word *kinesiology* is a combination of the Greek *kinein* meaning "to move" and *logos* meaning "discourse." Kinesiologists—those who discourse on movement—combine anatomy (the science of body structure) with physiology (the science of body function) to produce kinesiology, the science of movement of the body.

Kinesiology has long been used an umbrella term to describe any form of anatomic, physiologic, psychological, or mechanical human movement evaluation. Therefore, kinesiology has been used by several disciplines to describe many different content areas. A class in kinesiology may consist primarily of functional anatomy at one university and strictly biomechanics at another. Typically, a kinesiology course has been part of college curricula in physical education, exercise science, athletic training, and physical therapy programs. These courses usually focus on the musculoskeletal system, movement efficiency from an anatomic standpoint, and joint and muscular actions during simple and complex movements. A successful student in a kinesiology course could identify discrete phases in an activity, describe the segmental movements occurring in each phase, and then identify the major muscular contributors to each joint movement. Thus a kinesiologic analysis of the movement of a vertical jump would be as follows: The movements would be hip extension via the gluteus maximus and hamstrings, knee extension via the quadriceps femoris, and plantarflexion via the gastrocnemius-soleus complex. Such an analysis is considered qualitative because it involves the observation of movement and identification of the muscular contributions to that movement.

In the last 30 to 40 years, biomechanics has been developed as an area of study within undergraduate and graduate curricula throughout the world. The contents of biomechanics include a marriage of the areas of applied physics or mechanics and biology. Mechanics, the study of the effect of forces on an object and the resulting motions, is used by engineers to design and build structures or machines because it provides the tools for analyzing the strength of structures and methods for predicting and measuring the movement of a machine. Since it is natural to apply mechanics to the movements and structures of living organisms, the term *biomechanics* was created.

A biomechanical analysis evaluates the motion of a living organism and also may examine the forces responsible for the observed motion. Biomechanical analyses can be qualitative or quantitative, whereas a kinesiologic analysis would be strictly qualitative. Thus a biomechanical analysis of the vertical jump might include a qualitative description of the movement (similar to the kinesiologic analysis) in addition to the following: measurement of the forces between the person's feet and the floor: quantification of the joint angles at the hip, knee, and ankle; calculation of the joint forces acting at each joint; and the amount of muscle activity in specific muscles.

Each of the chapters in this book includes biomechanical analyses of a specific activity, since each describes certain movement characteristics and muscle activity *both* quantitatively and qualitatively, as available in the literature. More research is necessary before the biomechanics of every sport are fully understood. Clinicians today typically have several measurement tools—isokinetic/isovelocity dynamometers, electromyography (EMG) units, goniometers, and video systems—that enable them to conduct biomechanical analyses daily within the rehabilitation environment. A thorough understanding of the biomechanics of injury mechanisms, aspects of individual sports, and treatment interventions is crucial to providing the standard of care expected in today's sports medicine environment.

Core Areas of Study

FUNCTIONAL ANATOMY

Anatomy, the science of body structure, is a core component from which expertise about human movement is developed. Clinicians find it very helpful to develop a strong understanding of the regional gross anatomy of each joint. Specific knowledge of the bones, ligaments, tendons, muscles, innervation, blood supply, etc. and *how each work together to form a functional system* is a vital component in understanding the basic biomechanics of that joint. Simply knowing the detailed anatomy of a certain joint is not enough to effectively understand the biomechanics of that joint, however.

Additional knowledge such as how the lever arm and length of each muscle change with joint angle (due to joint morphology, for example) and the subsequent effect on potential torque output is important in understanding the normal function and capabilities of a joint. Appreciation of the difference in the functions of single- and two-joint muscles is also an important aspect of functional anatomy. Adjacent joints may be affected and functionally related to one another due to the effects of corresponding two-joint muscles.[21] Cadaver studies examining the physical and morphologic properties of muscle, bone, and connective tissue have proven to be especially valuable in our understanding of functional anatomy.[12,19]

For example, the length of the hamstrings is more affected by changes in hip angle than by changes in knee angle[13] because of the large change in the hamstring lever arm at the hip with increasing hip flexion. Thus the hamstrings, a two-joint muscle responsible for hip extension and knee flexion, are the largest contributor to hip extension torque at hip angles of greater than 50 degrees.[13] A good biomechanist may then realize that the hamstrings may be more susceptible to injury due to high forces and/or excessive stress during movements with excessive hip flexion. The authors of each of the chapters of this book provide excellent descriptions of the functional anatomy of specific joints related to each sport.

KINEMATICS

The term *kinematics* is used to describe analyses related to motion characteristics only. A kinematic analysis examines the motion from both a spatial and temporal perspective, without any reference to the forces causing the observed motion. Thus the components of interest in a kinematic analysis are an object's position, velocity, and acceleration. There are essentially two aspects of kinematic analysis—linear and angular kinematics. *Linear kinematics* deals with motion of an object or segment along a straight or curved pathway. An example of linear kinematics is the path of an athlete's center of mass during a high jump or the trajectory of a baseball following release from a pitcher's hand. Such a motion is typically termed a *translation* or *translational motion*. *Angular*

kinematics describes the motion of an object or segment around some point where different regions of that object or segment do not move through the same distance. A good example of angular kinematics is that of the tibia during knee extension. As the knee extends from 90 degrees of flexion to full extension (0 degrees), the medial malleolus (distal end, near the foot) travels a much greater distance than the tibial tuberosity (medial end, near the knee) because the malleolus is farther away from the knee, or point of rotation.

Almost all aspects of human motion and the motion of projectiles propelled by humans are a result of a combination of linear and angular kinematics. In fact, most linear movements of humans occur primarily as a result of different combinations and aspects of angular motion. For example, the angular kinematics of the hip, knee, and ankle during one stride of sprint running results in the linear motion of the center of mass of the body. Through examination of a movement kinematically, one can break a complex skill down into identifiable parts, compare certain aspects with a "normal" movement or that of an expert performer, and identify possible problems in the execution of that skill—even at the segmental level. Such a detailed analysis would not be possible with the human eye—even for a very trained observer. A detailed kinematic analysis of each sport becomes invaluable in gaining helpful insight into rehabilitation specific to that sport.

The complex skill of a baseball pitch is a great example of how kinematic analyses are necessary in developing a greater understanding of the biomechanics of pitching. Qualitative comparison of a high school pitcher versus a major league pitcher may reveal only a few differences in general motion. Even well-trained observers such as professional scouts use equipment such as radar guns and video cameras in evaluating the potential of a prospect. However, a detailed kinematic analysis of the high school and major league pitchers undoubtedly would reveal several differences. The angles of the shoulder, elbow, and wrist may differ dramatically in relation to each other. The angular velocity of the high school pitcher's wrist may not reach its peak at the moment of release of the baseball—as the major league pitcher's does—indicating an inability to transfer the momentum of the lower extremity, trunk, and proximal segments to the wrist at the optimal time. None of these subtle differences could be recognized without the use of an advanced kinematic analysis.

One of the important benefits of kinematic analyses is that the coordination of entire limbs and even the whole body can be examined in great detail. Kinematic analyses of a single joint typically are limited in their value to the clinician or health professional. Studies including multijoint kinematics are far more useful than those focusing on a single joint.[20] In almost all movements, the motion of one joint is closely related to and affected by the movement of its adjacent segments and joints. For example, some researchers have shown that the relative timing of movements between segments and joints is more useful in understanding injury mechanisms than certain discrete variables associated with the movement.[15] The genesis of most injuries and related rehabilitation problems can be identified by subtle changes in segmental, joint, or whole-body kinematics. Thus clinicians always should consider the interaction of adjacent segments and joints as well as the overall objective of the movement.

Finally, it should be stressed that kinematics typically is the most essential aspect of any biomechanical analysis. Although one also must consider the forces, muscle activity, and basic functional anatomy of the structures associated with the movement to fully understand the related biomechanics, none of the preceding parameters is useful without the kinematics. As you continue to read through the following sections on ki-

netic analyses and electromyography, be cognizant of the importance of the underlying kinematics in understanding these measures.

KINETICS

Force and Torque

Kinetics is a complex area of study that examines the forces acting on a system such as an object or the human body. Primarily using Newtonian physics (force = mass × acceleration), a kinetic analysis calculates the forces that must have been present to cause the observed movement. It must be remembered that forces cannot be seen; only the *effect* of forces can be observed. A kinetic analysis can provide a biomechanist with valuable information about how a movement was produced, the loads and stresses placed on the body or external objects at certain points in the movement, or how a certain position can be maintained.

Kinetic analyses, as with kinematics, have both linear and angular components. To review, forces are vectors in that they have both a magnitude and direction, and they may be applied to an object or segment at any point on its surface. If a force is applied directly through the center of mass of an object, then that object—depending on the magnitude of the force—may or may not undergo a translation or linear motion. If the force is not applied directly through the center of mass of the object, that object may undergo a rotation or torque. *Torque*, also referred to as a *moment of force* or *moment* by engineers and biomechanists, is not a force but simply the effectiveness of a force in causing a rotation. Mathematically, torque is expressed

$$T = F \times r$$

where T is torque, F is applied force, and r is the perpendicular distance from the point of force application to the center of rotation of the object. The *lever arm*, or *moment arm*, refers to term r in the preceding equation.

The concepts of torque and moment arm are especially important in biomechanics because almost all muscles are responsible for generating torque about a joint. In addition, a muscle's corresponding moment arm typically will change with alterations in joint position. Thus, it can be seen why the corresponding kinematics is such an important aspect of a kinetic analysis.

Work and Power

The concepts of work and power are also important to a better understanding of kinetic analyses. *Work* is essentially the product of force and the distance an object or segment moves as a result of the application of a force.

$$\text{Work} = F \times \Delta d$$

Thus, if a 100-newton (N) force (F) is applied to an object and that object moves a distance (d) of 1 meter (m), the work done would be 100 N · m, as expressed below:

$$\text{Thus } 100 \text{ N} \times 1 \text{ m} = 100 \text{ N} \cdot \text{m, or } 100 \text{ J}$$

The standard unit for work is joules (J) and 1 N · m = 1 J. It also should be remembered that work can be either positive or negative, depending on the direction in which the object or segment is moved. Specifically, if an object is lifted up or pushed forward (depending on your frame of reference) from its starting point, then positive work is done. In contrast, if an object is lowered or pushed backward from its starting point, then negative work is done. These scenarios are the same for angular work (more typically associated with musculoskeletal mechanics) in that if a torque of 100 N · m causes a positive angular displacement of 1 radian (rad), the resulting angular work would be 100 N · m or 100 J of positive work. Remember that radians are dimensionless and have no units (1 radian is equivalent to 53 degrees).

Power is simply the rate of change of work, or work done per unit time. The standard unit for mechanical power is watts (W), where 1 W = 1 J/s. Thus, if 100 J of work is done in 0.5 s, the resulting power output during that time is 200 W, as expressed below:

$$P = \Delta w / \Delta t$$

Thus: 100 J/0.5 s = 200 J/s, or 200 W

where w is the amount of work in joules, and t is the change in time in seconds. Another definition or way to express power is force × velocity, or

$$P = F \times v$$

which was derived from simply rearranging the power equation, as indicated below:

$$P = \Delta(F \times d)/\Delta t \text{ to } P = F \times \Delta d/\Delta t$$

Power is essentially the combination of force and velocity. In many sports, the ability to use the combination of force and velocity is highly correlated with success. Timely and rapid generation of muscular power is often exhibited in such sports as golf, baseball, and football, where the ability to effectively strike an object or person is a prerequisite for success.

Examples of Applications of Kinetic Analyses

The application of the concepts of work and power to human motion also provides insight into how muscles are being used during a specific motion sequence.[2] Specifically, if a net hip flexor torque and a hip extension velocity (negative hip flexor power) are observed simultaneously, then it is likely that the hip flexors are working negatively or eccentrically. In contrast, a net hip flexor torque coupled with a hip flexion velocity would correspond to concentric or positive hip flexor work. Equilibrium, or zero velocity at a joint, indicates either passive or isometric muscular use. The typical usage pattern of the hip musculature revealed by a power analysis of the swing phase of running (toe-off to foot-strike) are as follows: eccentric hip flexion as indicated by a negative hip flexor power, concentric hip flexion (positive hip flexor power), eccentric hip extension (negative hip extensor power), and finally, concentric hip extension (positive hip extensor power).[31]

Another example of a useful application of kinetics is in quantifying load thresholds for certain structures in the body. Cadaver studies and finite-element modeling have been combined recently to provide insight into the loads, stresses, and strains that certain tissues in the body can withstand.[27] Such investigations basically involve a battery of material tests performed on a tissue such as a ligament. Once the material properties of the ligament have been described, the results are then used to create a computer model of the tissue. The model is used to estimate what the strain on the ligament may be under certain simulated movement conditions. The results are painstakingly tested so as to optimize the model and make it as realistic as possible. The beauty of this approach is that once the model is determined to be accurate, the computer can be used to simulate a myriad of movement conditions and/or the effect of a prosthetic device of known material properties. Such analyses provide much insight into the development of certain rehabilitation techniques, surgical procedures, and possible prosthetic materials for the joint.

One interesting finding from these studies is that the forces and torques placed on ligaments and other connective tissues during a dynamic human motion such as a normal baseball throw approach or even exceed the failure loads of some of the involved tissues found during laboratory testing.[12] A small deviation from "normal" throwing mechanics could result in dangerous loads being placed on these connective tissues—enough to cause a major injury. These findings illustrate the importance of the clinician's thorough understanding of the biomechanics of such activities so that such potential problems can be circumvented. For example, recognizing abnormal kinematics and kinetics during an assessment or in the rehabilitation process could alleviate a major injury in many cases.

Limitations of Kinetic Analyses

One technique biomechanists use to estimate muscular work and power during different motion sequences is inverse dynamics using a linked-segment model. Inverse dynamics basically means that you work backward from what you are given—you know all forces acting on the system and the observed motion characteristics. Thus you are able to use Newtonian physics to estimate the torques that must have been present at each joint in the system in order to cause the observed motion. In order to perform an inverse dynamics analysis using this linked-segment model, certain assumptions are made to simplify some of the problems associated with applying the principles of mechanics to human tissue. There are some limitations to these assumptions, and a health professional must take them into consideration when interpreting the results of a work and power analysis.[37]

The first assumption is that all segments are considered rigid segments—which means that they are considered to be as stiff as steel. We know from experience that our skeletal segments are somewhat compliant and definitely not rigid; thus the values during an impact situation may be somewhat larger than probably occur during the actual motion. The next flawed assumption is that our joints are modeled as frictionless pin joints. This we also know to be a bit of a stretch. The healthy knee, although it probably does not have a significant amount of friction owing to the large amounts of synovial fluid, definitely is not a pin joint. Finally, the assumption that provides the largest limitation is that the model does not take into account the existence of two-joint muscles or the torques that each individual muscle is able to contribute to the movement. The model is only able to estimate the net torque that must have occurred about a joint to cause the observed motion. Thus, if the knee is extended, there may have been a net knee extensor torque of 60 N · m. This does not provide insight into how much torque was exerted by the hamstrings to oppose the observed knee extension. The main reason for highlighting the limitations in the assumptions of the link-segment model is to allow better understanding in interpreting the results of energy calculations and descriptions of muscular use during dynamic movements. Findings from such analyses can be especially useful if the limitations of the technique are fully understood.

There are also limitations in the kinetic analyses associated with cadaver studies and computer simulations. It must be remembered that cadaver specimens are not always well controlled for age, gender, health at the time of death, etc., so the tissues being tested may vary widely. Also, laboratory testing conditions sometimes do not resemble actual in vivo conditions in the least; e.g., a failure load of the medial collateral ligament may have been done with no other knee ligaments intact or no simulated muscle forces—both conditions are very unrealistic.

As pointed out in the preceding paragraphs, kinetic analyses are difficult to perform accurately and realistically. This is mainly due to the complexity of the human body and the tendency of its tissues and structures to behave in a nonlinear manner. However, the additional insight garnered from various kinetic analyses is much too valuable to ignore. Detailed study of the forces that may be causing the observed motions allows us a much clearer vision of the biomechanics of the human body.

ELECTROMYOGRAPHY

Electromyography, abbreviated EMG, is the recording of the electrical activity of a muscle. EMG as a biomechanics tool has become increasingly popular in the last 20 years. As with kinetic analyses, EMG provides additional insight into the biomechanics of a certain movement sequence by providing an idea of the associated muscle activity. Also, EMG is basically useless unless it is combined with at least a kinematic analysis and preferentially an analysis including both kinematics and kinetics. In a nutshell, EMG can provide meaningful data regarding the timing and relative amplitude of muscle activity.

There are essentially two basic types of recording systems for EMG—surface and needle.[1] It is important to have a general understanding of the type of information garnered from each recording system in order to perform meaningful interpretation of EMG results. Surface EMG electrodes are fixed to the skin surface and record a signal that is the sum of the action potentials within the measuring range of the electrode—typically much of the muscle and possibly weaker signals from adjacent muscles. Needle EMG electrodes are actually inserted directly into the muscle and are able to record action potentials only a short distance from the insertion point. One obvious advantage to surface EMG is the noninvasiveness of the measure. In addition, the signal is the sum of most of the action potentials occurring in the muscle of interest, and as such, it is a better representation of the signal given to the muscle by the central nervous system. A disadvantage of surface EMG is that the signal is susceptible to interference and crosstalk from adjacent muscles. The main advantage of needle electrodes over surface electrodes is the capability to record EMG from very small muscles with little possibility of crosstalk. However, there are several disadvantages to needle electrodes in that the measure is invasive, time-intensive, and also does not provide a good representation as to the overall activity pattern of that muscle. In addition, it is very difficult to control the depth of insertion of the needle electrodes, so the signal may vary widely between insertions in the same people.

An important aspect to remember about EMG is that muscle activity *does not* correlate directly with external force development of the muscle.[23] Larger amplitudes of EMG do not necessarily mean that there is greater force development by that muscle. In fact, EMG activity is typically less during eccentric contractions when muscle forces are at their highest levels. Increasing amplitudes of EMG do indicate that the central nervous system (CNS) is evoking a greater number of motor units within the muscle to accomplish the corresponding contraction.[23] There is also substantial evidence that elite athletes show more discrete "bursts" of activity during skilled movements because their EMG patterns are more definite and concise with less cocontraction.[23] Most important, EMG provides us with accurate depictions of the coordination of muscle contraction during a given movement.

Scientists and clinicians alike should exercise great caution in the interpretation of EMG data during movement sequences. We have seen several common mistakes in the interpretation of EMG data—in both the research and clinical settings. The following are some basic guidelines for meaningful interpretation of EMG data:

1. Amplitude comparisons should only be done *within* a muscle *between* movement conditions. Comparisons of differences in amplitude between muscles should not be attempted—the signals are from two different recording surfaces.

2. Extreme care should be exercised when attempting to "normalize" EMG to a standard or maximum voluntary contraction in order to facilitate between-subject comparisons of EMG amplitude for the same muscle. Such comparisons are not recommended.

3. Amplitude or timing comparisons of any kind should not be attempted if an electrode falls off or has been moved—especially if the electrodes have been taken off between testing sessions on different days.

4. Burst timing comparisons relative to an event such as foot-strike can be done between muscles and subjects.

For more detailed descriptions of EMG interpretation and analysis, please refer to the excellent paper by Kamen and Caldwell[23] or Basmajian's text.[1]

MUSCULOSKELETAL MODELING TECHNIQUES

In the last 10 years, the proliferation of computer models of the human musculoskeletal system has been impressive. However, most researchers would still consider these models very developmental at best. These models attempt to incorporate all core areas of study into an accurate model of the human musculoskeletal system.[5,6,22,35] Most models include the realistic surfaces of the bones, the kinematics of the joints, and the lines of action and force-generating parameters of the muscles. Once the models are defined, the function of each muscle and relative contribution to the movement sequence can be analyzed by computing its length, moment arms, force, and joint moments.[6,22] The effect of the resulting motions and muscle actions on the connective tissue and articular surfaces of each segment also can be calculated. These models are particularly useful in that existing kinematic, kinetic, and EMG data from a selected movement sequence can be used to drive the model and thus estimate the relative contribution of each muscle group. In addition, the graphic nature of the models provides an extremely valuable tool for visualization of the kinematic, kinetic, and muscle activity associated with the selected motion. The sophistication of these models indicates a significant advancement over conventional biomechanical analysis techniques and has tremendous benefits for the clinician.

The benefits of these computer-based musculoskeletal models to the health science professional are far reaching. One of the more interesting capabilities of the software simulating outcomes from surgical procedures such as tendon transfers has been demonstrated.[5] Better understanding of the loads experienced by different muscle groups during selected motion sequences should hasten the development of improved sports rehabilitation programs. More detailed assessment of the efficacy of existing rehabilitation equipment and programs also has now become possible. Improvements in techniques to enhance performance also should follow this progression. Most important, the ability to present complex data in a simple manner to athletes, coaches, and non-research-oriented clinicians is incredibly valuable to both researchers and health professionals. An example of the model's visualization capabilities is presented in Fig. 1.1.

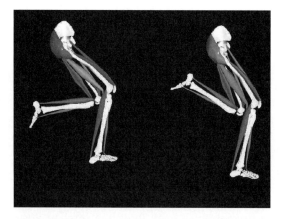

FIGURE 1.1

Musculoskeletal modeling software/visualization. Images generated using SIMM (Software for Interactive Musculoskeletal Modeling) Motion Analysis, Inc., Santa Rosa, CA.

As with the other areas of biomechanics, there are several limitations to today's musculoskeletal modeling techniques. The biggest challenges are in the areas of muscle mechanics. Muscle mechanics (and muscle modeling) has become a field of science in itself. Scientists specializing in muscle mechanics and muscle modeling have expertise in biomechanics, motor control, physiology, and computer science. One of their main goals is to develop more accurate computer models of human muscle. Although today's computer models of muscle do a fairly good job of simulating isometric and concentric contractions, there are few models that have been able to accurately simulate the mechanics of eccentric contraction.[22,25]

Clinical Biomechanics: An Integrated Approach

Just as Aristotle, da Vinci, and Borelli used biomechanics as a tool for improving their understanding of the human body, today's health professionals use their knowledge and the expertise of fellow colleagues in biomechanics to provide the best care possible to patients and athletes. Most sports medicine professionals are able to draw on the expertise of orthopedic surgeons, physical therapists, orthotists, kinesiologists, athletic trainers, exercise physiologists, and biomechanists to develop solutions to problems and provide the best care possible. Each of these professionals typically uses biomechanics as a tool to better understand the human body, much like some of the greatest scientists in history. The most effective professionals attempt to fully integrate and understand all aspects of the related biomechanics of the movement or skill of interest and effectively apply that knowledge to injury care, rehabilitation, and prevention.

The most insightful analyses of human movement are those that integrate all the core areas of biomechanics research. A thorough examination of the related kinematics, kinetics, and corresponding muscle functions associated with a movement or skill undoubtedly results in a more complete understanding of the biomechanics of the movement. However, there have been relatively few studies of biomechanics that incorporate such a full integration.[20–22,26,31] The musculoskeletal modeling, computer simulation, and motor control literature typically integrates the core areas well, but the movements are very basic and somewhat nonfunctional. Most of the biomechanics and related literature focuses on specific mechanisms or basic research. Although these investigations contribute much to the profession, the health professional is left to sort through an immense amount of research information just to decide what is relevant.

The authors of this book have done an outstanding job integrating the core areas of biomechanics of each sport of interest and provide an excellent foundation for improving rehabilitation methods and care.

RECENT ADVANCES IN BIOMECHANICS AND FUTURE DIRECTIONS

The field of biomechanics has gone through many metamorphoses during the last 30 to 40 years. The sophistication and accuracy of the measuring equipment have come a long ways since the days of Hill, Fenn, and Elftman. The accuracy of kinematic analyses approaches tenths of millimeters, and force measurements actually can reflect the beating of a person's heart while standing quietly on a force platform. Such accuracy levels have been available for over 10 years—a relatively long time in the young field of modern biomechanics.

The phenomenal growth of the computer industry and exponential increases in processing power over the last 10 years have particularly facilitated the proliferation of biomechanics literature. The computers on the desks of over 40 million people in the United States today have several times more processing power than the greatest supercomputers of the 1970s and early 1980s. Calculations that take today's biomechanists a few seconds would have a taken a few weeks to do in the 1970s on punch card–driven computers and possibly half a lifetime by hand, as Herbert Elftman did with his analyses. Such computing power allows us to examine a myriad of functional movement sequences and their associated muscular coordination patterns for much longer periods of time. Musculoskeletal modeling further facilitates this process by providing more insight into the actual functions of the muscles. Thus we are living in an exciting time for the field of biomechanics. In the following paragraphs we will outline some recent advances that we feel will have a substantial impact on the field of biomechanics.

Real-Time Motion Analysis

One of the most significant advancements in the field of motion analysis has been real-time capability. *Real-time motion analysis* basically means that the once laborious process of digitization, the computer-assisted process of converting the recorded motions of a segment or object into positional coordinates relative to a frame of reference, can be performed in a mere fraction of a second. As late as the early 1990s, biomechanists would have to examine each frame of a video or film recording and manually calculate the positional coordinates of each segment. A thorough kinematic analysis of one stride of motion sometimes would take weeks to complete. Advances in computer and optics technology eventually allowed the digitization process to become automated, but the actual kinematic analysis could not be performed until after a data-collection session.

The subsequent process was still very labor-intensive and time-consuming.

A combination of advanced computer software and algorithms, customized hardware, and high-speed processors allows these motion analysis systems to provide a researcher or clinician with the actual kinematic data and analysis as the data are collected. Some systems are even able to animate a computer model of the subject on a screen in front of the subject as he or she moves. The possibilities for enhanced biofeedback and virtual-reality training are phenomenal. da Vinci, Borelli, and Elftman would be thoroughly impressed.

A few of the high-end systems are able to fully integrate force measurements and EMG recordings, as well as musculoskeletal models, into the data-collection and analysis process. It is now theoretically possible to have the results of an integrated biomechanical analysis of a movement—kinematics, kinetics, EMG, even individual muscular force estimates—completed by the conclusion of the data-collection session. In addition, the improvements in data storage capacity and processing speed make it possible to collect integrated biomechanics data for extended periods of time—several minutes or even hours if necessary. For example, an integrated analysis of every footfall that occurs during a simulated 400-m—even a marathon—race could be examined. Thus more functional movements can be examined, and better insight into the intricacies of human motion can be gained.

Such technology has profound implications for biomechanics. Biomechanics finally can become the tool that clinicians and researchers have been waiting for—an efficient means of gaining insight into the complex nature of human motion. As more and more gait analysis laboratories and sports medicine facilities upgrade to this fascinating technology, the number of useful integrated biomechanical analyses undoubtedly will increase exponentially.

Field Studies

Another area of biomechanics that has benefited recently from improvements in technology has been the field of data-acquisition technology. It is now possible to perform fairly detailed integrated biomechanics analyses during actual field conditions. As you would imagine, there are several limitations to only performing research studies in the laboratory. For example, it is especially difficult to gain insight into the biomechanics of alpine skiing, skating, cross-country running, etc. in a laboratory. The nature of the movements cannot be replicated either accurately or at all in the laboratory. In the past, field studies were notoriously difficult to conduct—validity and accuracy of the investigation could always be questioned.

Several factors have resulted in improvements in the technology. They involve improvements either in sensing technology, related to miniaturization of a device without sacrificing accuracy, or in the means of data acquisition. Force, pressure, acceleration, and motion sensors have all been made portable. Telemetry, the method of transmitting data over long distances, allows for data from these sensors to be transmitted to a data-collection station with high fidelity. Thus patients or athletes do not have to be "wired" directly to the main acquisition system or actually carry a computer with them in the field. Telemetry vastly improves the freedom of movement of the subject and allows for a more realistic characterization of movement.

Another improvement related to but distinctly different from telemetry is the miniaturization of data-logging technology. As stated earlier, subjects would either have to be wired directly to the computer or carry the computer with them if telemetry were not possible. However, miniature data loggers (basically acquisition systems) have been developed that weigh only a few ounces. With the use of specialized storage devices, all the data basically can be collected into a "mini-computer" carried by the subject with little sacrifice in movement freedom. This technology even has some advantages over telemetry. Telemetered systems are sometimes subject to interference, their transmission distance can be limited, and the amount of data that can be transmitted can be inadequate.

A few examples of recent field studies that incorporate such data-logging technology are those of Greenwald et al.[14] and Strezing and Hennig.[30] Greenwald and his colleagues developed a portable system capable of collecting relative three-dimensional (3D) joint kinematics and EMG throughout an entire run of alpine skiing.[14] For the first time, 3D kinematic data were collected for more than one turn of alpine skiing—actually 40 to 50 turns per run. The sheer volume of data provides better insight into the actual coordination of skiing, since it is difficult to make conclusions from just one turn of data. Strezing and Hennig were able to using data-logging technology to collect rear-foot kinematics, in-shoe pressure, oxygen consumption, and shock-attenuation data at different intervals during a 10-km run on a track.[30] Their integrated analysis of the changes in foot mechanics, plantar pressures, and shock attenuation as the subjects became fatigued was particularly interesting.

Other technologies that are emerging into the world of field biomechanics are based on global positioning systems (GPSs). GPSs have been available to the public for quite some time and are particularly useful as a navigation aid. Using data from more than four satellites orbiting the earth, the GPS units provide users with their current position on the earth. The accuracy of the units available to the public was not good enough for even for basic biomechanics research (~50 ft due to military scrambling of the signal). In April 2000, the U.S. Department of Defense discontinued scrambling of GPS signals—improving the accuracy of a particular unit to 5 to 10

ft. Although this was a substantial and frankly amazing improvement, it is still not accurate enough to do more than very basic displacement and velocity calculations.[28] However, development is under way by several groups to integrate GPS units and other sensing technology such as gyroscopes and accelerometers that would improve the accuracy of the units to 1 cm. Although not yet available, a miniature GPS unit with such accuracy would mean that joint kinematics theoretically could be measured at any time anywhere on the earth. The implications for field research are obviously profound. Again, we are living in an interesting growth and maturation period for the field of biomechanics.

Dynamic Systems Approach

A relatively new approach to the analysis of biomechanical data is that of using techniques borrowed from the study of dynamic systems. These analysis techniques use higher-level mathematics (mostly calculus, differential equations, and chaos theory) to better understand, quantify, and predict the interactions of complex systems. These systems could be a complex machine, biologic habitat, or the basic coordination of human movement.[24] In relation to human motion, an analysis employing a dynamic systems approach will use measures that reflect the movement interactions between segments or between joint motions and a force measurement.[24,33,34]

One measurement approach, called *relative phase*, has been particularly useful in understanding the coordination of human movement. Relative-phase calculations take into consideration both the angular displacement and velocity of the segments or limbs of interest.[16,17,24,33,34] A relative-phase measurement can be either discrete (taken at a certain event) or continuous (taken throughout the movement sequence). The advantage of a relative-phase measure is that it reflects the interactions between the motion of different segments or joints throughout the movement sequence. Such a measurement technique has distinct advantages over traditional, more descriptive kinematic and kinetic analyses. A traditional biomechanics analysis will include discrete variables such as peak joint angle, peak joint angular velocity, time to peak joint angle, range of motion, etc. Often, it is very difficult for the researcher or clinician to interpret the physiologic meaning of these discrete variables. Also, these measures are sometimes not sensitive to subtle changes in coordination because they do not effectively take into consideration the movement characteristics of another segment or joint. Measurements based on relative phase are usually much more sensitive to these subtle changes because they incorporate the movement dynamics of multiple segments or joints.[16] In addition, examination of the variability of the relative-phase measures over prolonged periods (several minutes of running) is an elegant method of assessing coordination dynamics from volumes of data.

Over the last 15 years, studies incorporating dynamic systems analyses have become more prevalent.[24] However, most of these studies focused on basic coordination dynamics of novel tasks such as reaching, finger movements, or walking.[33,34,36] Recently, a few studies have been published that used dynamic systems to approach problems more related to sports medicine. Hamill et al. published a particularly interesting study comparing 10 individuals symptomatic with chronic patellofemoral pain versus 10 asymptomatic individuals.[16] Studies using a traditional biomechanics approach have had little success in finding biomechanical variables that correlate with patellofemoral pain or other pathologic problems.[15,29,32] Using a dynamic systems approach, the researchers were able to easily identify all 10 subjects with patellofemoral pain.[16] Heiderscheidt et al. were able to elucidate the influence of Q-

angle on running mechanics using this approach, another question that has been difficult to answer using traditional analyses.[17] These impressive results reveal the potent sensitivity and efficacy of the dynamic systems approach to kinematic analysis. A dynamic systems approach is a particularly elegant method of understanding and integrating all the core areas of biomechanics (kinematics, kinetics, EMG, etc.). As this analysis approach becomes more prevalent, it is likely that some of the more elusive answers to questions in biomechanics will be answered.

Summary

Beginning over 2000 years ago, scientists and artists in various disciplines have used biomechanics as an effective tool for better understanding human movement. The advent of more sophisticated measurement tools has particularly facilitated this process. Today's researchers and clinicians are able to effectively quantify subtle changes in the kinematics, kinetics, and muscular coordination patterns associated with a movement. The integration of these core areas of biomechanics and understanding of the limitations of each area are essential to a more complete understanding of human movement. The authors of this book have done an outstanding job of integrating these core areas of biomechanics and their particular application to each sport. It is important to keep the credo of integration of all areas in mind as you use this book. Finally, recent advances in technology should have profound implications for our ability to integrate and understand the biomechanics of human motion in sports. Clinicians and researchers undoubtedly will benefit from these advances over the next few years. It is an exciting time to be practicing sports medicine and sports biomechanics.

References

1. Basmajian JV, Deluca CJ: *Muscles Alive, Their Functions Revealed by Electromyography*. Baltimore, Williams and Wilkins, 1985.

2. Caldwell GE, Forrester LW: Estimates of mechanical work and energy transfers: Demonstration of a rigid body power model of the recovery leg in gait. *Med Sci Sports Exerc* 24(12):1396–1492, 1992.

3. Cavanagh PR: The mechanics of distance running: A historical perspective. In Cavanagh PR (ed.): *Biomechanics of Distance Running*. Champaign, IL: Human Kinetics, 1990, pp. 65–100.

4. Davidson PA, Pink M, Perry J, et al: Functional anatomy of the flexor pronator muscle group in relation to the medial collateral ligament of the elbow. *Am J Sports Med* 23(2): 245–250, 1995.

5. Delp SL, Loan JP, Hoy MG, et al: An interactive graphics-based model of the lower extremity to study orthopaedic surgical procedures. *IEEE Trans Biomed Eng* 37(8):757–767, 1990.

6. Delp SL, Loan JP: A graphics-based software system to develop and analyze models of musculoskeletal structures. *Comput Biol Med* 25(1):21–34, 1995.

7. Elftman H: The function of muscles in locomotion. *Am J Phys* 125:357–366, 1939.

8. Elftman H: The work done by muscles in running. *Am J Phys* 129:673–684, 1940.

9. Elftman H: The action of the muscles in the body. *Biol Symp* 3:191–209, 1941.

10. Fenn WO: Frictional and kinetic factors in the work of sprint running. *Am J Phys* 92: 583–611, 1929.

11. Fenn WO: Work against gravity and work due to velocity changes in running. *Am J Phys* 93:433–462, 1930.

12. Fleisig GS, Dillman CJ, Escamilla RF, et al: Kinetics of baseball pitching with implications about injury mechanics. *Am J Sports Med* 23:233–239, 1995.

13. Furasawa K, Hill AV, Parkinson JL: The dynamics of sprint running. *Proc R Soc Lond* 102(B):29–42, 1927.

14. Greenwald RM, Swanson SC, McDonald TR: A comparison of the effect of ski sidecut on three-dimensional knee joint kinematics during a ski run. *Sportverletz Sportschaden* 11(4):129–133, 1997.

15. Hamill J, Bates BT, Holt KG: Timing of lower extremity joint actions during treadmill running. *Med Sci Sports Exerc* 24(7):807–813, 1992.

16. Hamill J, van Emmerik RE, Heiderscheit BC, Li L: A dynamical systems approach to lower extremity running injuries. *Clin Biomech* 14(5):297–308, 1999.

17. Heiderscheit BC, Hamill J, Van Emmerik RE: Q-angle influences on the variability of lower extremity coordination during running. *Med Sci Sports Exerc* 31(9):1313–1319, 1999.

18. Hill AV: The air resistance to a runner. *Proc R Soc Lond* 102(B):380–385, 1928.

19. Hoy MG, Zajac FE, Gordon ME: A musculoskeletal model of the human lower extremity: The effect of muscle, tendon, and moment arm on the moment-angle relationship of musculotendon actuators at the hip, knee, and ankle. *J Biomech* 23(2):157–169, 1990.

20. Jacobs R, Van Ingen Schenau GJ: Intermuscular coordination in a sprint push-off. *J Biomech* 25(9):953–965, 1992.

21. Jacobs R, Bobbert MF, Van Ingen Schenau GJ: Function of mono- and biarticular muscles in running. *Med Sci Sports Exerc* 25(10):1163–1173, 1993.

22. Jacobs R, Bobbert MF, Van Ingen Schenau GJ: Mechanical output from individual muscles during explosive leg extensions: The role of bi-articular muscles. *J Biomech* 29(4): 513–523, 1996.

23. Kamen G, Caldwell GE: Physiology and interpretation of the electromyogram. *J Clin Neurophysiol* 13(5):366–384, 1996.

24. Kelso JA: *Dynamic Patterns: The Self-organization of Brain and Behavior*. Cambridge, MA: MIT Press, 1995.

25. Liu MM, Herzog W, Savelberg HH: Dynamic muscle force predictions from EMG: An artifi-

cial neural network approach. *J Electromyogr Kinesiol* 9(6):391–400, 1999.

26. Piazza SJ, Delp SL: The influence of muscles on knee flexion during the swing phase of gait. *J Biomech* 29(6):723–733, 1996.

27. Quapp KM, Weiss JA: Material characterization of human medial collateral ligament. *J Biomech Eng* 120(6):757–763, 1998.

28. Schutz Y, Herren R: Assessment of speed of human locomotion using a differential satellite global positioning system. *Med Sci Sports Exerc* 32(3):642–646, 2000.

29. Stergiou P, Nigg BM, Wiley PJ, et al: Tibial rotation, Q-angle and its association to PFPS in runners. In *Proceedings of the Ninth Biennial Conference of the Canadian Society for Biomechanics*. Vancouver, BC: Simon Fraser University, 1996.

30. Sterzing EM, Hennig EM: Tibial shock, plantar pressures, and rearfoot kinematics during a 10 k run. In *Footwear Biomechanics Symposium*. XVIIth ISB Congress, Canmore, Alberta, Canada. August 1999, p. 88.

31. Swanson SC, Caldwell GE: An integrated biomechanical analysis of high speed level and incline treadmill running. *Med Sci Sports Exerc* 32(6):1146–1153, 2000.

32. Tiberio D: Effect of excessive subtalar joint pronation on patellofemoral mechanics: A theoretical model. *JOSPT* 9:60–165, 1987.

33. Turvey MT: Coordination. *Am Psychol* 45:938–953, 1990.

34. Van Emmerik RE, Wagenaar RC: Effects of walking velocity on relative phase dynamics in the trunk in human walking. *J Biomech* 29:1175–1184, 1996.

35. Van Soest AJ, Bobbert MF: Effects of muscle strengthening on vertical jump height: A simulation study. *Med Sci Sports Exerc* 26(8): 1012–1020, 1994.

36. Wagenaar RC, van Emmerik RE: Dynamics of pathological gait. *Hum Move Sci* 13:441–471, 1994.

37. Winter DA: *Biomechanics and Motor Control of Human Movement*. New York: Wiley, 1990.

CHAPTER 2

Baseball

Karen J. Mohr
Clive E. Brewster

Baseball is a sport enjoyed by athletes spanning a wide range of age and skill levels. The participants in this sport range from very young children playing in community-based programs to professionals at the major league level. The act of throwing demands that the athlete maximally accelerate and decelerate the arm over a short period of time, repetitively, and through extreme ranges of motion. At the same time, the thrower must maintain precise control of the ball being thrown.

There are nine field positions in the game of baseball. The infield positions are pitcher; catcher; first, second, and third basemen; and shortstop. There are three outfielders located in right, center, and left field. While the overall dimensions of the field are variable, the distance between the bases and from the pitcher's mound to home plate are standardized. The distance between each of the bases is 90 ft. The distance from the pitcher's mound to the front edge of home plate is 60 ft 6 in.

There are few reports on the incidence of injury in baseball; however, the literature that exists documents that the upper extremity is more at risk for injury than other parts of the body because of the extreme demands that throwing places on it. In a prospective epidemiologic study, McFarland and Wasik reported a 19 percent injury rate over a 3-year period in Division I collegiate baseball teams.[1] Of these injuries, 58 percent of the injuries were to the upper extremity, 15 percent to the trunk/back, and 27 percent to the lower extremity. Upper extremity injuries accounted for 75 percent of the total time lost from the sport. It is essential that those working with baseball players have a thorough understanding of the mechanics of the sport to best prevent injury. When prevention fails, knowledge of the tissues at risk for injury will allow for early identification of injury so that the best treatment and rehabilitation programs can be implemented.

Biomechanics of Baseball

THROWING/PITCHING

Throwing is a high-demand activity that requires finely tuned coordination, efficiency, and conditioning. For the pitcher, control is also of the utmost importance, and even subtle alterations in form can affect the thrower's ability to locate the pitches successfully. Detection of these subtle alterations by the coach, trainer, therapist, and physician can result in identification of the early stages of injury to the thrower.

Anatomic Considerations

Since the shoulder is the joint most vulnerable to injury in the thrower, an understanding of basic biomechanics of the shoulder is tantamount to understanding the more complicated biomechanics of the throwing motion itself. Shoulder biomechanics are best described as a balance of extreme mobility with tenuous stability. The static and dynamic stabilizing structures of the shoulder provide the base from which control of the throwing motion can begin.

Static stability of the shoulder is provided by the skeletal coupling of the humeral head with the scapular glenoid. The glenoid is a shallow, concave-shaped structure that makes contact with about 20 percent of the humeral head. The glenoid labrum is a fibrocartilaginous structure that encircles the glenoid rim, deepening the concavity and doubling the contact area with the humeral head.[2] There can be much variability in the labrum in terms of size, appearance, and degree of attachment to the glenoid. Superiorly, the labrum closely resembles a meniscus with a loose attachment to the glenoid, whereas portions of the inferior labrum appear more like a rounded extension of articular cartilage. The labrum is thicker along the anterior and posterior margins, which correlates with its contributions to restraining translation. A close association between the superior labrum and the biceps tendon has been observed. Superiorly, there is an intermingling of collagen fibers from the labrum and the biceps tendon just distal to the biceps origin from the supraglenoid tubercle.[3]

The glenohumeral ligaments, which are thickenings of the joint capsule, provide the greatest amount of static stability. When the shoulder is in neutral rotation, the superior and middle glenohumeral ligaments provide an equal amount of restraint to anterior humeral translation. With abduction and external rotation, as in the throwing motion, the inferior glenohumeral ligament becomes the primary restraint to anterior translation, with minimal contribution from the other glenohumeral ligaments.[4] Additionally, negative intraarticular pressure has been proposed to contribute to static stability in the shoulder. The true contribution to stability from negative intraarticular pressure is not known, and its relative importance may be overstated.

Dynamic stability of the glenohumeral joint is provided by the scapular and rotator cuff muscles. The scapular muscles—trapezius, serratus anterior, levator scapulae, rhomboids, and pectoralis minor—are responsible for positioning the glenoid in relation to the humeral head to provide optimal contact of the joint and preserve the subacromial space. In 1944, Inman described the concept of muscle-force couple as it applied to the scapular muscles and their action in glenohumeral elevation.[5] This classic study of joint motion demonstrated that glenohumeral elevation in any plane depends on free motion in all four joints of the shoulder complex and that properly conditioned musculature was required for maintenance of smooth and coordinated movement.

Cadaveric studies have demonstrated four ways that the rotator cuff works to provide stability to the glenohumeral joint. First, the action of the rotator cuff muscles compresses the articular surfaces of the humeral head and the glenoid fossa together. The concavity-compression mechanism described by Matsen was reported to have a 40 percent efficiency of translational restraint relative to compression units.[2] Second, the motion of the humeral head serves to tighten static restraints. In neutral rotation, the inferior glenohumeral ligament lies inferior to the joint. As the humeral head is externally rotated, the inferior glenohumeral ligament is tightly drawn across the anterior aspect of the joint and becomes the primary restraint to anterior translation.[4] Third, by limiting the arc of motion, the contracted rotator cuff muscles provide a barrier effect to translation. Lastly, the bulk of the rotator cuff muscles is able to act as a passive restraint to translation.[6]

With a basic knowledge of the biomechanics of the shoulder joint, one can better understand the more complex mechanics of the overhead throw. The throwing motion can be broken down into six phases that take place as a continuum. These stages are windup, early cocking, late cocking, acceleration, deceleration, and follow-through[7] (Fig. 2.1).

Windup

The windup serves to balance the body in preparation for the beginning of the energy transfer that will take place from the ground up through the body to the ball. This phase begins when the pitcher starts the motion and ends when the ball is taken out of the glove. The pitcher initiates the throwing motion by stepping back with the stride leg. The contralateral leg is then placed laterally in front of the rubber. Weight is then shifted from the stride foot to the stance foot, the body is rotated 90 degrees, and the stride leg is elevated with the knee flexed so that the side of the body faces the batter. Since this is typically a balancing phase, little to no muscle activity is demonstrated in the upper extremity; therefore, minimal risk for injury exists.[7]

Early Cocking

Early cocking begins when the hands separate and the ball is removed from the glove. The lower extremities and trunk begin to re-

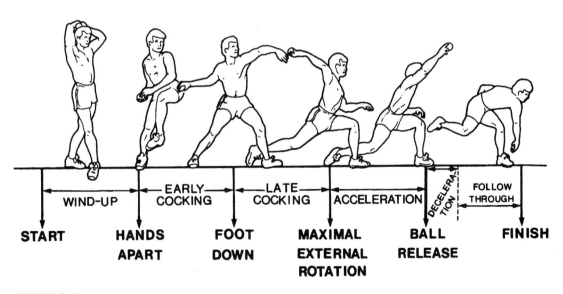

FIGURE 2.1

Phases of the baseball pitch. *(Reproduced with permission from DiGiovine et al.[7])*

lease stored energy that ultimately will be transferred to the ball. The stance leg is flexed, and the stride leg moves toward the plate. When the stride foot makes contact, it should be almost directly in front of the rear foot. If this foot is placed too far in either direction, the thrower will end up compensating with less than optimal mechanics, and energy will not be transferred optimally from the lower extremities and trunk to the upper extremity and, ultimately, the baseball. During this phase, the dominant shoulder rotates externally and reaches 104 degrees of abduction.[8] Rotation of the scapula is accomplished by coordinated activity of the scapular muscles to provide a stable platform that maximizes glenohumeral contact during the more stressful phases of the throw that follow. The trapezius and serratus anterior form a force couple that positions the glenoid, creating a stable base on which the humeral head can move. Elevation of the humerus is provided by a second force couple between the deltoid and supraspinatus. These muscles work together to maintain a congruent relationship between the humeral head and the glenoid as elevation occurs. The deltoid acting alone would cause significant shear forces along the superior glenoid margin and superior displacement of the humeral head. The synchronous action of the supraspinatus prevents this occurrence. This function of the supraspinatus distinguishes it from the other muscles of the rotator cuff that act as rotators of the humerus.

Late Cocking

Late cocking marks the start of hip rotation, which is then followed by trunk rotation. During late cocking, the humerus is brought into a position of abduction and maximal external rotation, stressing the anterior structures of the shoulder. This stress can lead to pathology that makes for a less efficient and less accurate throwing motion. The humerus should be in the plane of the scapula during this phase of the throw.

It is during late cocking that the infraspinatus and teres minor increase their muscle activity to provide external rotation of the shoulder. The thrower's shoulder may reach external rotation of up to 170 degrees.[8] The action of these muscles also serves to decrease the stresses on the anterior shoulder structures by pulling the humeral head posteriorly approximately 3 to 4 mm.[9] Strength and endurance of these muscles should be maximized to lessen the stress on the anterior capsule and labrum.

Late cocking is also the phase where significant forces begin at the elbow. These forces continue through the later phases of the pitch. During late cocking, elbow flexion increases from 63 to 74 degrees.[8] Muscle activity during this time is low to moderate in the elbow flexors probably because the elbow is already at or near its optimal position for energy transfer.[10] The extensor carpi radialis brevis and extensor carpi radialis longus demonstrate relatively high levels of activity at this point. Their function during this phase is to cock the wrist in preparation for the throw and final energy transfer.

Throughout the process of cocking the arm, a varus torque is produced at the elbow to prevent valgus. Fleisig and Barrentine reported that approximately 64 newton-meters (N · m) of torque is generated just before the arm reaches maximal external rotation.[11] This varus torque results in generation of a tensile force on the medial side of the elbow and a compressive force on the lateral aspect. The ulnar collateral ligament has been reported by Morrey and An to provide 54 percent of the resistance to valgus stress at the elbow.[12] Fleisig and Barrentine extrapolated this finding to the 64 N · m of varus torque generated and came to the conclusion that the ulnar collateral ligament therefore endures 35 N · m. The authors then compared this with the 32 N · m failure load of the ulnar collateral ligament as previously reported and determined that it is likely that with each pitch the ulnar collateral ligament is loaded at or greater than its normal failure load.[13] If this is indeed the case, then some reduction of force must be endured by the ulnar collateral ligament so that it does not rupture each time a pitch is thrown. This reduction in stress is likely caused by dynamic muscular contraction about the elbow. A cadaveric study demonstrated that the flexor carpi ulnaris and flexor digitorum superficialis anatomically overlie the anterior band of the ulnar collateral ligament and are therefore in the best position to offer dynamic stability.[14] This is supported by a biomechanical study that showed that these two muscles are capable of generating a varus moment about the elbow.[15]

Acceleration

The next phase of the throw, acceleration, begins with forward motion of the humerus and continues to ball release. At ball release, the thrower's trunk is flexed forward, and the lead leg should be extending at the knee. During this phase there is rapid internal rotation of the humerus, resulting in generation of significant torque and compressive forces about the shoulder and elbow. Peak angular velocity of internal rotation has been shown to reach 6100 degrees per second and occurs at approximately the instant of ball release.[8] During acceleration, the elbow experiences a rapid combination of valgus and extension forces. Extension occurs at a rate of 2200 degrees per second and proceeds to approximately 20 degrees of flexion.[8] The valgus stress to the elbow is secondary to the elbow lagging behind the rapidly internally rotating shoulder. This valgus load is transferred to the medial structures of the elbow, of which the ulnar collateral ligament carries the majority of the load.

During acceleration, the energy coiled within the lower extremities and trunk mus-culature is transferred to the ball by way of the shoulder and elbow. Most of the shoulder girdle musculature demonstrates increased activity. However, the only shoulder muscles thought to be able to contribute to the generation of velocity of the throw are the pectoralis major and the latissimus dorsi.[16] The strength of these two muscles has been shown to correlate with increased throwing velocity. The other shoulder muscles are working not as power muscles but rather to stabilize the head of the humerus in the glenoid. Scapular muscles also have been noted to increase muscle activity during acceleration.[7] This highlights the need for a stable scapula as the humerus rapidly rotates internally.

Throughout acceleration, three important force couples are noted. The posterior deltoid and the supraspinatus form the first, providing posterior restraint to the humeral head as it undergoes rapid internal rotation. Second, the pectoralis major and the teres minor work together. As the pectoralis major contracts, it adducts and internally rotates the humerus. The teres minor simultaneously fires to control internal rotation and keep the humeral head from translating anteriorly. Frequently, the teres minor and infraspinatus have been lumped together as having the same function; however, during the acceleration phase, these two muscles act independently of each other. The upper fibers of the subscapularis and latissimus dorsi form the last force couple of this phase. While the latissimus dorsi is active to powerfully and rapidly extend, adduct, and internally rotate the humerus, the subscapularis works to maintain the position of the humeral head in precise contact with the glenoid.

About the elbow, the pronator teres, flexor carpi radialis, flexor digitorum superficialis, and flexor carpi ulnaris demonstrate high activity during this phase in an attempt to stabilize the elbow against the large valgus stresses generated during the throw.[7] All these muscles should be targeted in a preventative or rehabilitation program designed for throwing athletes. As with the late cocking phase, acceleration requires precise coordination of muscle activity, and any alteration in mechanics may lead the athlete to an inability to throw effectively and efficiently and ultimately may result in pathology of the shoulder or elbow.

Deceleration and Follow-Through

The two remaining phases of the throw are deceleration and follow-through. These phases serve to dissipate any remaining energy that was not transferred to the ball, as well as position the thrower for fielding. The throwing arm should end up on the lateral side of the stride leg. The rear leg progresses forward to catch up with the stride leg and position the pitcher to be able to field the ball. During these phases, the posterior shoulder muscles are still active to control the position of the humerus during deceleration. The teres minor demonstrates the highest level of muscle activity of all the glenohumeral muscles. The elbow flexors demonstrate their highest level of activity at this time in an attempt to produce joint compression that decreases the force of olecranon abutment into the olecranon fossa.

BATTING

Little attention has been given in the literature to describing the mechanics of the baseball batting swing because it is thought to account for few of the reported injuries that occur during baseball. As with throwing, batting can be divided up into phases that occur sequentially. The four phases of batting include windup, preswing, swing, and follow-through[17] (Fig. 2.2).

Windup begins as the lead heel leaves the ground and ends as the lead toe reestablishes ground contact. During this phase, the batter's center of mass is shifted toward the trail leg.[18] Muscle activity is relatively low during this phase except for the trail leg hamstrings, which maintain hip extension as weight is shifted to the trail leg in preparation for the swing.

Preswing begins as the lead forefoot contacts the ground and ends when forward swing of the bat begins. During this phase, the hamstrings and lower fibers of the gluteus maximus are active to stabilize the hips and initiate the power of the swing. Erector spinae and abdominal muscles demonstrate high activity to stabilize the trunk and transmit power from the lower extremities to the bat.

The swing phase begins with forward movement of the bat and ends with ball contact. The lead leg extends at the knee, while the trail hip is pushed forward, creating a counterclockwise acceleration of the hips around the trunk. Rotational velocity of the hips during this phase is approximately 700 degrees per second. The shoulders and arms follow the hips, rotating at approximately 940 and 1160 degrees per second, respectively, at the instant prior to ball contact.[18] Dominant muscle activity during this phase is in the trunk muscles, demonstrating the important role of these muscles in the transmission of power from the lower extremities to the bat as it contacts the ball.[17]

Follow-through begins with ball contact and ends as the lead shoulder reaches maximum abduction and external rotation. Trunk muscle activity is decreased from the swing phase but still remains relatively high, maintaining rotation and stabilizing the trunk. Activity in the quadriceps is also high during this phase to control the flexing knees.

In summary, skilled batting requires coordinated transfer of energy from the lower extremities to the trunk, upper extremities, and ultimately, the bat as it contacts the ball. Large rotational forces are generated at the hips and trunk in this process. The muscles of the lower extremities and trunk should be

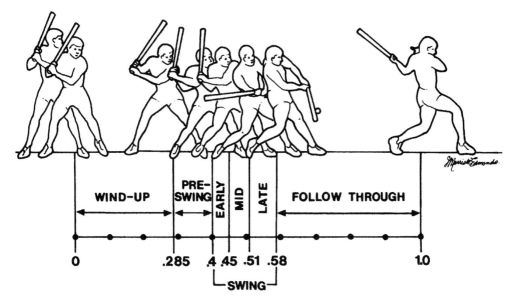

WIND-UP | **PRE-SWING** | EARLY | MID | LATE | **FOLLOW THROUGH**

0   .285   .4 .45 .51 .58   1.0

└─SWING─┘

FIGURE 2.2

Phases of the batting swing. *(Reproduced with permission from Shaffer et al.[17])*

highlighted in a prevention or rehabilitation program, as well as a program geared toward optimizing performance.

SLIDING

Since the slide enables the base runner to reach a base more quickly than any other method, it plays an important role in the offensive phase of baseball. Sliding can be performed using either the headfirst or the feetfirst technique. Regardless of the technique used, four distinct phases have been identified: sprint, attainment of the sliding position, airborne, and landing.[42]

Sprint

The first phase of the slide is the sprint. The sprint enables the base runner to achieve maximum speed by accelerating as quickly as possible in a horizontal direction. The sprint

is characterized by a forward body angle of approximately 25 degrees from upright.[43]

Attainment of the Sliding Position

Attainment of the sliding position is the next phase of the slide. In the headfirst sliding technique, forward body lean is increased during this phase, with the center of gravity remaining ahead of the striding foot. The knees are flexed, resulting in a lowering of the center of gravity. At the conclusion of this phase, when the sliding position for the headfirst slide is attained, the body is approximately 30 degrees from horizontal.[42] When performing a feetfirst slide, approximately 15 ft from the base the body becomes more relaxed and changes to a more erect position. The upper extremities then extend backward as the body moves into position for the slide. The body rotates clockwise, with the upper body moving upward and backward and the lower body moving downward and forward.

Airborne

While the airborne phase is distinct in the feetfirst slide, it is not always obvious in the headfirst slide. During the airborne phase of the headfirst slide, the arms are outstretched forward, and the remainder of the body is in a prone position with the trunk and lower extremities extended. The position during the airborne phase for the feetfirst slide is with one leg extended forward and the other leg flexed beneath the outstretched leg. Feetfirst sliders experience more vertical displacement than headfirst sliders, resulting in a greater impact force when they contact the ground.[42]

Landing

The final phase of the slide is the landing phase. During this phase, the body should be completely relaxed, and contact with the ground ideally should be made with as large a body surface as possible to aid in absorption of the impact. In the headfirst slide, the thighs and chest provide a large surface area for contact. However, in a biomechanical study of a limited number of sliders by Corzatt et al. the contact pattern was shown to be first with the hands and then with the knees.[42] In the feetfirst sliding technique, impact should be with both buttocks, the lower back, and the posterior thighs. The feetfirst sliders they studied made initial contact with the extended foot, the tucked-under foot, and the knee of the tucked leg. They observed the extended foot catching the ground at the heel, resulting in sudden and excessive plantar flexion.[42] This technique may slow forward progress and increase the risk for injury.

Sliding is an important aspect of an aggressive offense in the game of baseball. Both the headfirst and feetfirst sliding techniques have injury-causing potential related to impact with the ground after the airborne

phase. Keeping the body relaxed and maximizing the body surface that comes in contact with the ground can minimize the risk of injury during sliding.

Injury Prevention

In designing a program geared toward preventing injury in a baseball player, the focus should be on protection of the throwing shoulder and elbow because these are the most frequently injured joints in the sport. A comprehensive injury-prevention program should include proper warm-up, stretching exercises to maintain normal motion, and strengthening exercises specific to the muscles of the sport.

WARM-UP

There is ample evidence pointing toward the protective effects of warming up. It has been shown that passively warmed or isometrically preconditioned muscles can withstand greater length changes and greater force before failure.[19] Another study demonstrated that subjects who jogged for 10 minutes on a treadmill showed a decrease in muscle stiffness compared with subjects who did not warm up.[20] Electromyography (EMG) research has demonstrated decreased muscle activity in the calf muscles following warm-up on a stationary bicycle, implying increased relaxation in these muscles compared with before warm-up.[21]

Based on these findings, it is recommended that warm-up be incorporated into the athlete's exercise program to minimize the risk of injury. Warm-up should consist of a minimum of 10 to 15 minutes of cardiovascular exercise at 60 to 80 percent maximum age-predicted heart rate. Warm-up should precede any stretching or strengthening exercises as well as any competition.

STRETCHING

Stretching the shoulder of the throwing athlete is a balancing act. One must consider what is normal for these athletes. In both pitchers and position players, it has been demonstrated that there is increased external rotation and decreased internal rotation in the dominant arm compared with the non-dominant arm.[22] Due to the fact that these athletes already put tremendous stress on the anterior structures of the shoulder secondary to functional increases in external rotation, any further stretching of these tissues should be avoided.

Conversely, the posterior structures of the shoulder in the thrower are commonly tight, as manifested by decreased internal rotation. If the posterior capsule is allowed to remain restricted, it will force the humeral head to sit forward in the glenoid. Not only can this stress the anterior structures and contribute to instability and impingement, but it also causes the length-tension relationships of many of the shoulder girdle muscles to become less than optimal and perhaps leads to premature fatigue. This can then set up a cascade of effects that may lead to shoulder pathology.

Mobilization of the posterior capsule can be performed by a trainer or therapist or can be accomplished by the athlete through self-mobilization. The most commonly performed self-mobilization is performed by pulling the arm across the chest into horizontal adduction. If associated rotator cuff or bicipital irritation is present, this position may cause discomfort. An alternative stretching position is lying supine with the trunk slightly rotated toward the involved side with the shoulder abducted to 90 degrees (Fig. 2.3). The arm is then passively internally rotated, allowing the humeral head to stretch the posterior tissues. A therapist or trainer can effectively stretch the posterior capsule of the thrower by having the thrower lie on the uninvolved side

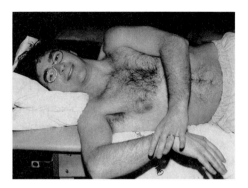

FIGURE 2.3

Alternative position for posterior capsule stretch.

with the shoulder horizontally abducted and the scapula adducted. The therapist or trainer fixes the axillary border of the scapula and horizontally adducts the humerus, stretching the posterior tissues.

Stretching of the elbow of a thrower should be approached cautiously. Many throwers and most pitchers have some degree of elbow flexion contracture that does not necessarily lead to significant pathology. The elbow can be gently stretched into extension but should be stretched to the point of the contracture only so as to avoid impingement in the posterior compartment.

Wrist flexor and extensor stretching should complete the stretching program for the upper extremity. The wrist should be stretched passively into a flexed position while maintaining elbow extension. Conversely, the wrist should then be stretched passively into extension with the elbow in extension.

STRENGTHENING

Strengthening exercises of the lower extremities and trunk should be the foundation of an injury-prevention program for throwers because this is where the power of the throw as well as the batting swing originates. Exercises should be included for trunk flexion, extension, and rotation. Lower extremity exercises should target the hip flexors and extensors, quadriceps, hamstrings, and gastrocnemius-soleus complex. The program should then be designed to optimize strength of the dynamic stabilizers of the shoulder—the scapular and rotator cuff muscles—as well as the positioning and power muscles. Muscles that are anatomically positioned to be able to attenuate the stresses imparted to the medial side of the elbow should be strengthened, as well as the flexors and extensors of the elbow. Finally, endurance cannot be ignored. The muscles of the shoulder and elbow must be able to contract pitch after pitch after pitch. We cannot expect an exercise that is performed for 3 sets of 10 repetitions to prepare muscles to contract as they need to in a game situation. Specific endurance exercises must be incorporated into the thrower's conditioning program. The most efficient exercises for targeting specific muscles are outlined in the rehabilitation sections of this chapter.

Etiology of Injuries

The most common injuries in baseball players involve the throwing shoulder and elbow. These injuries can be attributed to either intrinsic or extrinsic factors. Intrinsic factors that may cause injury in baseball players include decreased range of motion, impaired joint mobility, and decreased strength. All these factors can lead to compensatory throwing mechanics and, ultimately, injury. Alternatively, extrinsic factors that may contribute to injury include training errors and improper throwing mechanics.

INTRINSIC FACTORS

The common injury progression in the thrower begins with fatigue of the dynamic stabilizers of the glenohumeral joint. When

this occurs, greater than normal stresses are transferred to the anterior capsule and labrum. When subtle pathology exists, the thrower may develop compensatory mechanics such as moving the humerus out of the scapular plane and into the coronal plane during the late cocking and acceleration phases of the pitch (Fig. 2.4). This phenomenon is referred to as *hyperangulation*. If this situation goes unnoticed, the anterior structures will stretch out, and the shoulder will be subject to greater amounts of glenohumeral translation. With greater anterior translation of the humeral head, impingement of the posterior rotator cuff on the posterior glenoid, or *internal impingement*, can occur.

Asynchronous muscle firing patterns also can result in subtle biomechanical changes in throwing form to compensate for fatigued or damaged tissues. One change that often can be appreciated early on in the process leading to injury is scapular lag or winging. This is usually due to a weak or fatigued serratus anterior. Often the detectable change that can be seen in the throwing motion is a drop in elbow position in an attempt to accommodate for loss of scapular elevation. If this compensation is undetected and untreated, the thrower may begin to further compensate by moving the humerus out of the scapular plane and into the coronal plane during late cocking (hyperangulation), putting further stress on the anterior structures of the shoulder. It is critical to pick up these subtle changes in mechanics and start the thrower on the proper rehabilitation program early on to avoid more serious injury.

EXTRINSIC FACTORS

Throwing requires sequential, coordinated muscle activity; consequently, there is much opportunity for injury if mechanics are less than optimal. Poor technique in any phase of the throw can lead to the development of pathology. In many cases it is difficult to sepa-

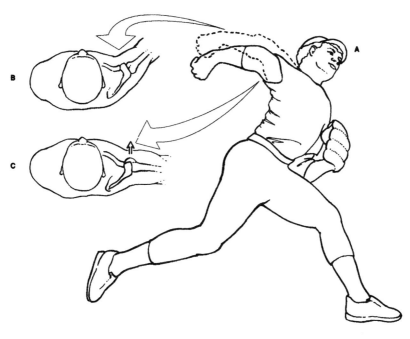

FIGURE 2.4

A. Baseball pitching with humerus moving from the scapular plane to the coronal plane. *B.* Overhead view of humerus in the scapular plane (correct). *C.* Overhead view of humerus in the coronal plane (incorrect). *(Reproduced with permission from Pink and Perry.[23])*

rate out whether a thrower's poor mechanics are a compensation for an inherent weakness or pathology or if it is the poor mechanics that lead to weakness, fatigue, and injury. The health care professional should work closely with the coaching staff to identify poor throwing mechanics and assess whether they are being caused by underlying pathology.

Common Injuries and Their Rehabilitation

SHOULDER

Rotator Cuff and Biceps Tendinitis

One of the most common findings in throwers is inflammation of the rotator cuff tendons and/or the tendon of the long head of the biceps. Coordinated control of humeral elevation and abduction combined with glenohumeral compression requires a specific sequential muscle firing pattern in order to maximize efficiency and avoid injury. Subtle alterations in biomechanics can cause the overuse or misuse of one or more muscles of the rotator cuff. Alternatively, overuse of improperly or inadequately conditioned muscles can lead to alterations in mechanics. If fatigue results, the other muscles of the rotator cuff attempt to compensate, and the alterations lead to dysynchronous action. Loss of the compressive effect of the rotator cuff leads to a change in the force vector across the glenohumeral joint from compression to shearing. This can affect the rotator cuff and/or the tendon of the long head of the biceps adversely.

The athlete with inflammation of the rotator cuff and/or the tendon of the long head of the biceps typically complains of pain that is localized to the area of irritation. Initially, the athlete may be able to play through the symptoms but will notice pain and stiffness afterwards. Examination of the athlete should demonstrate full range of motion with pain at the extremes in the irritated muscles. Strength is typically intact, with weakness perceived secondary to pain and/or fatigue. Treatment should focus on factors that interfere with or alter normal rotator cuff mechanics as well as associated conditions that contribute to impingement.

Treatment of tendinitis is aimed at decreasing inflammation through the use of modalities and anti-inflammatory medication. A period of relative rest from offending activities is required. The time period for relative rest should be adjusted on an individual basis according to continual reassessment of the athlete. During this time, it is essential that the athlete maintain the condition and strength of the trunk and lower extremity muscles as well as cardiovascular fitness.

Most cases of tendinitis will respond to a structured nonoperative program. It is unusual for these inflammatory conditions to warrant surgical intervention. If a case is resistant to conservative measures after at least 6 months, or if there is an underlying anatomic contributor to the pathology, then arthroscopic surgery may be indicated. A minimalist approach should be taken because studies have shown that overhead athletes do not necessarily respond favorably to subacromial decompression with anterior acromioplasty.[24]

Rotator Cuff Tears

Partial- or full-thickness rotator cuff tearing is often the next stage in the spectrum of conditions that affect the rotator cuff after prolonged inflammation. These injuries also can occur from a single traumatic event that placed excessive strain or tension on the rotator cuff insertion.

A full-thickness rotator cuff tear is rarely found in patients under 40 years of age. Conversely, partial-thickness tears are a common finding in overhead athletes. The cumulative effects of either internal or external impingement will lead to failure of rotator cuff fibers, most commonly along the undersurface. The significance of these partial-thickness tears is not fully known, but in the overhead athlete, if conservative treatment fails, they are usually debrided arthroscopically and then treated with an aggressive postoperative strengthening program. The rehabilitation program should emphasize restoration of the synchronous action of all components of the rotator cuff and scapular stabilizing muscles. It is extremely important to reveal any underlying or concomitant pathology such as glenohumeral instability. If anterior instability is found, it should be corrected so that the rotator cuff is not at further risk of damage.

In general, full-thickness tears are not compatible with optimal overhead performance and require operative repair in almost all circumstances. Attempts at conservative treatment through rehabilitation are made often, and success initially may be found, but invariably, the high demands of throwing wear down the remaining rotator cuff. Surgical options include an arthroscopic repair, mini-open repair, and a standard open repair. The time of healing following surgical rotator cuff repair is felt to be independent of the technique used and is on the order of 6 months.

Impingement

In throwers, a distinction must be made between external and internal rotator cuff impingement. External impingement consists of bursa-sided rotator cuff irritation resulting from any process that decreases the space between the rotator cuff and the acromion. These factors can be static or dynamic. Bursitis, tendinitis, and acromial spurring are all conditions that statically decrease the space available for the rotator cuff. Loss of precise rotator cuff control and compression of the humerus against the glenoid can arise when the rotator cuff muscles are fatigued. The result is that the humeral head migrates superiorly during glenohumeral elevation, which dynamically decreases the space available between the rotator cuff and the acromion. This is in contrast to internal impingement, where the injured portion of the rotator cuff differs. In this situation, rotator cuff fatigue leads to a cumulative effect of repetitive microtrauma to the anterior capsule and labrum, resulting in stretching of these structures and resulting anterior translation of the humeral head. This anterior translation causes the undersurface of the posterior rotator cuff to be brought against the posterosuperior surface of the glenoid and labrum, causing fraying and tearing.

Treatment of impingement depends on identifying the underlying cause of the impingement. External impingement must be treated by identifying and treating the cause of the subacromial impingement. In the throwing athlete, subtle instability is frequently the primary pathology, and internal impingement is the secondary pathology. In this case, the instability must be addressed through an aggressive rehabilitation program if the athlete is to return to pain-free throwing.

Glenohumeral Instability

Instability is found frequently in the shoulders of overhead throwers secondary to the high demands, repetitive stresses, and extreme ranges of motion to which these athletes subject their shoulders. Instability of the glenohumeral joint can fall anywhere along a continuum of pathology from subtle to gross instability. Often, the underlying pathology in throwers diagnosed with impingement or tendinitis is actually instability that has gone unrecognized.

In general, throwers with instability should be treated conservatively initially with rehabilitation. If the instability is recognized early, before pathologic changes in the tissues occur, a proper rehabilitation program can return approximately 95 percent of athletes to their prior level of competition without surgery. A minority of throwers with instability do not respond to a properly executed rehabilitation program and may require surgical intervention. Many procedures have been developed to correct anterior glenohumeral instability. However, because of the unique demands on the shoulder of the thrower, success (return to prior competitive level) has been less than satisfactory with these procedures. The ideal surgical procedure for the baseball player with glenohumeral instability is one that tightens the loose structures without significantly compromising the functional range of motion required for throwing. One procedure that meets the ideal criteria is anterior capsulolabral reconstruction (ACLR). This procedure aims to form a new capsulolabral complex by tightening the lax inferior glenohumeral ligament and capsule. Advantages of this procedure are that it addresses the primary pathology and does not require detachment, shortening, or transfer of any muscle. Since no muscles are detached during the procedure, range of motion can be initiated immediately postoperatively, and full range of motion can be achieved early in the rehabilitation process.

Recent advances in the surgical treatment of shoulder instability have come to include arthroscopic thermal capsular shrinkage. In this procedure, a probe is used to apply heat energy to the capsule and ligaments. Heating the tissue to a temperature of at least 65°C leads to alteration of the collagen fiber ultrastructure resulting in tissue shrinkage.[25–28] Capsular shrinkage has some advantages over the open stabilization procedures. Because it is performed arthroscopically, it is less invasive. Initially, there is a period of immobilization following arthroscopic capsular shrinkage, but then rehabilitation time and time to return to throwing are shorter than for the open capsular tightening procedures. There is little agreement among experts on the optimal amount of time of immobilization following capsular shrinkage to prevent restretching of the tissues. Despite the proposed advantages of capsular shrinkage, to date there have been no long-term clinical studies documenting outcome in patients or specifically throwing athletes. It is possible that over time these tissues may stretch out again, necessitating a second procedure.

Labral Injuries

Labral injuries are found commonly in association with glenohumeral instability, but they also can occur in the absence of obvious instability. Throwers with labral injuries usually complain of anterior shoulder pain, and a "click" is often associated with range of motion. Injury involving the superior aspect of the glenoid labrum beginning posteriorly and extending anteriorly (SLAP lesion) is often seen in throwers. It is thought that internal impingement of the rotator cuff against the superior rim during the throwing motion may be the cause of this condition. If a player is diagnosed with a labral injury that is causing problems with throwing, most likely it will be treated surgically. Labral lesions that involve an intact biceps tendon and labral attachment to the glenoid usually are treated with arthroscopic debridement of the torn labrum. Injuries that involve disruption of the labral attachment to the glenoid and the biceps tendon require reattachment of the biceps tendon and labral complex to the superior glenoid surface.

Rehabilitation of Shoulder Injuries

Rehabilitation of the injured shoulder in the overhead athlete requires not only an understanding of normal motion of all joints of the shoulder and elbow but also a thorough understanding of the sport-specific demands that throwing places on the upper extremity of the athlete. With this base of knowledge, an individualized rehabilitation program can be designed, with the goal being return of the athlete to his or her preinjury level of competition. Most injuries, if diagnosed in the early stages before significant pathology is present, can be treated conservatively. The rehabilitation goals for managing throwers are to restore normal flexibility to the involved structures and optimize the strength and endurance of the muscles about the shoulder and elbow.

For successful rehabilitation of throwers with shoulder instability and/or impingement, restoration of normal flexibility is essential. What is considered "normal" flexibility for an athlete is specific to the demands of his or her sport. Most competitive pitchers demonstrate external range of motion of their pitching shoulder that would be considered excessive in other populations. However, for pitchers, this motion is necessary to be successful in their sport. Since this extreme range of motion in external rotation leads to stretching of the anterior capsule, stretching exercises that put further stress on the anterior structures are discouraged. Conversely, tightness of the posterior capsule can contribute to anterior instability and exacerbate the symptoms of secondary impingement. In the presence of tight posterior structures and lax anterior restraints, the head of the humerus may be levered forward enough during shoulder motion to produce symptoms. Restoration of normal flexibility of the posterior capsule through stretching or mobilization will allow for normal posterior gliding of the humeral head, maintenance of maximal congruency of the glenohumeral joint, and optimal length-tension relationships of the muscles of the shoulder girdle. Mobilization of the posterior capsule either can be done by the athlete or can be performed by the therapist or trainer. Self-mobilization of the posterior capsule can be achieved by having the athlete pull the involved arm across the chest into horizontal adduction (Fig. 2.5). Sometimes the exact degree of elevation during this stretch must be modified so as to avoid a painful position. Posterior capsule mobilization can be performed by a therapist in either the supine or side-lying position. In the supine position, the arm is abducted to 90 degrees and passively rotated internally while the humeral head is stabilized. To perform mobilization of the posterior capsule in the side-lying position, the athlete lies on the uninvolved side, and the involved arm is passively adducted horizontally while the scapula is passively adducted by the therapist (Fig. 2.6).

Strength in the throwing athlete with shoulder instability should be addressed systematically. The first focus should be on the dynamic stabilizers—the scapular muscles and the rotator cuff muscles. Once adequate strength and proper synchrony of these muscles have been achieved, progression can be started toward strengthening of the deltoids,

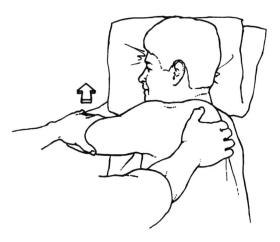

FIGURE 2.6

Mobilization of the posterior capsule in a sidelying position. *(Reproduced with permission from Brewster et al.[29])*

latissimus dorsi, and pectoralis major. Just as the order of muscle strengthening should be systematic, so should the progression of the types of exercises. The program should begin with isotonic exercises with a focus on synchrony of muscle activity. Progression can then be made to isokinetic exercises and, ultimately, to sport-specific drills. The timeline of progression is individual to each athlete and should be based on continual reassessment.

The scapular muscles are responsible for positioning of the glenoid and for providing a stable platform on which the head of the humerus can move. Additionally, proper positioning of the scapula enables optimal length-tension relationships of the rotator cuff muscles, allowing for efficient function. Since the scapular muscles attach to and control all aspects of the scapula, weakness or fatigue in one or more of these muscles can result in scapular asynchrony, thus contributing to the instability and/or impingement. Scapular muscles that should be included in a strengthening program are the upper, mid-

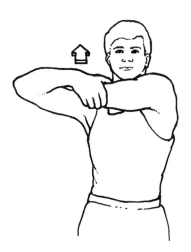

FIGURE 2.5

dle, and lower trapezii, rhomboids, levator scapulae, pectoralis minor, and serratus anterior. The serratus anterior requires special attention because it has been shown to demonstrate decreased activity in baseball pitchers with shoulder instability.[10]

EMG studies have been helpful in identifying exercises that most efficiently target specific muscles throughout their arc of motion.[30,31] Done in a prone position, horizontal rowing and horizontal abduction are effective exercises for targeting all parts of the trapezius, the levator scapulae, and the rhomboids. Shoulder flexion and scaption (scapular plane abduction) activate all the scapular muscles. Shoulder shrugs, press-ups, and push-ups with a plus (Fig. 2.7) are efficient exercises for the levator scapulae, pectoralis minor, and serratus anterior. The push-up-with-a-plus exercise is performed by having the patient do a push-up, and then when the elbows are maximally extended, the motion continues with additional scapular protraction (the plus). The plus maneuver similarly can be added at the end of the chest-press or bench-press exercise when the patient's

program has been progressed to include these exercises. Early in the rehabilitation process, this exercise can be performed with a wall push-up. As the patient progresses, the exercise can be performed on the knees and forearms, the knees and hands, and ultimately, in the standard push-up position with the legs extended and the weight on the toes. While performing this exercise, care must be taken not to allow the distal end of the humerus to go behind the plane of the body. If this were to occur, the humeral head would be levered forward in the joint, contributing to instability.

The muscles of the rotator cuff comprise the other group of dynamic stabilizers of the glenohumeral joint. The rotator cuff muscles are responsible for maintaining congruency of the humeral head in the glenoid fossa throughout the wide range of motion available to the shoulder. Because the tendons of these muscles insert close to the axes of motion of the shoulder, they are able to direct the position of the humeral head within the glenoid, thereby achieving optimal joint stability. Rather than being a true rotator of the

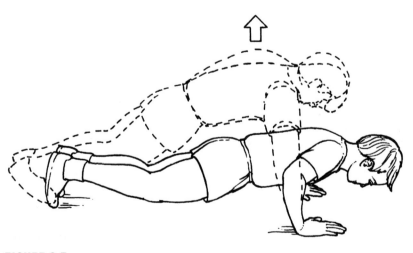

FIGURE 2.7

Push-up with a plus. *(Reproduced with permission from Pink et al.[32])*

glenohumeral joint, the supraspinatus forms a force couple with the deltoids to approximate the humeral head into the glenoid and compress and depress the humeral head during elevation by the deltoids. The supraspinatus is believed to be one of the first muscles of the shoulder girdle to fatigue, so endurance training of this muscle should be addressed.[33]

The supraspinatus can be strengthened effectively by performing scaption, or scapular plane elevation. Performing this exercise in a position of humeral internal rotation has been shown to maximize muscle activity in the supraspinatus, but care should be taken not to elevate the arm above 80 to 90 degrees while in the internally rotated position because this is the start of the range-of-motion arc for subacromial impingement.[31] An alternate position for strengthening of the supraspinatus is the prone position. The patient begins with the involved extremity hanging off the side of the table and, while keeping the arm in external rotation, abducts it horizontally. Care should be taken not to bring the humerus behind the plane of the body because this may lever the humeral head forward, compromising stability of the joint. Endurance of the supraspinatus should be addressed by having the patient perform many repetitions of these exercises with light weights.

External rotation of the glenohumeral joint is accomplished by the infraspinatus and teres minor. There has been some evidence that the infraspinatus has the major role of providing active external rotation at arm elevations below 90 degrees of abduction, whereas the teres minor takes over at elevations above 90 degrees of shoulder abduction.[7,34,35] This differentiation in function has not been observed consistently, which may be due to the fact that it is only seen when the shoulder musculature is maximally challenged, as in baseball pitching. In addition to providing active external rotation of the

humerus, the infraspinatus and teres minor work synergistically with the other rotator cuff muscles to provide maximum joint surface contact of the humeral head within the glenoid fossa.

As well as being an internal rotator of the shoulder, the subscapularis has been described as an anterior wall muscle that provides some protection against anterior translation of the humeral head due to its location across the front of the joint. However, it is important to note that the anatomic location of the structures of the glenohumeral joint change with differing degrees of abduction of the joint.[36] When the arm is at the side in neutral abduction, the supraspinatus is located superiorly and the subscapularis anteriorly. When the arm is moved up to a position of 90 degrees of abduction and 90 degrees of external rotation approximating arm position during throwing, the supraspinatus moves posteriorly and the subscapularis moves superiorly. Thus, in the cocking position of the throw, the subscapularis is not in an anatomic position to act as an anterior stabilizer.

In the early stages of rehabilitation, strengthening exercises for the external and internal rotators of the shoulder should begin in the side-lying position. For internal rotation, the patient is positioned on the involved side with the arm positioned slightly forward of the trunk. The arm is then rotated against gravity. To perform external rotation, the patient is positioned on the uninvolved side with a small pillow or towel roll placed between the involved arm and trunk to help maintain a position of slight abduction. The position of slight abduction allows for adequate blood flow to the rotator cuff while optimizing stability of the glenohumeral joint.[37] Internal and external rotation can be progressed by adding additional weight and then progressing to more challenging positions such as prone external rotation with the arm abducted to 70 degrees and, ultimately, isokinetic internal and external rotation. Since the teres minor has been shown to have high levels of activity in the later phases of throwing, it should be specifically targeted in the rehabilitation program. This can be accomplished by including exercises that are performed with the humerus elevated into the scapular or coronal plane rather than in adduction.

The optimal position for isokinetic strengthening of the rotators is controversial. Exercises performed in full adduction may compromise blood flow to the rotator cuff tendons.[37] This can be avoided by placing the humerus in approximately 30 degrees of abduction and 30 degrees of forward flexion when performing internal and external rotation on an isokinetic machine. Some physical therapists and trainers recommend progressing isokinetic strengthening of the internal and external rotators to a position of 90 degrees of abduction. While this position may appear to mimic the functional position of the thrower and also may allow for unrestricted blood flow, it is also a tenuous position for stability of the glenohumeral joint and should be approached with extreme caution.

As soon as sufficient strength and endurance have been achieved in the dynamic stabilizers of the shoulder, the rehabilitation program can be advanced to include the anterior, middle, and posterior deltoids, which function primarily to position the humerus in space. If strengthening exercises of the deltoids are initiated prematurely, the deltoids will be forced to function at a relative mechanical disadvantage because the proper glenohumeral relationship will not be maintained. This pathologic motion can cause the patient's symptoms to become exacerbated. Effective deltoid strengthening exercises are scaption, forward flexion, prone horizontal abduction, rowing, and the military press. Coronal plane abduction is a commonly performed deltoid exercise, but it should be avoided until the rotator cuff muscles are suf-

ficiently strengthened because impingement will occur if the humeral head is not depressed adequately.

The final group of muscles to be strengthened in a logically sequenced rehabilitation program is the power muscles—pectoralis major and latissimus dorsi. High activity has been shown in these muscles during throwing, and it has been demonstrated that these are the only two upper extremity muscles whose strength correlates positively with pitching velocity.[16] Again, caution should be taken not to include strengthening of these muscles prematurely before the dynamic stabilizers have achieved adequate strength and endurance.

Horizontal abduction, bench press, and latissimus pull-down exercises are good exercises to target the power muscles. Any position during these exercises that potentially can lever the humeral head forward in the glenoid should be avoided. With horizontal abduction and bench press, the arms should not go behind the plane of the body. When the latissimus pull-down is performed, the arms should remain in front of the body.

Toward the final stages of the rehabilitation program, functional activities and sport-specific drills should be incorporated. Care should be taken to initiate advanced activities only when the patient has achieved sufficient flexibility, strength, and endurance. Time should be taken at this point to reemphasize proper mechanics because compensatory mechanics may have been developed by the thrower prior to initiation of the rehabilitation program.

More challenging exercises for the shoulder complex that incorporate a variety of muscles include push-ups while balanced on a Swiss ball or balance board, stair-stepping in a push-up position, and plyometric throwing exercises. A graduated throwing program is begun when strength and endurance are deemed adequate and throwing can be accomplished painfree.

ELBOW

Overuse Injuries

Overuse injuries, usually involving the musculotendinous units, are among the most common conditions in the throwing athlete's elbow. Tendinitis can involve the flexor pronator mass on the medial side, the extensor supinator mass on the lateral side, or the triceps posteriorly. Because of the extreme valgus forces and terminal elbow extension required to complete a throw, medial epicondylitis and triceps tendinitis are much more common in throwing athletes than is lateral epicondylitis. The medial musculotendinous structures can be injured either by microtearing from the cumulative effect of repetitive throwing or by macrotearing from one overly forceful muscular contraction. If this injury goes undiagnosed or is treated improperly, the increased stress to the injured musculotendinous unit is passed onto the medially located ulnar collateral ligament and ultimately can result in attenuation or tearing of the ligament. If the ulnar collateral ligament is injured or becomes attenuated, the subtle instability that results has ramifications that affect all compartments of the elbow joint. Increased medial stress unable to be borne properly by the ulnar collateral ligament can subject the ulnar nerve to excessive traction. Also, compressive forces are transferred to the radiocapitellar joint. Overload to the articular surface can lead to cartilage damage and loose bodies. Posteriorly, this overload is borne by the posteromedial olecranon. With continued throwing, osteophytes form and can give rise to intraarticular loose bodies.

Treatment of throwers with overuse injuries of the elbow should begin with a structured, nonoperative program that includes measures aimed at reducing inflammation, relative rest from aggravating activities, and rehabilitation of the injured musculotendinous structures. The rehabilitation program should begin with range-of-motion exercises and progress to strengthening, endurance exercises, and coordination training. Also, the physician, therapist, trainer, coach, and athlete should work together as a team to address throwing biomechanics and make alterations as necessary. If conservative treatment has been unsuccessful after 6 to 12 months, and if other diagnoses have been ruled out, then surgical treatment may be considered.

The overuse syndrome can extend to involve the posterior compartment of the elbow. This condition, known as *valgus extension overload*, initially can involve the triceps insertion on the olecranon. Overuse, improper throwing mechanics, or poorly conditioned muscles lead to triceps strain with subsequent inflammation. Successful treatment depends on early diagnosis and initiation of proper modalities and rehabilitation exercises. Complete rupture of the triceps complex is rare in throwers; however, if it occurs, it requires surgical reconstruction to restore the elbow extensor mechanism.

Development of posteromedial osteophytes is a common entity resulting from chronic valgus extension overload. These osteophytes result in impingement in the posterior compartment of the elbow, which manifests as pain and decreased range of motion in extension. Continued throwing under this condition can cause the osteophyte to fracture and become a loose body within the elbow joint. The loose-body fragment can become a mechanical block to motion and can lead to irritation of the joint, swelling, and significant articular surface damage if it becomes lodged between articular surfaces.

Elbow arthroscopy is performed frequently to treat throwers with valgus extension overload. It can be used to debride fibrous tissue and posteromedial osteophytes or retrieve loose bodies that may have become entrapped in any one of the compartments of the elbow. Elbow arthroscopy is a technically demanding procedure and should be performed only by an experienced surgeon.

Elbow Instability

One of the most devastating injuries that throwing athletes can sustain is injury to the ligamentous stabilizers of the elbow. Injury to the ulnar collateral ligament is much more common than is injury to the lateral ligamentous complex. Surgical treatment is usually required to restore the athlete's ability to throw at the preinjury level.

Ulnar collateral ligament injuries can present as a gradual onset of medially located elbow pain that is noted during the more demanding phases of the baseball pitch—late cocking, acceleration, and deceleration. Conversely, ulnar collateral ligament injury can be associated with sudden, sharp medial pain associated with either an audible or appreciated pop that had its onset during one specific pitch. Diagnosis of the ulnar collateral ligament injury that occurs with sudden onset is more straightforward than that which comes on gradually because medial-sided tenderness also can be present with flexor pronator tendinitis. If it is determined that the ulnar collateral ligament is insufficient and does not respond to conservative treatment, surgical reconstruction is usually performed, with the palmaris longus being the graft of choice for reconstruction. Since the palmaris longus is absent in approximately 13 percent of the population, other potential graft sites include the plantaris tendon, long toe extensor, Achilles tendon, or an allograft. In this reconstructive procedure, the transplanted graft is a vascular tissue that relies on vascular ingrowth and cellular proliferation from the surrounding tissues. Overzealous rehabilitation and an aggressive return to throwing should be discouraged, even in a phase of asymptomatic throwing, because the natural healing response of the graft cannot be accelerated. It is believed by many that these grafts cannot resist the stresses of throwing in position players until 9 to 12 months postoperatively and possibly as long as 15 months for pitchers.

Rehabilitation of Elbow Injuries

The elbow is a less common site of injury for throwers than the shoulder due to the inherent bony stability. However, the elbow is subjected to tremendous stress during throwing that can result in an array of injuries to the musculoskeletal and ligamentous structures. The cumulative effect of these repetitive stresses can be devastating to the elbow and can render the athlete ineffective.

Since the elbow joint is one of the final links in the kinetic chain that is the act of throwing, optimizing strength of the lower extremities, trunk, and shoulder girdle muscles, as well as addressing proper mechanics during throwing, is tantamount to a successful rehabilitation program for throwers with an elbow injury. Specific to the elbow, there are four major areas that should be addressed during a rehabilitation program for throwers. These four areas are the elbow flexors, the medial aspect of the joint, the lateral aspect of the joint, and the posterior compartment.

Most of the forces encountered by the elbow joint immediately after ball release are absorbed by the flexors of the elbow—the brachialis, brachioradialis, and biceps. It is common for pitchers to develop stiffness and soreness within the flexor muscles after pitching. Over years of throwing, many pitchers develop flexion contractures of 20 degrees or more that do not interfere with performance. It is difficult to know how significant a problem this is or to determine which throwers with contractures will go on to develop more serious pathology. It is recommended that pitchers routinely stretch the flexors gently and ice the area down if it is symptomatic following a throwing session. If a contracture is present, the flexors should be stretched to the point of the contracture only. Forceful stretching may result in loose bodies within the joint because some of the bony overgrowth limiting motion may be broken off.

Large valgus forces generated at the elbow during pitching are responsible for causing injuries to the structures of the medial aspect of the elbow. Possible injuries include medial epicondylitis as well as the more devastating ulnar collateral ligament injury, which can be chronic or due to acute rupture. Rehabilitation is frequently not successful in returning a thrower with ulnar collateral ligament insufficiency to competition but should be attempted before surgery is considered. The rehabilitation program should include gentle stretching and strengthening of the elbow flexors and extensors, wrist flexors and extensors, and forearm pronators and supinators. Special attention should be given to strengthening the pronator teres, flexor carpi radialis, flexor carpi ulnaris, and flexor digitorum superficialis because these are the muscles that have been demonstrated as having high activity during the baseball pitch and are in the best anatomic position to offer dynamic stability.

As with rehabilitation programs for shoulder injuries, elbow rehabilitation programs should incorporate functional activities, sport-specific drills, and ultimately, a graduated throwing program in the final stages. At this point, emphasis should be placed on proper mechanics because compensatory mechanics may have been developed by the thrower prior to initiation of the rehabilitation program. The therapist, trainer, coaches, and player should work together during this critical phase of the athlete's rehabilitation.

POSITION-SPECIFIC INJURIES

Although the most common injuries in baseball players are to the throwing shoulder and elbow, other musculoskeletal injuries do occur and may be more common in certain players due to the specific demands of the position they play. To date, there are no reports in the literature describing baseball injuries as they relate to position, but several trends have been noted clinically.

Outfielders

Outfielders are commonly required to begin a run from a still position. In going from a dead start to a sudden sprint, tremendous stress is placed on the musculotendinous units of the lower extremities. It is not unusual for outfielders to be afflicted with musculotendinous injuries, especially to the gastrocnemius-soleus complex and hamstring muscle group. Outfielders should be educated in the importance of warm-up and stretching in helping to prevent these injuries. Additionally, traumatic injuries may be seen in outfielders as a result of running into the outfield wall to catch a fly ball.

Infielders

Each infield position has its own unique physical requirements. Of these positions, the middle infielders—the shortstop and second baseman—are at risk for low-back injuries. Their positions require frequent unsupported forward flexion, often with a torsional component. This places stress not only on the musculotendinous structures of the low back but also on the intervertebral discs as well. These athletes should be educated about the risk of these injuries and should incorporate additional trunk-stabilization exercises into their preseason and injury-prevention programs.

Catchers

Catchers are at risk for meniscal injuries of the knee, especially in the posterior horn of the meniscus, due to the amount of time they spend in a deep squat position. Catchers also may be at higher risk for elbow injuries because they are frequently throwing from their knees. Throwing from this position does not afford them the advantage of using their legs and trunk to optimally position the upper extremity for the throw and may increase the stress placed across the elbow.

Return to Sport

RETURN TO THROWING FOLLOWING INJURY

Below are sample throwing programs to be used to bridge the gap between the flexibility, strengthening, and endurance portions of the rehabilitation program and return to play. Emphasis should be on execution of proper mechanics and endurance. The number of throws and time spent throwing should be minimized initially and progressed only as tolerated. If pain occurs at any point in the program, the thrower should be returned to the previous level until painfree. Strength training should continue during the phase of transition back to throwing and should be performed after the throwing sessions.

Rehabilitation Program for Pitchers

Throwing Program[29]

Step 1

Toss the ball (no windup) against a wall on alternate days. Start with 25 to 30 throws, building up to 70 throws, and gradually increase the throwing distance.

No. of throws	Distance (ft)
20	20 (warm-up phase)
25–40	30–40
10	20 (cool-down phase)

Step 2

Toss the ball (playing catch with easy windup) on alternate days.

No. of throws	Distance (ft)
10	20 (warm-up)
10	30–40
30–40	50
10	20–30 (cool-down)

Step 3

Continue increasing the throwing distance while still tossing the ball with an easy windup.

No. of throws	Distance (ft)
10	20 (warm-up)
10	30–40
30–40	50–60
10	30 (cool-down)

Step 4

Increase throwing distance to a maximum of 60 ft. Continue tossing the ball with an occasional throw at no more than half speed.

No. of throws	Distance (ft)
10	30 (warm-up)
10	40–45
30–40	60–70
10	30 (cool-down)

Step 5

During this step, gradually increase the distance to 150 ft maximum.

Phase 5-1:

Distance (ft)	No. of throws
10	40 (warm-up)
10	50–60
15–20	70–80
10	50–60
10	40 (cool-down)

Phase 5-2:

Distance (ft)	No. of throws
10	40 (warm-up)
10	50–60
20–30	80–90
20	50–60
10	40 (cool-down)

Phase 5-3:

Distance (ft)	No. of throws
10	40 (warm-up)
10	60

15–20	100–110
20	60
10	40 (cool-down)

Phase 5-4:

Distance (ft)	No. of throws
10	40 (warm-up)
10	60
15–20	120–150
20	60
10	40 (cool-down)

Step 6

Progress to throwing off the mound at one-half to three-quarters speed. Pay special attention to proper body mechanics now that pitcher is throwing off the mound:

- Stay on top of the ball.
- Keep the elbow up.
- Throw over the top.
- Follow through with the arm and trunk.
- Use the legs to push.

Phase 6-1:

Distance (ft)	No. of throws
10	60 (warm-up)
10	120–150 (lobbing)
30	45 (off the mound)
10	60 (off the mound)
10	40 (cool-down)

Phase 6-2:

Distance (ft)	No. of throws
10	50 (warm-up)
10	120–150 (lobbing)
20	45 (off the mound)
20	60 (off the mound)
10	40 (cool-down)

Phase 6-3:

Distance (ft) (warm-up)	No. of throws
10	50
10	60
10	120–150 (lobbing)

10	45 (off the mound)
30	60 (off the mound)
10	40 (cool-down)

Phase 6-4:

Distance (ft)	No. of throws
10	50 (warm-up)
10	120–150 (lobbing)
10	45 (off the mound)
40–50	60 (off the mound)
10	40 (cool-down)

At this time, if the pitcher has completed phase 6-4 successfully without pain or discomfort and is throwing at approximately three-quarters speed, he or she may be progressed to step 7, "up/down bullpens." This step is used to simulate a game situation. The pitcher rests in between a series of pitches to reproduce the rest period in between innings.

Step 7

Up/down bullpens (one-half to three-quarters speed).

Day 1:

No. of throws	Distance (ft)
10 warm-up	120–150 (lobbing)
10 warm-up throws	60 (off the mound)
40 pitches	60 (off the mound)
Rest 10 minutes	
20 pitches	60 (off the mound)

Day 2:	*Off*

Day 3:

No. of throws	Distance (ft)
10 warm-up throws	120–150 (lobbing)
10 warm-up throws	60 (off the mound)
30 pitches	60 (off the mound)
Rest 10 minutes	
10 warm-up throws	60 (off the mound)
20 pitches	60 (off the mound)
Rest 10 minutes	
10 warm-up throws	60 (off the mound)
20 pitches	60 (off the mound)

Day 4:   *Off*

Day 5:

No. of throws	Distance (ft)
10 warm-up throws	120–150 (lobbing)
10 warm-up throws	60 (off the mound)
30 pitches	60 (off the mound)
Rest 8 minutes	
20 pitches	60 (off the mound)
Rest 8 minutes	
20 pitches	60 (off the mound)
Rest 8 minutes	
20 pitches	60 (off the mound)

At this point the pitcher is ready to begin a normal routine, from throwing, batting practice to pitching in the bullpen. This program can and should be adjusted as needed. Each step may take longer or shorter than the time listed, and the program should be monitored by the trainer, physical therapist, and physician.

Rehabilitation Program for Catchers, Infielders, and Outfielders

Throwing Program[29]
Note: Repeat each step three times. All throws should have an arc or "hump." The maximum distance thrown by infielders and catchers is 120 ft. The maximum distance thrown by outfielders is 200 ft.

Step 1

Toss the ball with no windup. Stand with your feet shoulder width apart and face the player you are throwing toward. Concentrate on rotating and staying on top of the ball.

No. of throws	Distance (ft)
5	20 (warm-up)
10	30
5	20 (cool-down)

Step 2

Stand sideways from the person you are throwing toward. Feet are shoulder width apart. Close up and pivot onto your back foot as you throw.

No. of throws	Distance (ft)
5	30 (warm-up)
5	40
10	50
5	30 (cool-down)

Step 3

Repeat the position in step 2. Step toward the target with your front leg, and follow through with your back leg.

No. of throws	Distance (ft)
5	50 (warm-up)
5	60
10	70
5	50 (cool-down)

Step 4

Assume the pitcher's stance. Lift and stride with your lead leg. Follow through with your back leg.

No. of throws	Distance (ft)
5	60 (warm-up)
5	70
10	80
5	60 (cool-down)

Step 5

Outfielders: Lead with your glove-side foot forward. Take one step, crow hop, and throw the ball.
Infielders: Lead with your glove-side foot forward. Take a shuffle step, and throw the ball. Throw the last five throws in a straight line.

No. of throws	Distance (ft)
5	70 (warm-up)
5	90

| 10 | 100 |
| 5 | 80 (cool-down) |

Step 6

Repeat the throwing technique as in step 5. Assume your playing position. Infielders and catchers do not throw greater than 120 ft. Outfielders do not throw greater than 150 ft (mid-outfield).

No. of throws	Infielders & catchers distance (ft)	Outfielders distance (ft)
5	80 (warm-up)	80 (warm-up)
5	80–90	90–100
5	90–100	110–125
5	110–120	130–150
5	80 (cool-down)	80 (cool-down)

Step 7

Infielders, catchers, and outfielders may all assume their playing positions.

No. of throws	Infielders & catchers distance (ft)	Outfielders distance (ft)
5	80 (warm-up)	80–90 (warm-up)
5	80–90	110–130
5	90–100	150–175
5	110–120	180–200
5	80 (cool-down)	90 (cool-down)

Step 8

Repeat step 7. Use a Fungo bat (a small bat used to hit during fielding practice) to hit to the infielders and outfielders while in their normal playing position.

Windmill Softball Pitch

Compared with the overhand baseball pitch, underhand pitching has received little attention in the medical literature. This may be due to the erroneous perception that compared with baseball pitchers, underhand pitchers are not susceptible to injury. In a survey of eight collegiate softball teams participating in the NCAA softball tournament, 80 percent of the participating pitchers reported injuries.[38] The upper extremity was involved in 82 percent of the time-loss injuries.

Like the overhand pitching motion, the windmill softball pitch can be divided into phases. Those phases are the windup, stride, delivery, and follow-through.[39]

WINDUP

The windup phase begins with the first motion of the ball and ends with the lead foot toe-off. This phase can be quite variable from pitcher to pitcher with regard to the amount of arm extension posterior to the sagittal plane of the body, elbow flexion, and forward trunk lean. Torques, forces, angular velocities, and muscle activity about the shoulder and elbow are of low magnitude during this phase.[35,39]

STRIDE

The stride phase starts with the lead toe-off and continues until lead foot contact. Kinematic and kinetic parameters remain low during this phase. In the first half of this phase, muscle activity is high in the supraspinatus and infraspinatus muscles, and the arm is raised overhead. The supraspinatus is active to centralize the humeral head in the glenoid as the deltoid elevates the arm. The infraspinatus may be assisting in the elevation of the humerus during this phase. A cadaveric study demonstrated that both the infraspinatus and subscapularis can contribute to humeral elevation in the plane of the scapula and that with the humerus positioned in internal rotation, the infraspinatus is more active in this role.[40]

DELIVERY

The delivery phase begins with lead foot contact and continues until the ball is released. This phase serves to accelerate the ball through a combination of trunk rotation, humeral flexion and internal rotation, and elbow flexion. The highest torques, forces, and angular velocities occur during this phase. Shoulder flexion and internal rotation velocities of 5260 and 4650 degrees per second, respectively, contribute to ball velocity.[39] While internal rotation velocity of the shoulder does not quite approach that of the baseball pitch, it is still of extremely high magnitude. These findings correlate with high muscle activity seen in the pectoralis major and subscapularis muscles during this phase.[35]

FOLLOW-THROUGH

The final phase of the softball pitch, follow-through, begins with ball release and ends when forward motion of the throwing arm has stopped. There has been some variation in mechanics described for this phase. Barrentine et al. have observed that the elbow flexes after the ball is released and the humerus passes forward of the trunk.[39] Maffet et al. reported that the pitching arm was decelerated by contact of the arm with the lateral hip and thigh at the instant following ball release.[35] This phase is characterized by maximum elbow flexion torque and maximum elbow compressive forces.[39] Extreme pronation of the forearm also has been observed during this phase and may be a factor that contributes to fatigue fractures of the ulna in softball pitchers.[41] Muscle activity in all shoulder muscles decreases with respect to the previous phases, with the teres minor maintaining the highest activity.[35] As in the overhand baseball pitch, the teres minor may be active during this phase to decelerate the internally rotating humerus.

Because the demands on the softball pitcher are not well understood, pitchers are often required to pitch more than one game in a day or pitch games on consecutive days throughout the season without adequate rest. Even the pitcher with perfect mechanics will be at risk for overuse injuries to the shoulder and elbow under these circumstances. Prevention of injury in fast-pitch softball pitchers should be addressed by understanding the biomechanical demands of the motion, strengthening the shoulder and elbow musculature, and ensuring adequate rest between pitching outings.

Summary

The shoulder and elbow are the joints most vulnerable to injury in baseball players as a result of the high forces and torques, extremes of range of motion, and large number of repetitions required during the throwing motion. There is a fine line between optimal performance and injury. Prevention, early recognition, and rehabilitation of injuries in baseball players depend on a thorough knowledge of the mechanics of the shoulder and elbow joints as well as the biomechanics of the throwing motion. The best approach to treatment of injuries in the baseball player is prevention through proper strengthening and conditioning that focuses on the lower extremities, trunk, shoulder, and elbow stabilizing muscles and performing with optimal mechanics.

References

1. McFarland EG, Wasik M: Epidemiology of collegiate baseball injuries. *Clin J Sport Med* 8(1):10–13, 1998.
2. Matsen FA, Harryman DT, Sidles JA: Mechanics of glenohumeral instability. *Clin Sports Med* 10(4):783–788, 1991.
3. Cooper DE, Arnoczky SP, O'Brien SJ, et al.: Anatomy, histology, and vascularity of the glenoid rim: An anatomical study. *J Bone Joint Surg* 74A(1):46–52, 1992.
4. Blasier RB, Guldberg MS, Rothman ED: Anterior shoulder stability: Contributions of rotator cuff forces and the capsular ligaments in a cadaver model. *J Shoulder Elbow Surg* 1:140–150, 1992.
5. Inman VT, Saunders DM, Abbott CL: Observations of the functions of the shoulder joint. *J Bone Joint Surg* 26A:19–30, 1944.
6. Morrey BF, An K: Biomechanics of the shoulder, in Rockwood CA, Matsen FA (eds): *The Shoulder*. Philadelphia: Saunders, 1990, pp 231–232.
7. DiGiovine NM, Jobe FW, Pink M, et al: An electromyographic analysis of the upper extremity in pitching. *J Shoulder Elbow Surg* 1(1):15–25, 1992.
8. Feltner M, Dapena J: Dynamics of the shoulder and elbow joint of the throwing arm during a baseball pitch. *Int J Sport Biomech* 2:235–259, 1986.
9. Howell SM, Imobersteg AM, Seger DH, et al: Clarification of the role of the supraspinatus muscle in shoulder function. *J Bone Joint Surg* 68A(3):398–404, 1986.
10. Glousman R, Jobe FW, Tibone JE, et al: Dynamic electromyographic analysis of the throwing shoulder with glenohumeral instability. *J Bone Joint Surg* 70A(2):220–226, 1988.
11. Fleisig GS, Barrentine SW: Biomechanical aspects of the elbow in sports. *Sports Med Arthroscopy Rev* 3:149–159, 1995.
12. Morrey BF, An KN: Articular and ligamentous contributions to the stability of the elbow. *Am J Sports Med* 11(5):315–319, 1983.
13. Fleisig GS, Dillman CJ, Escamilla RF, et al: Kinetics of baseball pitching with implications about injury mechanics. *Am J Sports Med* 23:233–239, 1995.
14. Davidson PA, Pink M, Perry J, et al: Functional anatomy of the flexor pronator muscle group in relation to the medial collateral ligament of the elbow. *Am J Sports Med* 23(2):245–250, 1995.
15. An KN, Hui FC, Morrey, BF, et al: Muscles across the elbow joint: A biomechanical analysis. *J Biomech* 14(10):659–669, 1981.
16. Bartlett LR, Storey MD, Simons BD: Measurement of upper extremity torque production and its relationship to throwing speed in the competitive athlete. *Am J Sports Med* 17:89–91, 1989.
17. Shaffer B, Jobe FW, Pink M, et al: Baseball batting: An electromyographic study. *Clin Orthop* 292:285–293, 1993.
18. Welch CM, Banks SA, Cook FF, et al: Hitting a baseball: A biomechanical description. *J Orthop Sports Phys Ther* 22(5):193–201, 1995.
19. Safran MR, Garrett WE, Seaber AV, et al: The role of warmup in muscular injury prevention. *Am J Sports Med* 16:123–129, 1998.
20. McNair PJ, Stanley SN: Effect of passive stretching and jogging on the series elastic muscle stiffness and range of motion of the ankle joint. *Br J Sports Med* 30:313–318, 1996.
21. Mohr KJ, Pink MM, Elsner C, et al: Electromyographic investigation of stretching: The effect of warm-up. *Clin J Sport Med* 8:215–220, 1998.
22. Bigliani LU, Codd TP, Connor PM, et al: Shoulder motion and laxity in the professional baseball player. *Am J Sports Med* 25(5):609–613, 1997.
23. Pink MM, Perry J: Biomechanics, in Jobe FW (ed): *Operative Techniques in Upper Extremity Sports Medicine*. St. Louis: Mosby–Year Book, 1996, p 116.
24. Tibone JE, Jobe FW, Kerlan RK, et al: Shoulder impingement syndrome in athletes treated by an anterior acromioplasty. *Clin Orthop* 198:134–140, 1985.
25. Hayashi K, Thabit G, Bogdanske JJ, et al: The effect of nonablative laser energy on the ultrastructure of joint capsular collagen. *Arthroscopy* 12(4):474–481, 1996.

26. Hayashi K, Thabit G, Massa KL, et al: The effect of thermal heating on the length and histologic properties of the glenohumeral joint capsule. *Am J Sports Med* 25(1):107–112, 1997.

27. Lopez MJ, Hayashi K, Fanton GS, et al: The effect of radiofrequency energy on the ultrastructure of joint capsular collagen. *Arthroscopy* 14(5):495–501, 1998.

28. Naseef GS, Foster TE, Trauner K, et al: The thermal properties of bovine joint capsule: The basic science of laser- and radiofrequency-induced capsular shrinkage. *Am J Sports Med* 25(5):670–674, 1997.

29. Brewster CE, Moynes Schwab DR, Seto J: Conservative and postoperative management of shoulder problems, in Jobe FW (ed): *Operative Techniques in Upper Extremity Sports Medicine.* St. Louis: Mosby–Year Book, 1996, pp 257–259.

30. Moseley JB, Jobe FW, Pink MM, et al: EMG analysis of the scapular muscles during a shoulder rehabilitation program. *Am J Sports Med* 20(2):128–134, 1992.

31. Townsend H, Jobe FW, Pink MM, et al: Electromyographic analysis of the glenohumeral muscles during a baseball rehabilitation program. *Am J Sports Med* 19(3):264–272, 1991.

32. Pink MM, Screnar PM, Tollefson KD, et al: Injury prevention and rehabilitation in the upper extremity, in Jobe FW (ed): *Operative Techniques in Upper Extremity Sports Medicine.* St. Louis: Mosby–Year Book, 1996, p 10.

33. Herberts P, Kadefors R: A study of painful shoulder in welders. *Acta Orthop Scand* 47:381–387, 1976.

34. Pink MM, Perry J, Brown A, et al: The normal shoulder during freestyle swimming: An electromyographic and cinematographic analysis of twelve muscles. *Am J Sports Med* 19(6):569–575, 1991.

35. Maffet MW, Jobe FW, Pink MM, et al: Shoulder muscle firing patterns during the windmill softball pitch. *Am J Sports Med* 25(3):369–374, 1997.

36. Turkel SJ, Panio MW, Marshall JL, et al: Stabilizing mechanisms preventing anterior dislocation of the glenohumeral joint. *J Bone Joint Surg* 63A(8):1208–1217, 1981.

37. Rathbun JB, Macnab I: The microvascular pattern of the rotator cuff. *J Bone Joint Surg* 52A(3):540–553, 1970.

38. Loosli AR, Requa RK, Garrick JG, et al: Injuries to pitchers in women's collegiate fast-pitch softball. *Am J Sports Med* 20(1):35–37, 1992.

39. Barrentine SW, Fleisig GS, Whiteside JA, et al: Biomechanics of windmill softball pitching with implications about injury mechanisms at the shoulder and elbow. *J Orthop Sports Phys Ther* 28(6):405–415, 1998.

40. Otis JC, Jiang CC, Wickiewicz TL, et al: Changes in the moment arms of the rotator cuff and deltoid muscles with abduction and rotation. *J Bone Joint Surg* 76A:667–676, 1993.

41. Tanabe S, Nakahira J, Bando E, et al: Fatigue fracture of the ulna occurring in pitchers of fast-pitch softball. *Am J Sports Med* 19(3):317–321, 1991.

42. Corzatt RD, Groppel JL, Pfautsch E, et al: The biomechanics of head-first versus feet-first sliding. *Am J Sports Med* 12(3):229–232, 1984.

43. McCord JD: Mechanical analysis of sliding. *The Ath J* 51:66–75, 1971.

CHAPTER 3

Tennis

Jane Jarosz-Hlis

Over the years, the game of tennis has made significant changes. Tennis has been influenced by advances in sports science and equipment technology.[12] Power, speed, strength, and physical conditioning have moved to the forefront of today's tennis game. This chapter will highlight current equipment choices, the physical demands of tennis, injury prevention, potential injury sites, and tennis-specific conditioning.

Equipment Design

Today's advancements in equipment design have played a significant role in changing the game of tennis. Racket materials, head size, racket length, and string type have all influenced the hard-hitting, aggressive game. In addition, advancements in footwear have developed such that a specific "tennis" shoe is recommended for play. Below, each of these areas will be described, as well as their influence on the current game style.

RACKET MATERIALS

Racket composition has evolved from wood and ceramic to composite, graphite, and carbon. A racket composed of graphite alone provides for a light and sturdy frame. This light material promotes increased racket speed and acceleration. Graphite also increases racket stiffness, thereby reducing the impact forces and vibration resulting from ball contact. A composite frame typically consists of a combination of graphite and ceramic materials. The composite frame achieves increased power over the graphite frame and is balanced by the control component of the ceramic ingredient. Carbon and titanium are the newest advancements in racket materials. They are lighter and stronger, promoting racket head acceleration and increased racket stiffness. The result is an increased force behind the ball.

RACKET DESIGN

Racket head size has evolved from the standard size to a midsized or oversized racket face. These larger racket heads increase the overall width of the racket. As a result, a greater "sweet spot" exists, thereby lessening the vibration transmitted to the wrist and forearm on off-center hits.[13] Recreational players who are new to the game will benefit from an oversized racket head because off-center hits are much more common in this population.

Overall racket length also has changed over the last few years. The new "extender" rackets have increased the overall length of the racket. Thus, the lever arm from the hand to the end of the racket is greater. This can lead to increased ball speed as compared with a standard-length racket accelerated at the same speed. However, significant strength in the forearm and shoulder girdle musculature is required to stabilize a longer racket throughout the entire stroke, especially at impact. Players who do not have well-developed forearm and shoulder girdle musculature must consider the increased potential for injury to the upper extremity with an "extender" racket.

GRIP SIZE

When choosing a grip size, it is important that a player feel comfortable gripping the racket. A grip that is too small often results in "wristy" strokes due to the inability to hold onto the racket adequately. A grip that is too big often results in a constant contraction of the forearm muscles, because the player fears letting go and having the racket fall out of his or her hand.

An arthropometric measurement technique has been developed to determine exact grip size. By placing a ruler from the distal palm line of the dominant hand to the tip of the fourth finger and reading the measurement in inches, the exact grip size can be determined.[25] Typically, if a player's measurement is between grip sizes, a smaller size is recommended because grip tape can be wrapped easily around the grip. This in-

creases the grip size to a comfortable circumference.

GRIP POSITIONS

The type of grip a player uses to hold the racket will vary according to the stroke hit. The grip itself can be broken down into eight separate bevels. The key anatomic points for the dominant hand include the heel of the hand and the base of the second knuckle. Below, the most common grip used for each stroke will be analyzed, and the hand position in relation to the grip's bevels will be discussed.

The eastern forehand grip is the most traditional of the forehand grips and results in relatively no ball spin. The racket face during the backswing is perpendicular to the ground. The heel of the dominant hand rests on bevel two or three, and the base of the second knuckle lies on bevel three.

The semiwestern forehand grip results in a topspin ball. The racket face during the backswing phase is slightly closed, facing the ground at approximately a 45-degree angle. The heel of the dominant hand lies on bevel three or four, and the base of the second knuckle rests on bevel three or four.

Extreme topspin is seen when the racket is held with a western forehand grip. The racket face on the backswing is very closed, typically parallel to the ground. During the western forehand grip, the heel of the dominant hand rests on bevel five or six, and the base of the second knuckle lies on bevel four or five.

The most common grip used for the one-handed backhand is the eastern backhand grip. This grip allows a player to vary the ball spin to flat or topspin. The heel of the dominant hand covers bevel one or eight, and the base of the second knuckle rests on bevel one.

The two-handed backhand can involve several combinations of grips because both the dominant and nondominant hands must hold onto the grip. It is important to note that during the two-handed backhand, the nondominant hand rests on top of the dominant hand, and they touch each other. This allows the two hands to work as one unit, optimizing forces at ball contact. Interlocking of the fingers is not recommended. Common hand positions include (1) dominant eastern backhand grip and a nondominant eastern forehand grip or (2) a dominant eastern forehand grip and a nondominant eastern forehand grip.

During the serve, the recommended hand position is the continental grip. This grip optimizes wrist motion, a firm hold, and variations in ball spin. The heel of the racket hand rests on bevel one and two, and the base of the second knuckle lies on bevel two.

RACKET STRING

Racket string is typically one of three types: nylon, composite, or gut. Nylon is inexpensive and durable. Composite string is a mixture of nylon and gut, combining durability and feel for the ball at contact. Gut string also promotes increased feel of the ball on the string. As a player's game develops, and touch, feel, and spin are emphasized, gut string may be more beneficial to enhancing performance.

The thickness of racket string, commonly known as *gauge*, also can affect ball feel. The standard gauge is 16. This promotes a balance between durability and ball feel. Fifteen-gauge string is thicker, resulting in more durability. Seventeen- and eighteen-gauge string is thinner and provides more control, touch, and feel for the ball. It is recommended that novice players initially consider a lower gauge string.

TENNIS FOOTWEAR

Tennis shoes today are specifically designed for tennis court play. Tennis footwear features include the following:

1. *Support insoles.* These provide optimal foot support and cushion.
2. *Heel counters.* These add stability and support, preventing the heel from shifting and slipping.
3. *Thick rubber outsoles.* These increase durability and typically are enhanced over the toe area.
4. *Reinforced midfoot support.* This provides optimal mediolateral stability, especially during dynamic directional changes.
5. *Wide toe box.* This allows players to spread their toes sufficiently.

Most tennis is played on one of two types of court surfaces: hard court or clay court. Thus the tread pattern of a tennis shoe's outsole may vary according to the court surface for which it is designed. An optimal tread pattern for clay court play is a small, shallow tread pattern. On the other hand, a wide tread pattern with deep flex grooves tends to provide better playability on hard courts.

Biomechanical Principles

NEWTON'S LAWS OF PHYSICS

Before discussing the biomechanics of the tennis stroke, the foundation on which these strokes rely must be established. Central to this foundation are Sir Isaac Newton's laws of physics, the principles of linear and angular momentum, the concept of the unit turn, and the kinetic-link principle.

Newton's first law of physics states that for every action, there is an equal and opposite reaction. Newton's second law states that an object at rest will stay at rest or an object in motion will stay in motion unless an outside force acts on it. Newton's third law of physics states that force equals mass times acceleration. As a player increases his or her racket speed, thereby increasing overall acceleration, the force generated to the ball increases as well. This increase in racket head speed has been a revolutionary process, contributing to the hard-hitting, power game of tennis today.

Efficient and effective use of the unit turn contributes to an overall increase in force generated by the body toward the ball. The unit turn occurs as the body moves as a whole unit during the backswing, contact, and follow-through phases of a ground stroke. Because of the dynamics of the game, the unit turn allows a player to optimally control his or her center of gravity and remain balanced throughout the stroke. Use of the unit turn also promotes optimal use of linear and angular momentum. Linear momentum occurs as a player transfers his or her weight forward to the front foot. A good example of this is a ground stroke hit with a square-stance position.

Angular momentum is generated as the body coils backward during the backswing phase, storing kinetic energy, and uncoils forward through to the contact and follow-through phases, using the stored kinetic energy. A rotational force results and is transferred to the ball. An example of angular momentum is the open-stance forehand. A key concept to the foundation of all tennis strokes is the kinetic-link principle. The *kinetic-link principle* can be defined as the summation of forces performed in a specific sequence resulting in an efficient and effective movement pattern. In tennis, the kinetic chain starts at the ground, moves up the lower extremity to the hips, and continues to the trunk and then to the upper extremity, including the shoulder, elbow, wrist, and hand.

Now that the foundation has been reviewed, the biomechanics of the basic tennis strokes, including the forehand, two-handed backhand, one-handed backhand, and the serve can be addressed specifically. Ground strokes are broken down into three phases of motion. They are the backswing, contact, and follow-through stages. The serve is composed of four phases, including the windup, cocking, acceleration, and follow-through phases. During all ground strokes and the serve, the primary goal of the lower extremities and trunk is to transfer kinetic energy to the racket by way of linear and angular momentum. If this is performed rhythmically and sequentially, optimal racket power and control result. Below is a detailed description of the joint motions during particular stroke phases.

FOREHAND BIOMECHANICS

The forehand is the fundamental stroke to the game of tennis today. Several variations in the biomechanics of this stroke are seen. This is primarily because several types of grips can be used, and some players use a two-hand forehand (Fig. 3.1). As a result, swing path and ball spin will vary greatly. The biomechanics of the forehand are described in Table 3.1.

Backswing

The backswing phase is designed to transfer kinetic energy from the ground upward through the body and store it in preparation for the contact phase. During the backswing phase of the forehand, some players will have a large loop, some a small loop, and some a straight takeback motion. Regardless of the type of backswing, all motions must have an external rotation component of the racket arm. Typically, the forearm and wrist positions of the dominant arm will vary according to the type of grip a player uses. The surrounding muscle groups of the forearm and wrist remain relatively quiet as the player submaximally grips the racket[23] (Fig. 3.2).

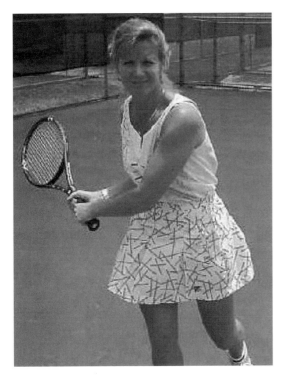

FIGURE 3.1

Two-hand forehand.

Contact Phase

After the backswing phase is complete, the contact phase begins. Acceleration of the body and racket toward the ball occurs during this phase. A transfer of weight to the front foot and ball impact are the two main actions highlighting this stroke phase.

The racket shoulder begins to internally rotate and horizontally adduct as the internal rotators, mainly the subscapularis and pectoralis major, of the dominant shoulder contract.[30] The scapula protracts as the serratus anterior shortens.[30] The dominant elbow extends as the bicep stabilizes forearm rotation.[23] Motion at the forearm and wrist of the racket arm will vary according to the type of grip a player uses. All players must achieve a near-vertical racket face at ball contact, no

matter what type of spin is desired.[12] At ball contact, a cocontraction of all the forearm, wrist, and hand muscles occurs in order to position and stabilize the racket, regardless of what type of grip is used during the forehand stroke. A firm grip acts as the final link to the body's kinetic chain, transferring optimal forces from the body to the racket.[23]

Follow-Through

Immediately after ball contact, the follow-through phase begins. Studies demonstrate continued electromyographic (EMG) activity of the anterior chest muscles during the follow-through phase, including the pectoralis, subscapularis, and serratus anterior.[30] In addition, after ball contact, the posterior shoulder girdle muscles, including the rotator cuff and scapular muscles, are eccentrically contracting to slow the arm down, particularly the infraspinatus.[30] The dominant elbow actively flexes, while the forearm and wrist muscle activity significantly decreases, except for the extensor carpi radialis brevis because it continues to assist in wrist stabilization.[23]

TWO-HANDED BACKHAND BIOMECHANICS

The biomechanics of the two-handed backhand are a combination of a dominant one-handed backhand and a nondominant forehand. The nondominant hand acts as a powerful addition as it moves in unison with the dominant upper extremity throughout the entire stroke. The biomechanics of the two-handed backhand are described in Table 3.2.

Backswing

During the backswing phase, forearm and wrist positions vary according to the preferred grip used for each hand. It is important to note that when gripping the racket during a two-handed backhand, the hands must touch each other but not interlock. This allows the upper extremities to move as one

TABLE 3.1

Forehand Stroke Analysis

Body Part	Backswing	Contact	Follow-Through
Front foot	Slight plantarflexion	Step into ball at 45 degrees	Dorsiflexion
Back foot	Foot parallel to net/dorsiflexion	Plantarflexion	Plantarflexion
Front knee	Flexion	Flexion	Flexion to extension
Back knee	Flexion	Flexion to extension	Extension
Front hip	External rotation (ER)	Internal rotation	Internal rotation
Back hip	ER to internal rotation (IR)	External rotation/ extension	External rotation/ extension
Trunk	Backward rotation	Forward rotation	Forward rotation
Racket shoulder	Horizontal abduction/ER	Horizontal adduction/ IR/protraction	Horizontal adduction/IR/ protraction
Racket elbow	Flexion	Flexion to extension	Flexion
Racket forearm/ wrist	Western—pronation Eastern—neutral	Vertical racket face	Flexion
Racket contact position		In front of lead foot	

link during the chain of events and the non-dominant hand to release quickly after shot completion (Fig. 3.3).

Contact Phase

After the backswing phase is complete, the contact phase begins. This is a very powerful stage because both hands are on the racket and the entire body is moving as one unit to generate power.

Follow-Through

The follow-through phase begins just after ball contact. The upper extremities continue to move in unison with the lower kinetic chain as the racket gradually decelerates. Both hands remain gripped to the racket until the follow-through phase is completed.

ONE-HANDED BACKHAND BIOMECHANICS

The second type of backhand to be analyzed is the one-handed backhand. The one-handed backhand is an extremely difficult shot to hit because it involves five separate links in the kinetic chain. These isolated links include the lower extremity, the hips, the trunk, and the proximal and distal upper extremity.[12] The biomechanics of the lower half of the kinetic chain of the one-handed backhand are

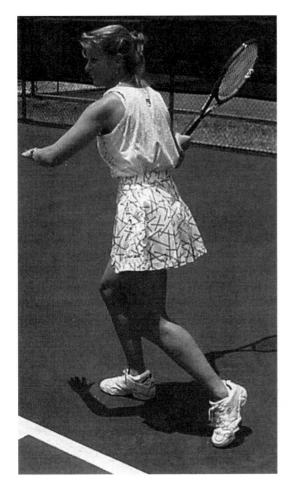

FIGURE 3.2

Forehand backswing.

similar to the motions occurring in the lower kinetic chain of the forehand and two-handed backhand during all phases. The biomechanics of the one-handed backhand are described in Table 3.3.

Backswing

During the backswing phase, the racket shoulder horizontally adducts and internally rotates, and the scapula protracts. The forearm and wrist remain fairly quiet during the preparation phase as the hand maintains an eastern backhand grip. The nondominant hand holds onto the racket to assist the racket arm during the backswing (Fig. 3.4A).

Contact Phase

As the contact phase begins, a forward step of the front foot and weight transfer toward the ball occur, generating linear momentum. Next, the oblique muscles contract as the trunk uncoils and rotates toward the ball. The scapula of the dominant upper extremity retracts.[12,30] The wrist extensors significantly

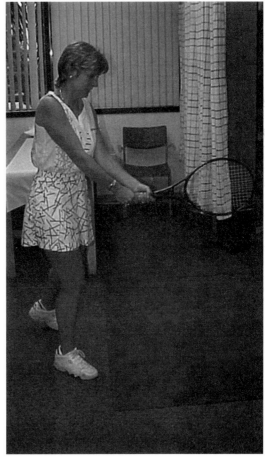

FIGURE 3.3

Two-handed backhand backswing.

TABLE 3.2

Two-Handed Backhand Stroke Analysis

Body Part	Backswing	Contact	Follow-Through
Front foot	Slight plantarflexion	Step into ball at 30–45 degrees	Dorsiflexion
Back foot	Parallel to net; slight dorsiflexion	Push off	Plantarflexion
Front knee	Flexion	Flexion	Flexion to extension
Back knee	Flexion	Flexion to extension	Extension
Front hip	External rotation (ER)	Internal rotation	Internal rotation
Back hip	ER to internal rotation (IR)	External rotation/ extension	External rotation/ extension
Trunk	Backward rotation	Forward rotation	Forward rotation
Racket shoulder	Horizontal adduction/ IR	Horizontal abduction/ ER/retraction	Horizontal abduction/ER
Nonracket shoulder	External rotation	Horizontal adduction/ IR/protraction	Horizontal adduction/IR
Racket elbow	Flexion	Flexion to extension	Flexion
Nonracket elbow	Flexion	Flexion to extension	Flexion
Racket forearm/ wrist	Varies	Varies; must achieve vertical racket face	Extension
Nonracket forearm/ wrist		Varies; must achieve vertical racket face	Flexion
Racket contact position		In front of lead foot	

increase their activity as the forearm and wrist position the hand for impact.[9,17,23] Increased EMG activity is seen in the wrist flexors during the late contact phase in uninjured tennis players.[9,17,23] This increased activity is most likely a stabilizing contraction of the forearm, wrist, and hand resulting from ball contact. Contact occurs approximately 12 inches beyond the front foot. In early contact phase, the nondominant hand releases the racket, and that shoulder begins to extend and abduct, counterbalancing the dominant shoulder's forward motion (Fig. 3.4B).

Follow-Through

The wrist flexors and extensors continue to stabilize the wrist in early follow-through, although their contraction lessens as compared with the contact phase.[9,17] Wrist flexor and extensor activity decreases significantly in

TABLE 3.3

Backhand Stroke Analysis

Body Part	Backswing	Contact	Follow-Through
Front foot	Slight plantarflexion	Step into ball at 30–45 degrees	Dorsiflexion
Back foot	Parallel to net in slight dorsiflexion	Plantarflexion	Plantarflexion
Front knee	Flexion	Flexion	Flexion to extension
Back knee	Flexion	Flexion to extension	Extension
Front hip	External rotation (ER)	Internal rotation	Internal rotation
Back hip	ER to internal rotation (IR)	ER/extension	ER/extension
Trunk	Backward rotation	Forward rotation	Forward rotation
Racket shoulder	Horizontal adduction/ IR/protraction	ER/horizontal abduction/retraction	Horizontal abduction/ ER/retraction
Nonracket shoulder	Extension	Extension/abduction	Extension/abduction
Racket elbow	Flexion	Flexion to extension	Slight flexion
Nonracket elbow	Flexion	Flexion to extension	Extension
Racket forearm/ wrist	Neutral	Neutral	Extension
Racket contact position		12–14 inches in front of lead foot	

the late follow-through stage. The nondominant shoulder and elbow complete their extension motions, maintaining body balance.

Tennis Serve Biomechanics

The tennis serve is a complex sequence of events demanding rhythmic muscle coordination and timing. The continental grip is used commonly for a topspin serve, whereas the eastern forehand grip is used for a flat serve. The serve can be broken down into four phases of motion: (1) windup, (2) cocking, (3) acceleration, and (4) follow-through. The biomechanics of the tennis serve are described in Table 3.4.

WINDUP

The windup stage begins as the serve is initiated and ends as the nondominant hand completes the ball toss. The body weight moves to the back foot. Linear momentum is then transferred forward, and angular momentum begins as the back, hip, and trunk rotate, and a coiling motion occurs.

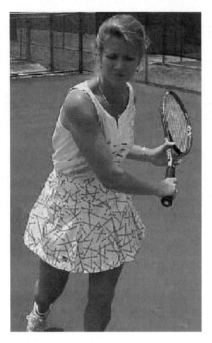 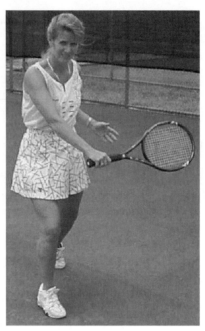

FIGURE 3.4

A. One-handed backhand backswing (1). *B.* One-handed backhand contact (2).

Assisted by the body's weight shifting backward, the dominant shoulder and elbow extend. The nondominant shoulder and elbow also extend, but only to the body's side or a neutral position. Once this neutral position is achieved, both shoulders elevate as the racket shoulder begins to abduct, and the nondominant shoulder flexes to complete the ball toss. The muscle activity of the shoulders, elbows, forearms, and wrists is minimal during the windup phase because the linear and angular momentum already generated assists in allowing these actions to occur[23,24] (Fig 3.5*A*).

COCKING

The cocking stage begins as the player completes the ball toss and finishes at maximum external rotation of the dominant shoulder. The supraspinatus actively contracts, and the external rotators shorten.[24,30] High activity in the serratus anterior muscle is needed for scapular stabilization in the racket arm.[30] The wrist extensors shorten.[23] Additionally, the trunk flexes laterally and extends in preparation to drive the hips and dominant shoulder upward for ball contact.[7] At this point, maximal potential energy has been stored, and acceleration is ready to begin (see Fig. 3.5*B*).

ACCELERATION

The acceleration phase starts as the racket shoulder begins to internally rotate and ends at ball contact. At this time, the subscapularis, pectoralis major, and latissimus dorsi are concentrically contracting.[30] The serratus anterior is also highly active because it stabilizes the scapula during this explosive movement. Effective scapular stabilization is a critical component to this stage because

TABLE 3.4

Serve Stroke Analysis

Body Part	Windup	Cocking	Acceleration	Follow-Through
Front foot	Approx. 45 degrees	Dorsiflexion	Plantarflexion	Dorsiflexion
Back foot	Parallel to slight angle to the net	Dorsiflexion	Plantarflexion	Plantarflexion
Front knee	Flexion to extension	Flexion	Flexion to extension	Flexion
Back knee	Slight flexion	Flexion	Flexion to extension	Flexion
Front hip	External rotation	External rotation	Internal rotation	Internal rotation
Back hip	Internal rotation	Internal rotation	External rotation	External rotation
Trunk	Backward rotation	Backward rotation/ extension	Forward rotation/ flexion	Rotation/ flexion
Racket shoulder	Flexion to extension	Abduction/ER	Horizontal adduction/IR	Horizontal adduction/IR
Nonracket shoulder	Flexion to extension	Flexion	Extension	Extension
Racket elbow	Flexion to extension	Flexion	Extension	Flexion
Nonracket elbow	Extension	Extension	Extension or flexion	Flexion
Racket forearm/ wrist	Neutral to extension	Extension	Flexion/ pronation	Flexion/ pronation
Nonracket forearm	Supination	Supination		
Racket contact position			In front of lead foot at peak ball toss	

forceful internal rotation can cause a anterior tipping of the scapula.[20,30]

The elbow of the racket arm extends as the triceps shortens.[6,30] The biceps eccentrically contracts during the late portion of acceleration, preventing hyperextension of the dominant elbow.[30] The pronators and wrist flexors of the dominant arm shorten, preparing for ball impact.[6] The lower legs, hips, and trunk produce 51 percent of the total kinetic

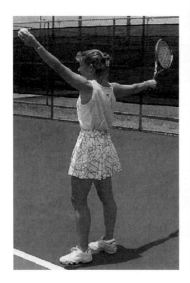 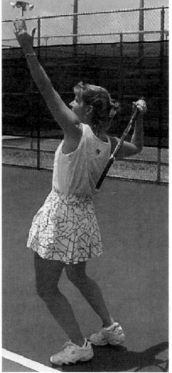 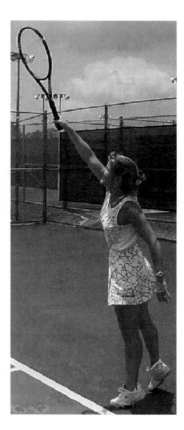

FIGURE 3.5

A. Tennis serve, windup. *B.* Tennis serve, cocking. *C.* Tennis serve, acceleration.

energy and 54 percent of the total force generated in the tennis serve[18] (see Fig. 3.5*C*).

FOLLOW-THROUGH

The final phase, follow-through, begins immediately after ball contact and ends at serve completion. This stage is characterized as a deceleration phase with primarily eccentric muscle contractions of the upper extremity occurring. In the dominant shoulder, the latissimus dorsi, subscapularis, and pectoralis muscle activity starts very high in the early stages of follow-through and decreases in the late stages.[30] The dominant shoulder completes its internal rotation as the rotator cuff muscles eccentrically contract to slow

the racket arm. Elbow flexion and forearm pronation of the racket arm occur as the upper extremity finishes its motion across the midline of the body. High EMG activity of the biceps occurs in late follow-through because it decelerates elbow extension and pronation movements during the acceleration phase.[23]

Injury Prevention

WARM-UP

Proper warm-up is a key factor in preventing injuries in any sport. When choosing components of a warm-up program, one must consider the dynamics of the sport, including the ranges of motion the body must achieve and the types of muscle contractions occurring during the sport. In tennis, the body moves through a variety of ranges of motion from a very short, compact range to a very broad, extreme range of motion. Therefore, it is important to warm up the entire body before a player hits the first ball on the court. A comprehensive step-by-step warm-up is described below.

First, hold a racket in the dominant hand during the warm-up to more closely simulate the true dynamics of the game of tennis. Start with a light jog. While continuing to jog, begin with small arm circles and gradually increase the size of the circles. Then raise the arms to shoulder height and move them side to side while continuing a light jog. Bring the arms to your sides and start to increase the height of the knees while jogging to a high march position. By this time, there should be a noticeable increase in overall body temperature and maybe some slight perspiration. If not, repeat the active warm-up until a light sweat appears.

In continuing with the active warm-up and becoming even more tennis-specific, a player can now begin to address the anaerobic aspect of the sport. Start at the center of the baseline and jog to the net forward, return backward, and then move side to side to each of the doubles sidelines and rest for 30 seconds. Make sure that the racket is in the dominant hand, and repeat this jog exercise two times while increasing speed on the second circuit.

Then, starting at the center of the baseline, run diagonally to the point where the service line meets the singles sideline, turn and run back to the starting point. Repeat to the opposite side. Both side-to-side running and crossover running (*cariocas*) should be performed. (See Chap. 13 for pictures of these.) After completing these running warm-up drills, perform 5 to 10 kangaroo jumps.

The kangaroo jump is a two-legged jump from a stand position, bending the knees to the chest in midair.

STRETCHING

After completing this warm-up, a player is ready to begin stretching exercises specific to tennis. Stretches can occur both statically and dynamically, the difference being with or without movement. An example of this is the groin stretch. To statically stretch, lunge out to the side, to approximately 50 to 75 percent of the end range of motion. Then lean further into the sideways lunge position to a comfortable stretch position and hold for 30 to 60 seconds. To dynamically stretch, lunge one leg out to the side to the end range of motion and then return to an upright position. Repeat to each side five times. Do not perform ballistic or bouncing movements. Stretching should not cause pain, only a pulling sensation.

Here are some recommended static stretches:

1. *Gastrocnemius-soleus stretch.* While standing, start with one foot slightly behind the other. Lean forward onto the front foot. Keep the back heel down on the ground and the back knee straight with the lower extremity in a neutral position. Feel the stretch in the calf area and hold for 30 to 60 seconds, repeating three times to each leg. In the same position, let the back knee bend, keeping the heel on the ground, and feel the stretch in the Achilles area. Hold and repeat three times to each leg. (See Chap. 9 for pictures of these stretching techniques.)

2. *Quadriceps muscle stretch.* While standing, bend the right knee backward and grab onto the lower leg area with the right hand. Make sure to maintain an upright standing position, and do not abduct the leg. To accentuate the stretch, posteriorly tilt the pelvis. This will increase the stretch on the rectus femoris by moving the origin away from the insertion. Feel the stretch in the front of the thigh. (See Chap. 9 for a picture of this stretching technique.)

3. *Hamstring stretch.* This is a very important stretching exercise for tennis players because the hamstrings are often in a shortened position as a result of maintaining a squat position during most of the match. In addition, the hamstring muscles must lengthen quickly when a player extends for far-reaching shots. To stretch the hamstrings, lie on the back with both legs out straight. Bring the right knee up toward the chest, achieving an approximately a 90-degree hip angle. Hold both hands behind the bent right knee. Then slowly straighten the right knee to a comfortable stretch position. Keep the left leg flat on the ground with the spine in a neutral position. This will prevent a strain to the low-back area. This stretch also can be performed standing. (See Chap. 9 for a picture of this stretching technique.)

4. *Hip and trunk rotator stretch.* Sit on the floor with the legs out straight, bend the right knee so that the foot is flat on the floor, cross the right foot over the straight left leg, turn the trunk toward the right, and hook the left elbow around the outside of the right knee. Simultaneously, push the right knee to the left with the left elbow and rotate the trunk to the right. Move to a comfortable stretch position, hold, repeat three times, and then perform to the opposite side. This stretch also can be performed sitting. (See Chap. 6 for a picture of this stretching technique.)

5. *Posterior shoulder capsule and rotator cuff stretch.* While standing, start with the dominant arm forward at shoulder height and move the dominant arm across the body. With the nondominant hand, grasp the elbow of the dominant arm and pull it further across the body to a comfortable stretch position while keeping the body straight forward. Often the dominant shoulder tends to elevate;

therefore, one must concentrate on keeping the shoulder girdle down during the posterior rotator cuff stretch. (See Chap. 2 for a picture of this stretching technique.)

6. *Inferior shoulder capsule stretch.* Start with both arms overhead, bend the right elbow, grasp the right elbow with the left hand, and gently pull the right arm over the head toward the left side. The player should feel a stretch on the underside of the shoulder (Fig. 3.6).

7. *Wrist flexor stretch.* In a sitting or standing position, start with the right arm

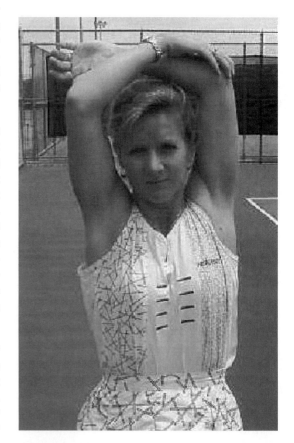

FIGURE 3.6

Stretching the inferior shoulder capsule.

forward at approximately shoulder height. Straighten the elbow completely, and keep the right palm upward. Bend the right wrist down while placing the left hand on top of the right, and gently pull the right wrist further downward until a comfortable stretch is felt in the forearm muscles. (See Chap. 6 for a picture of this stretching technique.)

8. *Wrist extensor stretch.* In a seated or standing position, start with the right arm forward at approximately shoulder height, straighten the elbow completely, and keep the right palm downward, bending the right wrist downward. Place the left hand on top of the right hand, and gently pull the right wrist further downward until a comfortable stretch is felt in the forearm muscles. If no stretch is felt, repeat with the hand in a fist. (See Chap. 6 for a picture of this stretching technique.)

Some of the recommended dynamic stretches include side-to-side lunges, forward lunges, diagonal lunges, trunk rotations in a diagonal lunge position, standing trunk rotations, and active wrist movements—up and down, side to side, and palm up and down—all performed with the racket in the dominant hand. Bouncing a ball to the ground with the racket is a great dynamic warm-up in preparation for ball contact.

STRENGTHENING

Because tennis is such a repetitious, dynamic sport, muscular endurance and the type of muscular contraction must be prioritized when designing a tennis-specific strengthening program. High repetitions (12 or 15) and low weight are recommended to most effectively simulate the sport of tennis. In addition, the type of muscle contraction, i.e., isometric, concentric, or eccentric, must be considered when performing tennis strengthening exercises.

Quadriceps strength is very important to the lower extremity because this muscle repetitiously contracts eccentrically while the body stops, starts, changes directions, and steps into the ball. Recommended strengthening exercises include lunge walks (Fig. 3.7), diagonal lunges, side lunges, and squats. Good posture and balance must be maintained during these exercises.

Trunk strength, especially the oblique muscles, is vital to transferring kinetic energy from the lower body to the upper body. Diagonal sit-ups, medicine ball trunk rotation exercises, and ground-stroke simulation using the medicine ball are effective exercises to building oblique trunk strength. These are mainly concentric-type exercises. The abdominals assist in maintaining trunk stability and good posture when playing tennis. Ab-

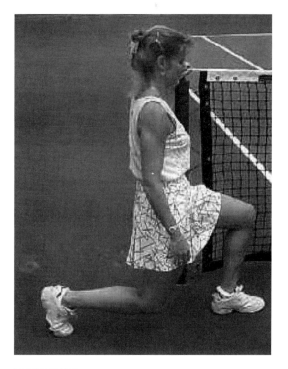

FIGURE 3.7

Strengthening, lunge walks.

dominal strengthening exercises include single leg raises, double leg raises, and bicycles while lying on the back. It is very important to remember to keep the spine neutral by maintaining an isometric contraction of the transversus abdominis and multifidus while dynamically moving the lower extremities.

Shoulder girdle stability and strength exercises must be included in all tennis-specific conditioning programs. The dynamic stabilizers of the scapula and the rotator cuff muscles are minimally active during the backswing phase, contract concentrically during the contact and acceleration phases, and contract eccentrically during the follow-through phase of all ground strokes and the serve.[26,30] Effective scapular stabilization exercises include prone rows, prone horizontal abduction, push-ups with a plus (the plus being an added push at the end of the push-up motion), (See Chap. 2 for a picture of this technique.) and push-ups with a turn (turning the body as a unit onto one arm as the opposite arm releases and rests at the body's side after performing the standard push-up). The body assumes a perpendicular position to the floor after the turn motion. Diagonal rubber tubing exercises and simulating ground strokes and serve motions are effective in simulating both concentric and eccentric muscle contractions. Strengthening can be performed at 0 to 90 degrees of shoulder abduction. These exercises can be performed slowly for control or plyometrically to optimize the concentric/eccentric transition of shoulder girdle muscle contraction.

Forearm strength and wrist strength are also critical components to develop in a tennis strengthening program. The muscle groups of the forearm and wrist frequently contract concentrically, eccentrically, and isometrically. Again, rubber tubing exercises are an effective tool to simulate slow, controlled motion or fast, rapid movements of the wrist and forearm. Recommended motions with the tubing include wrist flexion, extension, pronation, supination, and radial

and ulnar deviation. Wrist rollers, which involve rolling a weighted string around a stick, are very good for improving muscular endurance. Gripping a punctured or "dead" tennis ball is effective in simulating the cocontraction of the wrist muscles at ball contact as they control the racket face position.

Etiology of Tennis Injuries

Both intrinsic and extrinsic factors can lead to tennis injuries. Each of these areas will be highlighted below.

INTRINSIC FACTORS

Because the body is moving continuously in all directions while playing tennis, poor flexibility of the key muscle groups often leads to injury. Specific warm-up and stretching exercises are addressed in the warm-up and stretching section of this chapter.

In addition to flexibility, proprioception and balance are vital to maintaining a player's center of gravity when changing directions. Footwork must be addressed to maintain dynamic balance. Examples of footwork drills are discussed in the warm-up section of this chapter, and many different line and cone drills can be used.

Muscular strength and endurance must be considered when determining the cause of a tennis injury. Eccentric breakdowns often occur in both large and small muscle groups, resulting in tendinitis, a common overuse injury.

EXTRINSIC FACTORS

Poor stroke mechanics are the leading cause of tennis injuries. Rhythm, timing, and sequential movement from the ground upward are important factors to a smooth, linked system. Frequently, "kinks" occur somewhere in the chain, resulting in compensations and stresses to other links. One example is the "missing-link syndrome." This occurs when a player hits an "all arm" shot during the forehand stroke, failing to use the lower, more powerful links of the lower extremity and trunk. Virtually all angular momentum is lost. As a result, the upper extremity is overstressed because it must supply more force than normal in order to generate adequate ball velocity. The second type of breakdown in the kinetic chain can be a timing problem. This is often seen when a pause occurs during the serve motion. When transitioning from the cocking to the acceleration phase, a pause or hitch occurs, preventing a continuous motion and stopping the summation of forces throughout the entire body.

Another factor influencing stroke mechanics is grip position. It is important for a player to use a specific grip for each stroke in order to prevent injury. The proper grip positions for each stroke are outlined in the grip position section of this chapter.

Equipment design must be considered when addressing the cause of a tennis injury. Guidelines vary depending on the player's strength, coordination, and skill level. Specific recommendations are outlined in the equipment design and rehabilitation sections of this chapter.

Common Injuries and Their Rehabilitation

WRIST INJURIES

Because the wrist is a distal link in the kinetic chain, compensatory movements often are made at the wrist joint to nullify the adverse motions of the earlier links during tennis strokes. This compensation coupled with impact forces occurring repeatedly can result in a wrist injury.[27] Players may experience carpal tunnel syndrome, which is compression of the median nerve. The player may complain of tingling in the thumb, index, and middle fingers. A Phalen's special test can be useful to diagnose this condition. DeQuervain's tenosynovitis, inflammation of the extensor pollicus brevis and abductor pollicus longus, is also seen commonly. There is normally tenderness in these tendons, and a Finkelstein test will cause increased pain. Tendinitis of the flexor carpi ulnaris and extensor carpi ulnaris is typically caused by abnormal repetitive wrist motions.[14,27]

Cartilage tears in the wrist also may be seen in tennis players. The triangular fibrocartilage complex (TFCC) provides stability to the ulnar side of the wrist. In tennis, a tear may occur because of repetitive twisting motions of the wrist.[32] In this case, a wrist strengthening program, similar to the examples given earlier, is essential in preventing a TFCC injury. Once the tear occurs, attempt conservative treatment with modalities and strengthening. If the player is unable to return, surgery may be indicated.

Symptoms in the wrist can be minimized with wrist taping, which helps the player avoid excessive wrist motions. When establishing a tennis-specific wrist strengthening program, a low-weight, high-repetition regime of all the wrist motions, including gripping, is recommended. In addition, wrist exercises, both concentric and eccentric, are vital in simulating the specific muscle contractions of the wrist and forearm while playing tennis. For example, when performing the wrist curl exercise, stabilize the forearm on a fixed object such as a table, and place the hand palm up off the edge of the table. Holding a light weight in the hand, raise the hand upward slowly, a concentric contraction, and then lower it slowly to the starting position, an eccentric contraction. This same concept can be applied to all the active wrist exercises described earlier. Median nerve glides can be helpful in treating carpal tunnel syndrome. Ice should be applied after exercise and after playing tennis to prevent inflammation.

From a biomechanical standpoint, a stable wrist position is critical at ball impact. Ultimately, an equipment check and a stroke analysis must be considered to eliminate the potential source of a wrist injury. Key areas to address include the type of grip, grip size, swing path, and contact point.

A grip adjustment that moves away from a western grip and toward an eastern grip during the forehand stroke may promote increased wrist stability. The eastern backhand grip also promotes a stable position of the wrist during the one-handed backhand stroke. Measuring a player's racket hand for grip size, as recommended by Nirschl's arthropometric technique, is useful in determining appropriate grip size.[25]

Efficient and effective movement and timing of the lower links are critical in reducing the overload stresses on the most distal link, the wrist.[32] Stroke modifications such as altering the racket's swing path to a more horizontal plane of motion may reduce excessive wrist motion. The contact point for all ground strokes must be near or in front of the front foot to allow achievement of a vertical racket position at impact.

ELBOW INJURIES

Tennis elbow, medically described as lateral epicondylitis, occurs in 40 to 50 percent of average recreational tennis players, most of them greater than 30 years old.[21,25] Lateral epicondylitis is an inflammation of the soft tissue located on the outside of the elbow, commonly the extensor carpi radialis brevis muscle and its tendon. The area is tender to palpation, and pain will be elicited with a tennis elbow special test. Medial epicondylitis, commonly called *golfer's elbow*, involves the soft tissue on the inside of the elbow and is not a common injury in tennis, although it

can be seen with forehand dysfunctions. As a result, lateral epicondylitis will be the focus of this discussion.

The most common cause of tennis elbow pain is the one-handed backhand. From a biomechanical standpoint, five distinct body parts sequentially coordinate in hitting a one-handed backhand.[12] Rhythm, timing, and effective use of all five body parts are critical to an effective stroke. If coordination of these components fails, the result is a breakdown in the kinetic chain. The wrist often compensates, resulting in stress at the common extensor tendon. Ultimately, an overuse injury occurs due to the repetitive stresses to the outer elbow area.

Players also may experience lateral epicondylitis symptoms while performing the serve motion. It has been found that most players with tennis elbow pain during their serve lacked adequate wrist extensor flexibility and were hyperpronated with an exaggerated wrist snap during the acceleration phase.[25] Performed on a repetitive basis this can lead to excessive stress and an eventual injury to the extensor musculature.

Physiologically, the EMG activity of the forearm muscles of professional and collegiate tennis players during the forehand, backhand, and serve motions was studied as a percentage of a maximum manual muscle test (mMMT). It was found that there was a high level of EMG activity of the extensor carpi radialis brevis (ECRB) during acceleration of the racket in the contact phase (60 percent of mMMT) and moderate activity in the early follow-through phase (47 percent of mMMT) during the backhand stroke. A significant increase in EMG activity, 49 to 58 percent of mMMT of the ECRB during the acceleration phase of the forehand and serve motions, was found.[24] Thus, lateral epicondylitis may be a result of a continuous use of the wrist extensor muscle group throughout tennis play, not just impact forces during the one-handed backhand.

Equipment design is a consideration when evaluating contributing factors to lateral epicondylitis. Racket twisting occurs when a ball is struck off-center. This twisting occurs so quickly that it is rarely detectable. It is recommended that the player's grasp be firm enough to prevent excessive rotation of the racket handle in the gripping hand during off-center hits.[11] However, if these off-center hits occur frequently, the forearm muscles may fatigue more quickly, resulting in an overuse injury. For this reason, an oversized racket with a larger "sweet spot" may be beneficial.[29] This racket will be more stable, will decrease twisting, and will reduce arm vibration during off-center hits.[13] In addition, a stiffer racket frame reduces vibration forces by decreasing the amplitude of frame vibration and dampening the vibration forces more quickly.[29] Lastly, the application of a cushioned grip tape was found to increase racket dampening by up to 100 percent.[33] In summary, an oversized racket made of a stiffer material and use of a cushioned grip tape can assist in preventing lateral epicondylitis.

When analyzing string tension and its benefit to preventing tennis elbow, most manufacturers recommend a string tension range specific for each individual racket. Generally, a lower string tension will increase the time the ball stays on the racket, creating a trampoline effect, which, in turn, absorbs some of the shock resulting from ball impact.[12]

Common rehabilitation methods for tennis elbow include a flexibility program emphasizing the forearm extensor mass, as described in detail in the stretching section of this chapter. Activity modification is a must. This includes not only tennis but also any activity such as repetitive gripping or fine motor activity that involves prolonged forearm extensor muscle use.

Conservative treatment consisting of ice and anti-inflammatory medication is often prescribed. Soft tissue mobilization and modalities such as ultrasound, iontophoresis, and splinting of the wrist or forearm may be recommended. Radial nerve glides are also helpful. As the player's pain level decreases, a progression to a submaximal strengthening program consisting of isometrics, eccentrics, and concentrics of the forearm, wrist, and hand muscles is advised. Because all these types of muscle contractions occur in the distal upper extremity while playing tennis, a comprehensive sport-specific strengthening program can be established. Components of the elbow strengthening program include light gripping and releasing to simulate ball contact especially during the one-handed backhand, intrinsic strengthening of the hand using a rubber band around the fingers, wrist curls, reverse curls, neutral curls, and pronation/supination motions. It is important to perform these exercises in a slow, controlled manner to achieve the concentric and eccentric strengthening benefits. In addition, an evaluation of shoulder girdle range of motion and strength, in particular the rotator cuff and scapular stabilizers, is beneficial because this is the closest link to the distal upper extremity. Often, if the rotator cuff is inflexible or weak or the scapula is not adequately stabilizing the shoulder while playing tennis, the elbow, wrist, and hand must compensate, resulting in an overuse injury.[20]

Effective scapular strengthening exercises include prone horizontal abduction, supine scapular protraction, push-ups with a plus, and prone rows. Rotator cuff strengthening includes side-lying external rotation, prone external rotation in a 90-degree abducted position, and standing scaption in both an externally rotated and internally rotated shoulder position.

An analysis of the stroke mechanics causing the tennis elbow pain is crucial. Conservative treatment in combination with stroke correction has produced 90 percent excellent or good results when symptoms lasted for less than 6 months. Symptoms that lasted more than 6 months shows 82 percent excellent or good results, and for some players, stroke modification alone rectified the elbow symptoms.[16] Using a certified tennis teaching professional is often helpful in analyzing and modifying stroke mechanics.

The two-handed backhand is less stressful to the forearm extensor muscles of the racket arm as compared with the one-handed backhand because the swing mechanics are altered significantly.[21] Players who develop tennis elbow from the one-handed backhand stroke and continue to have difficulty mastering the stroke with recommended modifications may benefit from changing to a two-handed backhand. Conventional grip position, optimal contact point, and effective timing of the lower links in the kinetic chain are often biomechanical solutions to strokes that are producing lateral elbow pain.

SHOULDER INJURIES

Impingement is a common shoulder injury in tennis. It can be defined as a narrowing of the subacromial space as the upper extremity actively elevates overhead. The rotator cuff tendons lie in this space and are often "impinged" if abnormal biomechanics of the shoulder exist. The biceps tendon also can be impinged. (See Chaps. 2 and 6). Causes for these pathologic movement patterns of the shoulder may include poor flexibility, muscle imbalances, decreased scapular stability, and poor stroke mechanics. The player often will be tender over the supraspinatus and bicep tendons and will test positive on a Hawkins-Kennedy or Neers impingement test.

Dominant shoulder rotation range of motion is a major consideration in addressing an injury-prevention program for the shoulder in tennis players. The average total shoulder rotation in world-class players is 97 degrees for the forehand, 189 degrees for the backhand, and 165 degrees for the serve.[18]

Studies have confirmed that anatomic adaptations occur in the racket shoulder of tennis players. A significant loss of active and passive internal rotation range of motion has been found when compared with the nondominant shoulder, and a loss of total shoulder rotation is well documented.[3,5,19,31] These decreases in active dominant shoulder internal rotation and total rotation of the dominant glenohumeral joint are potential risk factors for an overuse shoulder injury.

An excellent preventative exercise includes stretching the posterior capsule and posterior muscles of the racket shoulder. A detailed explanation of how to perform this is outlined in the stretching section of this chapter. To test the functional range of motion of the shoulder rotators, the player can hold a tennis racket or towel behind the back and also can stretch the rotators by moving the racket up and down. (See Chap. 5 for pictures of these stretching techniques.)

During the serve motion, the major muscle groups of the shoulder girdle that play an important role in providing powerful motion and dynamic stability include the rotator cuff, the scapular stabilizers, and the biceps brachii.[26] Adequate strength and coordination of the shoulder girdle muscles are imperative to eliminating overuse shoulder injuries. Plyometric exercises for the shoulder girdle incorporate coordination training by emphasizing speed and change of direction. Specific upper extremity plyometric exercises for tennis include medicine ball forward, diagonal, and overhead passes. Dominant arm plyoball (2 lb) throws against a minitrampoline with the shoulder in 80 to 90 degrees of abduction with a takeback and diagonal follow-through simulates the shoulder motion during a serve. The same exercise performed in 0 to 45 degrees of abduction simulates the forehand and backhand motions.

In tennis players, muscle strength of the shoulder internal rotators in the racket arm was found to be significantly greater than in the nondominant arm, with the external rotators being equal bilaterally. External to internal rotation strength ratios in the dominant arm of elite junior male tennis players ranged from 51 to 70 percent. In female elite junior tennis players, a 67 to 70 percent ratio resulted. It is important to strive for a 2:3 ratio, or an imbalance in the dominant shoulder may predispose players to overload shoulder injuries.[1,2]

Positive objective and functional improvements have been documented in elite tennis players who underwent a shoulder internal and external isokinetic concentric and eccentric strength training program. Functional gains were seen in serve velocity as compared with a control group.[22] The internal and external rotators of the dominant shoulder contract concentrically or eccentrically depending on their function during the tennis stroke. Typically, when acting as an accelerator, the internal and external rotators shorten. When functioning as a decelerator, these muscles lengthen. As stated earlier, because of the strength imbalance of internal rotators to external rotators commonly seen in tennis players, concentric and eccentric strength training of the external rotators is vital to shoulder injury prevention. Eccentric training of both the internal and external rotators to effectively stabilize and decelerate the shoulder during the cocking and follow-through phases of the tennis stroke is recommended when developing a tennis-specific exercise program.[26] Exercises for shoulder internal and external eccentric training include the PNF patterns D1 and D2 flexion and extension motions performed plyometrically with tubing to mimic the ground-stroke and serve motions. When performing these exercises, variables such as intensity and frequency should focus on light resistance and high repetition to specifically simulate the physical demands of tennis.

The scapular muscles, including the serratus anterior, rhomboids, trapezius, and leva-tor scapulae, cocontract and provide a stable base on which the humerus rotates. They also allow the scapula to move from full retraction during the cocking phase of the serve to full protraction during the follow-through stage in a controlled manner.[20]

Thus, concentric and eccentric strength exercises of the serratus anterior, rhomboids, trapezius, and levator scapula will promote scapular stability. Push-ups with a plus, prone rows, and shoulder shrugs performed slowly as the muscles contract concentrically and eccentrically are excellent scapular stabilization exercises for tennis players.

The biceps brachii mainly acts as a dynamic stabilizer for the glenohumeral joint during the cocking phase of the serve and as a decelerator of the arm during the follow-through phase.[30] Thus, concentric and eccentric strength training of the biceps musculature is recommended. Bicep curls with shoulder flexion, with an emphasis on light weight during the eccentric phase, are beneficial.

From a biomechanical standpoint, early breakdown in the kinetic chain can lead to overload stresses in the later links, particularly the shoulder. Thus, a thorough analysis of the stroke(s) reproducing the painful shoulder symptoms should be performed. As a result of the tendency to achieve a greater than 90-degree shoulder abduction or flexion/internal rotation position, the common strokes that may lead to shoulder impingement include the topspin forehand and the serve.

Since the semiwestern and western forehands increase the low-to-high swing path, the follow-through position of flexion/internal rotation coupled with horizontal adduction is more likely to occur. If the dominant shoulder moves into this position forcefully and repetitively, impingement symptoms may result. It is recommended to finish the topspin forehand with the dominant hand at or below the nondominant shoulder, maximizing dominant shoulder flexion to 90 degrees while completing the internal rotation and horizontal adduction motion. In addition, a player must focus on generating energy and forces from the lower, larger, and stronger segments in the kinetic chain in order to decrease overload stresses to the shoulder complex. These biomechanical adjustments may assist in eliminating the risk for shoulder impingement.

In elite players, the actual shoulder abduction position during the serve is approximately 83 degrees, not above shoulder height as thought previously.[6] This is often deceiving when viewing the serving motion because while the arm is rising on one side of the body, the trunk is side-bending downward on the other side. From a professional tennis teacher's point of view, instructing a player to "reach higher" with the dominant shoulder to optimize racket height at ball contact may not be the answer to optimal ball contact position. Players literally may elevate the racket shoulder greater than 90 degrees and position themselves for an impingement situation. Instead, carefully analyzing the timing and sequencing of the kinetic chain prior to the acceleration phase may solve the optimal contact dilemma.

BACK INJURIES

Low-back strains and facet impingement syndromes are also common injuries in tennis players. A 21.1 percent incidence of injuries over a 6-year period at the U.S. Tennis Association's boy's tennis championships was reported. Back injuries were the most common injury, accounting for 16.1 percent of all injuries.[15] Several back injuries were found to be a result of high muscle and joint reaction forces, especially during the cocking phase of the serve when the spine flexes laterally and hyperextends.[7]

Both flexibility and strength must be addressed when developing a rehabilitation program for back injuries. Because the hip is the closest link in the chain and affects trunk movement, adequate flexibility of the hip internal and external rotators, flexors, and extensors is crucial. The hip rotator and back stretch outlined in the stretching section of this chapter is very beneficial.

Strengthening the abdominal muscles including the transversus abdominis and oblique abdominals provides the power and spinal stability necessary to generate adequate trunk force and control. A high-repetition, low-resistance strengthening program is emphasized for tennis players because the abdominal muscles are used on a repetitive basis throughout tennis play. Crunches, crunches with a turn, supine double leg raises, and medicine ball throws from overhead and diagonally, all while maintaining a neutral spine position, emphasize the upper, lower, and oblique abdominal musculature. Additional abdominal exercises are outlined in the strength section of this chapter. Extension exercises such as prone bilateral arm and leg raises will assist in stabilizing the lumbar spine.

KNEE INJURIES

Overuse knee injuries are seen commonly in tennis players because of the explosive, repetitive, and multidirectional movements made during match play. Common injuries include patellofemoral tracking syndrome and patellar tendinitis.[8]

Patellofemoral tracking dysfunction and chondromalacia may be caused by biomechanical problems, including a large Q angle, pronated feet, squinting patellae, or a tight lateral retinaculum. In treating this problem, emphasis is placed on flexibility, particularly the quadriceps, hamstrings, and gastrocnemius-soleus complex, as described in the stretching section of this chapter. In addition, stretching of the tensor fasciae latae and myofascial release of the lateral retinaculum are also recommended. Activity modification, including limiting prolonged tennis play and deep squatting, is advised.

Common modalities include ice, ultrasound, electric stimulation, and iontophoresis. Assessing patellar position and addressing abnormalities such as a lateral tilt or glide with taping are beneficial. Custom orthotics may be considered when addressing biomechanical dysfunctions as well. Commonly, inadequate strength or endurance of the quadriceps is present. Often a muscular imbalance of the vastus lateralis to vastus medialis is observed. Thus, emphasis on vastus medialis oblique strengthening is recommended.

Isometric strengthening of the quadriceps musculature is initiated with quadriceps setting. A progression to closed kinetic chain exercises such as one-quarter squats with isometric adduction to facilitate the vastus medialis is recommended. Wall sits with isometric adduction and a progression to multiangle lunges and plyometrics are used to emphasize the eccentric contraction repetitively performed by the quadriceps musculature during tennis play. During these activities, it is important to observe knee position and patella control.

Footwear must be evaluated to ensure adequate support and cushion. Additionally, a court surface change from hard to clay may be beneficial in reducing frictional forces to the lower extremities because players tend to slide on the forgiving clay courts.[28]

Patellar tendinitis also can be the result of abnormal patellofemoral tracking, poor lower extremity flexibility, and/or inadequate eccentric quadriceps strength and endurance. Additionally, a muscular imbalance of the vastus lateralis to vastus medialis may be present. Tenderness can be found near the inferior pole of the patella or at the tibial tubercle. Patellar tendinitis is treated similarly to a patellar tracking dysfunction in that a comprehensive lower extremity biomechanical evaluation, strengthening, and stretching are

also recommended. Activity modification is advised as well.

Conservative treatment consisting of ice and anti-inflammatory medication is often prescribed. Modalities and counterforce bracing to disperse the forces through the patellar tendon may be implemented. Once signs and symptoms have been resolved, a progressive eccentric training program should be started. Strengthening exercises include closed-chain squats, lunges, and the lateral step-downs. As eccentric strength increases, so should the progression to plyometrics. Footwear and court surface also must be addressed. Wearing a comfortable, supportive, and well-cushioned shoe and playing on a softer clay court surface is recommended.

Prior to returning the athlete to the tennis court, plyometric exercises and functional tests should be performed. Box jumps, a single leg hop test, or a shuttle run test can be helpful in determining if the athlete's lower extremities are ready for a return to the sport.

ANKLE INJURIES

Lateral ankle sprains are a common ankle injury to tennis players.[15] The quick changes of direction and the stopping and starting motions often cause this traumatic injury. Tenderness can be present over one or all of the lateral ligaments; with severe sprains, the deltoid ligament may be tender as well. An anterior draw test or talar tilt may be positive in these players. Initial conservative treatment for a lateral ankle sprain includes rest, ice, compression, and elevation (RICE). Depending on the severity of the sprain, activity modification is commonly recommended. Bracing or taping using stirrups and figure-eight and heel-lock techniques to support the lateral side of the ankle is beneficial. Modalities such as the whirlpool, contrast baths, and electrical stimulation are commonly used to decrease swelling. Flexibility exercises for the gastrocnemius-soleus complex are important in reestablishing normal range of motion and a normal gait pattern. A progression to balance and proprioception exercises, both static and dynamic, is critical for safe return to tennis play. Static exercises include single-leg balance on a stable surface with the eyes open and closed. Use of balance beams and unstable surfaces such as platform rockers or wobble boards can challenge the dynamic stabilizers of the ankle.

Strengthening of the entire lower extremity is recommended, with an emphasis on the lateral ankle musculature. Resisted eversion exercises isolate the peroneal muscle group. Beginning phases of rehabilitation include side-lying ankle eversion with resisted tubing or cuff weights. Eventually, pattern running laterally and diagonally with an emphasis on changes of direction over short distances to specifically simulate a game situation prepares the player for on-court activity. As with knee rehabilitation, prior to returning the athlete to the tennis court, plyometric exercises and functional tests should be performed. Box jumps, a T test for agility, a single-leg hop test, or a shuttle run test can be helpful in determining if the athlete's lower extremities are ready for a return to the sport.

Return to Tennis Program

When returning to the tennis court after an injury, it is recommended that a player initially return to a controlled environment such as a ball machine or professional instruction. In this way, a player can concentrate on his or her mechanics because the placement, height, and pace of the ball are more predictable.

Footwork must be emphasized first to optimize the lower kinetic chain, followed by

rhythm and timing. If the initial injury was the result of a particular stroke, begin with the asymptomatic strokes at 50 percent effort. For instance, if the one-handed backhand caused pain, start with the following and progress as outlined below:

Day 1

Stage 1 (50 percent effort): 20 forehands, 20 serves, and 20 volleys.
Stage 2: Mimic 10 one-handed backhands without hitting the ball.
Stage 3 (50 percent effort): Hit 10 one-handed backhands with a ball. Assess the effects. Repeat stages 1 through 3 two more times pain-free.

Day 2

Rest one day.

Day 3

Increase the repetitions of stage 1 to 30 and stage 3 to 20. Assess the effects, and repeat the pain-free sequence twice.

DAY 4

Rest one day.

Day 5

Repeat day 3, increasing effort to 75 percent.

Day 6

Rest one day.

Day 7

Increase repetitions of stage 1 to 40 and stage 3 to 30 at 75 percent effort for 15 to 20 balls and 100 percent effort for 15 to 20 balls.

Day 8

Rest one day.

Day 9

Rally with a partner and include serves and specialty shots for a total of 20 minutes.

Day 10

Rest one day.

Day 11

Rally 10 to 15 minutes; play four games.

Day 12

Rest one day.

Day 13

Rally 15 minutes; play six games.

Day 14

Rest one day.

Day 15

Rally 15 minutes; play one set.

All play days should be pain-free. No increase in injury pain should be noted on any day. If pain does occur, go back to the last pain-free day and restart. Progress to the next day only if injury symptoms are eliminated. It is common to experience muscle soreness, and this should not prevent a player from progressing through the return to tennis program unless this leads to previous injury pain.

Return to Tennis Guidelines

GENERAL CRITERIA TO BEGIN ON-COURT ACTIVITIES

1. Pain-free tubing simulation of strokes—forehand (FH), backhand (BH), serve.
2. Pain-free strokes using Nerf balls.
3. Pain-free strokes with racket cover on.

SPECIFIC CRITERIA TO BEGIN ON-COURT ACTIVITIES

Upper Extremity

1. Able to meet general criteria above.
2. Able to simulate serve motion throwing a ball over the net 10 to 20 times.

3. Pain-free simulation of forehand, backhand, and serve motions using a 4- to 6-lb medicine ball.

Lower Extremity

1. Able to perform pain-free lunges forward, backward, and diagonally.
2. Able to run forward, backward, side to side, and *carioca,* changing directions at moderate speed.

Always warm up and stretch. Good on-court warm-up activities include jogging around the court; jogging forward, backward, sideways; and touching the lines of the court; arm circles; and rapidly bouncing the ball downward and upward with the racket.

It is recommended that a player begin using a controlled environment such as a ball machine or tennis pro who can feed balls easily to the player. Then progress to using a wall or back board if desired.

Day 1	Day 2
Total time = 20–25 min 5–7 min forehand 5–7 min backhand Break 5 min 5–7 min second serves, light spin if any	Same as day 1
Day 3 Off	**Day 4** Total time = 24–30 min 8–10 min forehand 8–10 min backhand Break 5 min 5 min serve 5 min overhead
Day 5 Off	**Day 6** Same as day 4

Day 7
  Off

Day 8
  Total time =
  30 min
  Hit balls with
  another player
  Practice only for
  20 min
  Serve for 10 min

Day 9
  Off

Day 10
  Total time =
  40 min
  Same as day 8
  with hit time =
  30 min
  Serve for 10 min

Day 11
  Off

Day 12
  Play six games

Day 13
  Off

Day 14
  Play one set

Day 15
  Off

Day 16
  Off

Day 17
  Play one and
  one-half sets

Day 18
  Off

Day 19
  Off

Day 20
  Play one match

Day 21
  Off

Day 22
  Play one match

Day 23
  Play one match

References

1. Chandler TJ, Kibler WB, Stracener EC, et al: Shoulder strength, power and endurance in college tennis players. *Am J Sports Med* 20(4):455–458,1992.

2. Ellenbecker TS: A total arm strength isokinetic profile of highly skilled tennis players. *Isokinet Exerc Sci* 1:19–21, 1991.

3. Ellenbecker TS: Glenohumeral joint internal and external rotation range of motion in elite junior tennis players. *JOSPT* 24(6):336–341, 1996.

4. Ellenbecker TS: Rehabilitation of shoulder and elbow injuries in tennis players. *Clin Sports Med* 14:87–110, 1995.

5. Ellenbecker TS: Shoulder internal rotation and external rotation strength and range of motion of highly skilled junior tennis players. *Isokinet Exer Sci* 2:1–8, 1992.

6. Elliot BC, Marsh T, Blanksby B: A three-dimensional cinematographic analysis of the tennis serve. *Int J Sport Biomech* 2:260–217, 1986.

7. Elliott BC: Biomechanics of the serve in tennis: A biomedical perspective. *Sports Med* 6(5):285–294, 1988.

8. Gecha SR, Torg E: Knee injuries in tennis. *Clin Sports Med* 7(2):435–452, 1988.

9. Giangarra C, Conroy B, Jobe F, et al: Electromyographic and cinematographic analysis of elbow function in tennis players using single and double-handed backhand strokes. *Am J Sports Med* 21(3):394–398, 1993.

10. Glousman R: Electromyographic analysis and its role in the athletic shoulder. *Clin Orthop* 288:27–34, 1993.

11. Grabiner MD, Groppel JL, Campbell KR: Resultant tennis ball velocity as a function of off-center impact and grip firmness. *Med Sci Sports Exerc* 15:542–544, 1983.

12. Groppel JL: *High Tech Tennis*, 2d ed. Champaign, IL: Leisure Press, 1992.

13. Hennig EM, Rosenbaum D, Milani TL: Transfer of tennis racket vibrations onto the human forearm. *Med Sci Sports Exer* 24(10): 1134–1140, 1992.

14. Howse C: Wrist injuries in sport. *Sports Med* 17:163–175, 1994.

15. Hutchinson MR, Laparade RF, Burnett QM, et al: Injury surveillance at the USTA boys tennis championships: A six-year study. *Med Sci Sports Exerc* 27(6):826–830, 1995.

16. Ilfeld FW: Can stroke modification relieve tennis elbow? *Clin Orthop* 276:182–186, 1992.

17. Kelley J, Lombardo S, Pink M, et al: Electromyographic and cinematrographic analysis

of elbow function in tennis players with lateral epicondylitis. *Am J Sports Med* 22(3): 359–363, 1994.

18. Kibler WB: Biomechanical analysis of the shoulder during tennis activities. *Clin Sports Med* 14(1):79–85, 1995.

19. Kibler WB, Chandler TJ, Livingston B, Roetert P: Shoulder range of motion in elite tennis players. *Am J Sports Med* 24(3):279–286, 1996.

20. Kibler WB: The role of the scapula in athletic shoulder function. *Am J Sports Med* 26(2): 325–337, 1998.

21. Leach R, Miller J: Lateral and medial epicondylitis of the elbow. *Clin Sports Med* 6(2): 259–272, 1987.

22. Mont M, Cohen D, Campbell K, et al: Isokinetic concentric versus eccentric training of shoulder rotators with functional evaluation of performance enhancement in elite tennis players. *Am J Sports Med* 22(4):513–517, 1994.

23. Morris M, Jobe F, Perry J, et al: Electromyographic analysis of elbow function in tennis players. *Am J Sports Med* 17(2):241–247, 1989.

24. Moynes D, Perry J, Antonelli D, et al: Electromyography and motion analysis of the upper extremity in sports. *Phys Ther* 66(12): 1905–1911, 1986.

25. Nirschl R: Tennis elbow. *Orthop Clin North Am* 4(3):787–800, 1973.

26. Plancher K, Litchield R, Hawkins R: Rehabilitation of the shoulder in tennis players. *Clin Sports Med* 14(1):111–137, 1995.

27. Rettig AC: Wrist problems in tennis players. *Med Sci Sports Exerc* 26(10):1207–1212, 1994.

28. Renstrom AF: Knee pain in tennis players. *Clin Sports Med* 14(1):163–175, 1995.

29. Roetert P, Brody H, Dillman C, et al: The biomechanics of tennis elbow. *Clin Sports Med* 14(1):47–57, 1995.

30. Ryu R, McCormick J, Jobe F, et al: An electromyographic analysis of shoulder function in tennis players. *Am J Sports Med* 16(5):481–485, 1988.

31. Warner JJ, Micheli LJ, Arslanian LE, et al: Patterns of flexibility, laxity and strength in normal shoulders and shoulders with instability and impingement. *Am J Sports Med* 18: 366–378, 1990.

32. Werner S, Plancher K: Hand and wrist injuries. *Clin Sports Med* 17(3):407–421, 1998.

33. Wilson JF, Davis JS: Tennis racket shock mitigation experiments. *J Biomech Eng* 117(4): 479–484, 1995.

CHAPTER 4

Volleyball

David M. Drexler
William W. Briner
Jonathan C. Reeser

Volleyball continues to grow in popularity both in the United States and worldwide. It has become the world's most popular participation sport, according to the Federation Internationale de Volleyball (FIVB), which is volleyball's international governing body. Individuals of all ages and skill levels can enjoy the sport. Over 200 countries play volleyball, and almost half of these countries compete at the international level. The FIVB has 218 member nations, more than any other international sports federation. According to USA Volleyball, which is the national governing body for the sport in the United States, there were 34.1 million players in the United States in 1998. There were 122,968 players registered with USA Volleyball, and 65 percent of these players were less than 18 years of age. With respect to interscholastic competition, there were 12,896 high schools offering varsity girls volleyball to 370,957 participants. Girls' volleyball had more participants in 1998 than any other sport except basketball and track. There are 1441 schools offering boys' varsity volleyball to 32,375 students. Volleyball ranked as the eleventh most popular sport for boys in 1998 in the United States.

History

William G. Morgan invented volleyball at the YMCA in Springfield, Massachusetts, in 1895, under the recommendation of Dr. Luther Gulick, who believed that games should serve many participants rather than a few. Their goal was to create a game that would be less stressful than basketball on the bodies of young athletes. However, Mr. Morgan wanted the sport to be enjoyable, competitive, and challenging enough to keep people fit. He originally named the game *mintonette*. On July 7, 1896, Alfred T. Halstead of Springfield College remarked while watching a demonstration of the game that it looked like the men were "volleying" the ball back and forth over the net. When he suggested this to Mr. Morgan, he agreed, and the name was changed to *volleyball*. Over the years, the sport has flourished in both the United States and Europe. Perhaps some of the sport's success stems from the fact that a net and ball are all that are really needed to play the game, unlike some sports that require substantial financial resources for equipment. While volleyball was invented in the United States, it has become so popular in Asia, Europe, and South America that these continents now field many of the most elite national teams in the sport.

Volleyball was first recognized as an Olympic sport in 1964 in Tokyo, for both men and women. At that time, it was played on an indoor hard-court surface. At the 1996 Olympic games in Atlanta, beach (sand) volleyball was added as a full medal sport. Normally, there is a trial period during which a sport is presented as a demonstration. However, because of the overwhelming popularity of beach volleyball, it was contested as a full medal sport in its initial Olympic competition. Sand volleyball originated on the beaches of Santa Monica in southern California in the 1920s. Now there is a traveling professional beach doubles tour that allows elite players a reasonable income. Outdoor sand volleyball is played with two players per side, and the indoor game is contested with six players per side. Sand volleyball is officially referred to as *beach volleyball* (BVB) by the FIVB. *Park volleyball* is currently considered a new discipline of outdoor recreational (grass) volleyball, which was approved by the FIVB World Congress in 1998. Park volleyball is played by two teams of four players, is played under the rally point system, and is auto-refereed.

Levels/Types of Play

Many players participate in volleyball at a recreational level; others play frequently in locally sanctioned leagues. Players with a serious interest in the sport may wish to join USA Volleyball. This organization sanctions tournaments that are played both indoors and outdoors on all three surfaces (hard-court, grass, and sand). There are also many local volleyball clubs and amateur junior tournaments for young players. Interscholastic competition often begins at the high school level. There are currently more girls' than boys' volleyball teams at the high school level, but males are starting to field more teams as the sport's popularity grows nationally. Intercollegiate volleyball is also an option for those participants who excel at the high school level. At the intercollegiate level, 920 schools offer volleyball for women and 68 schools field teams for men. At the NCAA Division I level, 12 scholarships can be awarded to women volleyball players. For men that participate at the Division I level, 4.5 scholarships are available per team. In 1998, 3528 scholarships were awarded to women and 99 scholarships were awarded to men.

In the United States, there is a national team for men and for women. There are also professional indoor leagues for top players in Europe, Japan, and the United States. Professional beach (sand) volleyball has gained popularity in recent years with tournaments in cities across the country. USA Volleyball is the administrative body for all types of volleyball in the United States. The administrative body for the professional beach league in the United States is the Association of Volleyball Professionals (AVP). With substantial prize money at stake on the professional beach tour, many of the top players in the world participate in this format. There have been professional four-on-four volleyball tournaments for both men and women in the past. Sand volleyball is usually played with teams of two on the same size court that is used for the six-player indoor game. The court is 29 ft, 5 in (9 m) wide by 59 ft (18 m) long. The net is 39 in (1 m) in width and 32 ft (9.5 m) long and divides the court into two equal halves. The net for the men is 7 ft, 11⅝ in (2.43 m) high and for women is 7 ft, 4⅛ in (2.24 m) high. The official volleyball has 18 panels, a circumference between 25½ and 27 in (65 and 67 cm), a weight of 9 to 10 oz (260 to 280 g), and a pressure between 4.3 and 4.6 lb/in² (0.30 and 0.325 kg/cm²).[34]

Scoring/Side-Out

Volleyball scoring has gone through some changes in recent years. Different formats have been tried to speed up the game and/or allow it to fit consistently into a certain time period for the benefit of television. Traditionally, winning a game requires that a team scores 15 points, and the game does not end unless a team wins by 2 points. At the USA Volleyball Nationals this year, rally-point scoring was used. The FIVB World Congress has adopted the rally-point scoring system, which became effective January 1, 2000. Side-out scoring will most likely be abandoned in the United States. In side-out scoring, points are only awarded if a team successfully defends its serve. When the serving team fails to score, the opposing team is awarded a "side-out" and gets an opportunity to serve. In six-person volleyball, players rotate one position on the court in a clockwise fashion after each side-out. A second format is called rally scoring, in which points are awarded after each serve, no matter which team served the ball. In this format, the team that wins the point gets to serve the next point. In every other country except the United States, FIVB rules are followed. Volleyball matches use rally scoring for the best three out of five games. Games 1 through 4 are to 25 points, with game 5 being 15 points.

Additional Rules

After the serve, each team may contact the ball as many as three times. On the third hit, the ball must travel across to the other side of the net. Typically, the series of hits consists of a bump or dig, followed by a set and a hit or spike. Alternatively, a ball may be played across the net legally with a first or second hit. The centerline rule is the rule that has the largest impact on volleyball injuries. The centerline is a line immediately beneath the net in indoor volleyball that separates the court into two halves. Players are in violation if their foot crosses completely over the line. If any part of the foot remains in contact with the line, the player is not in violation. The most common injury occurs when a blocker lands on the foot of a spiker from the opposing team whose foot has come under the net.[1] The majority of the resulting injuries are inversion ankle sprains when the attacker's foot rolls over that of the blocker.

Some of the new rules that were adopted by the FIVB in January 2000 are

1. *The let serve is in play* (test period). If, when serving, the ball touches the net and goes to the opposite side, the play continues.
2. *Touching the net.* Touching the net is not a fault except when playing the ball or interfering with the play (i.e., an "incidental net" is legal).
3. *Time-outs.* In normal play, all time-outs are for 30 seconds; each team has two time-outs per set. In official FIVB and world competitions, all time-outs are for 60 seconds, except in the fifth set, where they are for 30 seconds. *In sets 1 through 4*, each team has the right to call only one time-out, and there are two technical time-outs, when the leading team reaches the eighth and sixteenth points. *In set 5*, each team has two 30-second time-outs, but there are no technical time-outs.
4. *Intervals between sets.* All intervals between sets are for 3 minutes. The interval between the second and third sets may be extended up to 10 minutes by the competition body at the request of the organizers.

Positions in Six-Person Volleyball

There are several different options for assigning position responsibilities to the six players on the court. Many competitive teams elect to use a single setter, and the other five players can all be used as hitters. This is referred to as a 5-1 formation. A brief overview would be that most teams have two middle blockers, a setter, an opposite hitter, and two outside hitters.

Ideally, the setter plays every second ball and sets it for a middle or outside hitter, depending on where the opposing blockers are positioned. Middle blockers jump at the net in the center of the court on each set.

Outside hitters attack sets from the far right or left side of the net. The opposite hitter plays in the position opposite the setter. Most elite teams elect to use two or three players who are the most proficient passers to bump or return all the serves. If the setter is in the front row at the time of the initiating serve, then two hitters jump at the net as potential front-row attackers. If the setter is in the back row, he or she has the option of setting three different front-row hitters.

One other recent change at the international level is the introduction of the libero position. This is a designated back-row player whose specialty is defense. This may allow players who are not as tall as "typical" national team players to participate at the elite level. Libero is played at all levels in other countries and is being adopted gradually in the United States.

Basic Skills

In general, all the players on a volleyball court engage in each of the various sport-specific skills during the course of a game. These skills have varying risks of injury. Play is always initiated with the serve, during which the player usually tosses the ball into the air and then strikes it with the hand overhead. Until recently, most players served with both feet on the ground. However, teams at the more competitive levels have come to realize that using the jump serve gives them an advantage to score points, so this serve has become more popular. Recreational players may be more likely to use an underhand serve. After the serve, the opposing team attempts to bump or "pass" the ball. This skill is almost always performed with the elbows extended and the hands below the waist. However, recently, an overhand pass has become more acceptable since passing rules have been liberalized. The overhand pass is the same skill as the set. The ball is passed to the setter, who usually sets it with the fingertips of both hands simultaneously and directs it toward the net, where it can be spiked by a teammate. In volleyball injury surveys, the skills of serving, passing, and setting have not been associated with high numbers of injuries.[3–9]

Biomechanics of Volleyball

SPIKING

The act of spiking or attacking the ball is quite similar to an overhand throwing motion. When spiking, the player jumps high into the air and contacts the ball at the highest point of his or her jump. There is a cocking period just prior to the point of contact when the shoulder is abducted and externally rotated with the elbow flexed. Then, as the ball is contacted, there is a forceful downward extension and internal rotation of the shoulder with concurrent elbow extension. This results in a whipping motion of the upper extremity. At the elite level, a spiked volleyball may travel at 80 to 90 mi/h.

A brief consideration of the kinematics of the spike follows. Note that although researchers have designated at least two styles of spiking (the backswing and elevation styles), we will discuss only the gross motor patterns that are similar to both styles. The interested reader is referred to the article by Oka et al. for further details.[33]

Phase 1: Approach

Although the slide attack (in which the athlete approaches the ball parallel to the net and employs a running, one-footed takeoff) is increasingly popular in women's volleyball, the traditional two- or four-step approach is far more common. In this technique, the athlete is roughly perpendicular to the net as he or she approaches the volleyball. A four-step approach results in more momentum than a two-step approach, thus enabling the athlete to jump higher. For either the two- or four-step approach, the final step is characteristically longer, as the athlete closes into the net in preparation for takeoff. It has been suggested that this "step close" technique permits optimal preloading of the lower limb musculature prior to jumping. At the conclusion of the approach phase of the jump, the athlete's hips and knees are flexed, and the ankles are dorsiflexed. The depth of this crouch is controlled by the eccentric action of the glutei, quadriceps, and gastrocnemius-soleus complex. In addition, the upper limbs are extended at the shoulders.

As the spiker prepares to jump, the arms swing downward and then forward into a position of flexion at the shoulders. This exaggerated pattern of upper limb rotation at the shoulders (arm swing) serves to increase the vertical ground reaction force and, in addition, may optimize force development of the hip and knee extensor muscle groups, thus increasing the athlete's vertical jump height.

Arm swing can contribute as much as 10 percent to the vertical jump height.

Phase 2: Takeoff

The takeoff phase of jumping is initiated by the explosive, sequential uncoiling of the hip, knee, and ankle—using predominantly concentric activation of the glutei, quadriceps, and gastrocnemius-soleus complex.

Phase 3: Cocking

While in the air, the spiker prepares to attack the ball. This has been referred to as "cocking the hammer." The trunk rotates toward the spiking side, and the lumbar spine extends while the knees flex. The spiking arm (typically the athlete's dominant arm) is brought into a cocked position (abducted and externally rotated at the shoulder, flexed at the elbow), and the opposite upper limb remains elevated (abducted and flexed at the shoulder, extended at the elbow).

Phase 4: Acceleration

The arm swing that will result in the spike actually begins when the athlete initially adducts and extends the nonhitting arm downward. Subsequently, counterrotation of the trunk and extension of the knees, combined with flexion of the lumbar spine (and occasionally of the hips), generates momentum that is "funneled" up the kinetic chain through the scapula on the hitting side to the upper limb.

Phase 5: Contact

The spiking arm is then sequentially adducted, internally rotated, and extended (both at the shoulder and the elbow) to bring the hand forcibly into contact with the volleyball. This position of full extension of the upper limb maximizes the moment arm and therefore the speed of the arm swing, enabling the spiker to impart greater velocity to the volleyball. A final rapid pronation of the forearm combined with flexion of the wrist imparts additional force to the volleyball. At the moment of contact, it has been estimated that the spiker's hand is moving at a speed of 20 m/s.

Phase 6: Follow-Through

After the ball is contacted, the arm decelerates as it follows through; this is the job of the rotator cuff musculature. In essence, the rotator cuff acts eccentrically to keep the humerus from dislocating after the spike.

Phase 7: Landing

Studies have shown that upon landing, the spiker initially contacts the floor with the foot opposite the hitting arm. The momentum of landing is rapidly dissipated through the eccentric action of the hip extensors, knee extensors, and ankle plantarflexors. Theoretically, single-leg landings place the athlete at greater risk for lower limb injury than do two-footed landings.

Spiking success depends in large measure on the athlete's jumping ability. The higher the point at which the athlete can make contact with the ball, the more easily the spiker can avoid hitting into the opponent's block. The jump employed with the step-close technique can best be described as a countermovement jump, in that the athlete preloads the lower limb musculature before takeoff. The skills of blocking, setting, and serving also demand jumping ability to a great extent, particularly at the elite level.

SERVING

Traditional Serve

The volleyball serve traditionally has been executed by striking the ball overhead so as to impart little (topspin) or no spin (floater) to it. The kinematics of these techniques are similar to the overhead arm swing of the spike, except that the athlete does not "snap" the wrist on contacting the ball and abruptly decelerates the arm thereafter (there is no follow-through). When contacting the ball, the center of gravity of the body is being shifted from the right rear foot to the front left foot for a right-handed player. The hitting arm's shoulder is rotating forward, and the elbow and wrist are extending. The ball is hit with the heel and palm of the hand. It looks like a throwing motion without the follow-through (Fig. 4.1). Performed correctly, the volleyball "floats" capriciously (much like a knuckleball in baseball), making it difficult for the receiving team to judge its flight and thus pass it effectively. Hitting the ball toward one side can create spin on the ball (Fig. 4.2). Spin will be toward the side where the least amount of pressure is applied. (See Fig. 4.3 for a topspin serve.) These traditional serves can average in the range of 33 mi/h.[34]

Jump Serve

The jump serve has become increasingly popular over the last decade, and the kinematics of this variety of serve are similar to those of the spike (Fig. 4.4). The jump serve has a lower trajectory and reaches speeds up to 52 mi/h (23 m/s). The jump serve also places the server in a better ready position for defense. The added power from the forward jump and arm swing creates the increased speed.[34]

Digging

The defensive player is usually in a low squat. This position is considered the ready position. The feet are slightly wider apart than the shoulders, the weight is distributed on the inside and balls of the feet, the knees are slightly flexed, and the arms and hands are waist to knee high in a neutral position.[34] Often, when the ball is spiked, the defensive player must dive to get the ball. This is called a *dig*. A properly executed dig is followed by a roll to return to the ready position.

Passing

The most common type of pass is the forearm pass (Fig. 4.5). Prior to contact with the ball, the player should be in the ready position with a

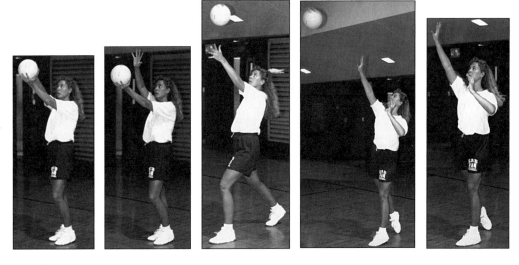

FIGURE 4.1

Overhead floater serve. *(Used with permission from Kluka and Dunn.[34])*

staggered, stable base of support. The elbows are extended, the shoulders are slightly flexed, and the wrists are deviated ulnarly. The forearms create a platform for the pass. The angle of the forearms and shoulders will change the rebounding direction of the ball. This allows the passer to direct the ball to another player. The ball contacts the distal portion of the forearms simultaneously. As the player contacts the ball, the body weight is shifted forward to the front

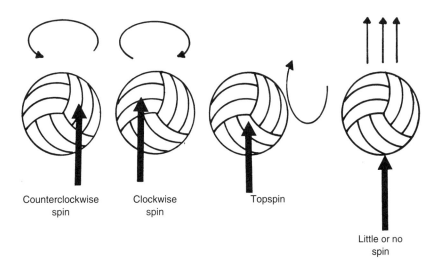

Counterclockwise spin   Clockwise spin   Topspin   Little or no spin

FIGURE 4.2

Spin on the ball. *(Used with permission from Kluka and Dunn.[34])*

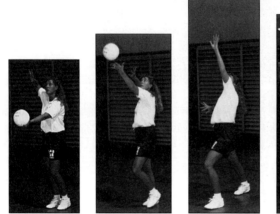
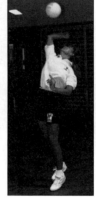
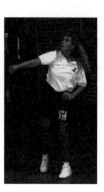

FIGURE 4.3

Overhead topspin serve. (*Used with permission from Kluka and Dunn.*[34])

foot to create an increase in speed on the pass. The knees also extend slightly as the ball is hit.

Setting

The role of the set is to place the ball for a spike. The overhead set can be directed to the front or the back. The accuracy depends on the absorption of force, redirection, and propulsion of the ball. Prior to contact, it is important to be in the ready position. The upper body is upright with the shoulders flexed to 90 degrees and the elbows flexed so that the hands are about 6 inches in front of the eyes. The fingers are spread apart, and the player views the ball between the spaces in the hands. The ball contacts the pads of the thumb, index, and middle fingers toward the sides of the ball. The wrists hyperextend and radially deviate as the force of the ball is absorbed. The absorption time ranges from 0.03 to 0.10 s. Following absorption and redirection, propulsion of the ball occurs via the lower extremities extending, shoulders flexing, elbows extending, forearms pronating, and wrists flexing (Fig. 4.6). The backward overhead set is the same (Fig. 4.7),

except that at contact, the hips and lumbar spine extend to create a backward trajectory on the ball.[34]

A front or back jump set can be used in combination with a quick middle attack (Fig. 4.8). There also can be a setter attack, where the setter hits the ball directly over the net (Fig. 4.9).

Blocking

Blocking is a skill highly dependent on a well-timed jump. Instead of the exaggerated countermovement jump used in the traditional spike approach, blockers frequently employ a squat jump. Since blockers (especially middle blockers) must make split-second decisions in response to the opponent's offensive strategy, they typically cannot afford the time required to perform a full countermovement jump. The squat jump, although it permits the athlete to get off the ground quickly, results in lower jump heights. Blocking places considerable demand on the athlete's trunk musculature and spine. The rules limit blocking to the three front-row players.

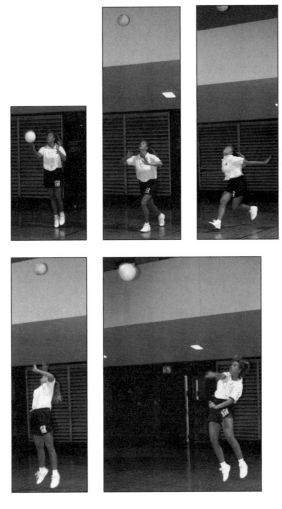

FIGURE 4.4

Jump serve. *(Used with permission from Kluka and Dunn.[34])*

Injury Prevention

WARM-UP AND SKILL DRILLS

A warm-up prior to practice or competition should last at least 15 minutes. Similar activities would be reasonable during a cool-down following volleyball activity, which again should last at least 10 minutes. A general warm-up should include activities that increase the core temperature, blood flow to the muscles, heart rate, and muscle extensibility. Good examples of this are fast walking/light jogging in a clockwise, counterclockwise, and diagonal direction around the court, jumping rope, and jumping jacks followed by active stretching. Following the general warm-up, the players begin skill-specific drills.[34]

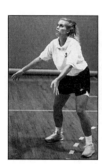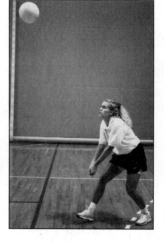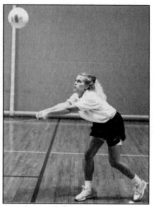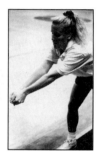

FIGURE 4.5

Forearm pass. *(Used with permission from Kluka and Dunn.[34])*

Most volleyball players warm up by hitting the ball back and forth by setting or passing it. This is usually performed in pairs and is referred to by players as "pepper." Next, players often practice spiking, with setters setting the ball to the hitters. Serving practice then immediately precedes the start of competition. While some repetitions of these sport-specific skills are undoubtedly beneficial, this warm-up regimen does not facilitate maximum flexibility, as a more comprehensive precompetition program might.

According to the FIVB 2000 rules, prior to a match, if the teams have previously had a playing court at their disposal, each team will have a 3-minute warm-up period at the net. If they did not have a court available to them, they may have 5 minutes each. If both captains agree to warm up at the net together, the teams may do so for 6 or 10 minutes. Following the game or practice, players need to incorporate a cool-down period that is similar to the warm-up period in reverse function with decreasing intensity.

Other sport-specific drills are self-passing drills. Players can practice passing the ball to a height 1 ft above the net and within a 5-ft cir-cle. In another passing drill, three players incorporate lateral movement and ball control.[34]

A setting drill can be accomplished using a volleyball on a basketball court, where a player is thrown a ball at the foul line and he or she tries to pass it into the basket. If the player misses, he or she needs to set the rebound into the basket.

A hands drill incorporates forward and backward movement and ball control. Three players begin on the end line, one at the right corner, one at the middle, and one at the left corner. An assistant tosses the volleyball to an area in front of a player. The player will move to the spot and then pass the ball to a predetermined area. Following the pass, the player will backpedal to tag the player standing at the end line. The players rotate in a clockwise manner after being tagged.[34]

STRETCHING AND STRENGTHENING

Unfortunately, the benefits of pregame stretching are difficult to quantify. However, there are data from animal models that demonstrate previously stretched muscles will lengthen to a greater extent before failure than those which

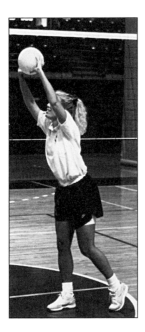
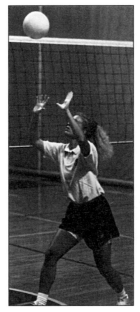
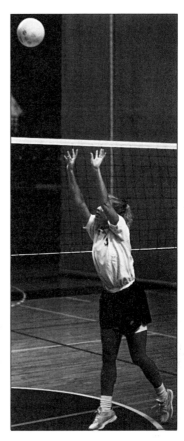

FIGURE 4.6

Overhead front set. *(Used with permission from Kluka and Dunn.[34])*

have not been stretched. Warm muscles are probably also more flexible than cold ones. A warm-up activity increases blood flow to the muscles so that they will be warmer and more likely to benefit from stretching activity.

Important muscle groups to stretch include the trunk rotators, quadriceps, and hamstrings, as well as the gastrocnemius. Upper extremity stretches should include forward flexion and abduction at the shoulder. Coaches may argue over which stretches are most appropriate, but stretches will be most effective if held for 10 to 30 s and repeated three to five times.

The vertical jump is an integral component in spiking and blocking. An off-season and in-season jumping program should include core strengthening and plyometrics. A shuttle press can be used for concentric or eccentric training as well as plyometric training. Low-impact hopping and bounding are good examples of plyometrics that can specifically help with vertical jumping. (See Chap. 13 for a jumping program.)

ENDURANCE AND PERIODIZATION TRAINING

Endurance and conditioning cannot be overlooked. There are several studies that suggest that fatigue results in abnormal muscular activation patterns, thereby placing the

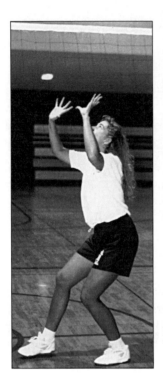
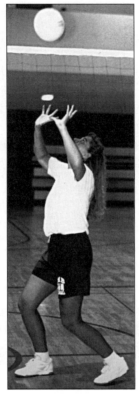
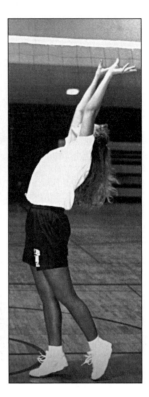

FIGURE 4.7

Overhead back set. *(Used with permission from Kluka and Dunn.[34])*

joint(s) acted on by those muscles (and the muscles themselves) at increased risk for injury. This is also borne out by the observation that the injury rate during competition increases as matches progress from the first through the third sets, according to NCAA Injury Surveillance System data for women's collegiate volleyball. Thus, in order to optimize performance and reduce the risk of injury, the volleyball athlete should participate in a structured volleyball-specific training program periodized to minimize the risk of overtraining, with appropriate attention to nutrition and rest. The conditioning program should include the following activities: static and dynamic balance, flexibility, strength, agility, aerobic and an-aerobic exercise, and muscular strength, endurance, and power.[34]

The following is an example of a full-year macrocycle subdivided into three mesocycles that covers the periodization training of a high school volleyball player.[35] The off-season runs from December 1 to August 1. Preseason training is from August 1 to September 15. From September 15 to November 1, the season begins, and two to three games are played per week. Championship play may extend until December 1.[35]

The first 21-week mesocycle begins with the off-season. It begins with a 1-month transitional period consisting of low-level cross-training activity. The next 17 weeks make up the preparatory period. The first 6 weeks of

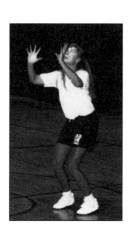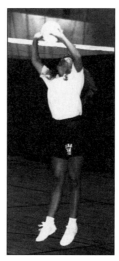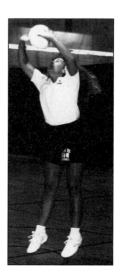

FIGURE 4.8

Jump set. *(Used with permission from Kluka and Dunn.[34])*

this are the *early hypertrophy/endurance phase*. This phase includes flexibility, strength, and endurance training. Flexibility exercises are performed during the warm-up and cool-down every day. The strength train-ing consists of 3 to 5 sets for 8 to 12 repeti-tions based on a 10-repetition maximum test. This is performed 3 days per week and in-cludes exercises such as squats, leg presses, calf raises, dead lifts, bench presses, and mili-

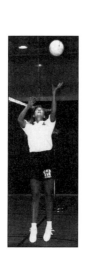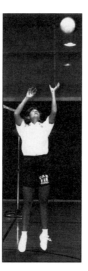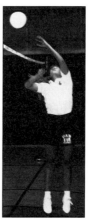

FIGURE 4.9

Setter attack. *(Used with permission from Kluka and Dunn.[34])*

tary presses. Endurance training is performed 2 days per week for 20 to 30 minutes. This is primarily a maintenance program because high-endurance training levels may be counterproductive to strength training.[35]

Following 1 week of active rest, the 4-week *strength phase* begins. This phase will include flexibility training, strength training, and skill drills. Flexibility exercises are still performed during every warm-up and cooldown. The intensity of the strength training increases to 3 to 5 sets for 4 to 6 repetitions based on a 5-repetition maximum for 3 days per week. Exercises should include the push presses, clean pulls, front squats, abdominal curls, pullovers, upright rows, and lateral shoulder raises. The same muscles as in the previous phase are the focus of this phase, but it is important to vary the exercises. The skill drills can include low- to moderate-level jumping exercises and serving drills as well as short-interval sprints. The workout should be performed 2 days per week and last 20 to 30 minutes.[35]

Following 1 week of active rest, the *power phase* begins and lasts for 3 weeks. This phase will include flexibility training, strength training, and skill drills. Flexibility exercises are performed with every warm-up and cool-down. The intensity of the strength training increases to 3 to 5 sets for 2 to 4 repetitions based on a 2-repetition maximum for 3 days per week. It is important to add warm-up sets to prevent injuries. Exercises should include squats, snatch pulls, push jerks, military presses, bench presses, dumbbell raises, leg presses, prone double leg lifts, and sit-ups. The intensity for each of the 3 days alternates from heavy to light to medium. The skill drills can include high-level plyometric sport-specific drills. These include box and depth jumping, bounding, push-ups with a clap in between, and medicine ball exercises for core strengthening.[35]

Following 1 week of active rest, maximal strength testing and assessment are performed for 1 week. This ends the first mesocycle.[35]

This is followed by a 2-week low-level cross-training transitional period. Then the second mesocycle begins. Intensity increases, more sport-specific and agility drills are performed, and there is an increase in anaerobic and aerobic training. This cycle incorporates the same three periods as the first mesocycle: a hypertrophy, strength, and power phase. Each phase includes flexibility, strength, endurance, and plyometric training. The strength training is performed 3 days per week with alternating heavy, moderate, and light days.[35]

The *hypertrophy phase* lasts 2 weeks. The strength training is performed 3 days per week with 3 to 5 sets of 8 to 12 repetitions of a 1-repetition maximum test. The endurance training is performed 2 days per week and includes anaerobic and agility drills. Low-intensity plyometrics are performed 2 days per week for 15 to 20 minutes with 200 to 300 foot touches.[35]

The *strength phase* last 2 weeks. The strength training is performed 3 days per week with 3 to 5 sets of 5 to 7 repetitions of a 1-repetition maximum test. The endurance training is performed 2 days per week and includes anaerobic and sport-specific agility drills. Moderate-intensity plyometrics are performed 2 days per week for 15 to 20 minutes with 150 to 250 foot touches.[35]

Following 1 week of active rest, the *power phase* begins and lasts 4 weeks. The strength training is performed 3 days per week with 3 to 5 sets of 2 to 4 repetitions of a 1-repetition maximum test. The endurance training is performed 2 days per week and includes anaerobic and sport-specific agility drills. High-intensity plyometrics are performed 2 days per week for 15 to 20 minutes with 100 to 150 foot touches. This ends the second mesocycle.[35]

After a 2-week transitional period of low-intensity cross-training, the third mesocycle begins. This correlates with the beginning of the preseason. The period is focused on maintenance of strength (2 days per week varying from low to high intensity over the 6 weeks), reduction in endurance and plyometric exercises to 1 day per week each, and the addition of daily volleyball practices, aerobic training, and sport-specific drills.[35]

The athlete is now ready to begin the last mesocycle, which includes in-season training. The volume is low. Weight training and plyometrics are alternated and performed once or twice during the week, depending on the number of competitions. Practices should include anaerobic training, and 90 percent of the athlete's schedule should be spent on skill and strategy development. Bench players need extra work following games to simulate game intensity and activity.[35]

PROPRIOCEPTION EXERCISES

Research has shown that attention to a program of ankle proprioceptive neuromuscular training exercises can reduce the incidence of ankle sprain injuries. Research regarding the use of rigid ankle orthoses suggests that they are also probably effective at reducing the risk of contact-related ankle sprains—particularly if the athlete has a history of a prior ankle sprain injury. The mechanism by which these orthoses are thought to work is not known with certainty but may involve simply enhancing proprioceptive awareness of the ankle joint. Furthermore, it appears unlikely that wearing an ankle orthosis increases the incidence of knee injuries, and most studies suggest that semirigid orthoses do not significantly impair athletic performance.

A Norwegian study demonstrated a twofold decrease in ankle sprains over the course of a season. There were two components to the study. The first component was the change in the centerline rule during practice. (No part of a player's foot may touch the centerline.) The second component was proprioception balance training. Proprioception is the ability to know where a body part is in space based on stimuli that the brain receives from muscles, tendons, and other tissues. It is believed that closed-chain balancing exercises can improve proprioception and strengthen muscles that arrest inversion.[15] In this particular study, balance training was taught to all the teams and continued for 10 weeks. Athletes balanced on an ankle disk each night. (See Fig. 4.10 for proprioception exercises.)

PROPHYLACTIC DEVICES

Many different ankle supports are available for athletes. A prospective study of air-stirrup ankle supports demonstrated this device to be effective for secondary prevention of ankle sprains.[10] Among athletes who had suffered a previous sprain, a fivefold decrease in ankle sprains was reported over one soccer season when the air stirrup was worn. However, it is important to note that there was not a significant difference in the number of sprains with the use of this device in ankles that had not been sprained previously.[10] Ankle taping has been shown to be beneficial in restricting inversion motion.[11,12] In addition, semirigid ankle supports have been demonstrated to decrease inversion range of motion during athletic activities.[13,14] It appears that ankle supports may be superior to ankle taping because ankle supports do not lose their ability to restrict inversion as tape does after several repeated cycles of vertical jumping.[12,14] These devices do not seem to restrict inversion in a substantial enough way to explain their prophylactic effect. Therefore, it might be that they are effective because they somehow enhance proprioception.

Etiology of Injuries

Volleyball has evolved from the recreational game of mintonette into a sport of explosive, powerful skills. A consideration of the volleyball injury epidemiologic data suggests that skills involving jumping and those requiring forceful contact of the volleyball with the

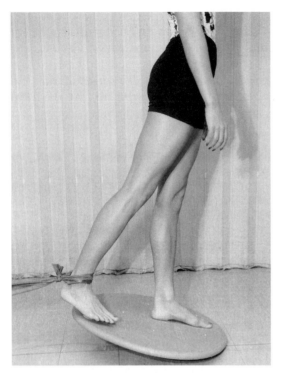 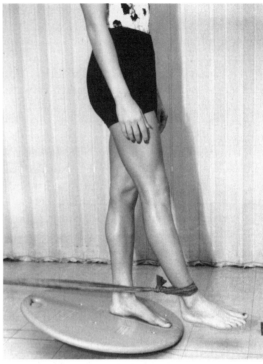

FIGURE 4.10

A. Elastic band for added perturbation for kicking while single-leg balancing on a balance board. *B.* Single-leg balance while plantarflexing with added challenge with Theraband. *(Used with permission from Prentice W: Rehabilitation Techniques in Sports Medicine, 3d ed. New York: McGraw-Hill, 1999, p 97.)*

upper extremity in an overhead position (spiking and serving) place the athlete at greatest risk for injury. Spiking, for example, requires the athlete to jump explosively and then "attack" the ball with a forceful overhead arm swing.

Not only is spiking a thrilling skill to perform and witness, effective spiking is essential to a volleyball team's success. However, spiking is a difficult skill to master. Consequently, significant emphasis is placed on developing the volleyball athlete's spiking capability. It has been estimated that an elite volleyball athlete, practicing and competing 16 to 20 hours per week, will perform 40,000 spikes in 1 year. Spiking places enormous de-

mands—both acute and chronic—on the musculotendinous structures of shoulders, knees, ankles, and low back. These structures need to be strong enough for repetitive use in the varying positions and with the various forces that occur. Often, injuries occur from trying to create spin on the ball. Consequently, these areas are at significant risk for injury in volleyball athletes.[4–6,8,9]

Players on the opposing team will attempt to block a spike by jumping and reaching with their hands overhead while their shoulders are maximally forward flexed. Blockers are attempting to force the ball back onto the hitter's side within the boundaries of the court. Two or even three players may jump simultaneously in attempts to block a spike. Blocking has been associated with the highest rate of injury in volleyball injury surveys. This is the most common mechanism of injury for ankle sprains.[3–6,8]

If the ball is spiked past the block, then the blocking team must play defense. This skill involves an attempt to bump or dig a spiked ball, similar to passing. The object is to keep the ball from touching the ground. Often the player is required to move quickly. Sometimes it is even necessary to dive to play the ball up into the air. Defense has been associated with a small number of volleyball injuries.[4,5,7,9]

In 1996, in Norway, Bahr et al.[2] studied a change in the centerline rule. A rule was instituted that made any contact with this line a violation. This change did reduce the number of ankle sprains. However, when the new rule was tested in tournament play, it was felt to be unacceptable by the players because of the number of centerline violations that resulted in stoppage of play. A reasonable option might be implementing this rule during practice to minimize injury risk.

EXTRINSIC FACTORS

Surface

Volleyball is somewhat unique among sports in that it is played on many different surfaces. There is evidence that when the game is played on softer surfaces, fewer injuries occur. In one study, patellar tendinitis was less common among players who played on wood surfaces than among those that played on harder surfaces such as concrete or linoleum.[31] Athletes in other sports are aware that harder surfaces may be more abusive on the body. Many distance runners train on dirt or gravel trails to avoid the pounding associated with training on asphalt. In a survey of elite college volleyball players, fivefold fewer injuries were reported on sand than on wood.[4] There are not much current data available regarding injury rates on grass.

Level of Play

It is often difficult to compare injury rates between groups because many variables may be at play. However, there does appear to be an association between higher level of play and increased frequency of injury. At the 1995 U.S. Olympic Festival, injuries occurred at a rate of one per 25 hours in training and/or competition.[4] These athletes had a mean age of 20 years and were elite college players. During the 1987 National Amateur Volleyball Tournament in the United States, the injury rate was one per 50 hours during competition.[7] This group of athletes represented a wide range of ages and skill levels. While it is difficult to draw conclusions from such a small subset of athletes, it does appear that higher skill levels subject athletes to greater injury risk. Elite athletes train for more hours, so the cumulative stress on their bodies may make them more vulnerable to injury. Another theory is that with increased intensity of play, injury risk increases.

Common Injuries and Their Rehabilitation

Volleyball injury epidemiology suffers from a problem common to many types of injury research—namely, the definition of injury has varied among different studies. Injuries during the course of one year have been examined retrospectively. Among 86 Scottish National League players, an injury rate of 53 percent was found. The definition of injury was "any condition resulting in 2 or more days missed from play." Most of these injuries were of mild severity, and only 26 percent resulted in more than 2 weeks missed from play.[9] The injury rate among 93 elite college-age volleyball players in the United States was 81.7 percent over one year. In this study, the definition of injury was "any condition resulting in at least 1 day missed from play." The majority of these injuries resulted in less than 4 days missed from play.[4]

The goal of rehabilitation is the restoration of function. In a sport-specific context, this means identifying the mechanism of injury, making an accurate diagnosis, and creating a treatment plan that will enable the athlete to return to competition and training while minimizing the risk of reinjury. Clearly, the treatment plan may differ based on the type of injury suffered—one does not treat an acute contusion or sprain injury in the same way one treats a chronic overuse injury. Thus, it is important first and foremost to make an accurate, complete diagnosis. This involves identifying factors that may have placed the athlete at risk for a particular injury and, if possible, characterizing the type of injury that has occurred. Kibler et al.[32] have identified several kinds of injuries based on the method of presentation, including acute injuries, chronic injuries, and acute exacerbations of chronic injuries.

The injured athlete may present with a variety of symptoms, including pain (either with activity or at rest), swelling, stiffness, erythema, or simply an inability to perform at the previous level. Kibler et al.[32] refer to this as the "clinical symptom complex." Symptoms generally are reflective of some sort of tissue alteration or damage that has occurred due to the mechanism of injury; this is referred to as the "tissue injury complex." As a result of this injury or as a consequence of the abnormal movement patterns that result from the injury, other tissues and structures are placed under increased stress. This is referred to as the "tissue overload complex." These structural deficits lead to deficits of function and biomechanics (i.e., technique), referred to as the "functional biomechanical deficit complex." This, in turn, causes the athlete to substitute new movement patterns in an effort to minimize the symptoms while attempting to compensate

for any dropoff in performance. This "subclinical adaptation complex," in turn, can lead to additional tissue overload, injury, symptoms, biomechanical deficits, and further (mal)adaptations. In this way, a "vicious cycle" is set up. Unless interrupted by a comprehensive rehabilitation program emphasizing strength, flexibility, proprioception, endurance, and proper technique, this vicious cycle can result in prolonged and often incomplete recovery from an injury, thereby placing the athlete in jeopardy of chronic or recurrent injury with long-term functional consequences.

Although the exact treatment protocol for different types of injuries varies, the process of treating injuries can be broken down into three phases: the acute phase, which is followed by the recovery phase, and finally, the functional phase. Different portions of the vicious cycle are addressed as the athlete progresses through treatment. In the acute period, the athlete's symptoms are treated, and the injured tissues are given an opportunity to begin healing. Common interventions include anti-inflammatory and analgesic medications, thermal modalities (i.e., ice and, in appropriate circumstances, heat), and protection and relative rest of the injured body part. During the rehabilitation phase of care, the athlete's injured tissues continue to heal. Biomechanical alterations and subsequent tissue overloads should be identified and treated through a program of progressive strengthening and conditioning, including flexibility and proprioceptive neuromuscular training throughout the kinetic chain. At the conclusion of the recovery phase, the athlete is ready to progress to sport-specific functional exercises, culminating in his or her return to participation. During this functional phase, the emphasis shifts from rehabilitation to "prehabilitation" in order to minimize the athlete's risk of reinjury. We will conclude the chapter with the most common volleyball-related injuries.

ROTATOR CUFF TENDINOPATHY

Biomechanics of Injury

Shoulder injuries account for 8 to 20 percent of volleyball injuries. The biceps and rotator cuff tendons are affected most commonly.[4,7,9] The shoulder (glenohumeral) joint is the most mobile joint in the human body. Unfortunately, this mobility comes at the cost of stability, of which the bony components of the joint provide very little. Ligamentous structures and the fibrocartilaginous glenoid labrum provide additional static stability, whereas the rotator cuff muscles dynamically stabilize the shoulder joint. These structures act in concert to control the motion of the humeral head within the glenoid fossa. The ligamentous structures provide stability at the extremes of glenohumeral motion, whereas the shoulder girdle musculature works through a precise system of force coupling and coactivation of agonists and antagonists to coordinate motion of the humerus and scapula throughout the shoulder's range of motion. The shoulder girdle musculature does not generate tremendous upper limb torque; roughly 85 percent of the energy required to spike or serve a volleyball is generated by the legs and back. However, when a proximal segment of the chain is injured, the more distal segments often attempt to "catch up" the deficit—placing them at higher risk of injury. By minimizing perturbation of the instantaneous center of joint motion throughout the shoulder's available range, the rotator cuff permits maximal transmission of energy from the proximal end of the kinetic chain to the upper limb. Because of the fine coordination needed throughout the entire kinetic chain to accomplish this task, optimal shoulder function depends on maintaining balanced strength and flexibility not only in the shoulder girdle but also in the hips and trunk.

If, through repetitive overload or acute trauma, the shoulder stabilizing system is compromised (tissue injury complex), the athlete will begin to substitute altered movement patterns in an effort to minimize symptoms and maintain performance (subclinical adaptation complex). Consequently, this increases the risk of injury to other structures within the kinetic chain (tissue overload complex). Pain, restricted range of motion, and muscle weakness/imbalance all can compromise glenohumeral joint function. One frequent sign of altered shoulder girdle mechanics is scapular dysfunction. One recent study of elite volleyball players with and without pain in the shoulder of their spiking arms documented nearly universal scapular dysfunction in those athletes who complained of pain. On examination, their scapulae were abducted (the "scapular slide"), and the musculature of the posterior shoulder girdle was tight, limiting internal rotation in the affected shoulder. This muscular imbalance can result in impaired glenohumeral control, with increased anterior translation of the humeral head in the glenoid fossa—in effect creating a "functionally unstable" shoulder. This places the athlete at risk for impingement of the supraspinatus and attrition of the glenoid labrum.

Rehabilitation

Rotator cuff injuries typically are overuse injuries. Of the four muscles comprising the rotator cuff, the supraspinatus is injured most frequently. The explanation for this observation is principally anatomic—the supraspinatus tendon travels in the space beneath the acromion and the coracoacromial ligament to insert on the humeral head and can become injured and inflamed as it is cyclically compressed with repetitive overhead motion. The mechanism by which the tissue injury occurs can be a primary phenomenon, wherein the rotator cuff simply deteriorates with time, age, and overuse. In athletes, however, tissue injury typically is a secondary phenomenon due to scapular dysfunction and the resulting dynamic instability of the glenohumeral joint. By the time the athlete complains of symptoms, the supraspinatus tendon shows little histologic evidence of inflammation, and thus it is probably more appropriate to diagnose the athlete with "tendinosis" or tendinopathy rather than tendinitis. The symptomatic athlete typically will complain of anterior shoulder pain with overhead range of motion, such as when spiking or serving. On physical examination, the athlete may be tender to palpation over the humeral head at the insertion of the supraspinatus tendon. Passive forward flexion or horizontal adduction with combined internal rotation of the shoulder will elicit pain—the impingement signs. Posterior capsular tightness results in restriction of both active and passive internal rotation of the affected shoulder. Although there may be pain inhibition of resisted rotator cuff activation, no true weakness should be present unless there is a rotator cuff tear or neurologic involvement. When inspecting the scapulae for evidence of abnormal positioning or motion, take note to rule out the presence of supraspinatus or infraspinatus atrophy that would suggest entrapment of the suprascapular nerve.

Acute management of rotator cuff tendinopathy should focus on relieving the athlete's pain through medication and the judicious use of thermal modalities, such as ice, ultrasound, electrical stimulation, and/or iontophoresis, promoting tissue healing, and minimizing the deleterious effects of rest and time off from competition. Once the athlete has minimal pain through a limited range of motion, he or she can progress to the recovery phase of rehabilitation. This stage emphasizes range of motion, strengthening, and scapular control. (See Chap. 6 for pictures of these techniques.) Sport-specific activities are reintroduced in the functional phase of rehabilitation. This third and final stage also seeks to identify and correct any underlying biomechanical deficits and subclinical adaptations that may have precipitated the rotator

cuff injury. Once the athlete can perform sport-specific skills through a pain-free range of motion, he or she can return to play. Table 4.1 summarizes a comprehensive rehabilitation program for rotator cuff tendinopathy.

SUPRASCAPULAR NEUROPATHY

Biomechanics of Injury

Suprascapular neuropathy (SSN) is a condition that is found in volleyball players and in players that participate in overhead sports.[22,23] A study of top-level German volleyball players revealed a 32 percent prevalence among 66 athletes.[23] In 1985, at the European championships, 13 percent of the 96 athletes evaluated had suprascapular neuropathy.[22] In volleyball players, the suprascapular nerve seems to be compressed at the spinoglenoid notch, where the terminal branch, an entirely motor nerve, passes to the infraspinatus muscle. From 1985 to 1996, Ferretti et al.[24] observed 38 cases of isolated atrophy of the infraspinatus muscle in volleyball players. At the time of the first examination, 35 of the 38 athletes were pain-free and were treated with strengthening exercises for the external rotators of the shoulder. Sixteen of these 35 players were contacted after a mean time of 5.5 years. At that time, 13 were still involved in volleyball, while 3 had retired symptom-free. The 3 patients who initially had pain and were treated with surgeries were all able to play at their preinjury level.[24]

SSN is believed to occur as a result of the "floater" serve.[22] When performing this serve, the player must stop the overhand follow-through immediately after striking the ball. This type of serve results in a forceful eccentric contraction of the infraspinatus muscle to decelerate the arm. This contraction is believed to result in traction from the myoneural junction to the spinoglenoid notch and compression of the nerve.[21] Infraspinatus strength should be tested during the preparticipation physical examination, particularly

TABLE 4.1

Rehabilitation for Rotator Cuff Tendinopathy

I. *Acute phase*

   Goals: Reduce symptoms, improve active range of motion, begin program of scapular control, maintain fitness

   Interventions: Passive modalities, active range of motion/stretching exercises, isometric exercises, closed kinetic chain exercises, relative rest

II. *Recovery phase*

   Goals: Increase strength, improve range of motion, improve scapular control, address flexibility imbalances

   Interventions: Active range of motion/stretching exercises, strengthen scapular stabilizers first, then move on to concentric and eccentric isotonic exercises isolating the rotator cuff, progress to sport specific movement patterns

III. *Functional phase*

   Goals: Increase power, increase endurance, restore sport-specific function (spiking and serving)

   Interventions: Exercises to strengthen the entire kinetic chain, upper limb plyometrics emphasizing specific movement patterns, analysis of technique

in volleyball players and especially those at the more elite levels. This site of compression is rare in athletes who are not volleyball players. A more common site is at the suprascapular notch, resulting in supraspinatus and infraspinatus weakness.

Rehabilitation

Since SSN is often painless, most players do not require medication. However, if deinnervation is not complete, then external rotator strengthening is important. See Figs. 4.11 through 4.15 for shoulder stabilization and rotator cuff strengthening exercises. If the patient is having pain, magnetic resonance imaging (MRI) should be strongly considered prior to surgical decompression, since up to 67 percent of affected individuals may have ganglion cysts compressing the nerve.[21]

One series of 27 patients with a space-occupying lesion compressing the suprascapular nerve showed that 21 were caused by ganglion cysts.[25] There is some controversy over surgical repair versus nonsurgical management in patients without a documented cyst.[21]

HAND INJURIES

Biomechanics of Injury

These injuries often occur while attempting to block a spiked ball. A series of 226 volleyball players in the Netherlands sustained 235 injuries to the hands.[26] The injuries occurred over 4 years. Sprains and strains were the most common injury (39 percent), followed by fractures (25 percent) and contusions (16 percent). Dislocations, mallet fingers, and open wounds made up the remaining 20 percent. Thirty-seven percent of hand injuries occurred while the player was playing defense, 36 percent during blocking, 18 percent as a result of falls, and only 8 percent while spiking the ball. The thumb and the little finger are the most vulnerable phalanges. The metacarpophalangeal joint of the thumb was

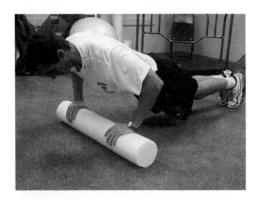

FIGURE 4.11

A foam roll can be used for push-ups for dynamic control while moving the roll forward and backward.

the most frequent location of ligamentous injury.[26] The radial collateral ligament of the thumb (metacarpophalangeal joint) is particularly vulnerable during blocking. However, this injury rarely results in significant disability, unlike injury of the ulnar collateral ligament or gamekeeper's thumb. One player was wearing a ring that got tangled in the net, resulting in a near amputation of the ring finger. This case emphasizes that players should not wear jewelry while playing volleyball.

Volleyball players can sustain other hand injuries such as a fracture of the pisiform bone. It is unclear if this injury is the result of contact with the floor or the ball.[27] Another injury that can occur is antebrachial-palmar hammer syndrome. This condition is caused by blunt trauma to the radial and ulnar arteries and may result in vasospasm of these arteries. There were three cases of antebrachial-palmar hammer syndrome among volleyball players in one series.[28] This condition presents with pain, distal cyanosis, and pulselessness. The "pancake" maneuver may be responsible for both of these types of injuries. This maneuver requires a defensive player to slide his or her hand under the ball

with the palm on the floor and the fingers extended. When performed correctly, the ball is kept from contacting the floor, thus keeping it in play. However, this maneuver leaves the hand vulnerable to injury because it is wedged between the spiked ball, which is traveling at high speed, and the floor.

Rehabilitation

Most finger sprains and closed fractures can be managed by splinting or "buddy" taping. With buddy taping, the injured finger is taped to the adjacent healthy finger, which acts as a functional splint. The thumb does not lend itself to buddy taping, but supportive taping may decrease the pain of a metacarpophalangeal joint sprain. Thumb spica taping usually gives enough support to allow return to play. (See Figure 6.19 in the diving chapter.) Ice is always useful in the acute phase.

ACUTE KNEE INJURIES
Biomechanics of Injury

Fortunately, acute knee injuries are rare, but when they occur, they can result in significant time lost from the sport before returning to play. The most frequent mechanism of injury is landing on another athlete's foot after jumping in the attack zone. The most common ligament injured in the knee is the anterior cruciate ligament (ACL), which is often accompanied by meniscus damage. In a series of 52 knee injuries involving the anterior cruciate ligament, more of the injuries were to women.[29] More data are needed regarding the relative risk of anterior cruciate ligament injury during volleyball in women as compared with men, but there is a great deal of anecdotal experience to suggest that women are more at risk for this injury in this sport. There has been much speculation as to the etiology of this apparent discrepancy in injury risk. Undoubtedly, the cause is multifactorial. Suggested factors have included

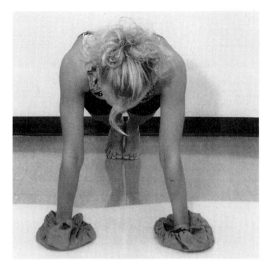
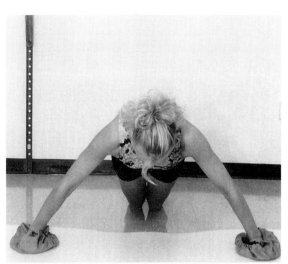
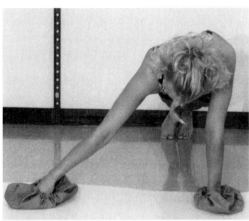
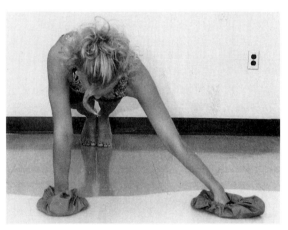

FIGURE 4.12

Dynamic stabilization for push-ups, shoulder horizontal abduction, adduction, and circular movements. *(Used with permission from Prentice W: Rehabilitation Techniques in Sports Medicine, 3d ed. New York: McGraw-Hill, 1999, p 97.)*

greater ligamentous laxity in women, increased recurvatum, greater valgus angle at the knee, narrower notch between the condyles of the femur through which the ACL passes, and variable firing of the hamstring and quadriceps muscles between the genders. For ACL rehabilitation, refer to Chaps. 10 and 14.

PATELLAR TENDINITIS, "JUMPER'S KNEE"

Biomechanics of Injury

Patellar tendinitis, or "jumper's knee," is the most common overuse injury in volleyball.[4,7,16] The knee joint connects the body's two longest lever arms: the thigh and the leg. It therefore must withstand high forces, ren-

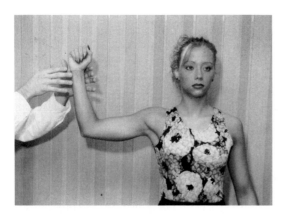

FIGURE 4.13

Rhythmic shoulder stabilization with external perturbations. *(Used with permission from Prentice W: Rehabilitation Techniques in Sports Medicine, 3d ed. New York: McGraw-Hill, 1999, p 97.)*

dering it vulnerable to injury. The patella plays a critical role in the biomechanics of the knee. By lengthening the moment arm on which the quadriceps acts, the patella increases knee extensor torque and enhances the mechanical advantage of the quadriceps muscle group, increasing extensor force production by approximately 50 percent. Some of the force generated during activation of the quadriceps is directed through the patella toward the knee joint's center of rotation. The patellofemoral joint reaction force is a measure of the compression of the patella against the femur and depends on the angle of knee flexion and the load applied. In general, with increasing knee flexion, there is increasing contact between the patella and femur, serving to distribute the increasing force—which with a deep knee bend can approach eight times the body weight. Maximal patellofemoral joint reaction force occurs at 60 to 90 degrees of knee flexion. Not surprisingly, research has shown that there is a correlation between knee joint kinetics and jumper's knee (also known as *patellar tendinopathy*). One study demonstrated that volleyball athletes who sustained the greatest ground reaction force during spike and block jumps were more likely to have symptoms of patellar tendinopathy. Similarly, those who developed the deepest knee flexion angle during landing from a spike jump were more likely to suffer from jumper's knee.[18] Other predictive factors included high knee extensor moments during landing, when the quadriceps are rapidly eccentrically activated in an effort to arrest momentum, and increased internal tibial torsion during takeoff.

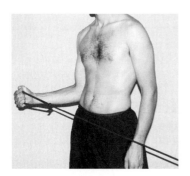 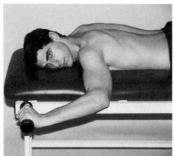 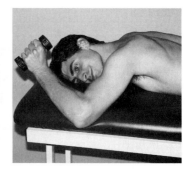

FIGURE 4.14

External shoulder rotation strengthening exercises with tubing and dumbbells. *(Used with permission from Prentice W: Rehabilitation Techniques in Sports Medicine, 3d ed. New York: McGraw-Hill, 1999, p 97.)*

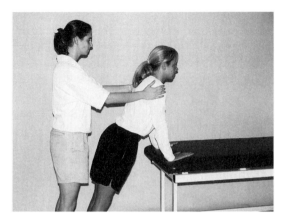
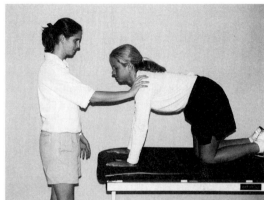
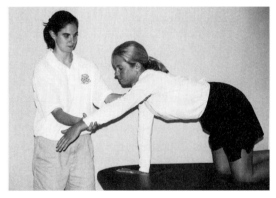
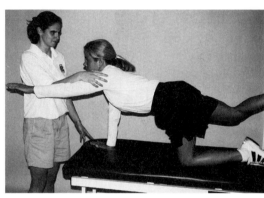

FIGURE 4.15

Closed-chain strengthening exercises. *(Used with permission from Prentice W: Rehabilitation Techniques in Sports Medicine, 3d ed. New York: McGraw-Hill, 1999, p 97.)*

Epidemiologic studies have shown that patellar tendinopathy is related to repetitive loading of the knee extensor mechanism. The prevalence of jumper's knee increases with the frequency of jump training and is higher among players who train or compete on hard, unforgiving surfaces. Interestingly, one study revealed that volleyball players with jumper's knee actually performed better than asymptomatic athletes in a standardized jump test emphasizing eccentric force generation.[17] This suggests that those athletes who jump well might be better able to eccentrically activate their knee extensor muscles, placing increasing load on the patellar tendon–bone junction. This can result in partial microscopic tearing of the tendon, which, if not treated adequately, can progress to complete tendon rupture.

Rehabilitation

The athlete with jumper's knee frequently complains of pain in the anterior aspect of the knee at the origin of the patellar tendon or at its insertion into the proximal tibia. Initially, symptoms may be present only after training or competition. As the condition worsens, however, pain may be present before and during participation and ultimately may become so severe as to prevent participation. Symptoms typically are provoked by jumping and also may be worsened by prolonged knee flexion (such as when sitting in a movie theater). The mechanism of injury typically is repetitive, chronic overload in athletes whose sports—such as volleyball—involve a great deal of jumping. Findings during physical examination may be few and subtle, depending on the stage of the condition. There may be focal tenderness to palpation at the tendinous insertion, and patellofemoral compression may prove painful. Hip external rotator weakness may be seen, as may tightness of the hip flexors, tensor fasciae latae and iliotibial band, hamstrings, and gastrocnemius-soleus complex. Inspection of the entire kinetic chain may reveal evidence of prior injury or predisposing factors, including a rigid cavus foot. Insufficiency of the medial quadriceps can predispose the athlete to abnormal patellar tracking, as can excessive pronation or a large Q angle. Rehabilitation therefore should focus on correcting strength and flexibility imbalances throughout the entire lower limb. Strengthening exercises should be performed initially at knee flexion angles that minimize patellar loading, beginning with isometric exercises and progressing through a functional continuum emphasizing eccentric strength training. Attempting to correct abnormal patellar tracking through bracing or taping can be therapeutic. Table 4.2 summarizes the principles of rehabilitation for jumper's knee.

ANKLE SPRAIN
Biomechanics of Injury

The lateral ankle sprain is the most common volleyball-related injury. It accounts for 15 to 65 percent of all volleyball injuries.[1,4,7,9] The true ankle joint consists of the talocrual (tibiofibular-talar) joint, but in a practical sense, the "ankle" also includes the subtalar joint. The typical volleyball mechanism of injury involves net play, most often a blocker landing on a teammate's foot or on the foot of the opposing spiker who has crossed over the centerline.[1] As the blocker lands, the ankles are typically plantarflexed in anticipation of accepting and dissipating the ground reaction force associated with landing. This is an anatomically disadvantageous position for the ankle, since the posterior talar plafond is narrower than the anterior aspect. When the foot is plantarflexed, there is inherently greater laxity in the true ankle joint. When landing on an uneven surface, unless the dynamic (muscular) ankle stabilizers can compensate, the ligaments that passively stabilize the ankle are suddenly overloaded. As the foot inverts and the subtalar joint oversupinates, a predictable pattern of ligamentous loading occurs that can lead to failure of one or more of the ligaments. The anterior talofibular ligament (ATFL) fails initially, followed by the calcaneofibular ligament and then the posterior talofibular ligament. In mild (grade 1) sprains, the ATFL simply may be stretched. In more serious injuries, one or more ligaments may be partially disrupted (grade 2), whereas a grade 3 injury indicates complete tearing of one or more lateral ligaments.

The athlete who has suffered an inversion ankle injury usually recalls a definite mechanism of injury with immediate functional disability proportional to the severity of the injury. The athlete may have felt or even heard a distinct "pop." On early examination, the amount of swelling typically correlates with the severity of the injury. If the injury has resulted in a complete ligamentous tear, the anterior drawer test will be positive in the absence of significant guarding. Comparison with the contralateral side should be made in order to rule out significant inherent ligamentous laxity. A history of prior injury may suggest preexisting instability. The athlete will be tender over the ligaments involved. Palpatory examination should include the entire leg and foot to rule out associated proximal fibular (*maisonneuve*) fractures or avulsion injuries of the peroneal tendons off their

TABLE 4.2

Rehabilitation for Jumper's Knee

I. *Acute phase*

    Goals: Reduce symptoms, restore pain-free range of motion, maintain fitness

    Interventions: Passive modalities (PRICE), active range-of-motion/stretching exercises, isometric quadriceps exercises, closed kinetic chain exercises (limit closed kinetic chain knee flexion to 50 degrees), relative rest

II. *Recovery phase*

    Goals: Improve lower limb and trunk flexibility (especially hamstrings), screen for and address lower limb and core imbalances of strength and flexibility, improve proprioception at the knee

    Interventions: Active range-of-motion/stretching exercises, eccentric quariceps exercises, closed kinetic chain exercises through a functional range of motion

III. *Functional phase*

    Goals: Restore sport-specific function (countermovement and squat jumping)

    Interventions: Therapeutic/prophylactic bracing as needed, sport-specific functional progression including plyometrics, analysis of technique

insertion onto the lateral aspect of the fifth metatarsal.

Rehabilitation

Grade 1 and 2 injuries are more common than grade 3 injuries and can be treated nonoperatively with aggressive early weight bearing and range of motion, progressing to strengthening and proprioceptive retraining exercises prior to return to play. As with all ankle sprains, the most important initial treatment is PRICE protection, (rest, ice, compression, and elevation). How long an athlete should use PRICE depends on the severity of the injury. Typically, the treatment lasts only a few days until the edema subsides. Often, nonsteroidal anti-inflammatory drugs (NSAIDs) are added to the regimen for a 2- to 3-week course. The ankle should be protected from weight-bearing activity until such activity can be done without increasing pain and swelling.

Ligamentous tissue heals in accordance with Wolff's law. Basically, this states that tissue heals in response to the stresses placed on it. Therefore, it makes sense to begin range-of-motion and functional resistance activity as soon as the injured ankle can tolerate it. At every stage of rehabilitation, progress can be gauged by whether or not there is recurrence of edema and ecchymosis. If these symptoms worsen, then rehabilitation is being "pushed too quickly."

After treatment of the initial inflammation, the next step in rehabilitation is to regain range of motion. Having the player write the letters of the alphabet with his or her big toe will put the ankle through a complete range of motion. Then gentle weight-bearing exercises can be initiated. Exercises to facilitate proprioception should be employed next. The athlete may begin simply by balancing on one leg at a time. Once the ankle is stronger, difficulty is increased by crossing the arms, and eventually, the athlete may close his or her eyes while balancing on one foot. By crossing the arms in front of the chest and closing the eyes, the athlete removes other balancing strategies, thus relying more exclusively on proprioception.

Another alternative proprioception ankle program may be to have an athlete stand in a doorway balancing on the injured ankle, then abduct both arms 90 degrees, and then "push off" the doorway from the right and left. When the athlete "catches his or her balance," he or she is strengthening the muscles of inversion and eversion while challenging their proprioception. The biomechanical ankle platform system (BAPS), tilt board, and ankle discs are used frequently in training rooms and physical therapy. Table 4.3 summarizes the principles of rehabilitation for an acute lateral ankle sprain.

Additional Injuries

BACK INJURIES

Back injuries account for up to 14 percent of volleyball injuries.[4,5,9] Jumping and repetitive loading of the posterior structures from extension and rotation are the primary cause of low-back pain secondary to the force that is exerted through the spine on landing. Patients may suffer from mechanical low-back pain and serious injuries such as disk herniations. It is probably helpful for all volleyball players to include lumbar flexion, extension, and rotation exercises in their training even before injury. However, once injury occurs to the low back and abdominals, such exercises are essential to rehabilitation. Players also may consider training and/or playing on softer surfaces such as sand.

CARDIAC INJURIES

There has been one reported case of myocardial infarction while playing volleyball. A 41-year-old man was struck in the chest by a spiked volleyball. It was felt that he sustained a traumatic coronary artery thrombosis resulting in an acute apical myocardial infarction.[30] However, this patient did have known coronary artery disease, and perhaps when the ball hit against his chest, it may have dislodged a plaque, resulting in obstruction.

TABLE 4.3

Rehabilitation for an Acute Ankle Sprain

I. *Acute phase*
   Goals: Reduce symptoms, improve active range of motion
   Interventions: Passive modalities (PRICE), support (tape or orthosis), active range-of-motion/stretching exercises, isometric exercises, open kinetic chain exercises, weight bearing as tolerated
II. *Recovery phase*
   Goals: Increase strength and endurance, improve proprioception at the ankle
   Interventions: Active range-of-motion/stretching exercises, isotonic exercises, closed kinetic chain exercises, proprioceptive exercises
III. *Functional phase*
   Goals: Restore sport-specific function (explosive jumping, landing, cutting)
   Interventions: Proprioceptive exercises, sport-specific functional progression, including agility drills and plyometrics

Return to Sport

Volleyball players need to have sufficient aerobic and anaerobic endurance as well as normal range of motion, strength, balance, and proprioception prior to returning to the court. The player needs to perform both upper and lower extremity plyometric exercises, working up to maximal intensity with 200 to 300 foot contacts per session before participating fully. Lower extremity plyometrics include double and single leg hops, bounding, and box jumping. Upper extremity plyometrics include weighted ball tosses and explosive push-ups with a clap in between each repetition. Agility drills such as the shutte run, T-running, and kariocas should be performed to test the athlete's readiness for play.

Volleyball players also need to practice spiking and digging drills. Once the player is able to complete these drills with control and accuracy, he or she can be returned to the game of volleyball. Ideally, the athlete is pain-free at this time.

References

1. Bahr R, Karlsen R, Lian O, et al: Incidence and mechanisms of acute ankle inversion injuries in volleyball. *Am J Sports Med* 22(5): 595–600, 1994.
2. Bahr R, Lian O, Bahr IA: A twofold reduction in the incidence of acute ankle sprains in volleyball after the introduction of an injury prevention program: A prospective cohort study. *Scand J Med Sci Sports* 7(3):172–177, 1997.
3. Briner WW, Kacmar L: Common injuries in volleyball: Mechanisms of injury, prevention and rehabilitation. *Sports Med* 24(l):65–71, 1997.
4. Pera CE, Briner WW: Volleyball injuries during the 1995 U.S. Olympic festival. *Med Sci Sports Exerc* 28(5S):738, 1996.
5. Goodwin-Gerberich SG, Luhmann S, Finke C, et al: Analysis of severe injuries associated with volleyball activities. *Phys Sports Med* 15 (8):75–79, 1987.
6. Schafle MD: Common injuries in volleyball. *Sports Med* 16(2):126–129, 1993.
7. Schafle MD, Requa RK, Patton WL, et al: Injuries in the 1987 National Amateur Volleyball Tournament. *Am J Sports Med* 18(6): 624–631, 1992.
8. Watkins J. Injuries in volleyball, in Renstrom PAFH (ed): *Clinical Practice of Sports Injury Prevention and Care*. Oxford: Blackwell Scientific Publications, 1994, pp 360–374.
9. Watkins J, Green BN: Volleyball injuries: A survey of injuries of Scottish National League male players. *Br J Sports Med* 26(2):135–137, 1992.
10. Surve I, Schwellnus MP, Noakes T, et al: A five-fold reduction in the incidence of recurrent ankle sprains in soccer players using the sport stirrup orthosis. *Am J Sports Med* 2(5): 601–606, 1994.
11. Hughes LY, Stetts DM: A comparison of ankle taping and a semirigid support. *Phys Sports Med* 11(4):99–103, 1983.
12. Laughman RK, Carr TA, Chao EY, et al: Three-dimensional kinematics of the taped ankle before and after exercise. *Am J Sports Med* 8(6):425–431, 1980.
13. Garrick JG, Requa RK: Role of external support in the prevention of ankle sprains. *Med Sci Sports Exerc* 5(3):200–203, 1973.
14. Greene TA, Hillman SK: Comparison of support provided by a semirigid orthosis and adhesive ankle taping before, during, and after exercise. *Am J Sports Med* 18(5):498–506, 1990.
15. Tropp H, Askling C, Gillquist J: Prevention of ankle sprains. *Am J Sports Med* 13(4):259–262, 1985.
16. Ferretti A, Ippolito E, Mariani P, et al: Jumper's knee. *Am J Sports Med* 11(2):58–62, 1983.
17. Lian O, Engebresten L, Øvreb RV, et al: Characteristics of the leg extensors in male volleyball players with jumper's knee. *Am J Sports Med* 24(3):380–385, 1996.
18. Richards DP, Ajemian SV, Wiley JP, et al. Knee joint dynamics predict patellar tendini-

tis in elite volleyball players. *Am J Sports Med* 24(5):676–683, 1996.

19. Brenneke SL, Morgan CJ: Evaluation of ultrasonography as a diagnostic technique in the assessment of rotator cuff tendon tears. *Am J Sports Med* 20(3):287–289, 1992.

20. Olive RJ Jr, Marsh HO: Ultrasonography of the rotator cuff tears. *Clin Orthop* 28(2): 110–113, 1992.

21. Briner WW, Benjamin HJ: Volleyball injuries managing acute and overuse disorders. *Phys Sports Med* 27(3):48–58, 1999.

22. Ferretti A, Cerullo G, Russo G: Suprascapular neuropathy in volleyball players. *J Bone Joint Surg* 69A(2):260–263, 1987.

23. Holzgraefe M, Kukowski B, Eggert S: Prevalence of latent and manifest suprascapular neuropathy in high-performance volleyball players. *Br J Sports Med* 28(3):177–179, 1994.

24. Ferretti A, De Carli A, Fontana M: Injury of the suprascapular nerve at the spinoglenoid notch the natural history of infraspinatus atrophy in volleyball players. *Am J Sports Med* 26(6):759–763, 1998.

25. Fritz RC, Helms CA, Steinbach LS, et al: Suprascapular nerve entrapment: evaluation with MR imaging. *Radiology* 182:437–444, 1992.

26. Bhario NH, Nijsten MWN, van Dalen KC, et al: Hand injuries in volleyball. *Int J Sports Med* 13:351–354, 1992.

27. Israeli A, Engel J, Ganel A: Possible fatigue fracture of the pisiform bone in volleyball players. *Int J Sports Med* 3:56–57, 1982.

28. Kostianen S, Orava S: Blunt injury of the radial and ulnar arteries in volleyball players: A report of three cases of the antebrachial-palmar hammer syndrome. *Br J Sports Med* 17(3):172–176, 1983.

29. Ferretti A, Papapndrea P, Conteduca F, et al: Knee ligament injuries in volleyball players. *Am J Sports Med* 20(2):203–207, 1992.

30. Grossfield PD, Friedman DB, Levine BD: Traumatic myocardial infarction during competitive volleyball: A case report. *Med Sci Sports Exerc* 25(8):901–903, 1993.

31. Ferretti A, Puddu G, Mariani PP, et al: Jumper's knee: An epidemiological study of volleyball players. *Phys Sports Med* 12(10): 97–103, 1984.

32. Kibler WB, Herring SA, Press JM: *Functional Rehabilitation of Sports and Musculoskeletal Injuries*. Gaithersburg, MD: Aspen Publishers, 1998.

33. Oka H, Okamoto T, Kumamoto M: Electromyographic and cinematographic study of the volleyball spike, in Komi P (ed): *Biomechanics of Volleyball*. Baltimore: University Park Press, 1976, pp 326–331.

34. Kluka D, Dunn P: *Volleyball, Winning Edge Series*, 4th ed. New York: McGraw-Hill, 2000.

35. Baechle TR, Earle R: Essentials of strength training and conditioning. Champaign, IL: *Hum Kinet* 2nd edition, 2000.

Selected References

Cian O, Holen KJ, Engebresten L, et al: Relationship between symptoms of jumper's knee and the ultrasound characteristics of the patellar tendon among high level volleyball players. *Scand J Med Sci Sports* 6(5): 291–296, 1996.

Ferretti A: *Volleyball Injuries*, 1st ed. Lausanne, Switzerland: International Volleyball Federation, 1994.

Ferretti A, Papandrea P, Conteduca F, et al: Knee ligament injuries in volleyball players. *Am J Sports Med* 20(2):203–207, 1992.

Kugler A, Krüger-Franke M, Reininger S, et al: Muscular imbalance and shoulder pain in volleyball attackers. *Br J Sports Med* 30:256–259, 1996.

Lucs J: *Pass, Set, Crush: Volleyball Illustrated*. Wenatchee, WA: Euclid Northwest Publications, 1993.

Richards DP, Ajemian SV, Wiley JP, et al: Knee joint dynamics predict patellar tendinitis in elite volleyball players. *Am J Sports Med* 24(5):676–683, 1996.

Thacker SB, Stroup, DF, Branchem CM, et al: The prevention of ankle sprains in sports. *Am J Sports Med* 27(6):753–760, 1999.

Whiting WC, Zernicke RF: *Biomechanics of Musculoskeletal Injury*. Champaign, IL: Human Kinetics, 1998.

CHAPTER 5

Swimming

Charles Shapiro

Swimming has become one of the most popular sports in the world. The level of swimming competition ranges from friendly races at the "old swimming hole" all the way up to world competition, including the Olympics. Swimming frequently begins at a very early age, with swimmers as young as 7 years old competing through local park and recreation programs and at YMCAs, Jewish Community Centers, and swim clubs throughout the United States. These swimming programs form the foundation of competitive swimming in the United States and produce many of the athletes who end up swimming for American colleges or the U.S. Olympic teams.[1] Most beginning athletes in the sport of swimming excel due to natural talents and inherent athletic ability. Athletes who advance through the ranks of competitive team swimming to become elite high school and college swimmers will find that natural talents alone are not enough to keep them competitive, and soon training and coaching become significant factors of success. Injuries are common in competitive swimming and can limit the degree of success achieved or the length of a swimmer's career.

Since the 1990s, swimming has increased in popularity among recreational athletes, as well as in high school and college sports. The number of athletes competing in recreational in multievent sports such as triathlons also has increased significantly since 1990, with competitors ranging in age from preteens to master-level athletes. Competitive swimming is well known for early morning and late afternoon practices in chilly water, with the highest level of competitive swimmers often participating in up to 10 to 12 two-hour training sessions per week. In addition, most of these athletes also participate in a weight training, running, or cycling program, which may involve 30-minute to 1-hour training sessions an additional three times per week.[2–4] This combination of intense dry-land and swimming training ultimately will have a cumulative effect on both the physical conditioning of the athlete and the propensity to injury due to the physical stresses on the body.

The majority of the injuries seen among swimmers are minor injuries such as bumps, bruises, and lacerations from slips and falls around the pool.[1] Swimmers are also subject to injuries to the face and head and fractures of the heels associated with accidental contact with the walls of the pool, especially when attempting flip turns.[2] These injuries are treated most frequently with common first aid and normally will not interfere with the swimmer's training or competition.

The most frequently seen problems that interfere with an athlete's ability to compete would be those musculoskeletal problems which stem from overuse or repetitive trauma.[5] Areas of the body most commonly affected are the shoulder, elbow, knee, ankle, neck, and back. This chapter will look at common injuries and illnesses seen in competitive swimmers. Through a review of biomechanics of the swim strokes, the chapter will associate common musculoskeletal injuries with the particular event or swimming stroke in which they occur most commonly. The various factors that influence swim training and injuries will be discussed.

Biomechanics of Swimming

HYDRODYNAMICS

Hydrodynamics is the science that deals with the motion of fluids, the forces acting on solid bodies immersed in fluids, and the motion relative to them. The science of human movement during exercise is *biomechanics*. In order to discuss injuries caused by swimming, we must consider both the hydrodynamic and biomechanical aspects of forces on the swimmer. The mechanical factors unique to the water environment include form drag, wave drag, and frictional drag.[4] These drag forces, when combined with the forceful movement of the swimmer in the water, play a dramatic role on performance during swimming. Streamlining and sculling are techniques used by swimmers to influence the mechanics of swimming.

FORM DRAG

Form drag is the resistance exerted on the body dependent on the position of the body as it moves in the water. The more horizontal the body is positioned in the water, the less the form drag will be. Any position in the water angled from horizontal will increase the surface area of the swimmer and will increase the form drag. Any lateral deviation of body position also increases form drag. It does this by increasing the frontal surface area of the swimmer and slowing the forward progression of the swimmer through the water. This, in turn, increases the demand on the muscles of propulsion. A streamlined horizontal position is most desirable for attaining speed through the water.

Swimming underwater meets less resistance than swimming at the surface, since form drag is greatest at the water's surface. This is why competitive swimmers stay underwater for extended distances on starts and turns. Rules have been established to limit the amount of time swum under water on starts and turns in the breaststroke, backstroke, and butterfly. The increased energy expenditure caused by holding the breath while underwater may offset any reduction of overall race times gained from underwater swimming, especially in the lower ranks of competitive swimming.

WAVE DRAG

Wave drag is the increased resistance of water caused by the wavelike movement of the water due to wind or turbulence created by the swimmers in the pool. In lake or ocean swimming, wave drag may result from wind, boats, and water currents. In pool swimming, wave drag is the result of the rebound of the water off the sides and bottom of the pool created by the movement of the swimmers through the water.

Wave drag can be decreased in pools by using wave-dispersing lane lines. The lane lines are devised not only to divide the lanes but also to control the movement of the water between lanes. The design and application of lane lines vary from pool to pool and can play an important role in the "speed" of the pool.

Wave drag is also decreased in deeper pools, where the water has less opportunity to rebound off the bottom and back to the surface. An official racing course must be at least 4 ft deep and is frequently deeper. Competition pools are built with these features in order to increase times in competition, with the top pools in the United States being 6 to 9 ft deep.

FRICTIONAL DRAG

The friction created between body hair and the water is referred to as *frictional drag*. Materials used in swimming suits are chosen because of their properties that decrease frictional drag of the body in the water. Swimming caps and shaving the body are also strategies used to decrease frictional drag.

STREAMLINING AND SCULLING

Two additional hydrodynamic principles that come into play in swimming are streamlining and sculling. *Streamlining* is the athlete's ability to stay horizontal in the water. Streamlining is important for efficient forward propulsion of the body through the water. This horizontal streamlined position is most pronounced during starts and turns. The movement of the extremities and trunk during the swim strokes causes deviation from this streamlined position.

Sculling is the term used to describe the movement of the hand in the water at an oblique angle to the direction of travel. This creates forward propulsion of the body in the water. The force produced by the hand during the pulling phase depends on the angle of the hand in the water and its speed or velocity. The surface area of the hand is also a factor in producing force, and webbed gloves are sometimes used in training to increase the surface area of the hand.

APPLIED HYDRODYNAMICS

Speed in swimming is achieved through the ability of the swimmer to produce power. Not all the power produced by the swimmer is directed toward forward propulsion of the body through the water. Due to the inherent properties of water, much of the power produced by the swimmer is dissipated in the moving water. This is similar to achieving a more powerful start in a running race when running on a solid surface such as turf than in sand. In swimming, pushing against still water allows a swimmer to generate more forward propulsive forces than pushing against moving water.

Biomechanics of Specific Strokes

It would not be possible to discuss swimming injuries without first looking at the different competitive swimming strokes and to describe the biomechanics unique to each. The biomechanics of swimming will be reviewed to the extent necessary to relate to the primary focus of this chapter—a discussion of the common injuries found in competitive swimming and their prevention and rehabilitation.

It is beneficial to first look at a general description of mechanics of the swim strokes by presenting the similarities between the different strokes before discussing the specific biomechanics of each stroke.

PHASES OF THE SWIM STROKE

A comparison of the four competitive swimming strokes reveals more similarities than differences with regard to the motion of the upper extremity. When observing the freestyle and backstroke events, one would see that the arms are used in an asymmetrical reciprocal pattern with an alternating pattern of water entry. In the butterfly and breaststroke, the arms are used in a bilateral symmetrical motion, entering and exiting the water simultaneously.[2,4] The pull-through phase is the underwater portion of the arm stroke that creates the forward propulsion of the swimmer through the water. The recovery phase of the swimming stroke is the out-of-water portion of the stroke.

The use of the lower extremities in swimming varies significantly between the different strokes. In both freestyle and backstroke, the swimmer uses an alternating *beat kick*, also called a *flutter kick*, to propel himself or herself through the water. A bilateral symmetrical undulating motion, referred to as the *dolphin kick*, is used in the butterfly stroke. The *breaststroke kick*, or *whip kick*, is performed by a bilateral symmetrical use of the lower extremities in which the legs are flexed toward the trunk and then forcefully thrust out, extended and adducted.

In the freestyle and backstroke, both the neck and trunk go through significant rotation in providing the mechanics necessary for breathing while swimming, as well as repositioning the body in the water to accommodate the asymmetrical motions of the upper extremities. In the butterfly stroke and breaststroke, no rotation of the torso about the longitudinal axis of the body occurs as the swimmer progresses through the water with a bilateral symmetrical use of the extremities. Consequently, breathing is accomplished as the head comes vertically above the water.

The phases of the swim strokes generally are divided into pull-through and recovery. The pull-through phase can be further divided into hand entry, catch, power phase/insweep, and finish (outsweep). The inclusion of hand entry in both the pull-through and recovery phases is due to the instantaneous transition where pull-through begins just as recovery is completed.

Pull-Through

Hand Entry   Hand entry is the beginning of the stroke where the hand enters the water prior to the catch. In the breaststroke, the hand remains in the water during recovery.

Catch   The catch phase follows hand entry. This generally consists of a hand sculling motion. This is the beginning of the propulsive phase of the stroke.

Power Phase   The power phase begins at the end of the catch phase and is the major propulsive force of the stroke. This may include the insweep and outsweep.

Finish   The finish is at the end of the pull-through phase and is the final emphasis and usually consists of a propulsive skull of the hand.

Recovery

The recovery phase is the period of time when the reposition occurs. This is not a propulsive phase of the stroke.

BUTTERFLY

The butterfly stroke can be described as a bilateral symmetrical simultaneous overhead motion of the arms combined with a simultaneous bilateral symmetrical undulating motion of the legs commonly known as a *dolphin kick*. Flutter kicking is not allowed in the butterfly stroke. As in the breaststroke, swimmers must touch the wall with both hands before turning (Figs. 5.1 through 5.4).

The butterfly stroke has significant biomechanical similarities to the freestyle stroke

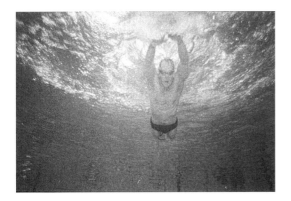

FIGURE 5.1

Butterfly stroke entry. (*Used with permission from Jager.*[20])

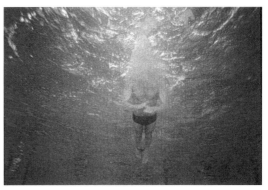

FIGURE 5.3

Butterfly stroke power phase. (*Used with permission from Jager.*[20])

in swimming with regard to the motion at the shoulders.[4] Butterfly is performed as a bilateral symmetrical motion, with the hips acting as a short axis for undulation. Body roll across the long axis does not occur as in freestyle and backstroke, making body roll unnecessary. The lack of rotation of the torso increases the need for scapular protraction and abduction in order for the arms to achieve the depth in the water necessary to create a powerful stroke. Other than the increased position of scapular abduction and

increased demand on the medial scapular stabilizing muscles, the muscles involved in pull-through and recovery are virtually the same as in freestyle.[4]

After the hands enter the water, the catch phase occurs as the forearms pronate, shoulders abduct, scapulae protract and abduct, and elbows flex slightly as the hands lead the pull phase of the stroke.

As in freestyle, the latissimus dorsi, subscapularis, teres major, and pectoralis major muscles forcefully adduct and internally rotate the glenohumeral joint during the pull-through phase to make the top of the "keyhole." The power phase and finish of the

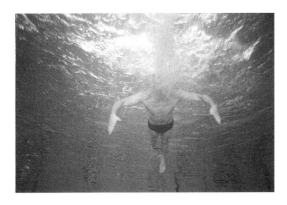

FIGURE 5.2

Butterfly stroke catch phase. (*Used with permission from Jager.*[20])

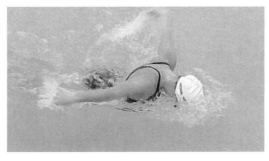

FIGURE 5.4

Butterfly recovery.

stroke consist of forceful shoulder and elbow extension creating the bottom of the keyhole. The anterior and medial deltoid, supraspinatus, infraspinatus, and teres minor bring the shoulder overhead into an internally rotated position during the recovery phase. The elbow flexes and extends during each cycle of the stroke, using the coracobrachialis and biceps brachii muscles for flexion and the triceps for extension. The wrist flexors, wrist extensors, and intrinsic muscles of the hand are also used in a sculling action in the butterfly.

The bilateral symmetrical use of the upper extremities requires a relatively stable trunk. An experienced butterflier will stay right along the water surface. The swimmer should stay in the same plane as the top of the water. The hips and shoulders rock up and down, but the shoulders should stay in relatively the same plane throughout the stroke. The mistaken emphasis on lifting the body out of the water causes swimmers to decreases efficiency and waste energy. The arms may clear the water on recovery, and then the shoulders drop back into the water immediately following the hand-entry phase. The trunk muscles are crucial for stabilization during propulsion of the trunk through the water.

As the hands enter the water, the swimmer presses the sternum (chest) toward the bottom of the pool. This causes the hips to rise. During the pull-through phase, the hips begin to drop, the feet will rise toward the surface, and the sternum rises up. As the arms reach the power phase of the stroke, the swimmer kicks the hands out of the water and then presses the sternum to the bottom of the pool. Staying lower in the water adds to the efficiency of pull-through in the butterfly, as well as decreasing form drag. In order to stay low in the water, vertical lift should be minimized. Driving the head forward will keep undulation to a minimum and convert upward lift to forward lift. The emphasis of the stroke should be for the head, shoulders, and arms to drive forward and not upward.

Positioning of the lower extremity is instrumental in creating an efficient kick in the butterfly stroke. The dolphin kick is performed as a bilateral symmetrical movement consisting of a downbeat and an upbeat motion. The legs kick in unison to a rhythm of two beats for every single arm stroke.

The downbeat motion begins with forceful trunk and hip flexion. The abdominals are the main driving force during this phase. The core muscles are developing the force, with the extremities following along. This is accompanied by knee flexion, followed by forceful knee extension until the knee reaches full extension at completion of the downbeat motion. The swimmer should imagine a whipping motion. During the upbeat motion, both knees stay extended, with the ankles held in plantarflexion to provide maximum surface area of the foot for propulsion. The muscles contributing to trunk and hip extension are the gluteus maximus, gluteus medius, gluteus minimus, erector spinae, and hamstrings. The ankles are held in plantarflexion by the gastrocnemius and soleus muscles, with the assistance of the tibialis posterior, peroneus longus, and peroneus brevis muscles. Resistance from the water during the downbeat also helps to plantarflex the ankle. The upbeat of the kick is created primarily by forceful contraction of the hip extensors and accessory muscles. Active contraction of the hamstrings during hip extension on the upbeat motion not only assists in the force of the hip extension but also acts to stabilize the knee toward flexion in order to avoid hyperextension stress to the anterior aspect of the knee.

A ratio of one arm stroke to two down beats of the dolphin kick is most efficient in the butterfly stroke. The first downbeat of the dolphin kick occurs during the entry and catch phases of the pulling pattern. The second downbeat (major power force) occurs during the finish phase of the pulling pattern. The timing of this is essential to efficiency in butterfly swimming. In addition, the relationship between vertical angle of the trunk will affect the ability to achieve the fully extended arm position.

BACKSTROKE

The backstroke is performed by an alternating overhead motion of the arms and a flutter kick of the legs while lying on the back in the water. The rules of the backstroke event dictate that the swimmer must swim in a supine position except during turns. There is no resting in a supine position, the backstroker mainly swims on his or her sides, rolling from side to side in a supine position (Figs. 5.5 and 5.6).

The motions and muscle recruitment patterns of the upper extremity for the backstroke show significant similarity to both the freestyle and butterfly strokes.[4] The stroke can be broken down into hand-entry, catch, pull-through, hand-finish, and recovery phases. The pull-though (underwater) phase of the backstroke can be divided into catch, pull-through, and hand finish. The recovery phase (above water) also can be divided into arm lift, midrecovery and hand entry.

The motion at the shoulder consists of flexion and internal rotation of the arm during the recovery phase of the backstroke

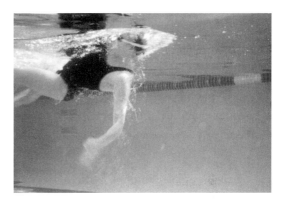

FIGURE 5.6

Backstroke power phase. (*Used with permission from Jager.[20]*)

along with elbow extension and forearm pronation. During the catch phase of the stroke, the glenohumeral joint abducts and externally rotates, and the elbow flexes. During the pull-through (power) phase of the stroke, the glenohumeral joint is adducted and internally rotated, leading with the hand, not the elbow. Also, during the end phase of pull-through, the elbow is forcefully extending. The hand finish demonstrates a sculling motion.

Body roll is most important in the backstroke in order to place the muscles of propulsion in a mechanically advantageous position without placing undue passive stresses on the glenohumeral joint and surrounding musculature. Body roll also reduces drag and resistance while decreasing the strain on the propulsive muscles. Swimmers are instructed to lead the stroke with the shoulder, trunk, and hips, which facilitates body roll for an adequate recovery phase and encourages the pull-through arm to reach deep into the water. The body roll of the shoulder, trunk, and hips needs to stay inline, with the head always looking up. If roll only occurs at the shoulders, frictional drag will increase along the torso and hips. Hip rota-

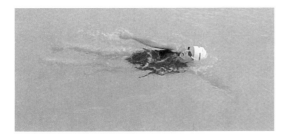

FIGURE 5.5

Backstroke recovery.

tion occurs to the opposite side with the pull-through (power) phase.

Backstroke incorporates a flutter kick using either a four- or six-beat kick. The kick is performed with mainly forceful hip flexion and extension combined with flexion and extension of the knee and plantarflexion of the ankle. The muscles primarily involved are the gluteals, quadriceps, hamstrings, tibialis posterior, peroneus longus, peroneus brevis, gastrocnemius, and soleus. The configuration of the talocrural joint lends itself to instability during plantarflexion and therefore requires cocontraction of the ankle dorsiflexors and plantarflexors to provide dynamic stabilization of the ankle so as to avoid overstretch of the ligamentous support of the joint during kicking.

BREASTSTROKE

The breaststroke is considered by many to be one of the most difficult strokes to master. The sequence of the breaststroke is a pull, breathe, kick, and glide. The breaststroke is performed with a bilateral symmetrical pattern of arm movement requiring simultaneous movements of the arms in the same horizontal plane. The hands, palms together, simultaneously reach forward through the water from the breast near the surface of the water and are then forcefully pulled back through the water, propelling the swimmer forward. The bilateral arm motion is alternated with a bilateral motion of the legs in performing a whip or breaststroke kick. Breaststrokers must touch the wall with both hands at the same time before executing their turn (Figs. 5.7 through 5.9).

The breaststroke pull-through phase can be divided further into the catch (upsweep and outsweep) and insweep. The catch begins with the arms fully extended and the hands outstretched forward in front of the body. The palms of the hands turn outward via pronation of the forearm and internal rota-

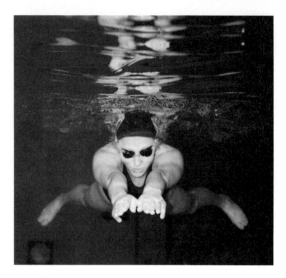

FIGURE 5.7

Breast stroke recovery. (*Used with permission from Jager.*[20])

tion of the shoulder. The hands are pitched approximately 40 degrees with respect to their line of motion.[4] The wrist flexes slightly through contraction of the flexor carpi ulnaris, flexor carpi radialis, and flexor digitorum profundus muscles. The arms begin to

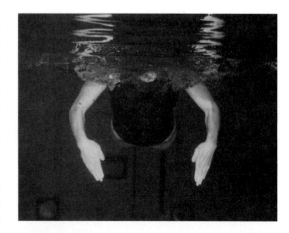

FIGURE 5.8

Breast stroke arm pull-through. (*Used with permission from Jager.*[20])

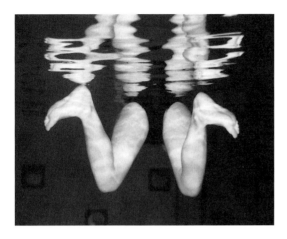

FIGURE 5.9

Breast stroke kick. (*Used with permission from Jager.*[20])

sweep outward and slightly upward as a result of the action of the posterior deltoid, infraspinatus, and teres minor muscles. This outsweep continues until the hands are 12 to 15 in wider than the shoulders. The triceps brachii are active to keep the elbow relatively extended.[4]

The insweep phase begins as the palms rotate downward and inward. The insweep motion is a lateral inward scull toward the shoulders with the hands pitched at approximately 40 to 50 degrees relative to the hand's line of motion. Supination of the forearm is performed by the biceps brachii and supinator muscles and assisted by the outward (external) rotation of the shoulder by the infraspinatus and teres minor muscles. The squeeze component of the pull-through phase, which begins with adduction of the shoulders (arms), is performed by motion at the shoulder and contraction of the pectoralis major, teres major, latissimus dorsi, and anterior deltoid muscles while the elbow is flexed by the biceps brachii and coracobrachialis. Adduction of the arms continues until completion of this phase, when the hands and elbows come together underneath the chest and abdomen.

The recovery phase consists of a forward reach of both arms, which is performed underwater and accounts for the difference in terminology as compared with the other strokes. Streamlining of the hands is critical during the recovery phase of the pulling pattern. As the hands meet at the end of the insweep phase, they begin to move forward together with the fingertips leading. This phase continues until the arms are fully extended out in front of the swimmer and are ready to begin the next outsweep.

Supination of the forearm continues from the end of adduction of the insweep into the beginning of the recovery phase to turn the hands toward each other. The forward recovery of the arms is accomplished partially by the anterior deltoid and the long head of biceps brachii for flexion at the shoulder, while the elbows are extended throughout recovery by the triceps brachii.

The breaststroke kick can be divided into the recovery and power phases (outsweep and insweep). In general, the swimmer is instructed to bend the knees, bring the feet apart, and then allow the knees to come apart. Then the swimmer kicks out and around and finally squeezes the legs together with the legs straight.

The outsweep (setup) phase of the kick begins with the knees flexed 90 degrees and the feet drawn up toward the buttocks. The feet turn outward (evert) so that the inside of the foot is facing away from the swimmer. This is accomplished through action of the peroneus longus and brevis muscles. Hip inward (internal) rotation occurs with eversion of the foot and is performed by the iliopsoas, tensor fasciae latae, and anterior fibers of gluteus medius and minimus. The outward rotation of the feet is critical at this point to maximize the propulsion from the kick by maximizing the surface area of the feet as they pass through the water. The feet push out, down, and back. The knees during the outsweep should be spread slightly wider than the hips. The key part of the outsweep is to spread the feet wider than the knees. In the frog kick, the knees are spread wider than the feet, which places less stress on the medial collateral ligament but produces a less powerful kick. The frog kick is not used in competitive swimming.

The insweep (propulsion) of the kick begins at the widest point in the kicking pattern. At the widest point of the outsweep of the kick, the knee undergoes a significant valgus stress as the lower leg begins the insweep phase. This is a common mechanism of injury for spraining the medial collateral ligaments of the knee. The path of the feet continues back, down, and now inward. This phase ends with powerful propulsion when the feet come together and the knees are straight. Hip extension by the hamstrings and knee extension by the quadriceps continue throughout the insweep. The legs are adducted from the hip through contractions of the adductor magnus, adductor longus, adductor brevis, pectineus, and gracilis muscles. This phase also includes slight hip outward rotation by the gluteus maximus, sartorius, and posterior fibers of gluteus medius and minimus muscles as the feet come together. To finish the kick in a streamlined position, the ankles are plantarflexed by the gastrocnemius, soleus, tibialis posterior, peroneus longus, and peroneus brevis muscles. The hamstrings also serve to lift the legs slightly to align them with the forward progression of the body.[4]

After the power phase of the kick, the swimmer will glide until his or her motion begins to slow. The swimmer then begins the recovery phase by flexing the knees to 90 degrees as the feet are drawn toward the buttocks (slight hip flexion occurs). This is accomplished by a combination of contraction of knee flexors, including hamstrings, gastrocnemius, sartorius, and gracilis muscles.

The tibialis anterior and extensor digitorum longus dorsiflex the ankle in preparation for the outward sweep, which is a combination of hip and knee extension accomplished by the hamstrings and quadriceps muscle groups, respectively.

Technique in the breaststroke has developed over the years to emphasize the importance of undulation of the body to improve efficiency of the stroke. Since the body is kept at the surface of the water during the breaststroke, form drag plays a significant role in speed. Surface resistance is greater at the water line than above or below the surface. A technique used by elite breaststrokers is to lift the upper body above the water's surface during each stroke cycle for breathing, followed by plunging the shoulders beneath the surface during the kicking phase. This motion is created as in the butterfly by the swimmer pressing the sternum toward the bottom of the pool at the end of the kicking phase and into the glide phase of the stroke. This is followed by a dropping of the hips as the legs prepare to kick and the swimmer takes a breath. This is thought to decrease the actual time of maximal surface form drag. In addition, this also simulates the undulations of the butterfly stroke, improving forward propulsion.

FREESTYLE

The freestyle event is named as such because the swimmer may choose to use any swim stroke desired. The most common stroke used is the *Australian crawl*, also referred to as simply the *front crawl stroke*. This stroke produces the fastest times and is performed by an alternating overhead motion of the arms accompanied by a bilateral alternating kicking motion of the legs (flutter kick). The flutter kick can range from a six-beat-per-stroke to a two-beat-per-stroke cycle rhythm. The two-beat kick typically is used in distance races because this technique conserves the energy necessary to complete the longer-distance races. The six-beat kick typically is used during sprinting in the shorter-distance events and during the finish of the distance events. See Figs. 5.10 through 5.12 for freestyle biomechanics.

Hand entry begins when the upper extremity makes its initial entry into the water with the fingertips and hand. The arm is outstretched in front of the head, midway between the head and the shoulder. The fingertips enter the water first, immediately followed by the hand with the thumb positioned slightly downward. This is accomplished by pronation of the forearm and internal rotation of the shoulder. Pull-through actually does not begin until the hand has entered the water. Having the fingertips enter the water first minimizes the water drag and creates a cavity in the water through which the hand, wrist, and elbow follow. As the wrist and elbow enter the water, the extremity continues to reach forward until the arm is extended fully in front of the swimmer.

The catch phase follows hand entry. The wrist flexes, and the palm rotates outward. The hand then pushes downward and outward, toward the outside of the shoulder, until reaching the lowest and widest part of this downward motion. The lowest point in the pulling pattern may be as much as 18 to 24 in below the surface of the water depending on the length of the arm and creates sig-

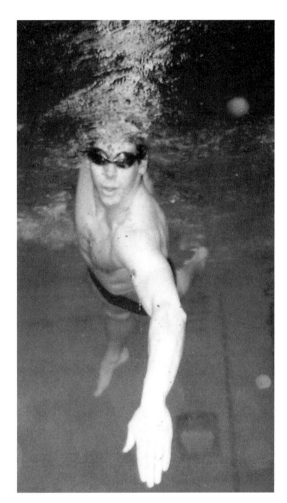

FIGURE 5.11

Freestyle pull phase. (*Used with permission from Jager.*[20])

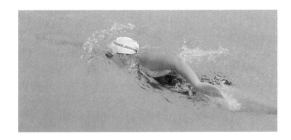

FIGURE 5.10

Freestyle recovery.

nificant leverage against which the shoulder extensors, internal rotators, and adductors must work.

Now the motion of the glenohumeral joint during the crawl stroke will be discussed. The motion at the shoulder during the stroke cycle can be broken down into components of abduction/adduction and internal/external rotation that produce functional flexion and extension through these motions. During the

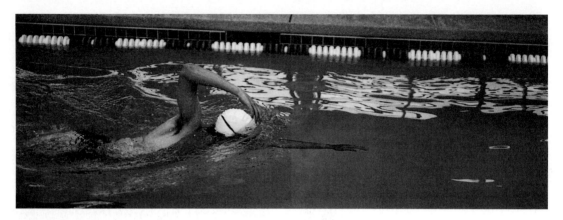

FIGURE 5.12

Freestyle high elbow position. (*Used with permission from Jager.*[20])

recovery phase of the stroke, the gleno-humeral joint is abducted and externally rotated. During the catch and pull-through phases, the glenohumeral joint is adducted and internally rotated.[6] The latissimus dorsi, teres major, subscapularis, and pectoralis major muscles forcefully adduct and internally rotate the glenohumeral joint during the pull-through phase. The deltoid, supraspinatus, infraspinatus, and teres minor bring the shoulder overhead into an externally rotated position during the recovery phase. Elite swimmers are taught to lengthen their body by leaving their extended arm in front of them until the recovering arm enters the water. This allows for a more streamlined approach.

This shoulder motion places a significant demand on the glenohumeral joint.[6,7] Efficiency of the stroke depends on greater than normal flexibility. This poses a significant challenge because this extreme degree of mobility comes at the expense of stability. Stability in most joints normally is achieved through the shape of the articular surfaces, normal length of the ligaments, and dynamic stabilization by active contraction of the surrounding musculature. Dynamic stabilization

of the glenohumeral joint is achieved in part by the rotator cuff muscles that centralize the humeral head in the glenoid fossa. The rotator cuff and deltoid muscles work together as a force couple. The rotator cuff muscles provide glenohumeral compression and a downward force to balance the upward sheer force generated by the deltoid muscles.[8] If the ligaments of the shoulder complex become lax via overuse, then the joint becomes increasingly dependent on the surrounding musculature for dynamic stabilization. Muscle reeducation will be necessary so that the muscles fire in a pattern adequate to stabilize the joint throughout the functional movement. In addition, stabilization of the scapulae on the thorax is necessary to achieve a normal scapulothoracic rhythm. Dynamic stabilization of the scapulae on the thorax is achieved by the levator scapulae, rhomboids, and trapezius muscles.[9,10]

At the elbow, flexion and extension occur in coordination with the motion of the shoulder during each phase of the stroke cycle. Elbow flexion during the catch phase is achieved by contraction of the coracobrachialis and biceps brachii muscles.[9] This motion accompanies the powerful outward motion of the hand and arm, creating the initial part of the pull-through. The triceps then forcefully extends the elbow, creating the outsweep part of the pull-through. The rotation of the torso through the stroke cycle creates what appears to be a S-shaped pattern as the hand pulls through the water. The S-shaped pattern of the pull-through promotes efficiency because the hand will constantly meet still water. The hand moves in a S-shaped pattern relative to the bottom of the pool, but the swimmers should feel like they are pushing the arm straight back. It is the body's rotation and not the swimmer's intent that creates this pattern. The elbow flexors and extensors are also active during the recovery phase as the elbow first flexes and then extends in reaching forward to begin the next stroke.

The wrist flexors, wrist extensors, and intrinsic muscles of the hand determine the position of the wrist and hand during entry and pull-through. Maintaining an appropriate pitch of the hand is crucial to creating the forward propulsive forces of the swimmer.

The finish phase starts with the hand being pulled out from underneath the swimmer's body in an outward and backward pulling motion, continuing upward and backward toward the surface of the water. The finish phase ends as the hand emerges from the water, where the recovery phase begins.

The recovery phase is that period of time the hand spends out of the water reaching forward to begin the next stroke. The elbow is kept high and flexed during the recovery phase, keeping the arm as relaxed as possible to provide a rest during the stroke cycle. Recovery may be further broken down into the components of elbow lift, midrecovery, and hand entry.

Trunk rotation is very important during the freestyle (crawl) stroke.[11] During each stroke cycle, the upper body will rotate between 60 and 80 degrees in each direction.[4,6] Adequate body roll provides for the shoulder

and arm of the pull-through side to drive deeper into the water, creating greater pulling power while simultaneously allowing the shoulder and arm of the recovery side to come further out of the water, decreasing resistance during the recovery phase. Body roll not only facilitates driving the arm down into the water but also is the movement that extends the arm forward before the catch and provides the impetus for finishing the stroke. Coaches usually emphasize finishing with triceps extension, but the triceps will fatigue if used this way. If the triceps are used as a stabilizer while power is provided by body roll, localized muscle fatigue is less likely to happen. Body roll also allows the head of the humerus to stay in a more neutral position relative to the scapula, providing a greater balance between the pectoral muscles and latissimus dorsi, thereby giving the swimmer the ability to create more power. Rotation of the torso depends on coordinated contractions of the trunk flexors, extensors, and rotators[10] (Fig. 5.13). The paraspinal muscles of the back, transversalis muscles of the trunk, and anterior abdominal muscles, including the internal and external obliques, all contribute to efficient freestyle swimming.[12]

The amount of cervical rotation needed to breathe is directly related to the degree of rotation of the trunk achieved during each stroke cycle. Decreased trunk rotation requires increased cervical rotation. Breathing to the right and left sides promotes balance of range of motion and strength of the cervical spine and the supporting musculature. Breaths can be taken every stroke cycle, or cycles can be skipped. Depending on the aerobic capacity of the swimmer, it is important to ensure an adequate intake of air during swimming to reduce the risk of fatigue due to dysfunctional sequencing of breathing. In considering head position, the swimmer should keep focus toward the bottom of the pool with the water hitting the top of the head. The head will roll with the body.

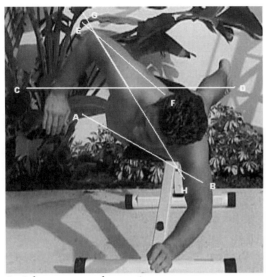

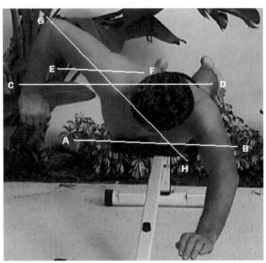

A: Adequate trunk rotation   B: Lack of adequate trunk rotation

FIGURE 5.13

Effect of trunk rotation on glenohumeral horizontal abduction and cervical rotation. With adequate trunk rotation (A) there is decreased horizontal abduction of the humerus against the posterior aspect of the glenoid fossa of the scapula while achieving the same amount of elbow lift out of the water. Also note the decrease in cervical rotation relative to the line of trunk rotation. AB represents the line of trunk rotation. CD represents the water line. EF represents the line of the scapula. GH represents the line of the humerus.

The leg kick is performed by the dynamic body roll, with the lower extremities stabilizing the force. The core muscles create the power in the two-beat kick. In the six-beat kick, there is a powerful contraction of the muscles of the hips, knees, and ankles. The sequencing of kicking is important to the efficiency of the arm stroke because it is what provides stability of the trunk in the water. If the trunk is not stabilized by a coordinated kick of the legs during any stroke, the trunk would tend to rise or sink in the water with each arm stroke. This would decrease streamlining and the efficiency of each stroke. Since the flutter kick is performed in an alternating pattern, the stabilization actually occurs in an alternating pattern. A well-executed flutter kick provides a stable base of support to allow the body to roll about the longitudinal axis in both the freestyle and backstroke.

Two common kicking patterns are used during the freestyle: the six-beat and two-beat flutter kicks. The six-beat kick pattern is performed with each leg performing three down-beats and three upbeats per stroke cycle. The two-beat kick pattern is performed with each leg performing one downbeat and one upbeat per stroke cycle.[13] The upbeat phase of the kick is considered the recovery phase for the legs. It is accomplished through active hip extension performed by the gluteals, biceps femoris, semitendinosus, semimembranosus, and gracilis muscles. The knee is in full extension, which is maintained by the resistance of the water on the upbeat. The ankle is kept slightly plantarflexed by the soleus, gastrocnemius, tibialis posterior, peroneus longus, and peroneus brevis muscles. Maintaining the ankle in plantarflexion creates continued forward propulsion during the recovery phase of the legs.

The downbeat of the kick is the most powerful phase of the kick and is responsible for propulsion. Powerful hip flexion initiates the downbeat, which is sequentially accompanied by forceful knee extension with the ankle maintaining a position of plantarflexion. This downbeat motion is produced by the iliopsoas and rectus femoris at the hip, the quadriceps at the knee, and the gastrocnemius, soleus, tibialis posterior, peroneus longus, and peroneus brevis muscles produce plantarflexion at the ankle. It is important for the swimmer to maintain ankle plantarflexion on both the upbeat and downbeat of the kick because this will provide forward propulsion forces in both directions. The resistance of the water assists plantarflexion on the downbeat but resists plantarflexion on the upbeat. An appropriate position of plantarflexion is necessary to maximize surface area of the foot during the kick.

Injury Prevention and Treatment

Swimming creates repetitive demands at the extremes of range of motion of the joints of the extremities and spine.[3,14,15] This stress at the end of the range of motion places an extremely high physical demand on the soft tissue structures of the musculoskeletal system, especially the ligaments and joint capsules. Each tissue will be required to function at its highest physiologic level to provide the coordination of joint mobility, dynamic stability, and execution of skill necessary to create a high level of performance while at the same time avoiding injury. This can only be achieved efficiently and effectively if there is a functional balance of the muscles, ligaments, and soft tissue that support and move the extremities and spine. The acceleration of the arm in one direction causes forces that must be controlled by muscles and ligaments on the opposite side of the joint in order to avoid injury.[9] The biomechanics of movement of the extremity in swimming is more complex than on dry land because of the resistance applied to the surface area of the extremities due to the hydrodynamics of the water, which actually changes the lever system of the joint. Most injuries in swimming are caused by an imbalance or failure of one or more of the anatomic soft tissue structures to perform their intended function, resulting in abnormal stresses on the synergistic structures.[3,5,14]

An injury prevention program proactively includes all the same elements of a thorough rehabilitation program. Prevention should be targeted at the anatomic, biomechanical, and physiologic properties of the body structures and systems as they specifically apply to swimming. This will include a specific program of stretching, strengthening, cardiovascular conditioning, technique development, and injury prevention education.[16-19] In order to meet the physical demands of swim training, these exercises need to be incorporated into a preseason and off-season conditioning program. All phases of conditioning need to be performed at least three times per week for 6 to 8 weeks prior to the start of swim training. Many athletes like to break their conditioning program down into a 6-day-per-week program, with each day being of shorter duration. This can be achieved easily by working different muscle groups on alternating 3-day cycles. If a 6-day a week program is chosen, the athlete should make sure that each major muscle group is addressed three times per week with 24 hours rest between workouts. Warm-up, stretching, and cool-down periods must be performed every day.[19] Routine icing after strenuous training can also be beneficial.

WARM-UP

A general warm-up is a good idea prior to any exercise. Getting the heart pumping and blood flowing prepares the muscles and joints for the stresses of swimming. In addition, the warm-up period gives the swimmer a chance to become mentally prepared for the upcoming workout. In some cases, land-based equipment may be available to use for a general warm-up but cannot replace the effectiveness of warming up via light swimming. Warming up by swimming at slow speeds with perfect stroke mechanics will prepare all the muscles to be used later when swimming for speed and conditioning. Incorporating the front crawl, backstroke, and breaststroke into the warm-up will provide a good, well-rounded warm-up. The arm strokes and leg kicks involved in these strokes will take the spine and extremities through a significant range of motion and muscle contraction to adequately prepare the swimmer for intense training. The butterfly stroke should be avoided during warm-up. The butterfly stroke is performed with such powerful strokes to maintain proper form that the demands on the muscles are considered to be beyond that of a warm-up level of intensity.

The warm-up should make up at least 20 percent of the total swim workout, with some coaches extending that to as much as 33 percent.[20] If a training session is broken up into a phase of kick-only laps, the swimmer must remember to take a few minutes to warm up the upper extremities through some light swimming using the arms, since the arms will tend to cool down during the kick-only sets. A cool-down period of light swimming similar to the warm-up should comprise approximately 10 percent of the overall workout.[20] The cool-down period is thought to help work out some of the metabolic waste products that accumulate during intense training, as well as replenishing the muscles with nutrients contained in the fresh blood supply brought to the muscles being exercised during this cool-down phase of the workout.[21,22]

STRETCHING

A program of stretching should begin prior to any thought of swimming for training or competition, regardless of the age of the swimmer. Traditional stretching routines seen in swimming emphasize stretching the musculature of the neck, shoulder, trunk, low back, and legs (hamstrings). Most other joints of the extremities used in swimming are used within the midrange of muscle length and therefore are less prone to injury or dysfunction from the stresses of swimming. Stretching is specifically targeted at increasing muscle length and flexibility (elasticity). Increased muscle length will allow a joint to go through more range of motion without restriction, and increased elasticity will allow muscles to lengthen during activity without tearing, providing a shock-absorbing property to the muscles.[23,24]

Stretching may be performed either in or out of the water. Stretching should be performed as part of a warm-up prior to any swim training, swim competition, or any other exercise program that will place high demands on the muscles and joints. Many trainers believe that performing light exercise prior to stretching "warms up" the muscle and improves their pliability, but many believe that this is more psychological than physiologic.[19]

A slow, sustained stretch is less likely to cause injuries than ballistic stretching.[19] A quick stretch to a muscle will cause the firing of the muscle spindle of that muscle, facilitating a contraction of the muscle being stretched. Through the principle of reciprocal inhibition (inverse stretch reflex inhibition), contracting a muscle of opposing action to the one being stretched will cause the stretched muscle to relax momentarily.[25] Relaxation of a muscle complements stretching of that same muscle. Coordination of breathing while stretching also can aid in relaxation of the muscle. Deep breathing in a pattern of "in through the nose, out through the mouth" targeting the exhalation to coordinate with an overpressure toward the direction of stretch is recommended to facilitate the stretch. The stretch should be maintained for 30 seconds, followed by a 10-second rest. Three to five repetitions of each stretch should be performed.[19] The following paragraphs will describe common stretches performed prior to swimming.

All standing stretches begin with standing erect with the feet hip width apart, knees held in neutral or "relaxed flexion," and a slight forward lean at the hips. The body should be positioned upright with a modest lumbar lordosis and slight axial extension of the head (minimal chin tuck). This is referred to as the *standing stretch position*.

The lateral trunk stretch is performed while in the standing stretch position. The athlete should reach toward the sky with both hands, alternately stretching one hand higher than the other. This position simulates the streamlining position of the body in the water and provides a stretch to the rib cage and lateral trunk musculature. This stretch can be modified by adding a lateral trunk flexion (sidebend) to both the right and left. If the alternate stretch is chosen, the athlete should take care to keep the head and trunk facing forward so as not to introduce a rotational component into the stretch.

Toe touching performed in the standing position will stretch the low-back extensors and hamstrings. This stretch is important in that it reproduces the flexibility needed while in the starting blocks. Low-back extensors often are found to be shortened in swimmers due to the extensive use of the back extensors in maintaining the head out of the water for breathing. This often results in an increased lumbar lordosis in swimmers. This standing stretch is most effective when implemented early in a swimmer's training. As tightness develops, the toe-touch stretch would not be specific to isolate the low-back extensors for stretching and is less effective. There is an inherent tendency for the athlete to bounce when performing the toe touch. This produces a quick stretch to the hamstrings, which is counterproductive to the goal of increasing muscle length.

Trunk rotation may be performed while standing by placing the hands on the hips and then rotating the trunk, alternating right then left. This will stretch the transversalis muscles used in rotation of the trunk. Care should be taken in keeping the pelvis pointed forward in order to isolate the stretch to the trunk rotators and decrease abnormal twisting forces at the hips and knees. Performing this stretch while seated will reduce the accessory rotation.

The shoulder rotator stretch is performed by reaching one hand behind the neck while simultaneously reaching the other hand behind the back and trying to touch the fingertips in the area between the shoulder blades. The arm reaching behind the neck will be stretching the internal rotators of the rotator cuff, whereas the bottom arm reaching behind the back will be stretching the external rotators of the shoulder. A towel can be used to assist with this stretch (Fig. 5.14).

The anterior chest stretch is performed by horizontally abducting the shoulder with the elbow either flexed or extended and holding onto a fixed object. Multiple angles of shoulder abduction should be used. The swimmer will rotate the trunk away from the side being stretched while trying to prevent anterior humeral glide. For swimmers who swim an upper extremity synchronous stroke, this stretch should be performed bilaterally at the same time. This can be performed in a doorway, where the swimmer holds onto the doorframe and steps or leans through the doorway (Fig. 5.15).

The posterior shoulder stretch is performed by reaching the arm across the chest at

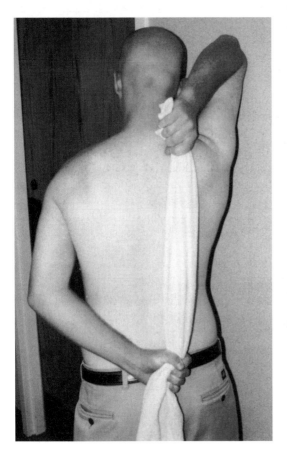 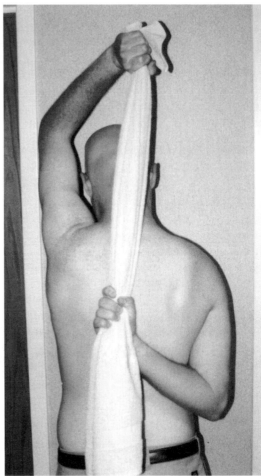

FIGURE 5.14

A. Towel stretch for shoulder internal rotators. *B.* Towel stretch for shoulder external rotators.

shoulder level and then reaching behind the elbow and pulling the arm into the chest. This position also will stretch the posterior deltoid.

The triceps stretch is performed by reaching up and behind the head, grasping the elbow with the opposite hand, and then applying pressure to pull the elbow toward the opposite side.

Partner stretching is often used in swimming and implies that a partner will be providing additional overpressure to increase the degree of stretching. Partners should be sensitive to the concept that "harder is not necessarily better." The pectoral stretch–anterior shoulder capsule stretch (Fig. 5.16) and an alternate low-back and hamstring stretch is best performed with a partner standing behind the swimmer to provide added effectiveness to the stretching. A moderate-intensity, longer-duration stretch will be more effective than a high-intensity, short-duration stretch. After working together over a few days of partner stretching, the athlete will learn to feel the muscle give way to the stretch. This

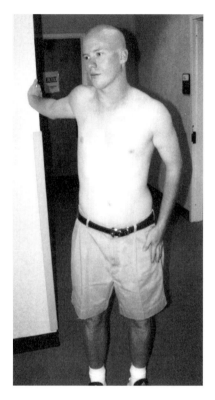

FIGURE 5.15

Pectoral stretch.

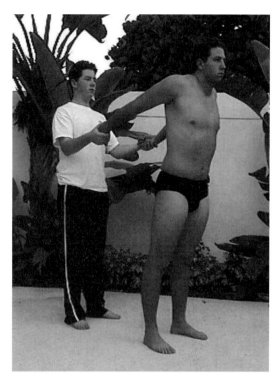

FIGURE 5.16

Partner stretch for anterior shoulder–pectoral stretch.

feeling of the muscle relaxing is in contrast to the muscle fighting the passive stretch. It is at this point that the most benefit is gained in actually lengthening the muscle.[25]

STRENGTHENING

Training for muscle strength, muscle power, and muscle endurance is an aspect of muscle conditioning that should be addressed in a well-rounded exercise program for swimmers. A combination of dry-land and pool-based exercises should be incorporated.

Weight training for strength should incorporate the overload principle of training. Each athlete should have a specific plan to address the major muscles of the extremities and trunk. These exercises can include traditional joint-specific free-weight exercises and exercise machines that isolate specific joint motions such as an arm curl, deltoid raise, or knee extension exercise. In addition, functional multijoint free-weight exercises such as squats, dead lifts, and clean and press exercises are appropriate to build strength and power.

Regardless of the exercise method used to build strength in swimmers, there is no evidence that muscle bulk has any correlation with success in swimming. Exercises that emphasize building muscle bulk should be avoided in swimmers. Overloading muscles through heavy-resistance, low-repetition exercise probably is not the best way to train for strength in swimmers. Training with heavy resistance without proper stretching promotes power and bound movements, which are opposed to the free-movement (mobility) demands of the sport of swimming. Overloading through exercises that employ moderate resistance through high repetitions addresses both the muscle strength and muscle endurance demands of swimming. Exercise regimes that emphasize negative work or eccentric contractions do not have the same level of functional importance in swimmers as in other athletes. The influence of the properties of the water eliminates most of the negative work of muscles during swimming other than in the above-water recovery phases of the strokes, in leaving the starting blocks, or in contacting the wall during turns. Alternative forms of resistance such as plyometrics, elastoresistive exercises, and isokinetic resistance exercises also can be used to develop muscle strength and endurance in swimmers. These types of exercise play an important role in preparing the swimmer for functional out-of-water activities, especially those high-demand activities involved in cross-training for conditioning the swimming athlete. Devices such as a swim bench or Vasatrainer also can be used to simulate the swimming motion while providing resistance to increase strength, power, and endurance. A swim bench allows the swimmer to perform and train the swim strokes biomechanically correctly in a prone or supine position while out of the water.

The concept of specificity of training is very important in conditioning swimmers. Because of the unique resistance of water, a significant amount of time in building strength, power, and endurance must be performed in the pool. Training in the event-specific stroke in which the swimmer will compete is essential in all muscle conditioning programs for swimmers. The use of hydrotherapy exercise aids as well as swim aids such as hand paddles and webbed gloves can increase the drag in the water, making it possible to use the water's resistance for strength training in the pool (Fig. 5.17).

CARDIOVASCULAR CONDITIONING

Cardiovascular conditioning should be developed through a combination of swimming and dry-land conditioning. Swimming as the primary method of cardiovascular conditioning is a great idea for nonswimming athletes and the general population but is not a good idea for competitive swimmers. The high demand of competitive swimming and structured training sessions dictates that the swimmer needs a fairly high level of both cardiovascular and muscle endurance prior to swim training. It has been demonstrated that upper extremity anaerobic power in young swimmers correlates with swimming performance. Research also has revealed significant changes in stroke mechanics associated with fatigue.[26,27] These changes in the stroke mechanics make the joints vulnerable to injury. Swimmers should participate in a cardiovascular conditioning program prior to a swim season to ensure that they have the endurance necessary to carry out the demands of swim training without injury. Once the swimmer has achieved the appropriate level of cardiovascular conditioning through dry-land exercise, swim training becomes a safe and effective method of taking this conditioning to a significantly higher level. A number of cardiovascular conditioning programs are readily available, including programs of running, cycling, and rowing. These programs can be performed outdoors as the activity would imply or indoors with equipment such as a cycle ergometer, treadmill, or rowing machine. The concept of cross-training may be particularly advantageous in training swimmers because some of the activities suggested, especially running, place additional stresses on swimmers who are used to exercising in the stress-free environment of water that they would not normally endure. Compressive forces through the lower extremity experienced during closed kinematic chain exercise such as running assist in the development of the long bones of the lower extremities.[9] The increased cocontraction of muscles

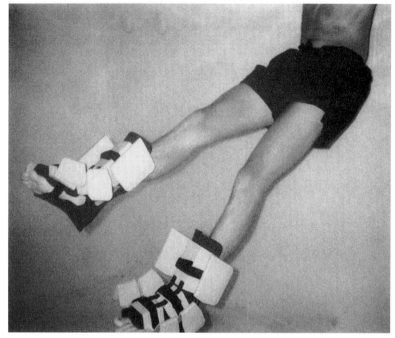

A

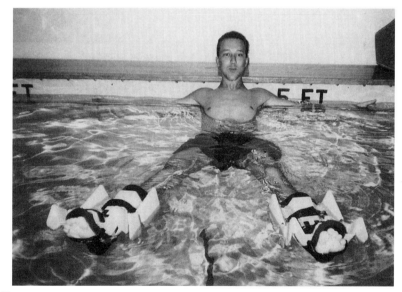

B

FIGURE 5.17

Aquatic exercises. *(Used with permission from Canavan PK: Rehabilitation in Sports Medicine. New York: Appleton and Lange, 19, Chap 11, Fig. 11-20A, B, p 284.)*

on both sides of the joints of the lower extremities required during running may add to the development of muscles as stabilizers around the ankle, knee, and hip joints.[10]

COACHING

Coaching is very important at every level of competition. Many of the flaws in stroke mechanics not only hurt performance but also cause abnormal stress on the muscles and joints. In most cases, the swim coach is the only source of feedback to the swimmer with regard to the successful application of proper stroke mechanics. Without this feedback, the swimmer only has speed as a gauge of success and will do whatever seems appropriate to increase speed. Since swim injuries tend to come from repetitive trauma, practicing poor technique is sure to meet with only limited success and short careers in swimming.

One goal of coaching is to teach safe, efficient stoke mechanics that have proven successful. This teaching can only be achieved by frequent observation of the swimmer performing each stroke during training. Faulty stroke mechanics need to be pointed out to each individual swimmer, and the swimmer should not be allowed to train or compete in a particular stroke until the mechanics have been mastered to a minimal level of proficiency. Coaches should refrain from entering a swimmer in an event where the athlete has not demonstrated proficiency. This can be especially tempting during a close meet for a team that lacks depth when it may be one swimmer short to swim a team relay or medley race. Coaches must remember that it may only take one injury swimming an unfamiliar event to ruin a swimmer's career.

SAFETY EDUCATION

Many injuries in swimming are inherent to the high physical demands of the sport. However, the most common injuries associated with swimming are also the most preventable. A commonsense approach to educating athletes about the hazards that exist around the sport of swimming can prevent many injuries. Signs warning the athlete of "No running" and "No diving" should be posted and enforced and can prevent injuries ranging from serious lacerations to spinal cord damage. A "Don't panic" sign may be a reminder to swimmers that frequently it is the panic that follows an incident in the pool that causes the swimmer the most significant problems, including drowning or near-drowning.

Swimming alone presents an inherent danger to the swimmer. A swimmer in distress in the water is obviously faced with the potential of drowning. This is particularly true of multievent athletes who swim in open waters. Drugs, including alcohol, and swimming do not mix. These substances may affect an athlete dramatically while swimming, since the intensity of exercise causes significant metabolic changes. The athlete should inform the coach of all medications he or she is taking. Medical professionals should inform the athlete of all precautions and side effects of medications prescribed, accounting for changes in dosage and method of delivery of the medication depending on the athlete's stage of training or competition.

TRAINING

Success in swimming is judged primarily on performance during competition meets. However, success in competition is directly related to the training leading up to these meets. The conditioning of swimmers involves training that usually includes strength and endurance achieved over several months. There are many ways to structure training programs, which may vary depending on what each coach believes produces the best results, but there are some general guidelines to use in establishing a good training program.

The swim season can be divided into different phases or periods, first from the perspective of levels training and second from the level of competition. It is important for members of the health care team to understand the terminology associated with the different phases of the swim season and the physical and psychological demands required of swimmers at different times of the year. This will assist health care practitioners in taking a history and ultimately making a diagnosis and outlining a rehabilitation or training program.

The over-distance period, the specialty period, and the taper period divide the swim season according to the intensity of training that the swimmer will go through. The *over-distance period* is the period at the beginning of each season when it is necessary for the swimmer to get a feel for the water and develop the basic techniques of the strokes. Speed is not emphasized during the over-distance period because speed and form tend to oppose one another. The philosophy tends to be that as strength and endurance develop while maintaining good form, speed will soon follow. Training too hard and too fast is likely to put the swimmer at unnecessary risk of injury.

The *specialty period* is the time in which swimmers focus on their specialty strokes. Training sessions are organized so that the intensity of workouts and stroke drills are specifically targeted to promote maximum performance within the specialty stroke of each individual swimmer. This period is most demanding on the swimmer as the intensity of swimming within each stroke reaches its peak. Due to the increased intensity of training, stroke specific injuries may be more common. Chronic fatigue and the associated musculoskeletal injuries are most common toward the end of the specialty training period.

The *taper period* is the time of the season during which the swimmer will cut back yardage in order to avoid cumulative trauma and chronic fatigue. Yardage is the total distance swum during each session. Dry-land ex-

ercises also should be cut back at this time because the detrimental physiologic effects of too much exercise.

The swim season is also divided into the precompetition, dual-meet competition, and championship-meet phases. The precompetition phase correlates with the over-distance period described earlier. The dual-meet competition phase is the time period in which swimmers will be perfecting their strokes and testing their skills. This correlates with the specialty training period described previously. Nearing the end of the season, teams enter into the championship-meet phase, at which time each swimmer's specialty events have been determined by performance during dual meets. As the championship-meet phase of the season approaches, coaches, swimmers, and health care practitioners need to communicate on a regular basis regarding the physical status of the swimmer. There will be a point at which the swimmer has reached a peak performance level, at which time the goal of training will be to maintain optimal performance. It is at this time that the taper period needs to begin to ready the swimmer for the championship meets. The actual timing of the tapering of training may differ from one swimmer to another depending on the season's prior events for an individual swimmer. Injuries, illnesses, total yardage swum, and total events participated in during dual meets must all be considered in determining the taper period leading up to the championship meets. Many coaches feel that the ability to effectively manage the taper period of the season is a primary factor in how well a swimmer will perform in the championship meets held at the end of the season.

PREVENTING SHOULDER INJURIES

As a result of the intensity of training in competitive swimming, a routine program of prevention is critical in maximizing performance and extending the careers of competitive swimmers. Continual reinforcement of proper stroke mechanics and adequate flexibility is essential. Distance and speed must be increased gradually at the start of each season, and warm-up and cool-down periods should be emphasized before and after each practice session or event. The swimmer must understand that each area of the body needs to be warmed up immediately before using the area. Kick-only sets are used in training to build up the endurance in the legs. During these kick-only sets, a swimmer does not use the arms and shoulders and will need to stretch and warm up the shoulders before swimming regular strokes at normal speed.[30] Both strength and flexibility imbalances have been associated with shoulder injuries.[33]

Stretching must be performed appropriately to be effective. The shoulder is particularly difficult to stretch because of the dependent relationship of the humerus, scapula, and ribcage. As an example, in order to stretch the posterior capsule and the lateral scapular musculature of the shoulder, the scapula must be stabilized on the thorax. Failure to provide stabilization will allow movement of the scapula toward protraction, resulting in a stretching of the rhomboids instead of the posterior capsule of the shoulder or the teres major and teres minor muscles. Swimmers and coaches must become familiar with proper stretching techniques to ensure that appropriate flexibility is achieved. Coaches should seek the advice of a licensed physical therapist or an athletic trainer in learning appropriate stretching techniques to incorporate into the training of their swimmers. Anterior inflexibility of the shoulder correlates with increased shoulder pain and can contribute to an impingement syndrome.[33,34] Posterior inflexibility of the shoulder may result in abnormal scapulohumeral rhythm causing decreased force-production capabilities of the rotator cuff musculature and possibly tendinitis.

Weight training should emphasize the same goals as rehabilitation. Strengthening must promote balanced strength around the joints of the extremities and trunk.[33] The sport of swimming inherently will create imbalances of musculature because of the fact that the underwater phases of the swim strokes force the muscles to work against heavier resistance than do the out-of-water phases of the stroke. This is particularly true for the muscles of the rotator cuff.[35,36] Hand paddles increase the surface area of the hands, thereby further increasing the resistance against which the shoulder and arm muscles must work. Introduction of hand paddles into the training regime should be done with caution and only at such time that the individual swimmer has demonstrated the strength and power necessary to use them properly. The distal resistance of the hand paddles can alter the swim mechanics at the shoulder significantly, and the swimmers form should be monitored at all times when using swim aides such as hand paddles. These prevention strategies can greatly decrease a swimmer's chances of shoulder overuse but will only be effective when implemented consistently. The intensity of training can overshadow good injury prevention strategies.

Cardiovascular strength and muscular endurance are equally important physiologic properties needed for injury-free swimming. A minimal level of endurance must be achieved prior to entering the pool for swim training. The quality of the mechanics of the swim strokes declines as a swimmer fatigues. If a swimmer tries to build endurance solely through increasing swim distances without already having the muscular and general endurance necessary to maintain good stroke mechanics, then every stroke is creating abnormal wear and tear on the muscles being used. Weight training with relatively light weights (60 to 70 percent of a 10-repetition maximum) for three to five sets of 10 repetitions performed three times per week over a 6- to 8-week period will help develop the muscular endurance in the extremities and trunk needed for swimming.[19] Athletes should balance their exercise program intensity to include an equal amount of exercise on each side of the joints (flexors and extensors, abductors and adductors, internal and external rotators) in order to create the necessary balance around the joints. Combining weight training with plyometric training, elastoresistive exercise, medicine ball programs, and aerobic exercises will provide a well-rounded endurance training program that will address the minimum needs for swimmers to begin swim training in the pool. Swim endurance training in the pool should progress over a period of weeks and should be progressed based on the individual swimmer's ability to maintain good stroke mechanics. Coaches should observe for altered stroke mechanics related to endurance and encourage a dry-land-based program targeting the muscle groups contributing to the poor stroke mechanics.

Etiology of Injuries

Several factors influence performance in swimming, ranging from the environment of the pool to the anatomic and physiologic factors of the athletes. Intrinsic risk factors that contribute to overuse injuries include dysfunctional alignment of joints, muscle imbalance, inflexibility, muscle weakness, and ligamentous instability. Extrinsic factors include poorly planned or executed training programs, technically weak swim stroke mechanics, swimming too many events, or a mismatch between a swimmer and events swum. These factors will be discussed in the context that they relate to performance and injury in competitive swimming.

EXTRINSIC FACTORS

Training errors can be one of the sources for injury in the swimming athlete. This includes the use of swim training aides such as hand paddles and kickboards to increase surface area and water resistance can exacerbate shoulder pain.[31] Excessive weight training, stretching exercises, and improper stretching technique may irritate an injured shoulder.[34,37]

Wet pool decks present an additional extrinsic factor that may lead to injuries in swimmers. In fact, survey research of the most common injuries in swimming reveal that slip and fall injuries in and around the pool deck account for the majority of injuries. These injuries are usually lacerations and contusions due to the contact with the pool deck but also can extend to more disabling injuries such as muscle strains, ligament sprains, fractures, and even head injuries.[1]

Swimming Pool

Competitive swimming pools are designed with specific standardized features. Competitive swim races that potentially can be counted for world records may only be set in 50-m long-course or 25-m short-course pools. In the United States, you also will find pools that have been built as 25-yd pools. The size of the pool used for practice and competition affects race times and can be a factor that influences the injury rate because a shorter pool requires more frequent turns to achieve the same swimming distance, therefore increasing the physical demands on the joints and muscles used during turning. Many practice pools vary in length, and sometimes teams are forced to use the width of a pool to accommodate more swimmers at one time during training sessions. A competition pool has a minimum of eight lanes, with each lane measuring from 7 to 9 ft wide. Competitive pools are equipped with starting blocks, with the front edge of the starting blocks measuring 30 in above the surface of the water.

The water temperature for official competitions must be between 25 and 27°C,[4] which is also a good range for training pools. Cold pools can cause muscles to be more prone to strain injuries due to decreased blood flow to the area and may require additional warm-up exercises to compensate for the cold temperature. Swimmers should be kept active in a cold pool to maintain the effects of the warm-up period. Warm pools may increase the core temperature of the swimmer and lead to fatigue and poor muscle performance, which also could lead to altered stroke mechanics, resulting in injury.

In order to control the pool water environment, most specifically bacteria, a number of chemicals are used. Typically, these chemicals are either chlorine or bromine used in conjunction with algicides and chemical stabilizers. Indoor and outdoor pools present their own unique challenges in managing the pool environment. Outdoor pools tend to require more chlorine and other chemicals due to the accelerated breakdown by the rays of the sun. Pool maintenance needs to be coordinated with coaches to make sure that chemicals have been added at such a time that they have mixed thoroughly throughout the pool. Chemicals in high concentration in areas of the pool can be hazardous to swimmers. Adequate ventilation in a natatorium is necessary to overcome the tendency of the room to trap humidity and chlorine fumes. Recent advances in technology have resulted in the development of devices used to maintain the water environment. These devices range from electrical devices that introduce chemicals into the water to totally passive devices such as rare-earth magnets. These devices are intended to decrease the amount of chemicals used in the pool and have the potential to decrease the detrimental effects that chemicals have on the skin, hair, and respiratory system. Proper ventilation is very important for maintaining the environment around an indoor pool.

Events in a Swim Meet

The events of a swim meet have significant effects on the training of swimmers and on the demands placed on them during a competition. The event being swum determines not only the type of stroke to be used but also the demands relative to the distance and speed that will be expected of the swimmer during competition.

A competitive swim meet is comprised of the four primary swim strokes, including the freestyle (Australian crawl), butterfly, breaststroke, and backstroke. Recreational swimming and multievent competitions such as triathlons would include these same four strokes in modification. Regardless of the event-specific stroke in which a swimmer may compete, a significant amount of the conditioning and training of all swimmers will be performed using the freestyle stroke. This is probably the most comfortable stroke for swimmers to perform biomechanically, allowing them to achieve the mileage necessary for conditioning. It is important for swimmers to train using the unique resistance created by the hydrodynamics working against the body and extremities while swimming. This unique resistance is sport-specific to swimming and cannot be emulated by dry-land exercises, regardless of the exercise device used. However, this does not negate the use of dry-land exercises for strengthening and conditioning.

Competitive swim meets are divided into events based on a combination of the type of stroke and the distance. A swim meet may include 14 individual events and 3 relay events, with divisions for both men and women in each event. The events are broken down into butterfly, backstroke, breaststroke, freestyle, individual medley, and medley relay. These events are organized into multiple distances to comprise the total number of events in a swim meet. In Olympic competition, there are only 13 individual events and 3 relays for men and women. Men do not swim an 800-m freestyle, and women do not swim a 1500-m freestyle. The freestyle events will include 50-, 100-, 200-, 400-, 800-, and 1500-m races. Backstroke, breaststroke, and butterfly race distances are 100 and 200 m.

In addition, swim competitions will include medley and relay races. The individual medley (IM) is a race that combines all four competitive strokes, and a single swimmer swims one-fourth of the race with each of the four strokes. The IM is organized in the order of the butterfly, backstroke, breaststroke, and freestyle. The IM is swum in 200- and 400-m distances.

The medley relay (MR) is an event where all four strokes are swum by four different swimmers. No swimmer may swim more than one leg of the relay race. The MR is swum in the order of backstroke, breaststroke, butterfly, and freestyle. The MR is swum in four legs, with each leg being 100 m, and is commonly referred to as a 4 × 100 m relay race.

There are two freestyle relays, the 400- and 800-m races. In freestyle relays, each of four swimmers swims one-fourth of the 400- or 800-m distance. As in the MR, no individual may swim more than one leg of the relay.

INTRINSIC FACTORS

Muscle Endurance

Muscle endurance is an important property of muscle performance in swimming. A study by Troup et al.[39] in 1991 demonstrated that muscle activity increases with the onset of fatigue as the athlete tries to maintain speed in the water. Muscle efficiency decreases as the rate of firing increases and the force output decreases.[4] Resistance to muscle fatigue can increase only through endurance training through high-intensity anaerobic conditioning. Both dry-land exercises and swim training may be modified to include aerobic and anaerobic conditioning of the muscles. In addition, the amount of time between morning

and afternoon practices is very important in avoiding fatigue. It may be necessary to have 8 hours of rest between practice sessions in order to replenish the glycogen levels in the body.[4]

Muscle weakness, muscle imbalances, or poor flexibility also will predispose swimmers to injury.[33,38]

Nutritional Concerns

Nutrition plays an important role in decreasing muscle fatigue. Prolonged swim training increases the carbohydrate requirement to maintain glycogen levels and exercise capacity.[4] The body depends on the intake of carbohydrates as an immediate source of fuel. Once exercise intensity uses up the carbohydrates taken in, the body turns to the glycogen stored in the body for fuel. Costill et al.[40] showed that glycogen levels fall to significantly low levels following short, high-intensity interval swim training. Once stored glycogen is depleted, the body is dependent on the breakdown of stored fats for fuel. Since the percentage of body fat of both male and female swimmers tends to be lower than that of the average person,[4] using stored fats for fuel is inefficient and places a high energy demand on the system that contributes to fatigue. Carbohydrate supplements are often recommended during intense training, and research[41] supports the intake of high-carbohydrate gels or drinks within 30 minutes of swimming.[4] A well-balanced diet including caloric intake sufficient to maintain the athlete's caloric expenditure depending on the intensity of training is recommended. Rapid weight loss has been shown to decrease muscle strength and power and should be discouraged in competitive swimmers.

TECHNIQUE ERRORS

Errors in stroke biomechanics combined with predisposing factors in the swimmer can also contribute to injury. For example, there is often a mistaken emphasis on forcefully accelerating the extremities against resistance instead of using the extremity as an anchor and allowing body roll to move the body past the anchoring point. The rotator cuff functions as a stabilizer, as it is designed, rather than accelerating the limb backward against resistance.

Swimmers may have increased shoulder laxity when compared with nonswimmers, especially in the anterior and inferior directions.[29] Swimmers with the greatest shoulder laxity will increase the use of their rotator cuff muscles in order to stabilize the humeral head in the glenoid fossa. This may overwork the rotator cuff muscles and increase the risk of tendinitis.[30] The freestyle arm stroke naturally strengthens the internal rotators. Most swimmers will have significantly stronger internal rotators of the shoulders than external rotators.[31] A 1992 study of men and women swimmers revealed a shift in torque ratios of specific shoulder muscles.[32] The study revealed an increase in shoulder adduction/abduction torque ratios and a decrease in shoulder external rotation/internal rotation. Since all shoulder torque values are greater in swimmers than in the mean population, it can be deduced that this shift in torque ratios can be attributed to the repetitive strengthening of the adductors and internal rotators of the shoulder. These muscles are most active during the pull-through or propulsive phase of the arm stroke in swimming.[32]

Lack of body roll in novice swimmers results in the need for excessive shoulder abduction in bringing the arm out of the water in freestyle swimming and in pull-through in the backstroke. With repetition, this may cause an anterior instability or posterior impingement syndrome of the glenohumeral joint. Carrying the elbow low during the recovery phase of freestyle and butterfly strokes places undue stresses on the muscles of the rotator cuff and can lead to tendinitis in these muscles.

In order to avoid excessive external rotation of the shoulder during the freestyle stroke, the elbow should remain well above the hand during the out-of-the-water phase (recovery) and catch phase of the stroke. Dropping the elbow during these phases may irritate the rotator cuff muscles by placing the shoulder at a mechanical disadvantage in creating the necessary torque to move the hand through the water.[3] The high elbow position on the recovery must be achieved through body roll or else the shoulder will be required to abduct and externally rotate excessively. A body roll of 60 to 80 degrees to each side is necessary to avoid excessive forceful abduction of the shoulder, which would result in repetitive impingement of the shoulders.[4,6,12,28]

In the entry and catch phases of the freestyle stroke, the hand and arm must reach forward close to the line of the torso, aligning the arm for a direct pull through the water. A common error is a deviation of the arms lateral or medial to the line of the torso, decreasing the efficiency of the pull-through. This lateral or medial deviation of the arms takes the arm out of a direct line of pull and causes torsional forces at the shoulder when the arm is extended during pull-through.

The whip kick used in the breaststroke requires forceful contraction of the quadriceps muscles while at the same time placing a significant valgus stress on the knee. This combination of forces makes any swimmer with a high Q-angle prone to patellofemoral pain syndrome.[5] Some swimmers may not be good candidates to become breaststrokers due to their inherent Q-angle. Exercises to emphasize use of the vastus medialis muscle should be performed by breaststrokers year-round to help control patellar tracking and decrease the chance of developing patellofemoral pain syndrome. Decreased hip flexion during the breaststroke kick places the lower extremities at a mechanical disadvantage so that additional valgus stresses are placed on the knee when the whip kick is used. Coaching the whip kick in breaststroke swimmers is of particular importance because the breaststroke is probably the most difficult stroke for swimmers to perform correctly.

These errors are common in poorly coached swimmers or when the swimmer is fatigued. Other fatigue-related errors in competitive swimmers such as breathing only to one side,[28] kicking poorly, and losing a buoyant body position may add to overuse stress. Coaches should observe for fatigue-related technique problems, and the training session should end at any point at which the swimmer is exhibiting poor technique. Coaches and athletes should keep in mind that practice makes perfect only when practice *is* perfect. Practicing inefficient swim strokes will only ingrain abnormal patterns of movement that will be very difficult to break.

Common Injuries and Their Treatment

OVERTRAINING SYNDROME

Swimmers are at risk for overtraining because they participate in long, intense two-a-day practices during the season. Masters-level swimmers may use the shoulders in an overhead position up to 11,000 times per week of training.[5,6,16] Some swimmers swim with more than one team, extending their season to virtually year-round training and competition. Overtraining is common among swimmers. Between 10 and 21 percent of swimmers experience signs of overtraining during the course of a competitive swim season.[2,15,41,42] Overtraining is so common that any swimmer experiencing any injury or pain should be questioned for signs of overtraining.[5]

General health questions should identify recurrent minor illnesses, changes in sleep pat-terns, nutritional habits, and overall mood states that may be indicators of early overtraining. Female swimmers are often susceptible to the *female athlete triad*. This triad consists of eating disorders, amenorrhea, and osteoporosis. Female athletes should be questioned about a history of stress fractures, menstrual abnormalities, and eating habits. Concerns about individual athletes should be referred to a physician because early intervention is key in decreasing the devastating effects of the triad.

Overtraining syndrome can develop when swim training outpaces rest and recovery.[41] This can occur as a result of flaws in the training program at several levels. At the stroke level, if a swimmer exhibits a stroke technique with an inefficient recovery phase, the muscles used during the stroke will be overworked, placing a higher physical demand on the swimmer and making the swimmer vulnerable to the effects of overtraining. If an athlete swims too many events during training or competition without adequate rest between events, overtraining may occur. Inadequate time between morning and afternoon practices also can cause overtraining. Overtraining can occur in as little as 10 days of increased training without adequate rest, resulting in decreased performance.[2,43]

Signs and symptoms of overtraining in swimmers would include behavioral changes such as difficulty sleeping, increased or decreased appetite, general fatigue, inability to concentrate, irritability, and loss of motivation. It also may include physiologic problems such as nausea, diarrhea, change in bowel habits, frequent colds or flulike symptoms, and increased resting heart rate. Weight may change according to whether the athlete's eating habits have increased or decreased. Musculoskeletal problems such as muscle strains, chronic muscle soreness, and minor ligamentous sprains may occur due to the biomechanical dysfunction caused by muscles performing suboptimally as a result of the overtraining.[4,44]

Treatment of Overtraining Syndrome

If an athlete exhibits signs of overtraining, he or she must be seen by a health care practitioner to rule out other disorders that may present with similar signs and symptoms. The diagnosis of *overtraining syndrome* is made through a process of elimination. Once other diagnoses relative to the presenting signs and symptoms have been ruled out, it may be concluded that the symptoms are due to overtraining. Treatment of overtraining consists of rest, hydration, and balanced nutrition. The length of rest may range from 2 or 3 days to several weeks. If symptoms are recognized early, a modification of training to a period of relative rest may be enough to keep the athlete from developing a true overtraining syndrome. Swimmers will return to training when symptoms subside. Overtraining syndrome can be prevented if both the coach and athlete understand that adequate rest is considered part of the training.[45] This includes both adequate rest between training events or strokes and adequate rest between practice sessions.

Prevention of injuries and illness, as well as injury rehabilitation, often requires alteration of a swimmer's training program. Communicating the need for these changes to both the athlete and the coach is instrumental in achieving compliance. Alteration in swim training in the area of biomechanical technique, speed, distance, and duration or frequency of training sessions may provide a period of "relative rest" adequate to achieve recovery or healing while keeping the swimmer swimming. Research has documented the negative effects on performance of taking a swimmer out of water for rest.[45] Nonetheless, injured tissue must be rested. If this can be achieved through modification of aspects of the training program, then keeping the swimmer in the water would be the approach of choice. Modification of training programs conducted in the water to provide relative rest to the injury will have better compliance than suggesting that the swimmer train only on dry land. Effective communication among the swimmer, coach, athletic trainer, physical therapist, and physician is instrumental to successful outcomes of rehabilitation.

OVERUSE INJURIES

The most common injuries seen in swimmers are due to overuse and cumulative trauma.[1] Cumulative, repetitive microtrauma can cause tissue damage that leads to overuse injuries. An important step to the successful treatment of swimming injuries is to have an organized approach to injury treatment regardless of the muscle, joint, or other tissue that is injured. First of all, it is important for the athlete to get to the appropriate health care professional as soon as possible. This means that the coach must put together the sports medicine health care team long before the season starts. Easy accessibility is the key to determining who will be on the health care team. A team physician would be the ideal professional to head the sports medicine team. However, in the managed care environment of today, some athletes may be excluded from seeing the team physician because the physician is not on their health plan. A physical therapist or certified athletic trainer may be more accessible to athletes in some circumstances and would have the ability to identify when physician's services are necessary.

All health care professionals on the team should be experienced in working with swimmers. Early intervention is the key to preventing acute injuries into chronic syndromes. Coaches should not try to diagnose painful conditions themselves. Early intervention is inexpensive and may even salvage the career of a swimmer. Many health care professionals volunteer time to sports teams as part of their commitment to the community.

Once the athlete is referred to the appropriate professional, there is a systematic approach to treating overuse injuries regardless of the location of the injury. This will include making an accurate diagnosis of the injury, controlling acute symptoms, promoting healing of involved tissues, improving function of the tissue involved, and preventing reinjury of the injured tissue.

Treatment of Overuse Injuries

Overuse injuries result from microtrauma. This trauma causes localized inflammation and/or local tissue damage in the form of cellular and extracellular changes. This tissue damage will manifest as overuse injuries such as arthritis, bursitis, capsulitis, tendinitis, myositis, impingement syndromes, neuropathies, and ligamentous laxity.[10]

These injuries are most likely to occur when a swimmer overloads a muscle, ligament, or joint in such a way that there is no chance for adequate recovery. This may be due to either the immediate intensity of the overload or the overload over time. Microtrauma may occur without any clinical presentation of pain. Over time, however, the microtrauma accumulates to the point of becoming symptomatic.

Differential Diagnosis   The first step in the treatment of overuse injuries is making a diagnosis. An experienced clinician often can make a preliminary diagnosis simply by taking a thorough history. The physical examination will confirm most overuse injuries involving soft tissue. In most cases, swimmers will not present with a history of overt physical trauma, and therefore, radiographs (x-rays) frequently are not beneficial in the differential diagnostic procedure. Radiographs may be necessary is some cases to rule out bony pathology such as fractures, intraarticular abnormalities, heterotopic calcification, and other pathologies such as tumors. In severe cases, magnetic resonance imaging (MRI) may be used to definitively diagnose specific pathology such as rotator cuff tendinitis with combined labral pathology or clinical evidence of major soft tissue disrup-

tion. Most overuse injuries in swimmers can be diagnosed solely on the results of the physical examination and special orthopedic and neurologic tests.

A specific diagnosis is key in the treatment process. A diagnosis of "swimmer's shoulder" does nothing to direct the treatment of the underlying condition because this diagnosis does not identify the tissue pathology. A diagnosis of "supraspinatus tendinitis" in a freestyle swimmer or "grade 1 sprain of the medial collateral ligament" in a breaststroker appropriately defines the problem and tissue at risk and qualifies what needs to be done.

As part of the diagnostic process, one must recognize that swimmers do not use their muscles and joints in isolation. Muscles and joints are used in kinetic and kinematic chains. Any movement dysfunction or painful condition must be examined thoroughly to include all interactive components of the movement. For example, any decreased or painful motion at the shoulder would warrant examination of the glenohumeral joint, the acromioclavicular joint, the scapulothoracic joint, and the sternoclavicular joint. Without normal function of each one of these joints and their corresponding ligaments and muscles, limitation of motion of the shoulder would be predictable. At some point, an assessment of the stroke mechanics in the pool would be a helpful diagnostic approach, especially in the return to swimming and injury prevention phases of treatment.

Control Acute Symptoms   The primary acute symptom following microtrauma is inflammation. Inflammation is required for proper healing of injured tissue. However, excessive or prolonged inflammation is not good, nor is it normal. Controlling inflammation is of the utmost importance in the treatment of overuse injuries. The most popular approach to the management of swelling incorporates the traditional formula rest, ice, compression, and elevation (RICE). The traditional RICE formula works well in the acute phase of injury or following active exercise of the injured tissue at any stage of treatment. In both cases, the traditional RICE formula will work to keep additional swelling out of the area. Once the swelling has reached the area, especially in the case of chronic recurrent swelling, the traditional RICE formula will not be adequate. Prolonged swelling deposits waste materials in the tissues that are counterproductive to efficient tissue function. Physical modalities such as electrical stimulation and ultrasound are useful in the treatment of overuse tissue pathologies.[10] These modalities can be used alone or together with steroids and local anesthetics. Oral or intramuscular injections of medications also may be part in the medical management of these injuries. Decreasing pain should not be a primary goal of treatment. Pain reduction should come as a result of successful management of the underlying pathology. Treating the pain may cause the swimmer to return to training prematurely, causing more damage to a partially healed tissue. Pain should be a guide to the athlete to encourage appropriate use of the injured tissue and should not be masked with pain medications.

Nearly all protocols for managing overuse injuries begin with curtailing the activities that stress the injured tissue. The "rest" in RICE means resting the tissue that is injured. Sometimes this may mean resting the entire extremity or body part, or it may mean using it in a manner that takes the stress off the tissue. A swimmer may rest a particular muscle by simply swimming slower. Research shows that slowing the stroke rate improves form. With the improved form, the muscle may not overwork, and therefore, relative rest is accomplished. Relative rest protects the injured area while avoiding the negative effects of deconditioning.

Although corticosteroids are potent anti-inflammatory drugs commonly prescribed in managing athletic injuries, many physicians are becoming more conservative in using them. Corticosteroids in oral and injectable forms are thought to decrease collagen and ground substance production, weaken the tensile strength of tendons, and ultimately retard healing. Injection of corticosteroids near a weight-bearing tendon may be accompanied by restriction of swimming for 2 to 3 weeks. Injecting into weight-bearing tendons is contraindicated. Many physicians use the guideline of no more than three corticosteroid injections per year for an athlete. However, this is just a guideline, and there are no definitive studies to support or contraindicate more or less frequent use.[19]

Promote Healing Many times an athlete returns to training or competition as soon as the symptoms of pain and swelling subside. This often results in reinjury. Health care professionals, coaches, and athletes alike must become aware of the fact that rest and controlling inflammation do not heal the tissue—they only position the tissue to heal. Tissue will heal best when activity is used as part of the healing process. Healing involves the proliferation of vascular elements and fibroblasts that create collagen deposition and maturation in injured tissue. Specific, therapist-directed exercise will best promote this revascularization. Aerobic conditioning complements the revascularization process by increasing the oxygen content of the blood, as well as by sending additional blood supplies to the general area for added nutrition. A general conditioning program will provide neurologic stimulus to injured tissue, reestablishes proprioceptive and feedforward/feedback mechanisms, minimizes weakness of surrounding uninjured tissue, minimizes negative psychological effects, and controls unwanted weight gain. In addition, progressive exercise can help align collagen fibers. Many of the body's tissues develop according to the stresses placed on them. Gradually loading the tissues in sport-specific exercises will strengthen the tissues toward the tasks that eventually will be required of them. The coach and the athlete need to be educated to these principles to ensure compliance with the program.

Conservative care is most often effective in the treatment of overuse injuries in swimmers. If a rehabilitation program is not successful, surgery may be a consideration. If rehabilitation is not successful and surgery is being considered, the athlete should seek a second opinion to make sure that all conservative approaches have been tried. Surgery is performed to remove or repair the injured tissue and restore maximum function. Surgery may be a consideration if the rehabilitation program has been unsuccessful (after 3 to 6 months), swim performance has declined significantly, swimming causes chronic reinjury of same area, or the injury has affected the quality of the athlete's life.

Avoid Reinjury Once the injured tissue has healed and is performing normally, the goal is to avoid reinjury. For a swimmer returning to training and competition, the only way to achieve this is through a swim-specific conditioning program targeted at filling in any of the gaps that may have predisposed the athlete to injury. Every aspect of swimming that has the potential to affect the previously injured tissue needs to be addressed. This includes exercises for achieving maximum flexibility, strength, power, muscular endurance, and cardiovascular endurance. Postural education and muscle reeducation will be instrumental in promoting a balance of the active and passive tissue structures that have to function in synergy during all aspects of swimming.

Promote a Healthy Lifestyle Adequate rest and good nutrition will round out the injury prevention and final phase of rehabilitation. In addition, the swimmer will make all modifications necessary to control stresses on the injured area. This will come from working on the efficiency and technique of the stroke mechanics; modifying the swim training program in speed, distance, duration, and time between practices; and swimming events that eliminate stress on the injured area. Improving the swimmer's stroke mechanics is critical because abnormal and improper biomechanics quickly promote reinjury.

COMMON UPPER EXTREMITY INJURIES

Intense daily training distance can average 10,000 to 15,000 yards over a 4- to 5-month season with virtually no breaks. In a single year, an individual swimmer may put his or her upper extremities through 2 million arm strokes.[3] This repetitive motion in and of itself would be considered traumatic from the aspect of normal wear and tear and often results in repeated microtrauma to the musculoskeletal structures, including muscles, tendons, ligaments, and joints. The shoulder in particular is put through its maximum range of motion during each swimming stroke, which causes microtrauma and frequently leads to mechanical breakdown of the biomechanics of the shoulder complex[42] and results in painful conditions of the shoulder.

Research has shown that the physical abuse to the shoulder is cumulative and that there is a positive correlation between the frequency of painful shoulder conditions and the years of participation in the sport of swimming.[5] Swimmers in the younger age groups show a high incidence of shoulder pain, although the average age of swimmers first seeking medical attention for shoulder pain is 18 years.[3] There is probably some merit to the common belief that "kids heal quickly," so a few days off from swimming frequently result in the pain subsiding, giving the swimmer the ability to return to competition. However, not changing the painful stimulus makes them vulnerable to reinjury. This reluctance to seek medical attention results in decreased access to health care professionals that could examine the athlete and assess the specific biomechanics of the shoulder. Based on this assessment, the therapist can prescribe a rehabilitation and training program that will improve the efficiency of the arm stroke to prevent further cumulative trauma to the shoulder. The lack of appropriate medical and physical therapy care may result in recurring musculoskeletal problems and may lead to career-ending injuries that could have been rehabilitated or prevented. Many injuries seen in elite college swimmers are the cumulative result of minor injuries first occurring several years earlier.

Shoulder pain is the most common musculoskeletal complaint among competitive swimmers.[5,6,15,43,46] Numerous reports have documented not only the basic impingement syndrome as the most common cause of shoulder pain in swimmers but also the underlying instability of the glenohumeral joint, which predisposes to inflammation of the subacromial bursa and tears of the glenoid labrum.[15,29,43,46]

Swimmer's Shoulder

The shoulder goes through the extremes of range of motion with each stroke. "Swimmer's shoulder" is an overuse injury resulting in inflammation in the supraspinatus and/or biceps tendons,[36,43] usually caused by multidirectional glenohumeral instability and/or impingement of the tendons between the head of the humerus and the acromion process of the scapulae. The normal scapulohumeral rhythm dictates a unique balance between movement of the scapulae on the thorax and movement of the humerus in the glenoid fossa.[9] Often during the final aspect of the pull phase of the butterfly stroke, the shoulder is taken into full adduction, causing a compression of the blood vessels in the area and a "milking" of the blood supply out of the

area. This will cause degenerative changes in the supraspinatus tendon over time.[28] Localized swelling also can alter the biomechanics of the shoulder joint. Localized inflammation of the glenohumeral joint secondary to trauma will manifest clinically as a restricted pattern of movements in abduction, external rotation, and internal rotation (a capsular pattern of restriction). Continuing swimming in the presence of an inflamed glenohumeral joint will require significant alteration of normal mechanics of the scapulae, neck, and trunk. Repeated irritation of the supraspinatus tendon may lead to repeated episodes of space occupying local inflammation that further decreases the subacromial space, causing secondary impingement and possibly leading to irritation of the subacromial bursa resulting in an acute bursitis. Inflammation of the bursa or tendons superior to the head of the humerus will present clinically as a painful arc on shoulder abduction.

Proper stroke technique greatly improves a swimmer's ability to train without injury. Technical flaws lead to increased shoulder stress and become more frequent and severe with fatigue.[47] Most competitive swimmers receive significant instruction in technique at younger ages, but work on stroke mechanics drops considerably after age 12.[3] Technical flaws in the freestyle stroke significantly stress the shoulder joints and can lead to overuse injuries. Dropping the elbow during recovery may injure the muscles of the rotator cuff. Decreased rotation of the trunk about the longitudinal axis of the body will encourage excessive cervical rotation for breathing, ultimately leading to possible cervical facet syndrome, subsequent muscle spasm of the trapezius and/or scalenes, and altered mechanics of the scapulae or clavicle. At the same time, decreased body roll will create the need to excessively abduct the glenohumeral joint, leading to a posterior impingement or possibly an anterior overstretch of the capsule of the glenohumeral joint.

Diagnosing Swimmer's Shoulder The accurate diagnosis of injuries in swimmers is essential to successful treatment outcomes. Injuries seen in competitive swimmers are not unique to the sport, even though the cause of the injury may be specific to the unusual demands of swimming, as discussed earlier in this chapter. The diagnosis of any musculoskeletal problem requires good listening skills combined with a thorough manual examination. Most injuries seen in swimmers involve soft tissue trauma and may not be diagnosed definitively through x-rays or high-tech scans. A series of manual examination procedures and special tests often use symptom reproduction as a diagnostic tool. Since the source of irritation of many maladies is related to the repetitive nature of the stresses of swimming, it is not uncommon for an athlete to present symptom-free at the time of examination. If a history of injury presents data such as "it only starts hurting after I swim 60 laps and feels better when I rest it," then the examiner should be prepared to examine the athlete poolside immediately following the sixtieth lap. Direct observation of the athlete swimming is probably the only accurate way to perform a biomechanical analysis to detect possible problems with the swimming stroke that may be contributing to the problem.

When evaluating a swimmer's shoulder pain, identifying the painful phases of the stroke through a good history will assist in the diagnosis and treatment of specific shoulder problems. Pain frequently occurs when the arm is pulling against the resistance of the water, which would be during the catch phase and early to middle pull portion of the pull-through phase of the freestyle stroke. These motions involve the latissimus dorsi, teres major, pectoralis major, and shoulder internal rotator muscles in forcefully adducting and internally rotating the glenohumeral joint. Posterior impingements and anterior instabilities also may present with increased pain during the elbow-lift phase of recovery,[37] as well as pain associated with the use of the deltoid, supraspinatus, infraspinatus, and teres minor muscles in bringing the shoulder overhead into an externally rotated position during the recovery phase. If the history reveals pain in these specific phases of the stroke, clinical examination of these same movements may confirm a diagnosis. Passive range of motion with overpressure may reveal strain or laxity of a joint, whereas a resistive isometric muscle contraction may reveal tendinitis. Multidirectional instabilities may be seen as excessive glides in the anterior, posterior, and inferior directions. This also will test positive on a sulcus sign special test.[48]

The examiner also should observe for patterns of pain behavior during range-of-motion testing. The *painful arc syndrome* and the *capsular pattern* are quite helpful in making a differential diagnosis. A painful arc on active abduction between 45 and 120 degrees suggests an impingement between the head of the humerus and the acromial arch. The structures being impinged may include the subacromial bursa and the tendons of the rotator cuff muscles inserting onto the greater tuberosity, especially the supraspinatus tendon. The clinician also should evaluate for joint inflammation; bursitis; impingement syndromes; internal or external rotator cuff muscle weakness; anterior, posterior, inferior, or multidirectional instability; and point tenderness over the supraspinatus and/or biceps tendons.[48]

Treatment of Swimmer's Shoulder All the diagnoses presented here most likely are related directly to overuse during swimming. This may be due to poor technique, too much training, or simply cumulative trauma over many seasons of swimming. Regardless, treatment of shoulder injuries begins with rest. It is important to understand that rest only applies to resting the structure that is injured. As discussed previously, one would anticipate the greatest compliance by minimizing the time out of the water. Modifying the stroke mechanics, the distance swum, the intensity or speed, or the stroke swum to non-aggravating strokes can be used to achieve rest of the injured structure. One should use caution in prescribing drills using kickboards because they present different challenges to the shoulder.[38]

The physical therapist and/or athletic trainer needs to communicate to the coach any need to modify the stroke mechanics to prevent reinjury. NSAIDs and ice are part of the standard treatment. Ice is most effective in keeping fluids out of the area following an acute injury or flare-up but does little to remove subacute and chronic swelling. NSAIDs probably are more effective in decreasing swelling once the swelling has reached the injured area. In severe cases, steroids may be used to treat persistent swelling. Icing of the shoulder following workouts is a good routine practice.[38]

Exercise should include strengthening of the internal and external rotators of the shoulder as well as periscapular muscle strengthening. Strengthening of the rotators should be performed in both arm abduction and adduction.[36,37] Achieving a balance of muscle strength around the shoulder is of primary importance because the muscles not only will need to produce large forces for speed of swimming but also must achieve the dynamic stabilization necessary to avoid abnormal shoulder mechanics. Steroid injections must be used with caution in all athletes. For swimmers, training load should be decreased for 3 to 4 weeks after injection.[30] In some cases, it is necessary to have the swimmer take a complete rest from swimming in order to allow the injury to heal.

Surgery is rarely needed in young swimmers.[36] However, surgery is sometimes considered for athletes with chronic shoulder problems after repeated attempts at conserva-

tive therapy have proven unsuccessful. Surgery to tighten the capsule of the shoulder may be considered for athletes with chronic instability. Subacromial decompression should be considered as a last resort for swimmers who have a hooked (type III) acromion.[36,48]

Thoracic Outlet Syndrome

Thoracic outlet syndrome (TOS) is a term given to a specific group of signs and symptoms resulting from compression of the subclavian artery, subclavian vein, and brachial plexus within the thoracic outlet. Symptoms relate directly to the structure that is compressed.

Because swimming involves so much repetitive overhead motion, one may expect a higher incidence of TOS in the swimming population. Differentiating between TOS and a typical "swimmer's shoulder" is a challenge and often is overlooked. However, the differential diagnosis of shoulder pain in swimmers should include TOS. Nevertheless, the diagnosis is difficult because there is no single reliable objective test that pinpoints TOS. Consequently, diagnosis of TOS is based on symptom history, symptom behavior, and physical findings supported and corroborated by several objective clinical tests.

TOS involves an entrapment of the neurovascular structures in the area of the neck and is some cases may involve the presence of an "extra rib." In reality, this "rib" is an anomaly involving extended growth of the transverse process of the cervical vertebrae into the anatomic first rib. This results in a narrowing of the space through which the neurovascular structures pass and compression by the overlying clavicle. Surgical removal of the cervical rib is sometimes necessary to eliminate compression of the neurovascular structures. The subclavian nerves and vessels also can be compressed by the normal first rib or the scalene muscles. Entrapment syndromes of TOS differ according to which structure is primarily compressed. This may be the artery, vein, or brachial plexus. The location of compression may be at the level of the anterior scalene muscle, the true thoracic outlet between the clavicle and first rib, or the area of the coracoid process.

Neurologic symptoms of pain, numbness, and tingling are the most common and have the most significant effect on swimmers. A swimmer with TOS may exhibit signs and symptoms during swimming. Freestyle, butterfly, and backstroke all require a well-timed powerful motion at the extremes of range of motion of abduction and external rotation of the shoulder. As pull-through begins at the end of range position, the muscles of the entire upper quarter must create significant power through shortening of the muscles via contraction. Complaints of tightness and pain about the shoulder, neck, and clavicle at the hand-entry position would be a definite clue that the athlete should be examined for TOS. The neurovascular structures pass under the arch of the coracoid process, and as the swimmer reaches hand entry, the neurovascular structures approximate the bony structures of the scapulae and clavicle. Size and insertion of the pectoralis minor muscle also can play a role in causing TOS.

Complaints will range from pain in the lower face and ear and possibly accompanying headaches. These may be combined with radiating pain into the shoulder, thumb, and index and middle fingers. It may be necessary in such patients to differentiate TOS from shoulder pain, "swimmer's ear," and simple headaches. Weakness and fatigue of the deltoid, biceps, triceps, or forearm muscles may occur with the upper type of TOS. Loss of strength of the intrinsic muscles of the hand may make grasping objects difficult, representing a compromise of the C8 and T1 nerve roots, the medial cord, and the ulnar nerve. This early fatigue syndrome of the intrinsic muscles of the hand may be the initial complaint of the swimmer. A common sign in swimmers is difficulty in keeping the fingers together and the inability to control movement of the hand during the sculling mo-

tion of the pull-through phase of any of the four swimming strokes.

Complaints of shoulder pain in TOS differ from those of classic "swimmer's shoulder" in that in TOS there are no findings of glenohumeral instability. However, some swimmers may exhibit the instability even though it is not contributing to the signs or symptoms of TOS. The pain of TOS typically is located both anterior and posterior to the clavicle, and there often are radicular symptoms, including numbness, tingling, and pain in the ring and small fingers. Compression of the subclavian artery can lead to complaints of coolness and pain, or compression of the subclavian vein can cause a feeling of fullness in the upper extremity.

Diagnosis of TOS A careful history from the athlete will elicit a symptom complex different from that of primary shoulder pain or cervical nerve root compression. Physical examination will include several special tests that may corroborate the diagnosis.

The Adson's maneuver is performed by assessing the radial pulse while the athlete rotates the head to face the test shoulder. The patient extends the head while the examiner laterally rotates and extends the patient's shoulder. The patient takes a deep inhalation with the head turned toward the affected side; diminution of the radial pulse is considered positive for the diagnosis of TOS. The reverse Adson's maneuver is the same test but with the patient's head turned away from the affected side, again resulting in a decrease in the radial pulse.[48]

The Roos test also tests for TOS. The patient stands while externally rotating and abducting the shoulders to 90 degrees and flexes the elbows to 90 degrees. The patient then opens and closes the hands slowly for 3 minutes. If the patient is unable to keep the arms in the starting position for 3 minutes or suffers ischemic pain, heaviness or profound weakness in the arm, or numbness or tingling in the hand, the test is considered positive for the affected side. The test is often called the *positive abduction and external rotation (AER) position test,* the *hands-up test,* or the *elevated arm stress test (EAST test).*[48]

Spurling's (foraminal compression) test for nerve root compression, as well as pain with hyperextension of the cervical spine, will help to differentiate TOS from cervical nerve root impingement. In the Spurling's test, the patient side bends and rotates the head toward the same side with extension, and the examiner applies compression to the head. Neck pain with radiation constitutes a positive test.[48]

The use of x-rays is necessary to diagnose the existence of a cervical rib. A radiographic contrast study may objectively show a constriction of the subclavian artery and confirm the diagnosis of TOS. High-tech imaging is of little use in diagnosing TOS. Electromyography (EMG) and nerve-conduction testing often are used in the diagnostic process of TOS. However, if the EMG reveals compromise of one of the nerves or nerve roots, a diagnosis of nerve root compression also must be considered.

A concept called the *double-crush theory* was introduced by Upton and McComas[49] in 1973. This concept states that proximal nerve compression will render distal portions of the same nerve less tolerant of compression forces. Under this generally accepted theory, carpal tunnel syndrome or cubital tunnel syndrome is more likely to occur in a patient with TOS. It also would imply that a swimmer with signs and symptoms consistent with a distal upper extremity numbness, tingling, or weakness should be evaluated for a proximal nerve compression problem as well.

Treatment of TOS   TOS can be managed conservatively or with surgery. A nonsurgical approach is always preferable because there are potential complications with any surgery and no guarantee of good results. A surgical solution is reserved for those athletes with severe symptoms in whom conservative therapies have proven unsuccessful.

Nonsurgical treatment begins by decreasing inflammation. Compression of the brachial plexus results in inflammation and swelling of the nerves. Anti-inflammatory measures should provide relief from symptoms. Relief from the swelling and inflammation of the nerves not only decreases pain but also actually decreases mechanical compression of the nerves under the clavicle or scalene muscles.

Muscle imbalances and poor posture can contribute to compression of the neurovascular structures. The typical slouching posture of swimmers contributes to a downward pressure of the clavicle on the first rib, causing TOS. Exercises are directed at correction of postural abnormalities. The large chest and shoulder muscles of swimmers present their own complications in postural training for relief of TOS.

Muscle and myofascial tightness contributes to TOS, so myofascial release and a stretching program of the muscles about the upper quarter should begin immediately. Stretching the scalenes, pectoralis major and minor, trapezius, levator scapulae, and sternocleidomastoid muscles may lead to a decrease in the symptoms of TOS. It is important to assess the mobility of the first rib, which often is hypomobile and requires mobilization. Injury or dysfunction of the cervical spine also may play a role in TOS. A condition such as a whiplash injury or a cervical facet syndrome may lead to spasm of the scalene muscles causing compression of the neurovascular structures in the thoracic outlet. The cervical spine must be cleared via examination, and any dysfunction must be addressed as part of the treatment of TOS.

Elbow Injuries

Swimmers are coached to use a high elbow position during the pull phase of the freestyle stroke. This position may predispose the swimmer to increased strain on the medial elbow that may overload the medial collateral ligament and place the elbow at risk for injury.[50] A swimmer may drop the elbow during the pull-through phase to compensated for painful weakness at the elbow. This decreases the efficiency of the stroke and increases the stresses on the shoulder and common wrist extensor muscles and tendons. This can cause an overuse of the extensor carpi radialis brevis and extensor communis aponeurosis at the lateral epicondyle and result in inflammation. Lateral epicondylitis is a common injury in swimmers.[30,38]

Diagnosis of Lateral Epicondylitis The diagnosis of lateral epicondylitis can be made by physical examination. A positive finding for lateral epicondylitis would be increased pain over the lateral epicondyle on resisted contraction of the wrist extensors. More specific localization of the inflammation may be achieved by differentiating medial and ulnar components of wrist extension. Any of the orthopedic special tests used for diagnosing tennis elbow also would be appropriate for diagnosing lateral epicondylitis in swimmers.[48]

Treatment of Lateral Epicondylitis Treatment of lateral epicondylitis begins by addressing the inflammation of the specific tendons. The use of ice, NSAIDs, and other anti-inflammatory agents is incorporated as needed. Stroke mechanics must be evaluated and modified. The swimmer should avoid all strokes that are painful at the elbow. If a history reveals a repeated pattern of increased pain with use and decreased pain with rest, the swimmer probably has a chronic recurring tendinitis. This pattern is indicative of a breach in the tendon caused by the irregular healing of the tissue following multiple repeated microtears of the tendon. This type of injury lends itself to treatment with deep friction massage. Deep friction massage will realign the fibers of the tendons so that they decrease the irritation at the site of the injury, therefore breaking the cycle of rest-activity-reinjury.[51] It is important to assess the athlete's shoulder strength and begin the athlete on a wrist isometric program progressing to progressive resistance exercises.

Once the inflammation has been resolved and the integrity of the tendon reestablished, the swimmer will return to swimming with improved mechanics, gradually building speed and distance in the water. It is important to assess the biomechanics in the pool.

Triceps Strain

Diagnosis of Triceps Strain Other overuse injuries of the elbow include triceps strains and synovitis, which result mainly from the force of the elbow going into full extension during the backstroke.[50] A triceps strain will present as pain on resisted contraction of the triceps during clinical examination. Synovitis will show a freely movable joint with pain, mild warmth of the elbow, and some limitation of full extension.

Treatment of Triceps Strain Management of the inflammatory process is of primary importance, as in the other overuse injuries described. The analysis and alteration of stroke technique are especially important in long-term management of elbow injuries. Elbow braces have been used to limit the amount of elbow extension used during the swimming stroke. These braces are useful in preventing further stress in training while the acute inflammatory stage of the injury is managed but have limited use in long-term management of the condition because braces do not address the necessary changes in stroke mechanics. Braces are not worn during swimming competitions.

COMMON LOWER EXTREMITY INJURIES

Breaststroker's Knee

The most common knee injury in swimmers is a strain of the medial collateral ligament of the knee and is commonly referred to as *breaststroker's knee.* This is related to the forceful whip kick used in the breaststroke.[31] Breaststroker's knee is a chronic medial collateral ligament (MCL) sprain that results from repetitive stress on the MCL.[30,52] Symptoms of breaststroker's knee are point tenderness along the MCL and pain or abnormal joint opening on valgus stress testing.

Diagnosis of Breaststroker's Knee Since the mechanism of injury is low impact as compared with mechanisms of injury found in contact and collision sports, a valgus stress test is frequently found to be positive for pain but negative for ligamentous laxity. All other special tests of the knee will be negative. Laxity is a possibility with repeated use, so early intervention is the key to good recovery. It is also possible for hip adductor and abductor muscle strength and flexibility imbalances to be a contributing factor.[30]

Treatment of Breaststroker's Knee Treatment begins by addressing any swelling that may exist. Relative rest must be implemented in order to take the repeated valgus stress off the knee. This may mean refraining from swimming breaststroke until the acute swelling is under control. Returning the swimmer to the breaststroke includes minimizing breaststroke distance by cross-training with other strokes, ensuring adequate warm-up, increasing training distance gradually, and limiting distance to pain-free yardage.[38] Breaststroker's knee results primarily from the abnormal stresses to the knee inherent in the whip kick. The breaststroke swimmer should be instructed to keep the knee in alignment with the hip, allowing the knees to separate only to the width of the hips. This will decrease the lever arm toward a valgus stress at the knee as the legs are brought toward midline.

Other Knee Injuries

Other knee injuries related to swimming include patellofemoral pain, medial synovitis, and medial plica syndrome.[28] Patients who have patellofemoral pain syndrome commonly present with anterior knee pain beneath the patella. Anteromedial pain suggests medial synovitis or medial plica syndrome. These syndromes are usually treated with correction of stroke mechanics, relative rest, anti-inflammatory medication, strengthening, and stretching. Patellar tracking problems may require muscle reeducation techniques including biofeedback or taping techniques to realign the patellae during exercise. A detailed history including an in-depth review of the swimmer's dry-land exercise program is necessary. The stresses of running and weight lifting are likely to contribute to knee pain in swimmers.

Foot and Ankle Injuries

The most common injury to the foot and ankle in swimming is tendinitis of the extensor tendons at the extensor retinaculum caused by repeated extreme plantarflexion in the flutter kick and dolphin kick.[47] On examination, crepitus can be felt and heard when the foot is passively dorsiflexed. Treatment includes stretching and relative rest, followed by strengthening of the ankle musculature. It is difficult to eliminate the foot and ankle from any of the swim strokes and still use the lower extremities for kicking. Arm-only sets can be performed by placing a floatation device such as a pull-buoy between the thighs to assist the body in maintaining the appropriate buoyant position in the water.[38]

Less frequent foot and ankle problems include foot contusions, heel bruises, and ankle sprains from contact with the pool wall on flip turns or slipping on a wet pool deck or ladder. It is again important to assess the dry-land training program to make sure that any weight-bearing activities contributing to the foot and ankle problems are eliminated.

BACK AND NECK INJURIES

Back pain is a common complaint among competitive swimmers.[53,54] Diagnoses of back pain include mechanical low-back problems, spondylolysis, spondylolisthesis, and Scheuermann's kyphosis.[30,38] Low-back injuries in swimmers are caused most often by repetitive stress during turns and the strain of poor head and body position in the water.[47]

Treatment includes relative rest of the back by avoiding diving and flip turns.[28] Abdominal strengthening often is indicated because it is common for a swimmer to show an imbalance in strength of the trunk musculature due to the imbalance in swim training involving face-down swimming, which emphasizes work of the trunk extensors. Flexibility of the hamstrings and back extensors is very important in ensuring normal movement of the pelvis to which they attach.[9]

Scheuermann's kyphosis is the typical "swimmer's back" found in adolescent swimmers. This condition comes from repetitive flexion of the thoracic spine and frequently is aggravated by the butterfly stroke due to the complexity of the stroke and increased stresses caused by bilateral symmetrical use of the arms. Pain frequently is relieved by avoiding the butterfly stroke during training.[38] The butterfly stroke also involves repetitive hyperextension of the back, which may predispose the swimmer to spondylolysis. Spinal trauma from diving accidents is a concern in shallow pools, and divers should be instructed to dive only into the deep end of the pool. Starting blocks should be located only at the deep end.

The typical swimmer's posture presents as that of increased thoracic kyphosis, abducted and/or protracted scapulae, and a positioning of the head forward. This posturing is further reinforced in swimmers who suffer from recurrent nasal and sinus problems. Nasal and sinus infections, inflammation, or congestion are common among swimmers because of the exposure to bacteria and chemicals common in swimming pools. Swimmers who suffer from these problems usually experience difficulty breathing comfortably through their nose. Often this results in these individuals becoming habitual "mouth breathers." This is often observed best at night during sleep when the muscle tone of the air passages is decreased. Mouth breathing is best facilitated by postural extension of the head and neck to open up the air passages to allow improved airflow during inspiration when sleeping. This prolonged posturing during the sleeping hours results in an adaptive tightening of the subcranial ligaments and fascia, resulting in a tendency for the subcranial region to seek out a comfortable resting position of subcranial extension during postural activities. Subcranial extension during erect posture is nonfunctional in that it results in staring up at the sky. Therefore, a compensatory lowering of the eyes to the horizon is achieved through neck flexion, resulting in furthering of the forward head posture.

Postural exercises to encourage full range of motion of the cervical spine, including the subcranial region, thoracic spine, and lumbar spine, must be addressed. Any problems with breathing difficulties need to be addressed simultaneously for the reasons discussed previously.

Cervical Facet Syndrome

Freestyle swimming requires rotation of the head and neck in order to facilitate breathing during swimming. This puts the cervical spine through repetitive rotation on each breathing stroke cycle. Technique plays an important role in maintaining muscular balance and normal range of motion in the cervical spine. Lack of body roll will *increase* the degree of rotation that the cervical spine must go through with each breath. In addition, swimmers who breath only to one side will create an imbalance in musculature and range of motion to the side to which they breathe. Over time, these repetitive stresses will overstretch the ligaments at one or more levels of the cervical spine, possibly resulting in a dysfunctional positioning of the vertebrae at the facet joint.

A facet dysfunction presents as a painful condition of the neck, frequently accompanied by protective muscle guarding or muscle spasm. The swimmer may complain of difficulty moving the neck, particularly noticeable during freestyle swimming. Clinical examination will reveal asymmetrical active and passive movement of the head and neck on flexion and rotation and possibly side flexion of the neck, depending on the level of dysfunction. Intervertebral joint mobility testing will confirm the specific level of dysfunctional movement. This should be attempted only by skilled physical therapists and health care professionals with training in spinal joint mobility examination.

Treatment of cervical facet syndrome consists of resting the area, decreasing the muscle guarding or spasm, and reestablishing the normal movement of the dysfunctional vertebral segment through specific joint mobilization. Stretching of all tight musculature in the area needs to begin simultaneously, and the swimmer must correct the techniques that are contributing to the problem. A program of postural reeducation and strengthening completes the treatment program and will help stabilize the cervical spine during activity.

Neck Pain and Spontaneous Pneumomediastinum

Spontaneous pneumomediastinum (SPM) is usually a benign, self-limiting condition in which retrosternal chest pain is the most common complaint and subcutaneous emphysema is the most prevalent physical finding.[55] SPM may be caused by several conditions that allow free air to enter the mediastinal tissues but may be caused in swimmers by the frequent prolonged breath holding or performing the Valsalva maneu-

ver. Risk factors to consider include diabetic ketoacidosis, marijuana smoking, anorexia nervosa, bronchial and pulmonary function testing, and the use of illicit drugs such as heroin, cocaine, "ecstasy," and "speed."[56–58] SPM is relatively uncommon, but its occurrence is well documented in athletes. SPM is also known as *mediastinal emphysema*. SPM is the second leading cause for hospitalization in healthy individuals under the age of 30 who experience sudden chest pain or shortness of breath,[59,60] with spontaneous pneumothorax being the leading cause.

SPM is most often asymptomatic and resolves spontaneously. In swimmers, however, SPM has the potential to progress to a symptomatic stage due to the repetitive nature of the swim stroke and the frequent occurrence of breath holding during swim training and competition. Common signs include dyspnea, neck pain, weakness, dysphagia, sore throat, back pain, shoulder pain, swollen neck, and abdominal pain.[59,61] The presentation of pain can be confused with soft tissue strains or sprains. SPM also may present with symptoms of shortness of breath and difficulty swallowing, particularly after exertion or swimming.

Diagnosis of SPM The differential diagnosis requires ruling out a number of other diagnoses, including pulmonary embolism, panic disorder, exercise-induced bronchospasm or asthma, pneumothorax, cervical or mediastinal tumor, drug abuse, carotid thrombosis, cervical radiculopathy, foreign body aspiration, and esophageal stricture or tear. Chest radiographs can confirm the diagnosis.

An x-ray may reveal free air along the side of the mediastinum, with possible free air tracking up the deep cervical tissues and fascial layers behind the trachea and larynx. Computed tomography (CT) should be performed to determine the cause of the patient's pneumomediastinum and to rule out progression. Pneumothorax should be ruled out.

Hamman's sign, also known as "mediastinal crunch," is a crunching, rasping, or popping sound heard over the precordium that is synchronous with the heartbeat and sometimes is heard at a distance from the chest.[62]

Treatment of SPM There is some controversy over the treatment and management of SPM, and there are no evidence-based medical guidelines for the treatment of SPM. Some authors state that activity restrictions and avoidance of predisposing factors are unnecessary.[56,57,59,63] Others suggest hospital admission because of the potential for complications.[58,64] Although hospital admission is routine, some physicians believe that it is probably unnecessary unless SPM is associated with significant complications. Ferro and McKeag[17] promote a less conservative return-to-sport approach that involves careful monitoring and outpatient management.

Pneumomediastinum has been reported to resolve within 4 to 10 days[56–59,62,63] and appears to have a low recurrence rate, approximately 1 in 14 to 23 patients.[57,59,60] It seems reasonable, therefore, to allow an asymptomatic athlete to slowly resume full activity 7 to 10 days after symptoms occur, but only as long as there is no recurrence of symptoms.

Swimmers should be advised to refrain from swimming and exercise requiring breath holding for at least 1 week. On return to swimming, the swimmer must build up gradually in both speed and endurance, and diving into the pool should be avoided. On any return or increase in symptoms, the swimmer must stop all athletic activity and return to the physician for reexamination. The swimmer will be required to stop all athletics until all symptoms resolve. Resolution of the pain alone is not sufficient for return to swimming. Signs such as dysphagia and anxiety are sufficient to suspect that the condition of SPM is not fully resolved.

A chest radiograph and CT scan might be considered for follow-up testing to ensure that the patient's condition has resolved fully and to definitively rule out any underlying pathology.

COMMON MEDICAL PROBLEMS IN SWIMMERS

Breathing Problems

Breathing problems associated with swimming include asthma, sinus irritation, and sinus infections. Asthma is seen more frequently in swimming than in any other sport. This is probably because children diagnosed with asthma frequently are encouraged to begin swimming for exercise since the high-humidity environment of the pool is good for their breathing difficulties.[65] Cold, dry environments aggravate the symptoms of asthma. Control of the pool environment is critical for swimmers with asthma, since a poorly ventilated indoor pool will result in a buildup of chlorine gases given off by the water, causing an exacerbation of the symptoms of asthma.[66] Coaches must be aware of swimmers' preexisting medical conditions because swimmers with asthma must have their medication inhalers readily available at the pool.

Chronic sinus irritation and repeated or chronic sinus infections are common among swimmers because of frequent contact of their nasal passages with the water. Chemical imbalances in the water environment can cause unnecessary infections or sinus irritation. If the chemical balance is too low, swimmers are exposed to a high level of bacteria, resulting in infections in the sinuses or other body cavities. An excessively high level of chemicals can irritate the sinuses, causing obstructive breathing problems. Swimmers who experience repeated or chronic breathing problems should be referred to a physician who specializes in ear, nose, and throat disorders. Breathing problems will have a significant effect on physical performance in and out of the pool and can lead to a multitude of physical and medical problems.

Dermatologic Problems

Swimmers incur a variety of dermatologic problems. Many swimmers shave their body hair to decrease their resistance in the water. This practice should be reserved for the championship phase of the season because repetitive shaving increase the swimmers' risk for folliculitis. Repeated shaving with a safety blade razor removes superficial layers of the epidermis and increases the risk of minor cuts from the razor. This exposes the athlete to skin infections from *Pseudomonas* or *Staphylococcus* organisms. Mild folliculitis may be treated with topical antibiotics, whereas more extensive cases may require oral antibiotics. Prevention of repeated skin infections should be taken seriously, especially if they result in the need to take oral antibiotics. Repeated use of oral antibiotics can disrupt the normal balance of bacteria in the digestive tract, resulting in intestinal tract problems.

Blonde swimmers are subject to "green hair syndrome" caused by copper-based algicides used in some pools. Using a swim cap, shampooing immediately after swimming, and applying 3% hydrogen peroxide lotion helps to prevent this syndrome.[65] Darker-haired swimmers may have problems with bleaching of their hair from repeated exposure to chlorine. Bleaching also may be minimized by using a swim cap and shampooing immediately after swimming. Special shampoos and conditioners are readily available that may provide further protection for the hair.

Foot Infections

Fungal skin infections are common in swimmers and are referred to as *tinea*. Tinea is most prevalent on areas of the body that are subject to dark, moist environment such as found on the feet and toes (tinea pedis), groin (tinea cruis), and under the nails of the fingers and toes (tinea unguium). Tinea will re-

sult in a reddened, scaling, peeling, or cracking area on the skin, often emitting a pungent odor. Fungal infections under the nails will result in a yellowing and discoloration of the nails. Athlete's foot and "jock itch" are most frequently treated successfully with over-the-counter antifungal medications. However, fungal infections of the nails may require a prescription-strength antifungal agent to reach the source of the problems. Many fungal infections can be prevented by drying between the toes, in the groin, and under the arms. Wearing sandals will prevent exposure to fungus transmitted from pool decks and locker room floors.[47]

Tinea versicolor is a common superficial fungal infection of the skin that is most common in warm, humid climates. Tinea versicolor is commonly found on the scalp, shoulders, and upper back but may occur anywhere on the skin. The swimmer may first notice symptoms of splotchy coloring and/or scaling of the skin that appears to get worse with tanning of the skin by the sun. The patches of fungus actually prevent the sun from tanning the skin evenly. Diagnosis via use of a Wood's light (black light) will reveal a yellow-orange fluorescence, indicating the presence of the fungus. Topical agents including shampoos containing selenium sulfide (Selsun Gold or Exsel) are successful in the treatment of tinea versicolor, although recurrence is common. The athlete should shampoo the scalp vigorously and then lather the shampoo onto all affected body areas, allowing the shampoo to dry. The athlete then scrubs the skin in the morning to help remove the scales of tinea versicolor.

Viral warts are also common in swimmers. Warts present as a small nodular lesion on the skin. Warts can occur anywhere on the skin but are common on the hands and feet. On the feet, it is difficult to distinguish a wart from a callus. Examination of the potential wart through a magnifying lens will reveal tiny dots or thrombosed capillaries and disruption of the skin lines, which would not be the case with a callus. Warts can be treated with over-the-counter topical agents, but if the wart persists more than 2 weeks, the swimmer should be referred to a dermatologist. The dermatologist will have a stronger topical agent to destroy the wart or may use cryotherapy, laser vaporization, or surgical excision to eradicate the wart. Warts should not be ignored or taken lightly because they can grow deep, necessitating a more radical surgical procedure. Warts are viral in nature and can spread from one area of the body to another and from one individual to another. Molluscum contageosum is highly contagious and can mimic the presentation of folliculitis.

Sun damage is the most common injury to the skin among swimmers and ranges from premature aging (including wrinkling of the skin) to a deadly form of skin cancer called *malignant melanoma*. Premature aging of the skin as well as less dramatic forms of skin cancer (basal and squamous cell carcinoma) are the result of excessive sun exposure over several years of swimming. Malignant melanoma is thought to be related to a history of burn and peel in the early teen years or even prior to puberty. Light-skinned, light-haired, light-eyed individuals are at particularly high risk for acquiring malignant melanoma. The use of sun screens of SPF-15 value or greater is thought to be of significant value in preventing sun damage and cancers of the skin. Be sure to choose a full-spectrum sun screen intended to screen out both ultraviolet A and ultraviolet B rays. Sun screens must be reapplied often because they wash off during time in the water. Clothing and hats with large brims should be made of tightly woven fabrics and worn at all times that the swimmer is not in the water. It is said that 1 in 100 Americans will develop malignant melanoma within their lifetime, and this number is expected to increase to 1 in 75 for individuals born in the year 2000. Coaches, trainers, and therapists should edu-

cate their athletes in the area of good skin care and skin cancer prevention.

Swimmer's Ear

Otitis externa, or "swimmer's ear," is a common infection found in swimmers. Swimmer's ear is usually caused by *Pseudomonas aeruginosa* or, occasionally, *Aspergillus* organisms. Swimmer's ear presents as pain and/or itching in one or both ears. The swimmer may report tenderness on touching the ear. Tragal tenderness and pain on auricle manipulation are noted on examination, and inflammation and erythema of the ear canal will be seen via otoscope. Treatment includes either colistin sulfate or polymyxin B-neomycin-hydrocortisone. The suspension forms of these medications are preferred because they have a more neutral pH than the solution forms and thus are less harmful to a perforated eardrum.[67] Occasionally, the pain may be severe enough to warrant pain medications.

The swimmer should avoid getting additional water into the ear. This may mean that the swimmer avoids swim training for 7 to 10 days. Swimmers may return to swimming in 2 to 3 days if the pain has resolved and the athlete can tolerate alcohol ear drops used after swimming. Recurrences of swimmer's ear are common but can be reduced through the routine use of eardrops of isopropanol and vinegar solution applied after swimming and showering.[67] Solutions containing boric acid found in common over-the-counter eardrops may remove the protective coating of cerumen in the ear, especially when use repetitively by competitive swimmers. This may make the swimmer vulnerable to more severe ear infections.

Swimmers tend to adapt to bacteria found in their home pool. Swimming in an "away" pool may expose the swimmer to different levels of bacteria that he or she is not used to, putting the swimmer at risk to contracting swimmer's ear.[67] Coaches and swimmers should take this into account and use additional precautions and preventative measures to avoid developing an infection.

Wax earplugs are sometimes used to prevent water from entering the ear. However, they may trap bacteria, further increasing the risk of infection. A tight-fitting swim cap may be the best method of keeping water out of the ear. Self-manipulation of the ear and use of cotton swabs to remove water actually may drive the water deeper into the ear and should be avoided. The use of cotton swab sticks may damage the inner surface of the ear and also should be avoided.[68]

Eye Problems

The most common eye problem seen among swimmers is conjunctivitis. Conjunctivitis is caused most often by chlorine irritation.[47] Goggles are often used by competitive swimmers to decrease the exposure of the eyes to the chemicals in the water. Use of goggles is complicated by an inherent tendency for the lenses to fog, which is often addressed by using antifog agents in coating the lenses prior to swimming. These antifog agents also can cause irritation to the eyes, resulting in conjunctivitis. Adenovirus types 3 and 4 have been reported to spread in pools and can result in viral infections of the eyes. Over-the-counter eye drops or ophthalmic cromolyn sodium works well to resolve infections of the eyes.[47] Redness or itching of the eyes that does not seem to be improving within 24 hours of the use of over-the-counter drops should be examined by a physician. Swim goggles are very effective in preventing exposure to the chemicals in pool water when fitted appropriately. Goggles must be worn by the swimmer as part of the treatment of eye infections. Continued exposure to the water's chemicals in the presence of an eye infection will be counterproductive to successful treatment of the infection. During treatment of an eye infection, the swimmer should avoid anything that would irritate the eye. This in-

cludes prolonged exposure to direct sunlight and the drying effects of the wind. Sun glasses that wrap around the sides of the eyes and are fitted with ultraviolet protective lenses will protect the eyes from irritation from the sun and the wind.

Returning to Swimming

Rest is an integral part of the healing and rehabilitation process. In most cases, total rest from all swim activities will meet with very poor compliance by both coaches and athletes. The detrimental effect of complete rest on athletic performance is well supported in the literature. In a 1985 study, Costill et al.[40] reported that a period of interruption from training had significant deconditioning effects on swimmers and showed metabolic changes in the muscles of such swimmers. The concept of *relative rest* outlines a program of rest in which the injured structure is rested, but the swimmer is kept active with alternative swimming activities and dry-land exercises that do not stress the injured structure. The injured athlete should return to a modified swim program as soon as possible so long as relative rest is achieved. This does not mean that the swimmer is ready to return to competition or even practice his or her specific event.

Swimmers may experience injuries such as meniscus or anterior crucial ligament tears, which occur in adolescents who engage in sports and recreational activities. Special considerations apply to returning these swimmers to a regular training program for swimming. If these swimmers are treated conservatively for these injuries, then the swimmers should go through a thorough muscle strengthening program prior to returning to swimming. Swimmers should return gradually to swimming workouts, within limits of their pain. Isokinetic strength testing may be used to document the strength of the injured extremity and to compare with the uninjured extremity. Once strength is at least 90 percent of the contralateral extremity, then return to full athletic competition may begin. Even though swimming is not a contact or collision sport, the strength demands are significant. The repetitive nature of the swim stroke and kick makes the swim athlete vulnerable to reinjuring the joints if he or she returns to swimming prematurely. In the early phase of return to swimming, the swimmer should avoid high loads on the knee, such as may occur during the breaststroke kick. Different strokes should be used, and the swimmer may use pulling sets with avoidance of kicking. The swimmer should be assessed carefully for signs of pain and instability related to the underlying injury.

Returning to swim training and competition following injury or illness depends on effective communication among the athlete, coaches, parents, and all health care professionals involved in the athlete's care. There is no real challenge in returning the athlete to competition quickly. The challenge to everyone involved is to return the athlete to competition quickly and *safely*.

Summary

The sport of swimming presents a unique challenge to athletes, coaches, and health care professionals alike. The unique environment of the water poses significant challenges to the human body as it moves in a race against the clock and results in a wide array of injuries and illnesses. It is very important for health care professionals to understand the specific demands of the sport of swimming in order to successfully diagnose and treat these injuries and illnesses. In turn, it is equally important for coaches and swim athletes to understand the nature of the healing and rehabilitation process in order to get compliance with therapeutic regimes in the management of these problems. When the athlete, coach, and health care professionals reach this understanding of each other's role in competitive swimming, a positive outcome will result. Competitive swimming is a sport that can be enjoyed by athletes over a period of many years at a number of competitive levels. The incidence of illness and injury in competitive swimming will be significantly reduced as a result of effective training, coaching, treatment, and rehabilitation.

Acknowledgments

We would like to thank Terry Laughlin and Judy Van Atta for their contributions.

References

1. Richardson AB: Injuries in competitive swimming. *Clin Sports Med* 18(2):287–291,1999.
2. Kammer CS, Young CC, Niedfeldt MW: Swimming injuries and illnesses. *Phys Sports Med* 27(4):51, 1999.
3. Ciullo JV, Stevens GG: Prevention and treatment of injuries to the shoulder in swimming. *Sports Med* 7(3):182–204, 1989.
4. Troup JP: The physiology and biomechanics of competitive swimming. *Clin Sports Med* 18(2):267–285, 1999.
5. Jones JH: Swimming Overuse injuries. *Phy Med Rehabil Clin North Am* 10(1):77–94, 1999.
6. Richardson AB, Jobe FW, Collins HR: The shoulder in competitive swimming. *Am J Sports Med* 8:159–163, 1980.
7. Richardson AB: Thoracic outlet syndrome in aquatic athletes. *Clin Sports Med* 18(2): 361–378, 1999.

8. Pink M, Perry J, Browne A, et al: The normal shoulder during freestyle swimming: An electromyographic and cinematographic analysis of twelve muscles. *Am J Sports Med* 19:569–576, 1991.

9. Levangie PK, Norkin CC: *Joint Structure and Function*, 3d ed. Philadelphia: FA Davis, 2001.

10. Prentice WE: *Rehabilitation Techniques in Sports Medicine*. New York: McGraw-Hill, 1999.

11. Piette G, Clarys JP: Telemetric EMG of the front crawl movement, in Terauds J, Bedingfield W (eds): *Swimming III*. Baltimore: University Park Press, 1979, pp 153–158.

12. Ferrell MC: The spine in swimming. *Clin Sports Med* 18(2):389–393, 1999.

13. Rodeo SA: Knee pain in competitive swimming. *Clin Sports Med* 18(2):379–387, 1999.

14. Ciullo JV: Swimmer's shoulder. *Clin Sports Med* 5(1):115–137, 1986.

15. McMaster WC: Anterior glenoid labrum damage: A painful lesion in swimmers. *Am J Sports Med* 14:383–387, 1986.

16. Miller JW: Injuries and considerations in master's aquatic sports. *Clin Sports Med* 18(2):413–426, 1999.

17. Ferro RT, McKeag DB: Spontaneous pneumomediastinum presentation and return-to-play considerations, in Harmon KG (ed): *American Medical Society for Sports Medicine Case Report Series*.

18. Simon LM: Aquatic Sports, in Sallis RE, Massimo F (eds): *Essentials of Sportsmedicine*. St. Louis: Mosby–Year Book, 1997, pp 592–601.

19. Baechle TR: *Essentials of Strength Training and Conditioning*. Champaign, IL: Human Kinetics, 2000.

20. Jager T: Swimming, in Roberts SO (ed): *Winning Edge Series*. New York: McGraw Hill, 1999.

21. Brukner P, Khan K: *Clinical Sports Medicine*. Sydney, Australia: McGraw-Hill Book Company, 1993.

22. Prentice WE: A comparison of static stretching and PNF stretching for improving joint flexibility. *Athl Train* 18(1):56–59, 1983.

23. Beaulieu JE: *Stretching for All Sports*. Pasadena, CA: Athletic Press, 1980.

24. Magnusson SP, Constantini NW, McHugh MP, et al: Strength profiles and performance in master's level swimmers. *Am J Sports Med* 23(5):626–631, 1995.

25. Corbin CB, Dowell LJ, Lindsey R, Tolson H: *Concepts in Physical Education*. Dubuque, IA: Charles C Brown, 1978.

26. Hawley JA, Williams MM: Relationship between upper body anaerobic power and freestyle swimming. *Int J Sport Med* 12:1–5, 1991.

27. Inbar O, Bar-Or O: Relationship of anaerobic arm and leg capacities to swimming performance of 8–12 year old children, in Shepard RJ, Lavalle H (eds): *Frontier of Activity and Child Health*. Quebec: Pelican, 1997, pp 83–292.

28. Kenal KA, Knapp LD: Rehabilitation of injuries in competitive swimmers. *Sports Med* 22(5):337–347, 1996.

29. Zemek MJ, Magee DJ: Comparison of glenohumeral joint laxity in elite and recreational swimming. *Clin J Sports Med* 6:40–47, 1996.

30. Fowler PJ: Swimming, in Fu FH, Stone DA (eds): *Sports Injuries: Mechanisms, Prevention, Treatment*. Baltimore: Williams and Wilkins, 1994, pp 633–648.

31. McMaster WC: Painful shoulder in swimmers: A diagnostic challenge. *Phys Sports Med* 14(12):108–122, 1986.

32. McMaster WC, Long S, Caiozzo V: Shoulder torque changes in swimming athletes. *Am J Sports Med* 20:323–327, 1992.

33. Warner JJ, Micheli LJ, Arslanian LE, et al: Patterns of flexibility, laxity, and strength in normal shoulders and in shoulders with instability. *Am J Sports Med* 18:366–375, 1990.

34. Greipp JF: Swimmer's shoulder: The influence of flexibility and weight training. *Phys Sports Med* 13(8):92–105, 1985.

35. Bak K, Magnusson SP: Shoulder strength and range of motion in symptomatic and pain-free elite swimmers. *Am J Sports Med* 25(4):454–459, 1997.

36. Koehler SM, Thorson DC: Swimmer's shoulder: targeting treatment. *Phys Sports Med* 24(11):39–50, 1996.

37. Stocker D, Pink M, Jobe FW: Comparison of shoulder injury in collegiate- and master's-level swimmers. *Clin J Sports Med* 5(1):4–8, 1995.

38. Fowler PJ, Webster-Bogart MS: Swimming, in Reider B (ed): *Sports Medicine: The School-Age*

Athlete, 2d ed. Philadelphia: Saunders, 1996, pp 471–489.

39. Troup JP, Hollander AP, Bone M, et al: Performance-related differences in the anaerobic contribution of competitive freestyle swimmers. *J Sports Sci* 9:106–107, 1991.

40. Costill DL, Flynn MG, Kirwan JP, et al: The effects of repeated days of intensified training on muscle glycogen and swimming performance. *Med Sci Sports Exerc* 20:249–254, 1988.

41. Ivy JL, Katz AL, Cutler CL, et al: Muscle glycogen utilization during prolonged strenuous exercise when fed carbohydrate. *J Appl Physiol* 65:1703–1709, 1986.

42. McMaster WC: Swimming injuries: An overview. *Sports Med* 22(5):332–336, 1996.

43. McMaster WC, Roberts A, Stoddard T: A correlation between shoulder laxity and interfering pain in competitive swimmers. *Am J Sports Med* 26:83–86, 1998.

44. Fry AC: Resistance exercise overtraining and overreaching, neuroendocrine responses. *Sports Med* 23(2):106–129, 1997.

45. Lehmann M, Dickhutn H, Gendrisch G, et al: Training overtraining: A prospective, experimental study with experienced middle and long-distance runners. *Int J Sports Med* 12:444–452, 1991.

46. McMaster WC: Painful shoulder in swimmers: A diagnostic challenge. *Phys Sports Med* 14:108–122, 1986.

47. Hammer RW: Swimming and diving, in Mellion MB, Walsh WM, Shelton GL (eds): *The Team Physician's Handbook,* 3d ed. Philadelphia: Hanley and Belfus, 1997, pp 718–728.

48. Magee DJ: *Orthopedic Assessment.* Philadelphia: Saunders, 1997.

49. Upton AR, McComas AJ: The double-crush in nerve-entrapment syndromes. *Lancet* 2:359–362, 1973.

50. Johnson DC: The upper extremity in swimming, in Pettrone FA (ed): *AAOS Symposium on Upper Extremity Injuries in Athletes.* St Louis: Mosby, 1984, pp 36–46.

51. Tappan FM: *Healing Massage Techniques,* 2d ed. Norwalk, CT: Appleton and Lange, 1988.

52. Kennedy JC, Hawkins RJ, Krissoff WB: Orthopaedic manifestations of swimming. *Am J Sports Med* 6(6):309–322, 1978.

53. Bak K: Injuries in swimmers, locomotor system injuries in competitive swimmers. *Ugeskr Laeger* 152:2220–2224, 1990.

54. Goldstein JD, Berger PE, Windler GE, et al: Spine injuries in gymnastics and swimmers. *Am J Sports Med* 19:463–468, 1991.

55. Ferro RT, McKeag DB: Spontaneous pneumomediastinum presentation and return-to-play considerations, in Harmon KG (ed): *American Medical Society for Sports Medicine Case Report Series.*

56. Morgan EJ, Henderson DA: Pneumomediastinum as a complication of athletic competition. *Thorax* 36(2):155–156, 1981.

57. Pittman JA, Pounsford JC: Spontaneous pneumomediastinum and Ecstasy abuse. *J Accid Emerg Med* 14(5):335–336, 1997.

58. Onwudike M: Ecstasy induced retropharyngeal emphysema. *J Accid Emerg Med* 13(5):359–361, 1996.

59. Abolnik I, Lossos IS, Breuer R: Spontaneous pneumomediastinum: A report of 25 cases. *Chest* 100(1):93–95, 1991.

60. Yellin A, Lidji M, Lieberman Y: Recurrent spontaneous pneumomediastinum: The first reported case (letter). *Chest* 83(6):935, 1983.

61. Munsell WP: Pneumomediastinum: A report of 28 cases and review of the literature. *JAMA* 202(8):689–693, 1967.

62. Hamman L: Spontaneous mediastinal emphysema. *Bull Johns Hopkins Hosp* 64:1–21, 1939.

63. Bouwen L, Bosmans E: Posttraumatic pneumomediastinum: Not always cause for alarm. *Acta Chir Belg* 97(3):145–147, 1997.

64. Joshi JM: Spontaneous pneumomediastinum: Cause and consequence. *J Assoc Phys India* 44(11):829–831, 1996.

65. Sarnaik AP, Vohra MP, Sturman SW, et al: Medical problems of the swimmer. *Clin Sports Med* 5(1):47–64, 1986.

66. Potts J: Factors associated with respiratory problems in swimmers. *Sports Med* 21(4):256–261, 1996.

67. Schelkun PH: Swimmer's ear: Getting patients back in the water. *Phys Sports Med* 19(7):85–90, 1991.

68. Eichel BS: How I manage external otitis in competitive swimmers. *Phys Sports Med* 14(8):108–116, 1986.

Additional Readings

Ackland TR, Mazza JC, Carter L, et al: A survey of physique of world champion aquatic athletes. *Sports Coach* 14:10–11, 1991.

Araujo CG: Somatotyping of top swimmers by the health-carter method, in *Swimming Medicine IV*. Baltimore: University Park Press, 1978, pp 188–199.

Arborelius M Jr, Balldin UI, Lilja B, et al: Hemodynamic changes in man during immersion with the head above water. *Aerospace Med* 43: 592–598, 1972.

Astrand PO, Rodahl K: *Textbook of Work Physiology*. New York: McGraw-Hill, 1986.

Bardzukas AP, Trappe TA, Jozsi AC, et al: The effects of hydrating on thermal load and plasma volume during high intensity swimming training. *Med Sci Sports Exerc* 25:S20, 1993.

Bergstrom J, Hultman E: Nutrition for maximal sports performance. *JAMA* 221:999–1006, 1972.

Berning JR: The effect of carbohydrate feedings on four-hour swimmers, in Troup JP (ed): *International Center for Aquatic Research Annual*. Colorado Springs, CO: US Swimming Press, 1992, pp 145–149.

Boening D, Ulmer HV, Meier U, et al: Effects of a multi-hour immersion on trained and untrained subjects: Renal function and plasma volume. *Aerospace Med* 43:300–305, 1972.

Burke RE: Motor units: Anatomy, physiology, and functional organization, in Brooks VB (ed): *Handbook of Physiology*, sec 1: *The Nervous System II*. Washington: American Physiological Society, 1981, pp 345–422.

Butterfield G: Amino acids and high protein diets, in Lamb DR, Williams MH (eds): *Ergogenics: Enhancement of Exercise and Sports Performance*, vol 4 of *Perspectives in Exercise Science and Sports Medicine*. Carmel, IN: Benchmark Press, 1991, pp 87–122.

Cappaert JM: The importance of propelling and mechanical efficiencies, in Troup JP (ed): *International Center for Aquatic Research Annual*. Colorado Springs, CO: US Swimming Press, 1991, pp 75–80.

Cappaert JM, Bone M, Troup JP: Intensity and performance related differences in propelling and mechanical efficiencies, in Mac Laren D, Reilly T, Lees A (eds): *Swimming Science VI*. London: E & FN Spon, 1992, pp 53–56.

Clarys JP: Human body dimensions and applied hydrodynamics: Selection criteria for top swimmers. *SNIPES J* 23:32–41, 1986.

Costill DL, Fink WJ, Hargreaves M, et al: Metabolic characteristics of skeletal muscle during detraining from competitive swimming. *Med Sci Sports Exerc* 17:339–343, 1985.

Costill DL, Maglischo EW, Richardson AB: *Swimming*. London: Blackwell Scientific, 1992.

Costill DL, Miller J: Nutrition for endurance sport: Carbohydrate and fluid balance. *Int J Sports Med* 1:2–14, 1980.

Counsilman JE: Hypoxic and other methods of training evaluated. *Swimming Techniques* 12: 19–26, 1975.

Counsilman JE: *The Science of Swimming*. Upper Saddle River, NJ: Prentice-Hall, 1968.

Craig AB: Summary of 58 cases of consciousness underwater during swimming. *Med Sci Sports* 8:171–175, 1976.

Craig AB: The fallacies of hypoxic training in swimmers, in Terauds J, Bedingfield W (eds): *Swimming III*. Baltimore: University Park Press, 1979, pp 235–239.

Craig AB, Dvorak M: Thermal regulation of man exercising during water immersion. *J Appl Physiol* 25:28–35, 1968.

Faulkner JA: Physiology swimming and diving, in Falls HB (ed): *Exercise Physiology*. New York: Academic Press, 1968, pp 415–416.

Galbo H, Houston ME, Christensen NJ, et al: Hormonal response of swimming man. *Acta Physiol Scand* 105:326–337, 1979.

Gollnick PD, Armstrong RB, Sawbert CW, et al: Enzyme activity and fiber composition in skeletal muscle of trained and untrained men. *J Appl Physiol* 3:312–319, 1972.

Gullstrand L, Holmer I: Physiological responses to swimming with controlled frequency of breathing. *Scand J Sports Sci* 2:1–6, 1980.

Gullstrand L, Lawrence S: Heart rate and blood lactate response to short intermittent work at race pace in highly trained swimmers. *Aust J Sci Med Sport* 19:10–14, 1987.

Hay JG: *The Biomechanics of Sports Techniques*. Upper Saddle River, NJ: Prentice-Hall, 1985, pp 343–394.

Hayward JS, Eckerson JD, Collis ML: Thermoregulatory heat production in man: Prediction equation based on skin and core temperatures. *J Appl Physiol* 42:377–384, 1977.

Hollander AP, Troup JP, Bone M, et al: Estimation of the anaerobic contribution to energy consumption in swimming different distances. *J Sports Sci* 9:87–88, 1991.

Holmer I: Physiology of swimming man. *Exerc Sports Sci Rev* 7:87–124, 1979.

Holmer I, Bergh U: Metabolic and thermal responses to swimming in water at varying temperatures. *J Appl Physiol* 37:702–705, 1974.

Huijing PA: Mechanical muscle models, in Komi PV (ed): *Strength and Power in Sports*. London: Blackwell Scientific, 1992, pp 151–168.

Kavouras SA: *Growth, Maturation and Performance Evaluation of Elite Age Group Swimmers: 1992 United States Swimming Camp Report*. Colorado Springs, CO: US Swimming Press, 1993.

Kavouras SA: *Developmental Stages of Competitive Swimmers: 1991 United States Swimming Camp Report*. Colorado Springs, CO: US Swimming Press, 1992.

Khosla SS, Dubois AB: Osmoregulation and interstitial fluid pressure changes in humans during water immersion. *J Appl Physiol* 51:686–692, 1981.

Lange L, Lange S, Echt M, et al: Heart volume in relation to body posture and immersion in a thermo-neutral bath. *Pfluegers Arch* 352:219–226, 1974.

Lavoie JM, Taylor AW, Montpetit RR: Histochemical and biochemical profile of elite swimmers before and after six month training period, in Poortmans J, Nisert G (eds): *Biochemistry of Exercise*. Baltimore: University Park Press, 1981, pp 259–266.

Lemon PW, Proctor DN: Protein intake and athletic performance. *Sports Med* 12:313–325, 1991.

Magel JR: Comparison of the physiologic response to varying intensities of submaximal work in tethered swimming and treadmill running. *J Sports Med Phys Fitness* 11:203–312, 1971.

Malina RM, Bouchard C: *Growth, Maturation, and Physical Activity*. Champaign, IL: Human Kinetics, 1988.

McArdle WD, Glaser RM, Magel JR: Metabolic and cardiorespiratory response during free swimming and treadmill walking. *J Appi Physiol* 30:733–738, 1971.

McArdle WD, Magel JR, Lesmes GR, et al: Metabolic and cardiovascular adjustment to work in air and water at 18, 25 and 33°C. *J Appl Physiol* 40:85–90, 1976.

McCally M: *Body Fluid Volumes and Renal Response of Human Subjects to Water Immersion*. AMRL-TR-65-115. Aerospace Medical Research Laboratories, Wright-Patterson Air Force Base, 1965.

McMurray RG, Horvath SM: Thermoregulation in swimmers and runners. *J Appl Physiol* 46:1086–1092, 1979.

Medbo JI, Burgers S: Effect of training on the anaerobic capacity. *Med Sci Sports Exerc* 22:501–507, 1990.

Medbo JI, Mohn A-C, Tabata I, et al: Anaerobic capacity determined by maximal accumulated O_2 deficit. *J Appl Physiol* 64:50–60, 1988.

Montpetit R, Duvallet A, Cazorla G, et al: The relative stability of maximal aerobic power in elite swimmers and its relation to training performance. *J Swim Res* 3:15–18, 1987.

Nadel ER: Thermal and energetic exchanges during swimming, in Nadel ER (ed): *Problems with Temperature Regulation During Exercise*. New York: Academic Press, 1977, pp 91–119.

Nadel ER, Holmer I, Bergh U, et al: Energy exchanges of swimming man. *J Appl Physiol* 36:465–471, 1974.

Newsholme EA: Basic aspects of metabolic regulation and their application to provision of energy in exercise, in Hebbelinck M, Shephard RJ (eds): *Principles of Exercise Biochemistry*. Basel: Karger, 1988, pp 40–77.

Nielsen B: Temperature regulation during exercise in water and air. *Acta Physiol Scand* 98:500–508, 1976.

Nygaard E, Nielsen E: Skeletal muscle fiber capillarisation with extreme endurance training in Man, in Eriksson B, Furberg B (eds): *Swimming Medicine IV: Proceedings of the Fourth International Congress on Swimming Medicine*. Baltimore: University Park Press, 1978, pp 282–293.

Olbrecht J, Mader A, Heck H, et al: Importance of a calculation scheme to support the interpretation of lactate tests, in MacLaren D, Reilly T,

Lees A (eds): *Swimming Science VI*. London: E & FN Spon, 1992, pp 243–249.

Prins J: Muscles and their function, in Flavel ER (ed): *Biokinetics Strength Training*. Albany, CA: Isokinetics, 1981, pp 72–77.

Rohrs DM, Mayhew JL, Arabas C, et al: The relationship between seven anaerobic tests and swim performance. *J Swim Res* 6:15–19, 1990.

Saltin B: Metabolic fundamentals in exercise. *Med Sci Sports Exerc* 5:137–146, 1973.

Schleihauf RE: A hydrodynamic analysis of swimming propulsion, in Hollander AP, Huijing PA, De Groot G (eds): *Swimming III*. Champaign, IL: Human Kinetics, 1979, pp 173–183.

Shamus J, Shamus E: A taping technique for the treatment of acromioclavicular joint sprains: A case study. *JOSPT* 25:390–394, 1997.

Sharp RL, Armstrong LE, King DS, et al: Buffer capacity of blood in trained and untrained males, in Knuttgen HG, Vogel JA, Poortmans J (eds): *Biochemistry of Exercise*. Champaign, IL: Human Kinetics, 1983, pp 595–599.

Strass D: Effects of maximal strength training on sprint performance of competitive swimmers, in Ungerechts BE, Wilke K. Reischle K (eds): *Swimming Science V*. Champaign, IL: Human Kinetics, 1988, pp 149–156.

Toussaint HM: Mechanics and energetics of swimming. Ph.D. dissertation, Vrije Universiteit Amsterdam, 1988.

Troup JP: *International Center for Aquatic Research Annual, 1989–1990*. Colorado Springs, CO: US Swimming Press, 1990.

CHAPTER 6

Diving

Brian J. Tovin
Megan Neyer

The roots of competitive diving can be traced to the seventeenth century, when gymnasts moved their equipment to the beaches, and acrobatics over the water became a part of their training.[1] Modern diving achieved international notice in the 1904 Olympics in St. Louis when the platform was included as an event on the men's swimming program. Three-meter springboard diving was added for the 1908 games in London. In the 1920s, the sport evolved from "plain high diving" to "fancy high diving" because the athletes performed more difficult dives.

Since 1904, Olympic diving has changed tremendously and is still progressing at a rapid pace. In the early days of the sport, 14 different dives were used on the platform, and 20 different dives were used on the springboard. Today, 63 different dives can be used in competition on the 1-m springboard, 77 dives on the 3-m springboard, and 97 dives on the platform. The degree of difficulty of each dive also has evolved. A double somersault performed from the platform was considered dangerous in 1904. Elite divers today perform reverse three and a half somersaults on a routine basis. Similar to gymnastics, the sport of diving continues to evolve as more difficulty is added to the dives.

Biomechanics of Diving

Six different groups of dives exist in competitive diving.[1] The first four groups are classified based on the position the diver is in when leaving the board or platform. In a *forward* dive, the diver is facing the front of the board or platform and dives or somersaults forward toward the water. In a *backward* dive, the diver stands at the edge of the board or platform and faces inward, with the back to the water. The dive or somersault moves backward to the water. A *reverse* dive, sometimes referred to as a *gainer*, begins the same way as a forward dive, but after the diver leaves the board or platform, the rotation of the dive is backward, toward the board. An *inward* dive begins the same way as a backward dive, but the diver rotates forward, toward the board or platform. The fifth group is comprised of dives that include a *twisting* motion added to the somersaults. The final group is only used on the platform and includes dives that begin with an *armstand* (handstand).

DIVE COMPONENTS

Several elements compose a dive: the approach/hurdle, press/take-off, flight, and entry.[1] The approach and hurdle are used only for forward dives, reverse dives, forward twisting dives, and reverse twisting dives on the springboard. On the platform, an approach and hurdle are only used for forward dives.

Approach/Hurdle

The approach for the forward and reverse groups of dives is similar on the springboard. The diver is positioned midway to three-quarters of the way back on the board, facing forward toward the water. The diver then takes a series of steps (usually no less than three and no more than five) prior to the hurdle. The arms are down to the sides and move into slight flexion and extension in conjunction with the contralateral lower extremity. When the diver is a few feet from the edge of the board, the diver performs the *hurdle*, which allows the diver to jump high into the air. The hurdle is initiated by lifting one knee toward the chest so that the hip is flexed approximately 110 to 120 degrees, the knee is flexed approximately 90 to 100 degrees, and the ankle is plantarflexed. The other leg pushes the board downward. The diver should remain straight at the waist, and the arms should be fully elevated above the head.

Press/Take-Off

The hurdle allows the diver to gain height in preparation for the *press* phase of the dive. After the hurdle is executed, the knee is straightened as both feet land on the end of the board simultaneously. When the body starts to descend from the top of the hurdle, both arms begin to swing downward and backward. Just before the diver makes contact with the board, the hips and knees are slightly flexed and the feet are positioned shoulder width apart with the toes extended so that the diver can land on the balls of the feet. Both hips and knees flex as the diving board is depressed to absorb the momentum of the diver. Propulsion off the board is accomplished by extension of the board, extension of the hips and knees, and a swinging motion of the upper extremities. When the arms continue to move past the legs in an upward direction, the lower extremities and trunk extend as the recoil of the board propels the diver into the air.[1]

The type of take-off is determined by the direction of the dive. To rotate forward, the arms, chest, and shoulders are thrown forward while the hips are pushed backward. To rotate backward, the arms and shoulders are thrown backward, while the hips move forward. After the diver has initiated the direction of spin and rotation during the take-off phase, the diver is ready to begin to perform the dive, or enter the flight stage.

On the platform, an approach generally is used only on forward dives and, with some rare exceptions, on reverse dives. The diver is positioned midway on the platform, facing forward toward the water. The diver then performs a skipping action that consists of usually about five steps; the knees are bent slightly, and the trunk is upright. Divers use different arm-swing patterns while walking or skipping to the end of the platform. Once a diver arrives at the end of the platform, the arms are kept fully elevated. The diver puts his or her feet together with the knees bent at about 60 to 80 degrees at the end of the skipping action and "hits" (loads his or her weight quickly to provide a stretch reflex to the muscles) the end of the platform to maximize jump and initiate the spinning action of the dive.

The back press is used when performing back and inward dives on the springboard and platform. The diver stands with his or her back toward the water with the heels off the edge of the springboard or platform. On the springboard, the diver stands straight up with the feet in plantarflexion for balance. As the arms are abducted to approximately 45 to 90 degrees, the diver dorsiflexes and plantarflexes the ankles. This motion causes the springboard to bounce in synchronization with the ankle movement. The arms circumduct downward and backward as the diver flexes at the trunk, hips, and knees to generate force for push-off. The arms are brought down to the sides to fully depress the springboard. As the board extends upward, the hips and knees extend. At this time, the arms swing either forward or backward, depending on the direction of the dive. This motion puts the diver into the flight phase of the dive. On the platform, the action is similar, without the benefit of the spring of the board. All the momentum for the jump on the platform is generated from the diver's legs and arms (similar to a standing vertical leap).

Flight

When each type of dive is performed, regardless of the direction of the dive, one or more of the following body positions are used. These body positions are based primarily on the position of the hips and knees. The four positions include the straight position, pike position, tuck position, and free position.

Straight Position   In a straight position, divers are fully extended at the waist and knees (Fig. 6.1). Depending on the dive, however, there may be an arch to the back. The upper extremities are usually placed at 90 degrees of abduction or down by the sides with full elbow and wrist extension.

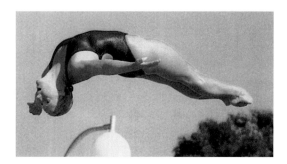

FIGURE 6.1

Diver in a straight position.

Pike Position   In a pike position, the hips are flexed to approximately 120 to 130 degrees, and the knees are maintained in full extension (Fig. 6.2). Arm placement is either at 90 degrees of abduction or wrapped around the knees, causing the chest to rest on the thighs of the diver.

Tuck Position   Divers using a tuck position appear to be rolled up in a ball, or the body is bent at the waist and knees, with the thighs drawn to the chest and the heels kept close to the buttocks (Fig. 6.3).

Free Position   The free position is not an actual body position but a diver's option to use any of the preceding three positions or

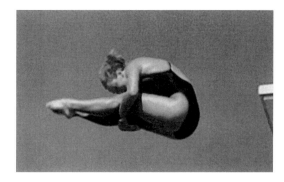

FIGURE 6.2

Diver in a pike position.

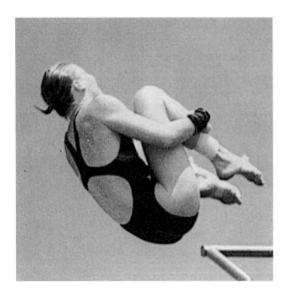

FIGURE 6.3

Diver in a tuck position.

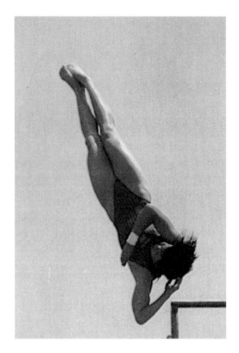

FIGURE 6.4

Diver in a free position.

combinations thereof when performing a twisting dive (Fig. 6.4). A combination of the straight and pike positions is used commonly, whereas the tuck is used rarely.

Entry

The goal of the entry is to maintain a vertical posture and produce as little splash as possible. During the entry, the arms are fully extended over the head with full scapular elevation, internal rotation of the glenohumeral joints, and full elbow extension. The forearms are pronated, and the wrists are extended and radially deviated (Fig. 6.5). The diver will clasp one hand on top of the other so that the palms of the hands hit the water in a flat position (called *flathanding*). The head and neck are nestled between the biceps, with the eyes looking up toward the hands. The position of the head and neck and upper extremities creates a hole in the water, through which the body passes. The ankles are plantarflexed, and the toes are pointed. During the entry,

the diver uses a technique called *swimming* as soon as the hands hit the surface of the water.[2] When the hands hit the surface of the water, the diver releases the grasp of the hands, and the arms are adducted rapidly to the side of the body with the wrists flexed and elbows extended. This action pulls the body through the hole created by the hands and enables the diver to enter the water with minimal splash.

Faults during any of the dive components can cause the need to slightly correct a dive at entry. To compensate for these faults, divers often make spontaneous adjustments of their bodies in order to "save" a dive. These spontaneous adjustments reduce the amount of overrotation or underrotation, allowing the diver to enter the water in a more vertical position and make less of a splash.

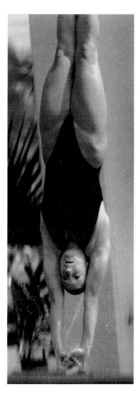

FIGURE 6.5

Position of upper extremities at entry.

When a diver comes out of a rotation too late or tilts past vertical, the diver "goes over" on a dive. When a diver underrotates a dive or comes out of a rotation too early, the dive is usually "short." Divers often perform a "save" as soon as the body is under the surface of the water to stop the rotation of the dive. During the entry for front- and inward-rotating dives, the diver quickly places the body in a piked position under the water as if doing a half somersault. In back- and reverse-spinning dives, the diver continues the same direction as the rotation of the dive and quickly draws the knees to the chest. Saves draw the feet through the water more quickly, which produces the *illusion* that the diver entered the water vertically.

Judging

Anyone observing competitive diving, especially by talented performers, may note that although several divers perform the same dive, it never looks quite the same. These subtle differences are the result of height, speed, and fluidity of movement. These unique mannerisms comprise an abstract but observable phenomenon called *style*.

The primary determinant of style is the personal choice of judges, which is why judging is difficult. Even though there are criteria of execution that all divers must meet, evaluation remains a subjective process. No matter how well a dive is performed, artistic likes and dislikes of the judges may influence the outcome of any contest. The subjectivity of the judges raises differences of opinion among coaches, competitors, judges, and spectators about the accuracy of the results.

Each judge scores a dive on a scale between 0 and 10 points, in ½-point increments.[3] A table of the scores and how they should be awarded appears below:

0	Completely failed
½–2	Unsatisfactory
2½–4½	Deficient
5–6	Satisfactory
6½–8	Good
8½–10	Very good

To judge a dive, the components of each dive must be analyzed and evaluated to determine a composite score. From a judging perspective, the different parts of a dive that are assessed include the approach or backpress, hurdle, take-off, elevation, execution, and entry. The approach or backpress should be smooth but forceful, and the diver should show good form, as described earlier. The take-off must show control and balance, with the body of the diver in the correct angle in relation to the board or platform. The elevation of the dive greatly affects the appearance of the dive and the judges' scores. The height is determined by the amount of spring or lift a diver receives from the take-off and is influenced by height of the hurdle and the amount of downward force applied to the board. A diver who attains great height has more time to execute the dive, making the dive more accurate, smooth, and less rushed. The execution of the dive in the air is the most important component of a score. A judge watches for proper mechanical performance, technique, form, and grace. The entry into the water is the second most important component because it is the last thing the judge sees. The two criteria to be evaluated for the entry are the angle of entry, which should be near vertical with the toes pointed, and the amount of splash, which should be as little as possible. Divers try to achieve a type of entry referred to as a *rip entry*. This type of entry refers to the sound that is made when the diver enters the water, similar to a piece of paper that is being rapidly ripped in half.[2] This entry and sound usually indicate that the diver entered the water with little or no splash. The quest for the rip entry is a source of potential injury, particularly to the shoulder capsule, because the diver must use the arms to accelerate through the surface of the water as quickly as possible.

Scoring

Seven judges are used in major competitions.[3] When the judges' awards are given, the high and low scores are eliminated, and the remaining five scores are totaled. This number is multiplied by the degree of difficulty (DD) rating assigned to the dive. The DD is predetermined with a mathematically computed table ranging from 1.2 to 3.6 in 0.1 increments. The DD is then multiplied by 0.6 to obtain the final score on a dive. A scoring example is shown below:

Awards from seven judges are 6, 5, 5, 5, 5, 5, and 4.
Subtotal: 25—because the highest (6) and lowest (4) are dropped.
Multiplied by the DD of 2.0: 50 points.
Total score: 50 × 0.6 = 30 points.

In synchronized diving events, nine judges are used because two judges will rate one individual diver, two other judges will rate the second individual diver, and five judges will rate the synchronization of the pair. The high and low individual scores will be thrown out, placing an emphasis on the synchronization scores. The final score is then determined using the formula just illustrated.

Competition Requirements

Specific requirements must be met in the springboard, platform, and synchronized diving events.[3] In the women's 1-m springboard, each diver must perform five dives from different groups (forward, back, reverse, inward, twisting) without a DD limit. In the women's 3-m springboard, each diver must perform a dive from each of the five different groups with the total DD not exceeding 9.5 and a dive from each of the different groups without a DD limit. In the men's 1-m springboard, each diver must perform six dives without a DD limit. These dives must include a dive from each of the five groups and an additional dive that may be selected from any group. In the men's 3-m springboard, each diver must perform a dive from each of the five different groups with a limit of 9.5 on the composite DD. In addition, the diver also must perform six dives without a DD limit, and these dives must include a dive from each of the five groups plus a dive selected from any group. In the women's 10-m platform event, each diver must perform a dive from four different groups, with the total DD not exceeding 7.6, and one dive from each of the five groups without a DD limit. In the men's 10-m platform event, each diver must perform a dive from four different groups, the total degree of difficulty of which shall not exceed 7.6, and a dive from six different groups without a DD limit.

In each of the men's and women's synchronized 3- and 10-m platform events, each pair must perform two voluntary dives with an assigned DD of 2.0 per dive, followed by three dives without DD limit. In the five rounds of dives, there must be at least one round with a forward take-off by both divers, at least one round with a backward facing take-off by both divers, and at least one round with a combination forward and backward facing take-off.

Injury Prevention

Several issues need to be addressed when designing an injury prevention program for competitive divers. If some of these issues are ignored, serious injury may result. A basic checklist for injury prevention in competitive diving should include

1. Equipment is in proper working order.
2. Coaches are certified professionals.
3. Divers are advanced at a rate that parallels their ability.
4. Divers have had a complete medical physical examination and are cleared for competitive diving.
5. Divers perform a warm-up routine consisting of stretching and flexibility exercises.

6. Divers participate in an individualized strength and conditioning program.

The following section on the etiology of diving injuries will provide more detail on items 1 through 4 as they relate to injury prevention.

Flexibility is the range of motion through which the joints of the body can move within the limits of pain. Active stretching in divers enables them to move a body segment against gravity and/or the opposing stretch of the antagonist muscles. Diving requires wide ranges of joint motion for both function and aesthetics. The functions of take-off require dorsiflexion in the ankle, flexion and extension in knees and hips for squats and jumps, shoulder circumduction in arm swings, and flexion and extension of the spine to initiate somersaults. In general, the more somersaults initiated, the greater is the degree of flexion or extension of the spine required. A functional hollow shape to create a rip entry requires shoulder girdle flexibility along the long axis with the arms overhead. Aesthetics require an elongated, rigid body with knees locked and ankles and feet plantarflexed during entry.[8] The objective of a stretching program is to achieve joint capsule flexibility so that the diver's optimal strength and power may be applied throughout the full range of motion. For injury control, the diver should demonstrate flexibility at the extremes of the range used during the competitive activity.[10] (See Fig. 6.6A–C for commonly used stretches and Chap. 5 for shoulder and anterior chest stretches.)

IMPORTANCE OF STRENGTH AND CONDITIONING IN DIVERS

Preparticipation screening evaluations effectively can help to determine potential problem areas in divers so that they are able to adequately address such areas in their strength and conditioning programs. Diving motor skills are very high in intensity and are per-

A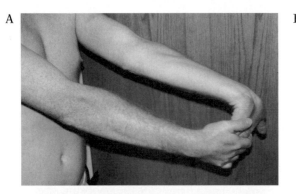

B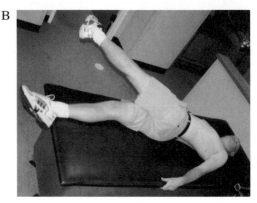

C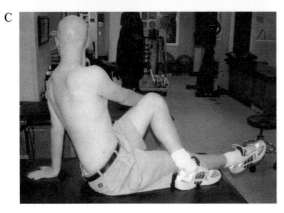

FIGURE 6.6

A. Self-stretching of the wrist flexor and forearm musculature. *B.* Self-stretching of the lumbar spine for rotation in the supine position. *C.* Self-stretching of the lumbar spine for rotation in a sitting position.

formed over an extremely short duration.[7] Strength and power fitness is characteristic of diving. Divers can increase their strength and power levels through a combination of strength and power training in the weight room and through plyometric exercises.[8]

Strength is defined as any maximal force production.[9] Strength is important in diving for holding armstands on the platform, holding specific muscles tight against gravity on entering the water, and holding tuck and pike positions while somersaulting. Power is required in diving when a muscular force must be exerted quickly. *Power* is defined as force times distance per unit time, which includes the component of movement or speed.[7] The

rate of application of muscular force varies for springboard and platform take-offs. Squatting movements are trained without emphasis on speed at first but with great attention to detail, beginning with no or light resistance. Form and strength are developed before shifting training emphasis from strength to power. Divers should follow a regular resistance program. The program should be based on the diver's age, physical development, and a periodic assessment of the diver's strengths and weaknesses. A resistance program should provide for "balance" in one's strength such that the diver is not strong in certain muscle groups and weak in others. Divers must be physically prepared to withstand the impact of water entry unique to this sport. Rubber tubing (e.g., Theraband) exercises have been especially useful in diving programs for shoulder rotator cuff injury prevention and rehabilitation.[8] Scapular stabilization is essential in order for the shoulders to tolerate the demands placed on them in this sport. Abdominal strength is necessary for prevention of back injuries, as well as for control of movement.

A periodized strength and conditioning program is necessary to ensure physical readiness of divers.[11] Plyometric exercises in diving usually consist of jumping drills and medicine ball work.[7] Plyometric training also should use the concept of periodization, and correct technique and progression are very important to avoid injury. Flexibility training is a daily requirement in the sport of diving.

Etiology of Diving Injuries

Because divers reach speeds of approximately 35 mi/h before hitting the water,[4] diving can be classified as a contact sport. Common musculoskeletal injuries in competitive diving involve numerous areas of the body and occur for several reasons.[4] Like most sports, the specific etiology of diving injuries can be attributed to external and internal factors. External factors that may contribute to injury include training errors, poor technique, or equipment malfunction. Internal factors may include impaired range of motion (ROM), joint mobility, muscle performance, motor control, and kinesthetic awareness.

EXTRINSIC FACTORS

Training Errors

Examples of training errors include overtraining, attempting dives that are too difficult, and inadequate progression of dives.[5] Overtraining can occur from performing too many dives in a practice, too many practices in a week or too much training on the 10-m platform. The amount of repetitions from the 10-m platform needs to be regulated closely because of the high compressive forces encountered when entering the water. High speeds result in impact forces between 2.0g and 2.5g (force of gravity), which can lead to musculoskeletal injury.[6] Therefore, the number of dives from the 10-m platform should be limited based on age, ability, and individual tolerance.

Attempting dives that are too difficult is a training error that is easily avoided if proper coaching is available. This training error often leads to "missed" dives, where the diver enters the water in faulty alignment. To prevent misses, divers go through a dive progression referred to as *lead-ups*. For example, if a diver is going to perform a front 3½-somersault dive from a 10-m platform, he or she may first perform a front double-somersault from the 3-m platform followed by a front 2½-somersault from the 5- or 7½-m platform. This progression gives the diver an opportunity to warm up in a steplike fashion.

Dry-land training is also responsible for several overuse injuries because of the number of repetitions performed. Most injuries associated with dry-land training involve the low back and lower extremity. Divers do a great deal of plyometric training to increase power. Overtraining can lead to inflammation of the quadriceps tendon, patellar tendon, and achilles tendon and also can lead to shin splints. These external factors usually are addressed by the coach but must not be overlooked by the therapist.

Poor Technique

Poor technique can occur during all phases of a dive, including the approach, hurdle, press, in the air, or at the entry. Poor technique on the approach phase of the dive can be a result of inexperience of the diver or poor coaching.[5] Poor technique on the hurdle and press also can be caused by inexperience of the diver, poor coaching, lack of strength or flexibility, or lack of kinesthetic awareness.

Poor kinesthetic awareness in the air can lead to an inability to visually "spot" the water. A diver must be able to spot the water or other landmarks to know when to assume the entry position. Because all phases of a dive are interrelated, an error in one phase usually will result in errors in the other phases. For example, a diver that misses a hurdle may not land in the appropriate position on the board or platform and may be leaning too far forward or backward. This altered position may result in decreased push-off force, leading to decreased dive height and altered direction. The end result is often a missed entry or the diver landing flat on the stomach or back. Landing in a flat position can result in bruised muscles, internal bleeding, or fractures.[4] If a diver lands on the side of the head, a ruptured eardrum may result.

As described earlier, experienced divers can make compensatory movements to save a dive. Although saving a dive is not a poor technique, these quick adjustments in body position can lead to injury. For example, when divers know that they may be short on a dive, a position where the body is less than vertical, they often compensate by reaching their arms back into hyperextension and arching the lumbar spine into greater lordosis. This position can lead to injuries of the neck, shoulder, and lumbar spine.

Equipment Malfunction

Equipment malfunction is rarely the cause of diving injuries. All organized competitive diving programs in the United States must meet certain safety standards that ensure that equipment is safe and coaches have the proper credentials. One piece of equipment that can lead to injury if it is not operating correctly is the air sparging system, referred to as the "bubble machine" or "bubbler."[12] This device operates in the water and consists of a compressor, which produces a combination of air and water to create turbulent bubbles at the surface. Use of this device can break the surface tension of the water by approximately 80 percent, providing a "softer" surface for divers. This machine is particularly useful for divers learning a new dive. The bubbler is turned on before the diver leaves the board or platform and is turned off just prior to or as soon as the diver makes contact with the water. The amount of turbulence must be regulated according to the size of the diver and the height of the dive. If too much turbulence is created and the diver enters the water in a straight vertical alignment, injury to the cervical spine or upper extremities may result from the increased upward forces of the bubbles.

Other equipment problems may be related to dry-land training. Devices such as trampolines and Port-o-Pit diving boards allow a diver to practice aerial maneuvers out of the water.[4] A Port-a-Pit is a cushioned landing area mounted under a diving board, allowing feet-first landings. Sprains of the ankle or knee are injuries that may occur on this equipment if divers do not land correctly. In some dry-land training, divers are strapped into a spotting belt. This belt is actually a harness with ropes attached to a pulley system so the coach can support the diver in the air. If the diver is spotted incorrectly or if the mechanism fails, serious injury may result.

INTRINSIC FACTORS

The relationship between tissue pathology and impairments is reciprocal. For example, tissue pathology such as a torn rotator cuff often *leads* to impairments such as decreased shoulder range of motion (ROM), decreased shoulder strength, and decreased motor control of the shoulder girdle. Conversely, tissue pathology can be *caused* by impairments, particularly with repetitive activities. For example, a diver who does not have adequate strength of rotator cuff and scapular musculature to counteract the forces of hitting the water may develop subacromial impingement, glenoid labrum pathology, or a traction tendinitis. To reduce the risk of injury, divers should be on an exercise program that emphasizes strength, endurance, and flexibility to meet the demands of diving.

The goal of the rehabilitation specialist is to identify specific impairments, determine the level of associated tissue pathology, and plan a treatment program. In some cases, the degree of tissue pathology may warrant a surgical consultation to determine if the injury is appropriate for rehabilitation. In these cases, preoperative rehabilitation may focus on resolving impairments prior to surgery. The following section will discuss the common musculoskeletal injuries that occur in competitive diving. This section also will review the potential causes of injury, methods of intervention, and functional progression for return to diving. Although traumatic injuries such as lacerations, contusions, or head injuries occur in competitive diving, these injuries are treated with first aid and will not be reviewed in this chapter. The intent of this section is not to present specific rehabilitation for each injury but to review the common injuries, offer treatment guidelines as they relate to diving, and discuss a functional progression for return to diving.

Common Diving Injuries and Their Rehabilitation

CERVICAL SPINE

Assessment of Common Cervical Spine Injuries

Sprains and Strains Cervical sprains and strains are common in competitive diving.[4] The most common cause of cervical injury is excessive loading of the cervical spine as the diver hits the water, particularly if the head and neck are positioned improperly.[4] When a diver hits the water with the cervical spine in excessive flexion, extension, or sidebending, the force of the water may accentuate the movement. Resulting injuries may include sprained ligaments and/or strained muscles on the side where traction forces are greatest. For example, hyperflexion injuries may lead to sprains and strains of the posterior structures, whereas hyperextension injuries lead to sprains and strains of the anterior structures. Entering the water with the head in lateral flexion can cause sprains and strains of the structures on the contralateral side. Improper head and neck position also can lead to injuries other than sprains and strains.

Common examination findings in divers with muscular strains of the cervical spine include limited active range of motion in directions that stress the injured tissues, painful resisted tests, and tenderness to palpation for the involved tissues. Pain also may be accompanied by weakness as a result of pain inhibition, depending on the severity of the injury. If muscle guarding continues, decreased intervertebral mobility also may be detected. The diver should have no referral of symptoms to the upper extremity that extend beyond the shoulder, and neurologic testing is negative.

Because few examination procedures exist to assess ligamentous integrity in the cervical spine, sprains of the cervical spine are difficult to diagnose. The clinician should be most concerned with assessing the ligamentous integrity of the upper cervical spine. Stability of C1 and C2 depends on the alar and transverse ligaments.[13,14] The alar ligaments are two ligaments that are comprised of two portions each.[13] The occipitoalar ligaments attach to the sides of the dens from C2 to the condyles of the occipital bone in the shape of a Y. The atlantoalar ligament connects the anterior aspect of the dens to the atlas. The transverse ligament is attached to arch of the atlas and stabilizes the dens against the anterior aspect of the vertebrae. The alar ligament restrains against rotation and sidebending, whereas the transverse ligament restrains against flexion. To test the stability of the alar ligament, the clinician places the diver supine and palpates the spinous process of C2 while the head is moved into slight lateral flexion.[14] This movement will tighten the alar ligament on the contralateral side, and movement of C2 is detected. Absence of movement warrants immediate referral to a medical specialist. To test the stability of the transverse ligament, the head is brought into slight flexion with the patient supine. An apprehension sign or considerable guarding warrants further investigation by a medical specialist. These physical tests should be followed with a magnetic resonance imaging (MRI) scan to document specific ligamentous, disk, or other soft tissue injury.

Brachial Plexus Traction and Nerve Root Compression Injuries If the neck is positioned in lateral flexion at entry, excessive forces will create compression on the ipsilateral structures and distraction of the contralateral structures. Compressive forces, which also occur in hyperextension injuries, can cause encroachment of the nerve roots, whereas traction forces can stretch the brachial plexus, referred to as a "burner" or "stinger."

Common examination findings in divers with nerve root compression injuries include the referral of symptoms to the upper extremity in the dermatome that corresponds to the vertebral level. Range of motion may be limited at the end range of each movement due to muscle guarding. Muscle guarding also may result in decreased intervertebral mobility and tenderness to palpation over the involved level. Symptoms may be reproduced when the head is put in an extension quadrant on the ipsilateral side. An extension quadrant is a combined movement of cervical

extension with rotation and sidebending to the same side. This position causes the neural foramen to narrow and usually will elicit symptoms. Resisted isometric testing may reveal weakness of the associated myotomes.

Conversely, divers with brachial plexus traction injuries will experience referred symptoms to the upper extremity in areas that correlate with peripheral nerves or a nerve trunk. Range of motion may be limited in sidebending or rotation away from the involved side. Unlike a nerve root injury, motor changes usually are not confined to one level. These divers also may have a positive upper limb tension test,[15] which is similar to a straight leg raise for the upper extremity. Palpation may elicit tenderness over the scalene triangle.

Cervical Facet Injuries In addition to nerve root compression, a diver may experience an injury to the facet joints when entering the water if the neck is in excessive extension or sidebending. These positions cause a compression of the joint surfaces, and impingement or inflammation of the joint capsule may result. In extreme cases, hyperextension injuries can lead to vertebral fractures or spinal cord compression.

Divers with facet injuries usually will have pain localized to the involved segments. Symptoms usually are not referred beyond the neck and shoulder area. Range of motion is usually restricted, particularly for extension, sidebending, and rotation. Hypomobility of the involved segments is detected when testing intervertebral mobility (see ref. 18). Changes in strength or sensation of the upper extremities are not normally detected with an injury isolated to the facet joints.

Disk Injury As a result of the large, repetitive compressive forces experienced by divers over several years, cervical degeneration is often observed.[16] Although a diver can receive a disk injury on one specific dive, disk pathology in these athletes is usually a cumulative effect. Disk herniation and disk degeneration can lead to nerve root encroachment.

Patients with disk pathology usually have cervical hypomobility and increased symptoms with prolonged positioning, particularly in flexion. Decreased intervertebral mobility and muscle guarding may be noted at the involved level. In some cases, patients with disk pathology may have changes in myotomes and dertmatomes.[17] These changes may be detected with sensation and motor testing of the upper extremities. A thorough history and physical examination that suggest a disk injury should be followed up with an MRI scan.

Prevention and Treatment of Cervical Spine Injuries

Preventing cervical spine injuries is accomplished through good coaching, diver education, and exercise.[4] Coaches should assist the diver in spotting the water by using verbal cues while the diver is in the air. Verbal cues let the diver know when to "come out of a dive" and assume the entry position. Divers also must be aware of the importance of head and neck position. Even if a dive is going to be missed, the diver should make an attempt to keep the head and neck in a neutral position. Lastly, when performing dry-land training, divers must spend considerable time on cervical strengthening exercises.

When treating cervical injuries related to diving, the therapist must first decide if the condition is appropriate for rehabilitation. If considerable changes are noted in myotomes or dermatomes, as evidenced by upper extremity weakness or sensation changes, the clinician should make sure that the patient has been evaluated by a physician. Once serious pathology has been ruled out, all impairments caused by the injury must be addressed. Regardless of the involved tissue pathology, rehabilitation is predicated on resolving the impairments. The degree of tissue pathology and level of inflammation will influence how fast or how slow to progress

treatment. Initial treatments may include cryotherapy, electrical stimulation, and thermal modalities to control symptoms. Manual therapy may be used to reduce pain,[18] enhance soft tissue mobility and flexibility, and increase intervertebral mobility. As the symptoms resolve, stabilization exercises for the upper quarter can be added to the rehabilitation program. Specific exercises and functional progression will be discussed at the end of this chapter.

SHOULDER

Assessment of Common Shoulder Injuries

The shoulder is the most commonly injured joint in competitive diving.[19] The primary reason for this high frequency is the fine balance between shoulder mobility and stability needed for the sport.[19] Divers must possess enough hypermobility at the shoulder girdle to reach full elevation with full upward rotation of the scapulae. This mobility must be balanced by static and dynamic control, accomplished through the neuromuscular and ligamentous systems. This control is vital to offset the large forces experienced at entry. Without this control, shoulder injuries often result.

Instability Glenohumeral instability is a common shoulder disorder experienced in competitive diving.[19] Although divers with excessive glenohumeral joint laxity may have hypermobile shoulders, they are not always unstable. Unlike hypermobility, instability is characterized by symptoms that develop from the inability of the neuromuscular system to compensate for excessive ligamentous laxity.[20] The resulting effect of instability is excessive humeral head translation and an inability of the humeral head to stay centered within the glenoid fossa during movement. *Macrotraumatic* instability usually results from a single traumatic dislocation, whereas *microtraumatic* instability results from an accumulation of repeated stress to the shoulder. Both types of instability are common in competitive diving.

Macrotraumatic instability or dislocation can result when the diver enters the water with the upper extremities posterior to the cervical spine (Fig. 6.7) or when divers "miss" their hands and cannot hold an entry.[4] Entering the water with the arms posterior to the cervical spine or frontal plane can push the arms further into abduction and external rotation. This position occurs when a diver is

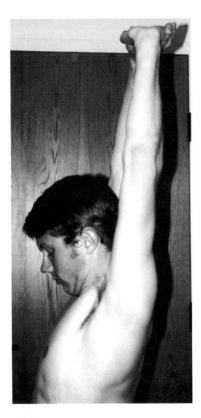

FIGURE 6.7

Faulty position of the head in relation to the upper extremities. When the diver hits the water in this position, the head is forced into excessive flexion while the upper extremities are pushed into flexion.

"short" and reaches posteriorly to save a dive and attain a vertical position at entry. As reviewed earlier, most divers hold one hand with the other during entry. This position, in conjunction with full elbow extension and full shoulder girdle elevation, is referred to as a *lock-out position* of the upper extremities and provides stability to the upper extremity. If divers "miss" their hands, they are unable to maintain the stable position and may not be able to hold their entry. The end result is that the upper extremities can be pushed in several different directions as the diver hits the water. Microtraumatic instability may result from repetitive small subluxations that are due to missed entries, inadequate neuromuscular stabilization, or lack of muscular endurance. In either case, common tissue pathologies that result from instability include rotator cuff tears or tendinitis, bicipital tendinitis, and glenoid labrum tears.

Examination findings in divers with instability include a positive sulcus sign, apprehension sign, load and shift test, and relocation test.[20,21] A detailed explanation of these special tests can be found elsewhere.[20] Although a diver may have a positive sulcus sign or a positive load and shift, these tests by themselves are not enough to diagnose instability. The clinician should correlate multiple tests with the presence of symptoms to distinguish hypermobility from instability. Patients with instability also may have a positive impingement sign, positive tests for rotator cuff pathology, and positive tests for glenoid pathology.[20]

Impingement Syndrome   *Subacromial impingement* is a term given to encroachment of the structures between the greater tuberosity and anteroinferior surface of the acromion. The pathomechanics of this condition are attributed to different impairments that can be divided into primary and secondary impingement.[20,22] *Primary impingement* of the subacromial space occurs when the superior aspect of the rotator cuff is abraded by the surrounding bony and soft tissue structures because of decreased subacromial space.[20] Neer[23,24] differentiated outlet from nonoutlet primary impingement. *Outlet impingement* is attributed to mechanical changes in the outlet of the coracoacromial arch, through which the rotator cuff passes. Impingement in this condition may be due to abnormal acromial morphology (abnormal tilt or slope), the coracoacromial ligament, acromioclavicular joint arthritis, or a tight posterior capsule.[25–30] *Nonoutlet impingement* is defined as rotator cuff pathology due to an otherwise normal outlet. Possible causes of this condition include poor motor control, rotator cuff weakness or fatigue, and a thickened rotator cuff bursa. *Secondary impingement* of the subacromial space occurs from glenohumeral instability and is more common in competitive diving than primary impingement.[20] Excessive superior translation of the humeral head may cause encroachment of the subacromial space, as well as a traction force on the capsule, rotator cuff tendons, and long head of the biceps. Consequently, capsulitis and traction tendinitis are common findings in divers with secondary impingement.

When making a diagnosis of impingement, the clinician also should make a secondary assessment of impairments. After a positive impingement sign is noted, the clinician should assess for the existence of a hypomobile posterior capsule, weakness of the rotator cuff and scapular muscles, poor motor control, and lack of upper quarter flexibility. Successful treatment of impingement is predicated on resolution of the impairment that led to the impingement.

Tendinitis and Rotator Cuff Tears Tendinitis and rotator cuff tears in the shoulder usually are secondary to either instability or impingement. To compensate for instability, the rotator cuff attempts to stabilize the glenohumeral joint by centering the head of the humerus in the glenoid fossa. The rotator cuff is assisted by the long head of the biceps, which acts to restrain superior migration of the humeral head. The biceps are also functioning while the diver is in the air in a tuck or pike position and holding the legs to the chest. As the muscles fatigue and the head of the humerus continues to translate, a traction force is placed on the tendons. This traction force can trigger an inflammatory response in the tendon. Conversely, tendinitis associated with primary impingement is a result of compressive forces. Divers with tight posterior capsules or abnormally shaped acromions are at risk for compressive tendinitis or rotator cuff tears.[25–30] In either case, chronic tendinitis can lead to tears of the rotator cuff or long head of the biceps.

Divers with tendinitis usually present with a painful arc of movement. The area of pain is usually localized to the insertion on the head of the humerus. Resisted isometric muscle testing is painful and may be weak as a result of pain inhibition or secondary to a tear of the tendon.

Prevention and Treatment of Shoulder Injuries

Prevention of overtraining is a key factor in avoiding shoulder injuries in divers. Overtraining can lead to muscular fatigue, decreasing the stability of the shoulder girdle. Prevention of shoulder injuries also can be accomplished by a comprehensive upper-quarter flexibility and strengthening program that emphasizes the rotator cuff and scapular stabilizers. Postural impairments also can lead to shoulder dysfunction. Common postural impairments observed in divers include a forward head, rounded shoulders with internal rotation of the glenohumeral joints, scapular protraction, and increased thoracic kyphosis. This posture may be due to tightness of the anterior chest musculature and weakness of the interscapular musculature. These postural impairments can predispose a diver to subacromial impingement because the greater tuberosity is moved in closer proximity to the anterior acromion. Maintaining the flexibility of the anterior chest musculature should be part of a diver's dry-land program. Figure 6.8 illustrates one way of stretching the anterior chest musculature without overstressing the anterior capsule of the glenohumeral joint.

If instability is diagnosed, the clinician must determine whether associated tissue pathology exists. Involvement of the rotator cuff or glenoid labrum may warrant surgical intervention. Patients with instability who are not surgical candidates should be involved in an upper-quarter flexibility program complemented by an exercise program that emphasizes strength and endurance of the shoulder girdle musculature, focusing on the rotator cuff and scapular stabilizers (Figs. 6.9 through 6.13). Patients with anterior instability may have tightness of the posterior capsule, which should be addressed with mobilization (Fig. 6.14). (See Chaps. 2 and 10 for additional rehabilitation approaches for shoulder instability.)

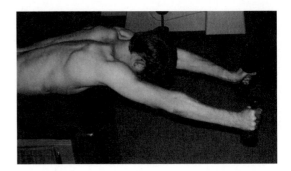

FIGURE 6.9

Bilateral shoulder flexion in the prone position.

When a diver presents with subacromial impingement, the primary goal of the clinician should be to identify the impairments that lead to the condition. Treatment of patients with outlet impingement may include joint mobilization and stretching of the posterior capsule (see Fig. 6.14). In some cases, these patients may require surgery for a subacromial decompression. Treatment of patients with nonoutlet impingement and secondary impingement due to instability usually requires dynamic stabilization through rotator cuff and scapular strengthening (see Figs. 6.9 through 6.13). Patients who have a subacromial decompression when the underlying impairment is instability usually have a poor outcome because the instability

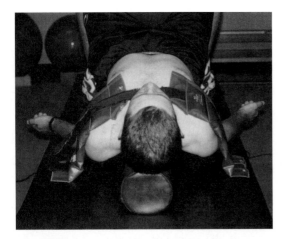

FIGURE 6.8

Stretching the anterior chest musculature over a foam roll.

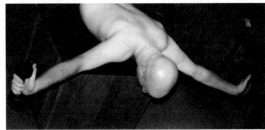

FIGURE 6.10

Bilateral shoulder horizontal abduction with external rotation in the prone position.

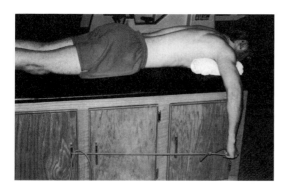

FIGURE 6.11

External rotation in the prone position at 90 degrees of abduction. The treatment table provides stabilization of the shoulder girdle.

is not addressed. If surgical intervention is indicated in these patients, a stabilization procedure is most beneficial. (See Chaps. 2 and 10 for additional rehabilitation for shoulder impingement.)

ELBOW

Assessment of Common Elbow Injuries

Hyperextension Injuries Elbow hyperextension may occur at entry as a result of the forces from hitting the water at fast speeds.[4] Recurvatum of the elbows is a common finding in divers because of the emphasis placed on maintaining elbow extension at entry. When divers are young, they are taught the importance of "locking out" their elbows to achieve a vertical entry. Maintaining elbow extension also prevents the arms from collapsing at the elbows when the diver hits the water. Failure to maintain elbow extension can result in the dorsum of the wrist and hand colliding with the head and causing injury to either area. Divers must rely on strength and endurance of the triceps to prevent these injuries. Patients with elbow hyperextension injuries usually will have pain when overpressure is applied to the end range of passive elbow extension.

Triceps Tendinitis Eccentric loading of the triceps is needed to counter the flexion forces that occur at entry. Overuse of the triceps can result in tendinitis where the muscle inserts on the olecranon process. If triceps tendinitis is present, the patient will have pain with resisted elbow extension or pain with compression applied through the hands when the upper extremities are in an entry position (Fig. 6.15). In addition, the patient may be tender to palpation over the triceps tendon at its insertion.

Medial Instability and Ulnar Neuritis When a diver enters the water, the first movement of the upper extremities is to adduct the arms rapidly to the side, with the elbows extended. This movement is known as a *swimming maneuver* and is done to "pull" the diver down through the water. This motion creates a valgus stress to the medial aspect of the elbow. Because of the repetitive nature of this movement, divers can develop laxity of the medial collateral ligament, which could lead to instability and traction of the ulnar nerve.

Divers with medial instability will have normal ROM but may report pain at the end range of extension. Valgus stress testing will elicit symptoms, and laxity may be noted. Strength testing is usually strong and painless. The diver will be tender to palpation over the medial collateral ligament. If the ulnar nerve is involved, divers will have radiating symptoms into the fifth finger and half of the ring finger and will be tender to palpation over the ulnar groove.

Prevention and Treatment of Elbow Injuries

Preventing elbow injuries in diving is accomplished through a progressive resistive training program that emphasizes strength and endurance. The diver and coach also must recognize the importance of avoiding overtraining. Overtraining usually leads to triceps fatigue and decreased stability around the

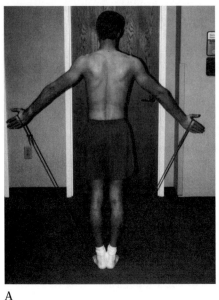
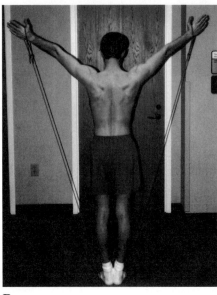
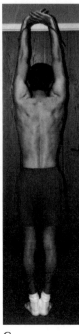

A   B   C

FIGURE 6.12

A. Start position for bilateral abduction in the standing position using resistance tubing. *B.* Bilateral horizontal abduction in the standing position using resistance tubing. *C.* Finish position of bilateral abduction in the standing position using resistance tubing. This position simulates the position of the diver at entry.

elbow. Following injury, a taping technique that limits elbow hyperextension can be worn by a diver during the transition back to diving (Fig. 6.16). However, external supports should not replace a comprehensive strength and flexibility program.

WRIST AND HAND

Assessment of Common Wrist and Hand Injuries

The wrist is another common area of musculoskeletal injury in diving.[31] When a diver enters the water, the palmer aspect of one hand grasps the dorsal surface of the other hand, and both wrists are in an extended position (Fig. 6.17). The wrist flexors must offset the forces of the water pushing the wrists into more exten-

sion. This repetitive action, as well as the repetitive handstands that divers perform, can lead to several different musculoskeletal injuries.

Sprain and Strains A strain of the wrist flexors occurs from the eccentric activity needed to counteract the extension forces when hitting the water. Physical examination reveals pain with active and resisted wrist flexion. Passive wrist extension may be painful at the end range, and the diver may be tender to palpation over the muscle belly. Hyperextension of the wrist also can lead to strained ligaments on the volar aspect of the proximal and distal carpal rows. Divers with ligamentous injuries may have pain at the end range of all wrist movements that stress the ligament. Accessory testing of the carpal bones may reveal

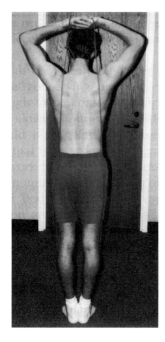 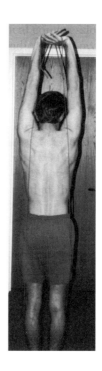

FIGURE 6.13

A. Start position of upper extremity press into entry position. This exercise emphasizes scapular, glenohumeral, and elbow muscle strengthening. *B.* Finish position of upper extremity press into entry.

hypermobility. Divers usually are tender to palpation over the involved ligaments. Resisted testing usually does not elicit symptoms.

Lunate Instability If wrist strains persist and become chronic, the acquired ligamentous laxity may lead to instability of the intercarpal joints. Subluxation of the lunate is a common complication of wrist instability in divers. As the wrist is forced into hyperextension, the lunate is pushed to the volar aspect of the wrist and may not relocate. On physical examination, decreased wrist flexion ROM is noted, and tenderness over the lunate is noted on palpation. If the lunate is palpated during passive wrist flexion-extension, the clinician may note the lack of dorsal translation during flexion. Divers with subluxations of the lunate may have a weak pincer grasp between the thumb and fifth finger.

Dorsal Impact Syndrome When divers hit the water with a flat-hand entry, the wrist and hand are forced in a dorsal direction. This repetitive force can lead to overuse injuries of the structures in the wrist, referred to as *dorsal impact syndrome*. Additionally, if divers fail to maintain elbow extension and "swim" their entry, the force of the water can push the dorsal aspect of the wrist and hands into the top of the head. The result of this collision is a contusion to the soft tissues on the dorsal aspect of the wrist and hand and, in some cases, a fracture of the metacarpals. Divers with this macrotrauma may present with swelling and bruising on the dorsum of the wrist and hand. This area will be tender to palpation, and ROM may be limited at the end range due to pain. Clinicians must test the strength and endurance of the triceps and

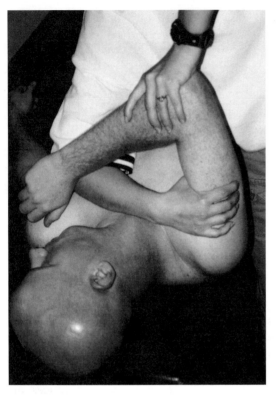

FIGURE 6.14

Mobilization of the posterior shoulder capsule.

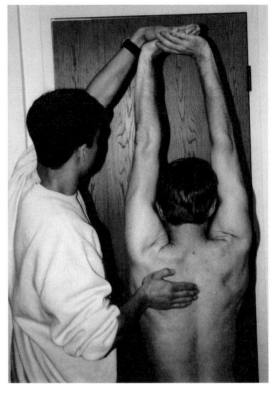

FIGURE 6.15

Resisted testing of the triceps with the diver in an entry position.

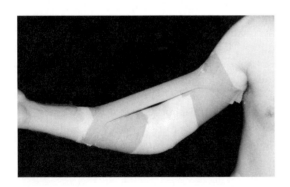

FIGURE 6.16

Use of athletic tape to limit elbow hyperextension.

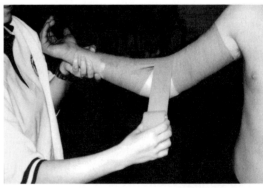

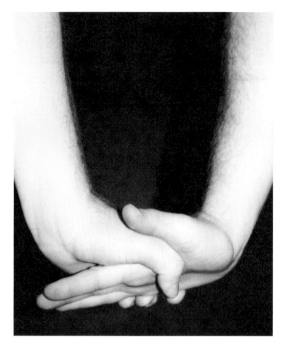

FIGURE 6.17

Close-up of the hands at entry position.

rule out the cervical spine as a possible source of triceps dysfunction in case it is the underlying cause of the problem.

Stress Fractures The repetitive compressive forces exerted on the carpal bones during entries and when doing handstands can lead to stress fractures. Divers who present with a painful wrist that does not respond to traditional treatment and activity modification after 2 to 3 weeks should be evaluated for a stress fracture. Divers with tenderness over the scaphoid may need to have a medical assessment sooner because of the risk of avascular necrosis. Because x-rays may be negative initially, a bone or MRI scan may be a more accurate diagnostic method.

Skier's Thumb When divers grasp one hand with the other prior to entry, the movement has to happen quickly to prevent divers

from "missing" their hands at entry. As a result of this quick maneuver, the web space between the thumb and index finger from one hand is forced against the web space of the other hand (Fig. 6.18). If a diver hits the ulnar aspect of the thumb instead of the web space, the thumb is forced into abduction and extension. The resulting injury could be a sprain or tear of the ulnar collateral ligament. The diver will present with pain and tenderness over the ligament. Increased laxity also may be noted with stress testing of the ligament.

Prevention and Treatment of Wrist Injuries

Preventing wrist injuries in diving is accomplished by avoiding overtraining and maintaining a comprehensive strength and flexibility program for the muscles of the upper extremity. Prophylactic taping of the wrist and thumb (Fig. 6.19) and the wearing of wrist guards (Fig. 6.20) may help prevent injuries similar to the way knee braces are worn by football players. Wrist guards can be

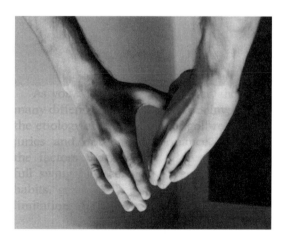

FIGURE 6.18

Mechanism of injury for damaging the ulnar collateral ligament of the thumb.

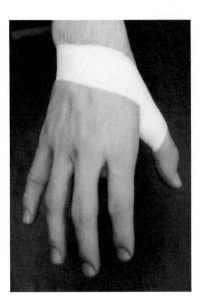

FIGURE 6.19

Spica taping to the thumb.

fabricated by folding athletic tape several times into a rectangular piece that is taped to the dorsum of the wrist, designed to limit extension (Fig. 6.21). In divers with lunate instability, tape can be used as a splint when out of the water to restrict a volar glide during wrist extension (Fig. 6.22). (See Chap. 10

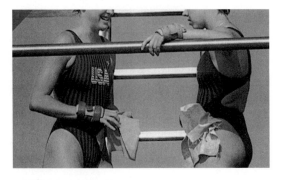

FIGURE 6.20

Divers wearing prefabricated wrist guards.

for additional rehabilitation approaches for ulnar collateral ligament injuries.)

LUMBAR SPINE

Assessment of Common Lumbar Spine Injuries

Injuries to the lumbar spine are common in divers because of the combined forces that are transmitted through the spine.[4] For example, consider the forces involved in a forward 1½-somersault in the pike position with 2½ twists from a 10-m platform. This dive involves a quick flexion movement into a pike position while the diver is rotating the body. The diver completes the dive by extending the spine into a neutral position and discontinuing the twisting just prior to encountering the compressive forces of the water. These movements, as well as heavy plyometric dry-land training, performed on a repetitive basis often lead to musculoligamentous injuries.

Sprains and Strains Divers with sprains and strains typically present with generalized pain in one region of the lumbar spine. Postural deviations, such as a lateral shift, usually are not present with these injuries. Symptoms may be reproduced with active motion testing in the directions that stress the injured tissue. Additionally, ROM may be limited in directions that stress the injured tissues. Palpation will elicit tenderness over the injured tissues, and intervertebral mobility may be limited secondary to muscle guarding. If inflammation is present, the symptoms may be constant.

Facet Injury The large extension and rotation forces also can result in injury to the lumbar facet joints. These types of injuries can be distinguished from sprains and strains because symptoms from facet joint injury usually are unilateral and localized to a specific level. ROM usually is most limited and painful in directions that compress the joint. For example, injury to the right facet joint at L3–4 will produce pain during joint compres-

A

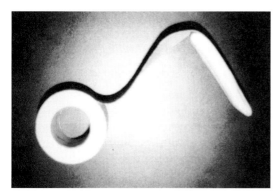

B

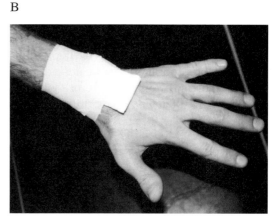

FIGURE 6.21

A. Use of athletic tape to make an extension block for the wrist. *B.* An extension block applied to a diver's wrist.

sion with right rotation, right sidebending, and extension. Movements in the opposite direction cause distraction of the joint capsule and also may elicit pain. Although muscle guarding may be present around the region, palpation will elicit localized tenderness and decreased intervertebral mobility.

Disk Pathology Disk injury in divers can be the result of cumulative microtrauma or a single macrotrauma. Compression of lumbar disks occurs from different forces. The forces from bouncing on the board or platform, entering the water, and rapidly flexing and extending the spine can cause disk compression. Twisting dives and entering the water in a nonvertical position also can create shear forces on the disk. These forces may lead to degenerative changes in the disk and, in some cases, disk herniation. Divers with disk pathology may present with unilateral or bilateral pain in the lumbosacral area. Any radiating symptoms usually are unilateral and can involve the buttock, thigh, calf, and foot. Symptoms that are referred to both lower extremities at the same time require immediate medical attention. Additionally, loss of sensation in the sad-

dle area, loss of any lower extremity motor function, and alteration of bowel or bladder function require immediate medical attention to rule out spinal cord compression.

Depending on the level of severity and whether the disk is compressing a nerve root, divers with disk injuries may present with a lateral shift of their trunk. Symptoms from a disk usually are related to prolonged positions and make changes in position difficult. The symptoms also may be aggravated by anything that changes intraabdominal pressure such as coughing or sneezing. Active movements may be painful and restricted at the end range, with backward bending or extension being the most limited. If dural tissue is involved, performing a straight-leg-raise test may aggravate the symptoms. If the disk is encroaching on a nerve root, changes in sensation, strength, and deep tendon reflexes of the lower extremity may be noted.

Spondylolysis and Spondylolisthesis Repetitive flexion and extension movements that occur in diving put high stress on the vertebral segments. These repeated forces could cause a stresslike fracture of the pars interar-

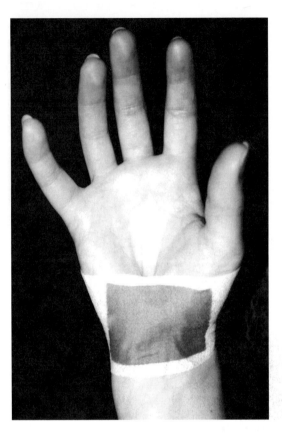

FIGURE 6.22

Use of tape to restrict volar movement of the lunate.

ticularis, the piece of bone between the facet joints. This condition is referred to as a *spondylolysis*. If the anterior shear force from one vertebra causes anterior slippage, the condition is called *spondylolisthesis*. In both conditions, the symptoms usually are localized to the lumbosacral area and are reproduced or aggravated by extension of the lumbar spine. Protective guarding may be noted in the paraspinal musculature, and spring testing over the spine may elicit symptoms. Intervertebral mobility also may be limited in adjacent segments to compensate for the instability.

Prevention and Treatment of Lumbar Injuries

Prevention of low-back injuries in divers is accomplished by maintaining flexibility and developing lumbopelvic stabilization. Most divers are involved in comprehensive flexibility programs and spend adequate time warming up prior to diving. However, with the exception of abdominal strengthening, many divers do not emphasize strengthening of the other muscles around the lumbar spine and pelvis in a way that promotes dynamic stabilization. These exercises are done in a manner that simulates functional positions for the diver (Fig. 6.23).

When planning a treatment program for a diver with lumbar dysfunction, the clinician should have an understanding of the medical diagnosis to know what activities to avoid. For example, knowing that a diver has a grade II spondylolisthesis alerts the clinician to avoid hyperextension movements during rehabilitation. However, a successful rehabilitation program is predicated on resolving impairments. Because specific tissue pathology may not be known and the findings of an MRI scan may not have high correlation with symptoms, clinicians should categorize patients by clusters of signs and symptoms.[32] For example, although a diver who presents with a lateral shift may have a disk injury, the role of rehabilitation is to correct the lateral shift and resolve any referred symptoms. This goal may be accomplished through an extension program, mechanical traction, manual therapy, or stabilization exercises. For a review of more specific rehabilitation strategies for the treatment of low-back pain, the reader is referred to other sources.[32]

KNEE

Assessment of Common Knee Injuries

Most knee injuries in diving involve the extensor mechanism and patellofemoral joint. Because of the high repetition of jumping involved in diving, the extensor mechanism is susceptible to many overuse injuries. Although the symptoms may be located in the same area, the symptoms may be caused by different impairments. The clinician must determine if the symptoms are due to impaired flexibility, impaired motor control, or biomechanical problems.

Patellofemoral Tracking Dysfunction
Divers with patellofemoral tracking problems usually present with symptoms around the patella. This diagnosis is often classified inappropriately as *chondromalacia*. Although patellar tracking problems can lead to bony changes, chondromalacia refers to degenerative changes of the articular cartilage, which cannot be made without arthroscopic observation. Female athletes with a large Q-angle may be predisposed to lateral patellar tracking. Altered patellar tracking also can be the result of tightness of the lateral retinaculum or secondary to impaired motor control of the quadriceps. Restricted mobility of the lateral retinaculum and iliotibial band may cause the patella to track laterally during a quadriceps contraction.[33,34] Due to the angle of the muscle fibers, the vastus medialis oblique (VMO) also has a role in preventing the patella from gliding laterally. Decreased activity from the VMO or an alteration in timing between the VMO and vastus lateralis (VL) also can lead to lateral patellar tracking.[35,36]

Divers with tracking problems may present with malalignment of the lower extremities, including pronated feet, tibial torsion, and "squinting" patellae. Static assessment of patellar position may show a lateral tilt and lateral glide if a tight lateral retinaculum is present. This condition is exacerbated by repetitive knee flexion and extension movements, and the diver usually will report discomfort during the eccentric (loading) phase of jumping or when going up the ladder. The diver also may report symptoms with prolonged positioning in flexion. Crepitus may be palpated during active motion, and lateral tracking of the patella usually is noted during an active quadriceps contraction. Restricted patellofemoral mobility may be noted.

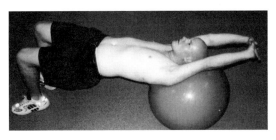
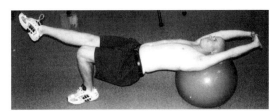
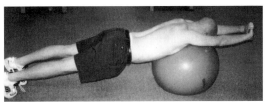

FIGURE 6.23

Stabilization exercises for the lumbar spine.

Tendinitis   Tendinitis is an overuse condition that affects several areas around the knee in competitive divers as a result of repetitive jumping. Patellar tendinitis and quadriceps tendinitis also may be due to abnormal patellofemoral tracking, lack of lower extremity flexibility, muscle imbalance, patella baja, or a deficit in quadriceps femoris muscle performance. In younger divers, increased stress on the patellar tendon may cause inflammation at the insertion site on the tibial tuberosity. This increased stress also can trigger increased bone growth, resulting in Osgood-Schlatter's disease.

Divers who present with quadriceps tendinitis usually have symptoms near the superior aspect of the patella, whereas divers with patellar tendinitis have symptoms over the patellar tendon, either at the apex of the patella or at the insertion on the tibial tuberosity. In these patients, the symptoms usually are aggravated by contraction of the quadriceps femoris, usually going up the ladder to the diving board or platform, as well as during the press phase of the dive. Patellofemoral mobility may be restricted, and tightness of the muscles in the lower extremity may be noted.

Iliotibial Band Friction Syndrome   Poor flexibility of the iliotibial band (ITB) or abnormal lower extremity alignment, such as genu varum, also can lead to an overuse condition referred to as *iliotibial band friction syndrome* (ITBFS). In this condition, repetitive knee flexion and extension cause the iliotibial band to glide over the lateral femoral condyle and perpetuate an inflammatory response.[37]

Divers with ITBFS present with symptoms over the lateral aspect of the knee. Symptoms usually are reproduced during physical assessment when the examiner palpates the lateral femoral condyle while passively flexing and extending the knee. Pain is experienced at 20 to 30 degrees of knee flexion, when the ITB is in contact with the lateral femoral condyle. Unlike a sprain of the lateral collateral ligament, which also causes lateral knee pain, symptoms are not reproduced with varus stress testing. Although a tear of the lateral meniscus also can refer pain to the lateral aspect of the knee, meniscus pathology usually results in joint effusion and pain with compressive forces. These symptoms are not associated with ITBFS.

Prevention and Treatment of Extensor Mechanism Dysfunction

Although different tissue pathologies may be associated with extensor mechanism dysfunction, treatment must focus on the resolution of impairments that may have lead to the tissue pathology. Treatment begins with management of inflammation, through medication, modalities, and activity modification. Activity modification for divers with extensor mechanism dysfunction should focus on decreasing the amount of dry-land training. Unlike upper extremity injuries, knee problems in diving usually are caused by dry-land training. If modification of dry-land training is not successful, the diver can decrease the number of dives in a practice. Only extreme cases of extensor mechanism dysfunction should cause a diver to completely miss practice.

Divers should emphasize flexibility of the hamstrings, ITB, quadriceps, and gastrocnemius-soleus muscle groups. Maintaining quadriceps strength, specifically the VMO, is another important factor for preventing or treating these knee injuries. Many studies have analyzed effective ways of training the VMO in patients with extensor mechanism dysfunction of the knee.[38–40] Although no one exercise has been shown to be consistently better than another for selected recruitment of the VMO, most research concludes that the VMO function is critical to function of the patellofemoral joint and overall knee stability. If biomechanical factors such as pronated feet are contributing to the knee symptoms, the rehabilitation program should incorporate motor control training. Motor control training can help the diver learn to control the degree of pronation when landing on the diving board or platform. Patellofemoral taping is another method of controlling symptoms[41] by allowing the diver to train and exercise in a painfree manner.

ANKLE

Assessment of Common Ankle Injuries

Sprains Although ankle sprains in divers can occur on the diving board or platform, these injuries usually are more prevalent with dry-land training. Divers practice dry-land techniques landing on a foam cushion, called a *Port-o-Pit*. This surface is designed to reduce impact forces when landing from heights. However, divers do not wear shoes and can lose their footing on landing, which can result in an ankle sprain.

Divers with an ankle sprain usually present with swelling and ecchymosis over the lateral and/or medial ligaments. If the foot is in extreme plantarflexion during an eversion or inversion injury, the anterior tibiofibular ligament may be involved in addition to the lateral ligaments or deltoid ligament. A diver with this injury usually has excessive translation with an anterior drawer test. A diver who sustains an inversion or eversion injury with the foot in dorsiflexion also can have involvement of the interosseous ligament. A diver with this injury usually has pain radiating into the distal third of the lower leg.

Achilles Tendinitis Achilles tendinitis is another overuse injury that can occur in diving due to the high demand placed on the calf musculature during push-off from the diving board or platform. Repetitive concentric-eccentric contractions without the shock-absorbing mechanism of a shoe and repetitive pronation can lead to acute inflammation.[42] Divers with achilles tendinitis report pain over the achilles tendon during the push-off phase of gait or during jumping. Palpation of the achilles tendon may reveal tenderness and some thickening of the tendon.

Fracture of the Fifth Metatarsal Divers put a tremendous amount of stress through the forefoot when pushing off from a diving board or platform. Eccentric loading of the ankle takes place after the hurdle and is followed by a rapid transition to a concentric contraction for push-off. Weight is distributed along the lateral aspect of the foot and over the metatarsal heads during this motion, but the bare foot has no support. If the diver lands incorrectly, a fracture of the fifth metatarsal can result. Repetitive stress over a prolonged period of time also can result in a stress fracture of the fifth metatarsal.

Tendinitis of the Tibialis Posterior (Shin Splints) Because divers are barefoot during most forms of training, they have no arch support during eccentric loading of the foot. To meet the demands of this loading, the tibialis posterior contracts to prevent a collapse of the longitudinal arch.[43] Overuse of the tibialis posterior or soleus can lead to tendinitis, sometimes referred to as *medial shin splints*.[44] Divers with tendinitis of the tibialis posterior may have pain with resisted inversion and may be tender to palpation over the tendon or over the muscle belly near the medial aspect of the tibia.

Prevention and Treatment of Ankle Injuries

To prevent and treat overuse injuries such as shin splints and achilles tendinitis, overtraining must be avoided. If these overuse injuries develop, activity modification is the first form of treatment. If a diver has had ankle injuries in the past, the use of ankle taping to restrict inversion and eversion may prevent future injuries. Although ankle taping can be used during regular training, the tape should not be applied if it compromises a diver's footing. Prophylactic ankle taping is used more commonly for dry-land training. Taping also can be used for injuries as an adjunct to treatment. Different taping methods can be applied for divers with an ankle sprain, achilles tendinitis, or shin splints.[45]

If a diver does experience an ankle sprain, treatment of this injury is not vastly different from treating ankle sprains in other athletes. Traditional treatment methods of reducing pain and swelling through anti-inflammatory modalities and medicine, restoring ankle strength, restoring ROM, and restoring proprioception should be incorporated into the rehabilitation program. In addition, rehabilitation must focus on restoring plyometric strength and proprioception so that the diver can return safely to jumping activities. (See Chap. 9 for additional rehabilitation strategies.)

Return to Sport

Many clinicians are familiar with the primary goals of rehabilitation that focus on resolving impairments.[46] Rehabilitation of most musculoskeletal injuries involves the restoration or resolution of one or more of the following impairments: pain, swelling, decreased ROM, decreased joint mobility, decreased muscle performance, and decreased motor control. However, clinicians must have a specific plan for returning a patient to the previous level of functional activity. To accomplish this goal, the clinician must understand the biomechanics of the sport and training methods to determine a safe progression.

In divers with upper extremity injuries or surgeries, the return to training can occur as soon as the impairments are resolved. Dryland training with a spotting belt allows the diver to go through the mechanics of diving putting minimal force on the upper extremity. When a diver is ready to return to the pool, training is initiated on a 1-m springboard or platform. From this low height, the diver can practice dives using feet-first entries. After participating in several practices without any residual symptoms, the diver can progress to simple front dives with a regular entry. The speed of this progression will be determined by the degree of injury or the type of surgery. As confidence is gained and symptoms are monitored, the degree of difficulty for the dives is increased. To prevent reinjury or an exacerbation, divers also should be instructed not to attempt to "save" dives during the initial training sessions.

After training for several weeks on the 1-m springboard without symptoms, the diver is advanced to the 3-m springboard. Forces on the upper extremity during entry from this height are considerably greater than on the 1-m springboard. Initially, the diver should attempt feet-first entries to ensure that the force of hitting the water from this height does not exacerbate the injury. After training with feet-first entries, the diver can progress to normal entries, beginning with easier dives first. Prior to returning to the 10-m platform, divers should go through a similar progression on the 5- and 7-m platforms, if they are available.

References

1. O' Brien R: *Diving for Gold*. Champaign, IL: Leisure Press, 1992.
2. Brown JG, Abraham LD, Bertin JJ: Descriptive analysis of the rip entry in competitive diving. *Res Q* 55:93–102, 1984.
3. US Diving, Inc: *1998 and 1999 Official Rules of Diving and Code of Regulations*. Indianapolis, IN: US Diving, Inc, 1998.

4. Kimball RJ, Carter RL, Schneider RC: Competitive diving injuries, in Schneider RC, Kennedy JC, Plant ML (eds): *Sports Injuries: Mechanisms, Prevention, and Treatment*. Baltimore: Williams and Wilkins, 1985, p 192.

5. Christina RW, Davis G: Principles of teaching skill progressions, in Gabriel J (ed): *United States Diving Safety Manual*. Indianapolis, IN: US Diving, Inc, 1990, p 89.

6. Stevenson JM: The impact force of entry in diving from a 10-meter tower. *Biomechanics* 9B:106, 1993.

7. Gater D, Rubin B: Strength and conditioning programs for sports of the Olympic Games. *Natl Strength Condit Assoc J* 10(4):7–25, 1998.

8. Brown M: Physical readiness, in Gabriel J (ed): *United States Diving Safety Manual*. Indianapolis, IN: US Diving, Inc, 1999, pp 127–136.

9. Sale DG, Norman RW: Testing strength and power, in MacDougall JD, et al (eds): *Physiological Testing of the Elite Athlete*. Ithaca, NY: Movement Publications, 1982, pp 7–38.

10. Mangine R: Preventative exercises for the back in the competitive diver, in Golden D (ed): *Proceedings of the US Diving Sports Science Seminar*. Indianapolis, IN: US Diving, Inc, 1982, pp 91–99.

11. Sands WA: Performer readiness, in George GS (ed): *USGF Gymnastics Safety Manual*, 2d ed. Indianapolis, IN: The USGF Publications Department, 1990.

12. Flewwelling H: Sparging systems, in Gabriel J (ed): *United States Diving Safety Manual*. Indianapolis, IN: US Diving, Inc,1990, p 57.

13. Panjabi M, Dvorak J, Crisco JJ, et al: Effects of alar ligament transection on upper cervical spine rotation. *J Orthop Res* 9:584–593, 1991.

14. Dvorak J, SchneiderE, Saldinger P, Rahn B: Biomechanics of the craniocervical region: The alar and transverse ligaments. *J Orthop Res* 6:452–456, 1988.

15. Butler DS: *Mobilisation of the Nervous System*. Melbourne: Churchill-Livingstone, 1991.

16. Anderson SL, Gerard B, Zlatkin M: Cervical spine problems in competitive divers, in *Proceedings of the US Diving Sports Science Seminar*. Indianapolis, IN: US Diving, Inc, 1993, p 144.

17. Cloward RB: Cervical discography: A contribution to the etiology and mechanism of neck, shoulder, and arm pain. *Ann Surg* 150:1052–1064, 1959.

18. Maitland GD: *Vertebral Manipulation*, 5th ed. Sydney: Butterworths, 1986.

19. Carter RL: Prevention of springboard and platform diving injuries. *Clin Sports Med* 5:185, 1986.

20. Jobe CM, Pink MM, Jobe FW, et al: Anterior shoulder instability, impingement, and rotator cuff tear, in Jobe FW (ed): *Operative Techniques in Upper Extremity Sports Injuries*. St. Louis: Mosby–Year Book, 1996.

21. Hawkins RJ, Hobeika PE: Physical examination of the shoulder. *Orthopedics* 6:1270–1278, 1983.

22. Tibone JE, Jobe FW, Kerlan RK, et al: Shoulder impingement syndrome in athletes treated by an anterior acromioplasty. *Clin Orthop* 198:134–140, 1985.

23. Neer CS II: Anterior acromioplasty for the chronic impingement syndrome of the shoulder: A preliminary report. *J Bone Joint Surg* 54A:41–50, 1972.

24. Neer CS II: Impingement lesions. *Clin Orthop* 173:70–77, 1983.

25. Matsen FW, Arntz CT: Subacromial impingement, in Rockwood CA, Matsen FA (eds): *The Shoulder*. Philadelphia: Saunders, 1990.

26. Morrison DS, Bigliani LU: The clinical significance of variations in acromial morphology. *Orthop Trans* 11:234, 1987.

27. Vaz S, Soyer J, Pries P, et al: Subacromial impingement influence of cora coacromial arch geometry on shoulder function. *Joint, Bone, Spine: Revue du Rhumatisme* 67(4): 305–309, 2000.

28. Mudge MK, Wood VE, Frykman GK: Rotator cuff tears associated with os acromiale. *J Bone Joint Surg* 66A:427–429, 1984.

29. Neer CS II: The relationship between the unfused acromial epiphysis and subacromial impingement lesions. *Orthop Trans* 7:138, 1983.

30. Neer CS II: Anterior acromioplasty for the chronic impingement syndrome of the shoulder: A preliminary report. *J Bone Joint Surg* 54A:41–50, 1972.

31. Le Viet DT, Lantieri LA, Loy SM: Wrist and hand injuries in platform diving. *J Hand Surg* 18:176, 1993.

32. Delitto A, Erhard RE, Bowling RW: A treatment classification approach to low back syn-

drome: Identifying and staging patients for conservative treatment. *Phys Ther* 75:470–485, 1995.

33. Puniello MS: Illiotibial band tightness and medial patellar glide in patients with patellofemoral dysfunction. *J Orthop Sports Phys Ther* 17:144–148, 1993.

34. Desio SM, Burks RT, Bachus KN: Soft tissue restraints to lateral patellar translation in the human knee. *Am J Sports Med* 26:59–65, 1998.

35. Souza DR, Gross MT: Comparison of vastus medialis obliquus: Vastus lateralis muscle integrated electromyographic ratios between healthy subjects and patients with patellofemoral pain. *Phys Ther* 71:310–320, 1991.

36. Boucher JP, King MA, Lefebvre R, Pepin A: Quadriceps femoris muscle activity in patellofemoral pain syndrome. *Am J Sports Med* 20:527–532, 1992.

37. Gose JC, Schweizer P: Illiotibial band tightness. *J Orthop Sports Phys Th*er 11:399–407, 1989.

38. Mirzabeigi E, Jordan C, Gronley JK, et al: Isolation of the vastus medialis oblique muscle during exercise. *Am J Sports Med* 27:50–59, 1999.

39. Laprade J, Culham E, Brouwer B: Comparison of five isometric exercises in the recruitment of the vastus medialis oblique in persons with and without patellofemoral pain syndrome. *J Orthop Sports Phys Ther* 27: 197–204, 1998.

40. Salzman A, Torburn L, Perry J: Contribution of rectus femoris and vasti to knee extension. *Clin Orthop* 290:236–243, 1993.

41. Gilleard W, McConnell J, Parsons D: The effect of patellar taping on the onset of vastus medialis obliques and vastus lateralis muscle activity in persons with patellofemoral pain. *Phys Ther* 78:25–32, 1998.

42. Reynolds NL, Worrell TW: Chronic achilles peritendinitis: Etiology, pathophysiology, and treatment. *J Orthop Sport Phys Ther* 13: 171–176, 1991.

43. Root ML, Orien WP, Weed JH: *Normal and Abnormal Function of the Foot*, vol 2. Los Angeles: Clinical Biomechanics, 1977, pp 151–152.

44. Cibulka MT, Sinacore DR, Mueller MJ: Shin splints and forefoot contact running: A case report. *J Orthop Sports Phys Ther* 20:98–102, 1994.

45. Arnheim DD: *Modern Principles of Athletic Training*. St. Louis: Mosby, 1985.

46. Guide to physical therapy practice: I. Description of patient/client management; II. Preferred practice patterns (2nd ed.). *Phys Ther* 81(1): 1–768, 2001.

CHAPTER 7

Golf

Paul R. Geisler

History of Golf

To many modern golfers, St. Andrews, Scotland, is considered to be the birthplace and home of the game of golf. However, historians have been able to date the game's origins to other European locations before the fifteenth century. In those days, a similar stick-and-ball game called *paganica* was played in Holland and France. Other historical records have shown that university students were playing this social game as early as 1415 in St. Andrews in Fife, Scotland. Origins aside, the game became popular in the early fifteenth-century Scotland and gained a large portion of its current shape, structure, and rules as a result of Scottish participation and infatuation. At that time, golf was mostly a game for the kings, queens, and noblemen, hence the reason for the familiar moniker, *The Royal and Ancient Game.*[25]

Golf did not become popular in the United States until the 1600s, and the first course on record was not built until 1888, in Yonkers, New York. Appropriately, it was named the *St. Andrews Club* and originally consisted of a crude three-hole layout. As a testament to the game's appeal and growing popularity as a game for everyone, over 1000 courses were built in America by the year 1900, with each state possessing at least one golf course.[25] Today, the United States possesses almost 17,000 golf courses and boasts a playing population of 26.5 million golfers.[20] To give the reader some perspective on the immense popularity of the game today, consider the following: (1) 503 new golf course construction projects were completed in 1999, (2) golfers spent over $30 billion on golf-related products and services in 1998, and (3) 60 percent of golfers reported that they have played golf with partial snow cover.[20]

To the casual observer, golf may be perceived as just a game, not a sport requiring high physical skill and athletic ability. However, those who have earnestly attempted to play this game will attest that golf is a sport that requires specific athletic abilities. Attributes traditionally reserved for other athletic endeavors, such as strength, agility, coordination, and endurance, are required in order to play high-performance, painfree golf. Each of these athletic components is woven into an integrated and complex motion that requires chronic repetition and diligent attention to detail to produce an efficient and accurate golf swing. As you will see in coming sections of this chapter, the game of golf can contribute significant musculoskeletal strain and injury to its participants.

Equipment Considerations

A golfer typically uses two distinct types of equipment that may help or hinder his or her game depending on his or her physical makeup and history: clubs and shoes. Today, golf clubs are available in a variety of sizes, shapes, styles, and weights. It is beyond the scope of this book to consider the multitude of technical differences between clubs and how each can be customized and personalized to suit an individual golfer. However, there are some general recommendations that the clinician should be aware of when considering the potential implications of equipment on the well-being of the patient.

GOLF SHAFTS

One of the recent technological advances in golf equipment is the ability to economically make the golf shaft out of graphite, titanium, and other "space age" polymer fibers. The golf shaft, once only available in steel, is responsible for transferring the energy created by the body through the hands and the club face and hence into the golf ball. Modern shafts made out of alternative materials are lighter and more flexible and are reported to be capable of absorbing more vibratory forces than steel. Lighter shafts also can be beneficial to those desiring greater club head

speed and greater distance on their full shots. Several companies are now marketing shafts with vibration-dampening devices built into the shaft for those golfers wishing to minimize the stresses transferred into the upper extremities. Golfers with degenerative arthritis and other upper extremity pathologies may be able to reduce the stress to their joints by using graphite, titanium, and other force-dampening shafts. The average golfer probably will not notice much reduction in the amount of vibration and force transmission to the upper extremities with graphite shafts without taking a look at his or her golf swing mechanics and practice habits.

Many golfers (typically the higher handicappers) tend to take large divots when striking golf balls off the ground. Taking large divots when striking the ball off the ground is usually representative of a major swing flaw know as *coming over the top*, which means that the downswing plane is too steep, or vertical. This type of swing pattern usually produces the familiar slice ball pattern in which the ball travels drastically from left to right for a right-handed golfer. More details on this concept will be covered in subsequent sections. Large, deep divots are usually the result of a very steep, sharp angle of attack of the club into the ball (in contrast to more skilled players, who take thin, smaller divots as a result of a proper swing plane and an improved ball-striking component). As you can imagine, taking these large divots (resembling a "pork chop") increases the amount of force transferred directly into the hands, negating any dampening effects that a high-tech golf shaft might possess. Finally, it is also important to be cognizant of the fact that lighter and more flexible shafts are also much more expensive and typically do not perform as consistently as do their steel counterparts (the technical shaft characteristics that skilled players prefer are more variable among different graphite shafts).

Another aspect of golf equipment that can be adapted for different people is the length of the golf shaft. The concept of using long-shafted putters is a fairly common practice today, as represented by the many long putters available on the market currently. There are also many successful golfers on the professional tours (particularly the Senior PGA Tour) using long-shafted putters in an effort to alleviate stress to the lumbar spine while putting. It is very common for golfers to complain of increased lumbar spine discomfort when practicing their putting and chipping skills. Typically, their discomfort is due to the prolonged periods of time they sustain a forward flexed and somewhat rotated position. Long-shafted putters should be a serious consideration for golfers with significant postural deficiencies and/or lumbar pathologies, but be aware that the putting stroke and joint kinematics required to putt also change significantly when incorporating such a drastic change.

The length of the shafts for the driving and striking clubs (woods and irons) also can be adapted to the individual golfer. It has been a popular trend for golfers to be *custom fitted* for their clubs. Many times golfers who are over 6 ft tall have had their clubs lengthened in order to accommodate for their increased height. Although this is done with good intention, simple analysis of physics shows that longer levers, although capable of producing greater force and speed, require greater muscular effort and control in order to move.

GOLF SHOES

The last piece of equipment modification that should be considered by the clinician is the golf shoe. In particular, the types of spikes used on the shoe need to be addressed. Shoes with metal spikes are designed to create more friction and torque between the ground and the golfer. As a result, they also can produce more torque in the knee and hip joints of the golfer. Thus golfers with joint instabilities, injury, pain, and/or degenerative conditions of the knee and/or hip joints should experiment with soft-spike shoes and the newer "sneaker" type of golf shoes that have molded, nonspike soles.

Biomechanics of the Golf Swing

The purpose of this section is to describe the general biomechanics of the full golf swing so that you can understand how the body needs to work and react while performing the maneuvers necessary to swing a golf club at a high-performance level. Learning to implement these concepts in real time and learning how to actually play golf are not the focus of this section. The assistance of a qualified and experienced Professional Golfers Association (PGA) or Ladies Professional Golfers Association (LPGA) teaching professional should be sought for further elaboration and clarity on specific swing-skill development and other aspects of playing the game. An attempt will be made here to differentiate between the proper swing mechanics of more skilled players and some of the more common swing faults seen in players with lesser skill. All references to the full swing will be based on the actions of a right-handed golfer (unless otherwise noted). Practical implications for injury, performance, rehabilitation, and exercise will be developed according to the mechanics outlined within the upcoming section.

KINESIOLOGY OF THE GOLF SWING

Kinesiologists have classified the motion of hitting a golf ball as being a *reverse underarm pattern*, a modification of traditional underarm patterns such as bowling or softball pitching.[5] This classification was based on the movement of the left arm from a horizontal position above or at shoulder level at the top of the backswing downward to a position parallel with the trunk at impact. The golf swing originally was termed a *reverse underarm pattern* because it was felt that the left arm contributed the primary force during the downswing (in a right-handed golfer). We now know that the golf swing varies from the traditional underarm pattern. Recent muscle electromyographic (EMG) studies have shown that both arms are active throughout the entire swing and that both arms contribute significantly to the development of club head speed during the downswing.[4,12]

The model swing has been described as having a single fixed center hub of rotation with a two-lever, one-hinge moment arm to impart force on the ball.[4] This center hub actually lies somewhere in the middle of the sternum and represents the player's dynamic center of gravity. The hub of the swing acts as the fixed center of the golfer, around which the moment arm rotates on a specific plane. This system works much like the hub and spokes of a bicycle or wagon wheel. The role of this hub and its component moving parts is crucial in full swing success.[4] In order to produce an efficient and accurate golf shot, the golfer should keep his or her center hub within the base of support during the entire golf swing. To further understand this concept, visualize a wagon wheel that is moving at high speed with the center axis (axle) also moving randomly and constantly, as if it were independent of the wheel itself. This model of two randomly moving parts would eliminate the solid, stable base needed to produce a stable rotating perimeter.

Perhaps a more appropriate analogy is the relationship known to exist between dynamic scapular stability and glenohumeral joint movement, precision, and function. A scapulothoracic joint that has the proper balance of rhythm, movement, and stability during complex overhead motions allows for the glenohumeral joint to move efficiently and with minimal stresses. A golfer with a stable center hub has a better chance of executing an accurate, powerful, and efficient golf swing with his or her upper extremities.

A skilled golf swing requires the same stability, balance, and coordination that a wagon wheel, a baseball pitcher or hitter, and a world-class tennis player require to perform properly. The athlete's hub should be kept centered so that the lever arms (spokes) can position themselves properly with minimal compensatory movements or unnecessary physical stress. Unnecessary lateral movement of the center hub will change the timing and joint action requirements of the subsequent motion. This results in an increased demand on the distal segments of the kinetic chain movement—the arms and hands.

The second fundamental concept of the perfect model golf swing is a two-lever action of the moment arm (Fig. 7.1). The left arm in a right-handed golfer forms the upper lever of the moment arm, whereas the club shaft forms the lower lever. The wrist joints serve as the hinge that controls the action of the two levers. When the wrists release just prior to impact, the club approximates its original position at setup and forms one straight lever arm from the ground up to the lead-arm glenohumeral joint. This action consequently produces what is known as the *final moment arm* at impact. During the downswing, it is thought that the left arm dictates the plane of the club, whereas the right arm follows this preset pattern and later provides substantial power to the downswing.[4] Successful utilization and coordination of these two principles is a characteristic of many highly skilled players and a cornerstone fundamental of many teaching professionals. Many less successful golfers fail to use these mechanical principles in their swings and end up losing significant power, accuracy, and repeatability.

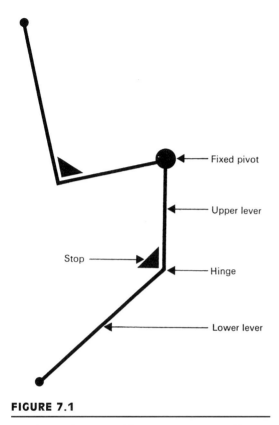

FIGURE 7.1

The two-lever, one-hinge system proposed by Cochran and Stobbs. The upper extremity and the golf shaft form the levers, while the wrist joints serve as the hinge. (*Used with permission from Cochran and Stobbs.*[4])

PHASES OF THE FULL GOLF SWING

The full golf swing can be broken down into four major phases: setup (or address), backswing, downswing, and follow-through.[4] The following biomechanical analysis will be given using a right-handed golfer as a model, whereby the right side of the golfer is referred to as the *back*-side, and the left side is called the *lead*-side.

The Grip

Although it is beyond the scope of this book to delve into the many complexities of the golf grip, its importance in the swing war-

rants some investigation so that the reader will be able to understand the action of the hands and wrists during a live swing. The proper grip also must be established during the setup phase, and although there are many schools of thought concerning the "proper" way to grip a golf club, the classic *Vardon grip* (or *overlap*) is the most popular and productive grip among touring professionals (Fig. 7.2). The *interlock* and the *baseball* grips constitute the other commonly used golf grips. In addition to the type of grip employed, grips are also characterized as being *neutral, strong,* or *weak* depending on the rotational position of the hands on the grip. Accomplished players usually rotate their lead hand to either a neutral or strong position while keeping their back-side hand relatively neutral, whereas lesser skilled players generally tend to rotate both hands to a typically strong hand position on the club.

As a right-handed golfer looks down at his or her hands on the grip, a strong grip is one whereby the hands are rotated more clockwise, showing much of the dorsal aspect of the left hand. This grip is considered strong because of the increase ability to release the hands during the downswing and impact phases, thus producing more speed as well as greater chances for mishits and off-line shots. Freddy Couples, John Daly, and Paul Azinger are some of the more popular professional golfers employing very strong grips. In contrast, weak grips consist of the hands being rotated more counterclockwise so that more of the dorsal aspect of the right hand can be seen. Weak grips decrease the amount of hand speed that can be contributed to the swing but allow for a little more club-face control. Although this grip is not very widely employed, Nick Faldo and Curtis Strange are probably the best examples of popular players with moderately weak grips. As you would suspect, neutral grips lie somewhere subjectively in the middle, and a majority of world-class players fall into this rather nebulous category.

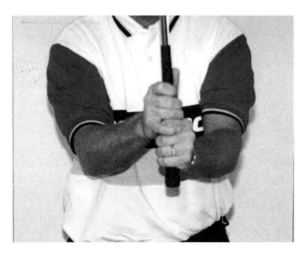

FIGURE 7.2

The classic Vardon or overlapping golf grip employed by the majority of professional tour players.

Regardless of the type of grip chosen, there are two distinct characteristics that should make up an effective and functional golf grip. An effective golf grip, regardless of style or personal choice, performs two functions: (1) it allows the club to hinge and unhinge during the golf swing, and (2) it controls the angle of the club face during the swing. The hinging and unhinging function of the grip is the primary physical mechanism whereby club-head speed is transferred from the body into the club, linking the two lever arms of the golf swing (lead arm and club shaft). The club-face control aspect of the grip is responsible for the directional and trajectory qualities of the golf shot, producing shots that may go left, straight, right, high, or low depending on the angle of the club face at impact.

In order for the chosen method of gripping the club to be deemed an effective golf grip, it must have great stability and adequate mobility. It is of little value to have an exaggerated hinging motion with the hands, wrists, and club and consequently lose control of the club and club face throughout the actual golf swing. Likewise, it is generally not very productive to have an extremely tight grip with maximum control of the club at the expense of an effective hinge and lever system. These mechanical grip flaws are two of the many common mistakes made by novice and intermediate golfers.

The natural structure and resulting mobility of the hands, wrists, and thumbs will strongly dictate the most effective grip for most golfers. In particular, the amount of radial deviation available in the lead hand of the golfer will dictate whether a golfer can use a neutral or strong grip position. Unpublished data collected by me have shown that among accomplished golfers, those with limited radial deviation (≤ 10 degrees) tended to favor using a strong left-hand grip, whereas those with more normal levels of radial deviation (approaching 20 degrees) were more comfortable with a neutral left-hand grip. Golf professionals who work on an individual basis and understand this elementary concept can work to custom fit a functional golf grip for each individual golfer through a fairly scientific trial-and-error process.

Setup Position

The setup phase (more appropriately, a position) is the first and most important phase in the golf swing. Often it is also the most neglected aspect of a golfer's practice and focus that can lead directly to poor performance, increased levels of physical stress, and eventually injury. As with other dynamic sports activities requiring precision and accuracy, the initial starting position for executing a full golf swing should align the golfer properly with the target, establish his or her dynamic and static balance, and place the golfer in a biomechanically sound and advantageous position from which to execute the ensuing golf swing.

When the movement of the backswing begins, the quality and sequence of moving body segments are going to be influenced directly by the initial setup position. If the golfer's position is biomechanically sound and balanced, the swinging motion has a better chance of being executed properly with higher efficiency. Likewise, if the setup position is biomechanically disadvantaged (i.e., the golfer's weight is on his or her heels, or he or she assumes a postural position characterized by cervical and lumbar flexion), the motion most likely will be forced, stressful, and of a compensatory nature. In effect, golfers who initiate their swinging motion with compromised setup positions are increasing the complexity of their movement as well as their chance for injury. More details on these principles will be covered in sections on the backswing and downswing.

Weight distribution at setup will vary from golfer to golfer and teacher to teacher, but scientific studies show that the golfer should be positioned with 50 to 60 percent of his or her weight on the back foot.[1] The knees should be flexed about 20 to 25 degrees, while the golfer must form and maintain two angles with his or her trunk in order to establish the proper position from which to rotate into the backswing.[21] The first angle is created by hinging the hips to perform forward trunk flexion called the *primary spinal angle* (Fig. 7.3A). The hip joints serve as the axis of rotation, whereas the midtrunk and thigh lines serve as the lever arms to form the angle. When a golfer fails to use a hip hinge to achieve the primary spinal angle, stress on the spine increases and free rotation decreases (Fig. 7.3B).

The second "angle" is created with a combination of lateral bending to the right in the spinal segments and slight depression and downward rotation of the arm and scapula and is termed the *secondary spinal angle* (Fig. 7.4). This position is a result of the necessary hand placement on the club grip, whereby the right hand is placed lower than the left. This functional hand position causes the right shoulder to tilt lower than the left. High-speed video analysis of professional golfers indicates that at setup, the average primary angle is approximately 45 degrees, whereas the average secondary angle measures 16 degrees.[21] Naturally, these values will vary according to the overall position assumed by each individual golfer during setup and his or her individual postural tendencies.

Backswing Phase

The exact timing, sequencing, and kinesiologic details of the golf swing (both downswing and backswing) have been, and will continue to be, the source of much debate among golf professionals and scientists. To complicate matters even further, very few scientific details exist today concerning the exact muscle firing patterns and/or joint activities during the golf swing. These next sections on the backswing and downswing will attempt to give the reader a detailed synopsis of the data and thoughts that do exist concerning the biomechanics and dynamics of the full golf swing.

Much like other sports motions (throwing, kicking, and striking), the backswing phase initiates movement in certain body segments to create maximal kinetic energy production with minimal effort. The purpose of the backswing is threefold. First, a skilled

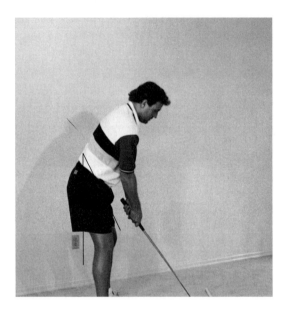

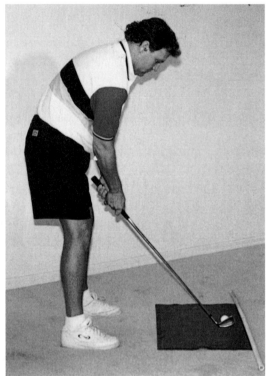

FIGURE 7.3

The primary spine angle achieved during the setup phase. This angle should be maintained throughout the entire backswing also. *B.* A golfer failing to use a hip hinge to achieve the primary spine angle. This position increases spinal stress and decreases free rotation.

backswing will position and align the golfer's center hub and club head in an optimal position from which to execute a powerful and accurate downswing.[4] Second, it provides the initial base link for the downswing's kinetic chain and summation of force principles to work. Third, the preparatory motion of the backswing places a stretch load on the muscular elements and joint structures involved in executing the downswing, creating greater potential energy and momentum.

It is widely believed that the backswing movement should be initiated with a "one-piece takeaway" of the club and the golfer's hands and arms.[9] The triangle that is formed with the two arms and chest at setup ideally should be maintained throughout the first 1 to 2 ft of the backswing to constitute a one-piece takeaway (Fig. 7.5). A proper one-piece takeaway is initiated by an active linear movement of the arms and hands along a line across the golfer's toes and parallel to the target line (an imaginary line running through the ball toward the target). In reality, rotation of the thoracic spine actually will work in concert with the abduction and adduction movements of the arms to initiate this movement. In effect, the first 2 ft of the golf swing

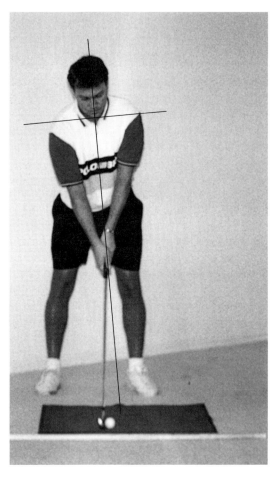

FIGURE 7.4

The secondary spine angle achieved during the setup phase. This angle is produced as an indirect result of the right hand being lower than the left on the grip.

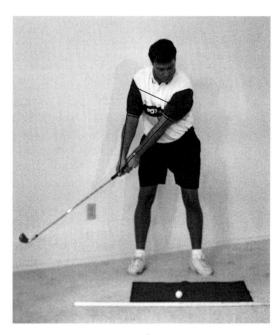

FIGURE 7.5

The one-piece takeaway recommended by most golf professionals. Note the triangle formed by the arms and torso.

should be identical in motion to that for a long putt or a short chip shot. Many golf instructors feel that critical swing flaws develop here during the first 2 to 3 ft of the takeaway and thus are directly responsible for many of the common downswing flaws seen in amateur golfers. Errors made here in skilled golfers will require an "equal and opposite force," or compensatory motion, during the downswing to correct the error and ensure

maximal accuracy and club-head speed development.

After this critical takeaway move, the thoracic cage (shoulders) continues to rotate and eventually pulls the pelvic girdle (hips) into rotation in synchronization with the arm movement. At about the time the hands reach hip level, the right arm will begin to abduct slightly from the body's midline, outwardly rotate, and flex at the elbow joint, whereas the left arm will adduct and inwardly rotate somewhat. This combined movement of shoulder rotation, adduction, and simultaneous slight arm flexion is a critical yet unnatural move for most people and is another source of swing mechanics error.[4] As noted previously, it is commonly believed that it is within the first 1 to 2 ft of movement that the plane of the backswing will be dictated. Following the lead given by the early backswing movement of the thoracic cage and arms, the remaining backswing actions either will follow the proper lead or will have to compensate to get back on track before the downswing begins.

A highly efficient swing will keep the club on plane throughout the entire swing and reduce excess off-plane movements.[4,9] The *swing plane*, a somewhat vague and often misinterpreted geometric and spatial concept, is merely the plane in which the club will move as it is manipulated by the golfer during all phases of the full swing. Instructors can complicate the concept by using terms such as *shaft plane, swing plane, club plane,* and even *club path* interchangeably. Significant controversy exists among teaching professionals today on the ideal swing plane and, more important, on how the club should work to get on and stay on plane. Ben Hogan described the swing plane as one traveling from the ball to the shoulders of the golfer and presented an image of a plate of glass with a hole cut out for the head running from the ball and resting on the golfer's shoulders.[9] He suggested that the club shaft ought to move up and down slightly on the inside (golfer's side) of the plate of glass and never come into contact with it. Contacting the plate of glass with the club, hands, or arms would result in a shattered sheet of glass and an over-the-top swing plane.

Still others draw, or imagine, a line running through the golf shaft and continuing up through the golfer's legs to indicate the shaft plane. Advocates of this viewpoint are more concerned with the plane of the club during the early takeaway phase of the backswing and then again during the late preimpact downswing phases and are subsequently less concerned with the plane of the club at the top of the swing. Others firmly believe that there are actually two planes in which the club travels: one fairly shallow plane that is parallel to the shaft at setup during the early and middle backswing and a sharper, more

vertical plane that mirrors Ben Hogan's model during the latter half of the backswing as the club nears the top.[9]

Observation of high-level golf swings reveals that this latter viewpoint is probably the most accurate of the lot. However, most experts agree that the downswing plane should be slightly more shallow than the backswing plane in order to strike the ball with maximum energy and precision.

Because the swing plane is probably the most influential factor in determining the quality of the golf shot, and because all serious golfers are concerned with and/or working on their swing plane at some point in their training, it is important for the clinician to gain an understanding of the swing-plane concept. One can gain a visual conception of the swing plane by observing the *swing-plane zone* that is formed by making a triangle when the golfer and the club are addressed to the ball (Fig. 7.6). In a very simplistic sense, the more that the club can stay in this swing-plane zone, the more successful the golf shot will be, and the more that it travels outside this zone, the more complicated the kinesiologic movements need to be to execute the shot. Because of differences in club length, lie angles (angle created between the club head and the shaft), setup postures, and other technical factors, each golfer's swing-plane zone is determined and preestablished at setup by the position of the club and that of the golfer when the club is placed behind the ball.

As the backswing continues, the shoulders will pull the pelvic girdle into right rotation, forcing the pelvis to turn clockwise away from the target line. This motion is accompanied by a change in the position of the center of gravity (COG). If the golfer has good rotary flexibility and maintains his or her secondary spine angle during this motion, the COG will translate primarily in a rotary fashion, staying well within the base of support (BOS). Because of certain rotary limitations and

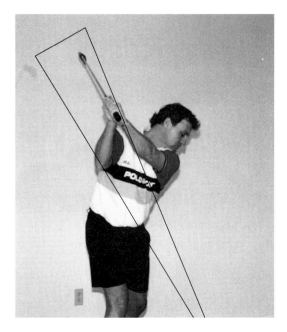

FIGURE 7.6

The swing-plane-zone concept represents the plane in which the back- and downswings should occur within. Note the shaft plane going through the shaft and the longer line going through the shoulders.

swing mechanic faults in many golfers, this rotary movement often produces a lateral shift in the center hub of rotation. In turn, this lateral motion tends to produce a concurrent loss in the secondary spine angle. This lateral weight shift is often a by-product of poor mechanics, misinterpreted teaching, or preexisting physical limitations (the consequences of an excessive lateral weight shift are discussed in the ensuing downswing section, whereas the specific physical limitations applicable to this problem will be discussed in the evaluation section).

There is a great deal of controversy surrounding the weight-shift principle in golf, with many teachers and players feeling that the large muscles of the buttocks, hips, and legs are responsible for producing the majority of club-head speed in the downswing. Perhaps the greatest ball striker ever, Ben Hogan, was a firm proponent of this principle, as published in his historic golf instruction text.[9] He felt that a very significant and active weight shift to the right side in the backswing, followed by an aggressive shift back to the left side to initiate and carry out his downswing, was critical to his success. Simple visual analysis of the greatest players today, including Hogan, reveals that most high-level players have very little true lateral motion of their base of support during the backswing. In contrast, a majority of the backswing motion in today's players is a result of rotation around a fixed base of support rather than an aggressive lateral weight shift.

I feel that a more appropriate term for the *weight-shift phenomenon* is *weight transfer*. This term allows for the existence of both a weight rotation and a slight lateral weight shift while not overemphasizing either. An efficient golf swing keeps the center hub of rotation more stable and consistent, which allows for an easier coordination of the moving parts during the swing. A significant lateral weight shift during the backswing can move the golfer's COG outside the base of support and consequently make it anatomically and kinesiologically difficult to keep the secondary spine angle. When a golfer overshifts his or her weight and or attempts to overrotate into the backswing, he or she often produces a reverse weight shift or pivot (Fig. 7.7). A reverse weight shift is characterized by having too much weight on the front foot at the top of the backswing and is usually a direct attempt to maintain swing balance. Furthermore, the notion of the hips and legs providing the speed in the downswing is challenged by scientific data indicating that the hips and torso produce approximately 10 percent of the total linear velocity in the downswings of skilled players[19] (Table 7.1).

Data generated from professional golf swing analyses indicate that the average

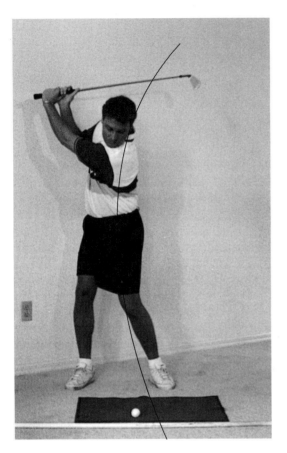

FIGURE 7.7

A reverse weight shift or pivot during the
backswing. This golfer has too much weight on
the front foot and has increased the stress on the
spine significantly. To initiate the downswing from
this position, the golfer must aggressively shift
the lower body toward the target in order to
reestablish the original position.

ranges of shoulder girdle and hip girdle rotation at the end of backswing are 102 and 47
degrees, respectively.[21] Other studies with
different assessment techniques have reported varying degrees of segmental rotation
as well as differences between golfing populations. One study found that PGA players averaged 87 degrees of shoulder rotation and
55 degrees of hip rotation, Senior PGA Tour
players averaged 78 and 49 degrees, and amateurs averaged 87 and 53 degrees for shoulder and hip-turn values, respectively.[18] Overall, these figures seem to concur with the
generally accepted notion of attempting to
turn the shoulders 90 degrees and the hips 45
degrees, or in an approximate 2:1 ratio. The
major empirical limitation of these studies
lies in the lack of control in measuring these
values with respect to the dynamic changes
in other critical motion variables such as the
spine angles (primary and secondary) and
the rear knee flexion angle. In effect, the
amount of perceived or measured hip and
shoulder rotation needs to be considered in
relation to other important swing characteristics. Much more research needs to be conducted to truly understand the complex relationships between all the kinetic links in the
golf swing and the associated "domino effect"
that occurs as a kinetic chain reaction un-
folds.

With the majority of golfers, it is important to realize that the relative amounts of
hip and shoulder rotation accessible during
the golf swing depend on specific physical
limitations and postural influences. In most
cases, the amount of hip and shoulder rotation "observed" usually is accompanied by
some form of physical or mechanical compensation that is undertaken in an effort to
achieve a "full backswing turn" in exchange
for maximal club speed and distance. The
consequences associated with this maneuver
are complex and have many physical and mechanical implications.

At the top of the backswing (Fig. 7.8), the
left elbow remains extended but not locked,
whereas the left shoulder joint has inwardly
rotated and horizontally adducted across the
chest. This action also causes the left shoulder blade to abduct, elevate, and rotate outwardly. As a result of the left arm position
during the backswing phase, a stretch load
is being placed on the posterior rotator cuff
and scapular muscles of the left shoulder,

TABLE 7.1

Linear Contribution of Joints in the Full Golf Swing[13]

Wrist	70%	Fastest acting joint, most distal link in chain
Shoulders	20%	The longest moment arm/lever
Spine	5%	Contribute energy and pass along to shoulders
Hips	5%	Fire in response to movement initiated by LE; transfer energy into torso/spine
	100%	

whereas the glenohumeral joint is forced into an impingement position.[26] Improper functioning, rhythm, and flexibility of shoulder and scapular muscles during this movement can contribute to shoulder impingement signs and symptoms, particularly in older golfers and those with a history of past shoulder problems.

While thoracic cage rotation to the right is nearing its end point, the right elbow passively flexes as the right shoulder joint is extremely rotating and abducting. The degree of the motions in both shoulders and arms will vary depending on physical limitations and swing philosophies, but the arm should be abducted approximately 75 to 90 degrees and externally rotated 90 degrees in order to maintain a consistent swing plane. It generally has been considered that the backswing is completed when the club shaft is at or near a position that is parallel to the ground when using a driver or number 1 wood. Observation of many of today's professional golfers will reveal a great deal of variance with regard to backswing length (John Daly versus Tom Lehman or John Cook). Anatomically, the available range of motion in the left shoulder complex, combined with the amount of spinal rotation, will be the deciding factor in determining the height of any one particular golfer's backswing (this will be covered in more detail in the following sections). Additionally, there is currently no scientific re-

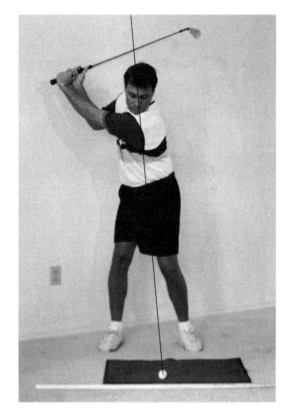

FIGURE 7.8

The top of the backswing. Note how the golfer has maintained the spine angles and the two-lever, one-hinge system.

search supporting the claim that *parallel with the ground* is the ideal position for the end of the backswing.

Depending on the instructor, the timing and mechanism by which the hands and wrist cock the club during the backswing will vary somewhat. Regardless of the precise cocking mechanism and timing of such a mechanism, most instructors attempt to get their golfers to cock their wrists and hands so that the dorsum of the left hand is parallel with its respective forearm and with the club face. This position is considered to be *square*. The ability to achieve this position depends directly on the amount of radial deviation present in the lead wrist. Golfers with adequate radial deviation of approximately 20 degrees should be able to achieve a wrist-cock position with minimal wrist extension. In contrast, golfers possessing limited lead-hand radial deviation must use a significant amount of wrist extension to cock the club. Many think that a square hand and club face position at the top of the backswing simplifies the releasing (uncocking) mechanism of the club during the downswing. Looked at from another perspective, an extension cocked hand and wrist position requires the golfer to actively eliminate the degree of wrist extension during the downswing if he or she wishes to return the club face to a square position just prior to impact.

At the end of the backswing, the lead leg is now bearing approximately 40 percent of the body weight[1] and has passively rotated externally as a result of the active pelvic rotation right. Although it is more a function of available range of motion and overall body posture, many golf instructors feel that the left patella should be pointing at or slightly behind the ball at the end of the backswing.[9] Although very difficult to quantify, and research has not yet addressed the subtlety of the motions, some degree of lead tibial internal rotation and foot pronation also will occur during the backswing phase of the full swing. As such, golfers with limited external hip rotation or tibial rotation in the lead leg might produce unwanted swing compensations and/or produce unwanted physical stresses to various components of the lower kinetic chain. Typically, this swing compensation takes the form of the lead heal leaving the ground (a combined plantarflexion-eversion maneuver) during the backswing move (i.e., Jack Nicklaus).

Continuing with the joint movements associated with the backswing phase, pelvic rotation forces the back-side femur to internally rotate within the acetabulum. Adequate amounts of internal rotation in the back-side femur allow for the pelvis to rotate fully and evenly, as indicated by level anterosuperior iliac spine (ASIS) landmarks, and for the right knee flexion angle (20 degrees) to be maintained as it was during the setup position. These dynamic abilities and swing references have a direct influence on the golfer's balance, hip levels, body position (including spine angles), and ability to properly initiate the swing move.

Anatomic and physiologic factors (retroverted or anteverted hips or capsular flexibility patterns) may play a role in the amount of lead heel lift employed by certain golfers and/or the ability to maintain the rear knee angle during the backswing phase. The amount of back-side hip internal rotation (IR) has a direct influence on the ability to maintain the same-side knee flexion angle. In effect, golfers with limited back-side internal rotation (<30 degrees) have difficulty keeping their rear knee flexion angle during the backswing, which causes a chain reaction of compensations to occur during the remaining swing movements. When the rear knee flexion angle decreases (knee extends) because of limited hip IR, the back-side ASIS will raise up and move laterally toward the back-side. If significant enough, this can cause a loss of secondary and primary spine angles and set the golfer up for more pronounced problems during the downswing. A golfer with limited hip internal rotation may be better off setting up to the ball with the feet flared outward approximately 10 to 20 degrees in an attempt to create more freedom of movement in the acetabulum. This will help the pelvis rotate more freely during both the backswing and downswing motions by creating a small degree of "false" hip internal rotation.

In order for the golfer's center of rotation to remain stable, both spinal angles need to be maintained as close to the original angles at the top of the backswing.[9] Maintaining both spine angles and achieving a full 90-degree shoulder turn and a 45-degree hip turn requires the golfer to have excellent hip, shoulder, and torso flexibility with minimal lateral weight shift. In addition, keeping the secondary spine angle during the backswing allows for a natural and uninhibited path during the downswing because it effectively prevents the body from getting in the way of the arms and club during the downswing. In contrast, losing the secondary spine angle (reverse pivot) places the player's body in the way of the downswing path and will require a very complicated and stressful maneuver during the downswing to get the body "out of the way." Skilled players generally do an excellent job of maintaining their spinal angles using true rotation and maintaining balance throughout their swings, whereas many high handicappers tend to increase the complexity and stress production by using a greater amount of lateral motion within their swings.

Downswing Phase

The function of the downswing phase is to return the club back to its original position, at the proper time, and with maximum speed in an effort to produce a crisp, powerful, and accurate golf shot. Although the speed and forces created are much greater, the kinetic sequence of the backswing is relatively reversed during the downswing. The down-

swing actually has two subphases that blend together to initiate movement of the body and generate club-head speed.[12] These subphases are known, respectively, as the *forward swing* and *acceleration*. The movement responsible for initiating the forward swing has been a chronic topic of debate among golf professionals. Some golf teachers feel that the hands initiate the forward swing, whereas others believe that hip turn and an aggressive weight transfer are primarily responsible.[3,9] However, scientific research supports the notion that the downswing motion starts from the ground up. Bechler[3] studied EMG output of the hip and knee muscles during the golf swing and found that the back-side hip extensors and abductors, in conjunction with the lead adductor magnus, initiated pelvic rotation during the forward swing. Although data are not available regarding the contribution of the lead foot and ankle, it is my belief that a subtle supinatory movement in this most distal link is responsible for producing a slight lateral rotation of the patella prior to the documented hip and pelvis activity.

Once initiated from the distal segments close to the ground, swing momentum and kinetic energy travel in a logical kinetic sequence. High-speed analysis actually has shown that this downswing sequence starts just before the backswing actually has finished its respective motion. Research has shown that the skilled performer initiates pelvic girdle rotation to the left before the shoulders and wrists have completed their respective backswing movements.[4,7] Bechler's work also supports the notion of the sequential firing pattern of the hip and knee muscles that take place during the competitive golf swing.[3]

Once the forward swing has taken place and acceleration has begun, the hips and shoulders continue their left sequential rotational pattern while the arms and hands gradually flow into the swing in an effort to generate club-head acceleration. The downswing in golf is a perfect example of the human kinetic chain principle in action. The legs and hips initiate the kinetic chain movement; pass it sequentially through the core, trunk, and shoulders; and then pass it into the hands and wrists. If executed properly, an amount of energy far greater than the sum of the parts is passed from the body into the club head. Proper coordination of this process allows for a gradual and natural summation of forces to occur so that a tremendous amount of kinetic energy is transferred into the club. This process is a very large component of the "effortless" characteristic used to describe many of the professional golf swings seen today.

During the downswing, the golfer must position the club on the proper swing plane (established at setup by the club position) before impact if he or she wishes to produce an accurate and repetitive shot pattern.[9] The resulting position of the club face as it is about to strike the golf ball largely depends on two primary factors: (1) the plane that the club took during the downswing and (2) the action the golfer has been forced to use at that precise moment in order to correct or compensate for other previously committed faults. If the downswing has remained on plane and its motion has been natural and efficient, the release of the hands, wrists, and club is a fairly simple and natural process. However, the actual mechanics employed during the release and impact phase is often directly influenced by any previous mechanical mistakes that were made by other body segments (off-plane backswing, improper sequencing of kinetic links, excessive wrist extension employed for the wrist cock, loss of secondary spine angle, and excessive flexion of the lead-side elbow are the most common early flaws). Uncoordinated and off-plane movements that produce exaggerated hip, torso, or hand positions can negatively influence the ability of the golfer to get the club face "square" at just the right time. This scenario is quite common in unskilled swings and can contribute heavily to the development of unnecessary stresses to vulnerable body segments. On the other hand, there are many accomplished golfers with tremendous eye-hand coordination and highly skilled hands that allow them to "recover" with remarkable consistency and accuracy (Lee Trevino, Freddy Couples, Corey Pavin, and Laura Davies are just a few).

Beginners often attempt to initiate the downswing too early and/or too fast with the hands and arms to generate immediate club-head speed, whereas more experienced players effectively use certain physical laws to their advantage. In general, skilled swings use centrifugal force and the law of conservation of angular momentum to gradually build maximum club-head speed at impact.[4,19] Centrifugal force is developed as the club head is completing its rotary motion toward the ball, seeking to impact its force in a linear direction at any one given moment in time. The connection of the club head to the body, via the club shaft and the player's hands, acts as the radius of the circle going toward the golfer's center hub of rotation and becomes the moment arm at impact.[4]

The law of conservation of angular momentum is applied to the golf swing as speed is being transferred from the hands to the club head. Remember that energy can neither be created nor destroyed; it is always conserved—angular momentum is no exception to this rule. At the beginning of the downswing, the hands are moving their fastest, whereas the club head is moving its slowest. As the club head nears impact, the hands begin to decelerate and transfer the angular momentum to the club head, which will then accelerate. The total angular momentum is maintained throughout. Smooth and efficient operation of this process requires a well-coordinated kinetic chain and proper action of the two levers and the one hinge to produce one effective moment arm at impact with maximum angular velocity.[4] Skilled players are effectively able to coordinate the action of the different body segments to allow these physical laws to occur naturally, whereas many amateurs try to force these laws to happen too early in the downswing.

As touched on earlier, another common theory in golf teaching circles is that the larger muscles of the legs, buttocks, and torso perform most of the work and therefore provide most of the club-head speed in the golf swing.[9] This theory is accompanied by the notion that using the entire body for power and endurance will decrease the demand and stresses placed on the smaller muscles and bones of the upper extremities. However, golfers who follow this theory tend to have too much lateral movement in their base of support and less rotary movement in their swings. The result is the tendency to attain the "reverse-C" swing pattern throughout the downswing and into the follow-through position. In fact, the greater the lateral weight shift, the greater is the extent of the reverse-C attained at the finish position. As most clinicians are aware, prolonged exposure to this position can produce significant hyperextension stresses to the vertebrae, disks, and soft tissues of the spine. Fortunately, most golf instructors have become aware of this relationship and have since abandoned it as a teaching method of choice.

Although it is true that all body segments must work together in a well-timed and well-coordinated sequence (kinetic chain and summation of forces) to produce a sound golf swing, we have not yet uncovered the true source of actual speed in the golf swing. In contrast to the weight-transfer school of thought, some teachers believe that shoulder and arm actions are responsible for a majority of the club-head speed and that the lower body segments and trunk merely contribute the base of support and some initial movement. Keeping the lower body balanced and

stable allows the arms and club to accurately repeat the backswing and downswing planes with minimal interference. Scientific experiments and current kinesiologic information tend to support this school of thought. Unfortunately, this also places greater physical demands on the anatomic structures of the shoulders, arms, and hands. Any individual golfer's true source of speed often will dictate the overall swing characteristics, the level of consistency, and the potential for injury. In general, golfers with a greater degree of rotary motion require greater shoulder, upper back, and arm strength and control, whereas golfers with more lateral movement require greater abdominal and lower-back strength and stability.

Golfers working on keeping their spine angles throughout the backswing need to be aware that it is very difficult to maintain both spinal angles when the hips move laterally in an effort to produce power. Likewise, golfers who are working to eliminate their lateral maneuver and the dreaded reverse-C finish during the downswing need to focus on keeping their secondary spine angle throughout their backswing. As one may suspect, significant spine angle changes can have drastic effects on the precise action, quality, timing, and rhythm of the swing, as well as on the physiologic well-being of the golfer. The physiologic implications will be discussed in more depth in the upcoming section on improper swing mechanics.

Although in-depth data regarding the precise sequence of joint and muscle action are not yet available, information regarding the segmental velocities during the downswing has been described in the literature. High-speed video analysis of professional golfers shows that average angular velocities for hip rotation, shoulder rotation, arm speed, and club speed were 498, 723, 1165, and 2090 degrees/s, respectively.[21] Maximum club velocity for the sample tested measured 2581 degrees/s, whereas other authors have reported the average club-head speed for top golfers to be approximately 100 to 110 mi/h.[5] About 60 percent of the linear club-head velocity is directly attributable to the action of the hands, with smaller amounts coming from the larger body segments (arms, shoulders, hips, etc.; see Table 7-1).[19] These studies support the kinetic chain and summation of forces concepts by showing how speed is generated over time and eventually passed to the most distal segment (hands) with the greatest kinetic energy.

As the hands and club are approaching the impact position, the arms, hands, and club should approximate their initial starting positions. The left arm is quickly externally rotating and moving toward the midline from a horizontally adducted position, while the right arm is internally rotating and adducting. The left elbow should remain fully extended, while the right elbow gradually extends to approximately 170 degrees. It is generally believed that the wrists should remain cocked until the last possible instant if maximum speed is to be achieved, in effect creating a "lag" effect (Fig. 7.9). It has been suggested that premature uncocking of the wrists (golf professionals refer to this action as "casting" the club, in reference to the action of casting a fishing rod) dismantles the effective two-lever, one-hinge system and creates a one-lever, no-hinge system. This action effectively decelerates the golfer's arm speed, thus decreasing the angular speed of the entire swing.

If the club is returned to its original starting position at impact, the left elbow will be fully extended, and the right elbow will extend to approximately 175 degrees. Meanwhile, both wrists should be released to approximate the starting position[9] (Fig. 7.10). During the release of the hands and wrists, the left wrist will uncock via a passive ulnar deviation movement while sustaining approximately 35 degrees of flexion (45 degrees of extension at setup). Some degree of left forearm supination and right forearm pronation are also involved as the hands release, but the significance of these actions has not yet been thoroughly investigated secondary to the speed and subtlety of the movement. However, the force that is created during a live swing will cause both wrists to ulnar deviate slightly and the left wrist to "bow" into flexion as the hands near the contact zone.

Recent EMG studies have helped to understand and dispel an old golf teaching myth concerning muscle activity and power generation. It has long been thought that the left side of the body provides the power to hit a golf ball, while the right side acts as a guide to help control the club and contributes very little of the effective energy to the overall

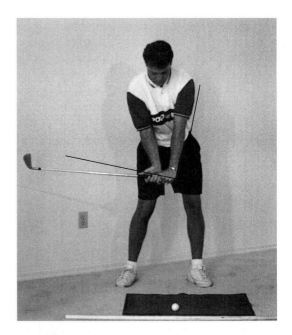

FIGURE 7.9

The *lag* created by swinging on plane in the late downswing. This is the essence of the two-lever, one-hinge system that provides significant energy and speed to the downswing. Golf instructors refer to this position as *maintaining the angle.*

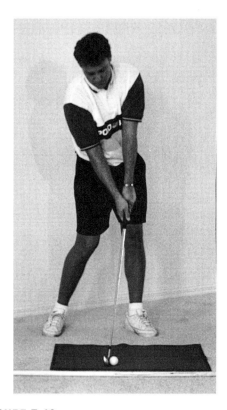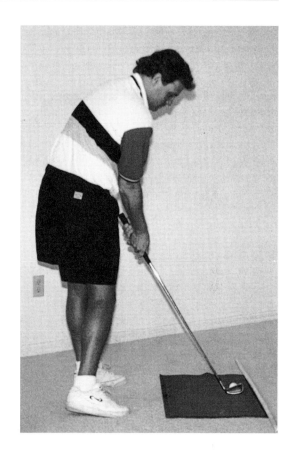

FIGURE 7.10

The impact position. Note how the club is basically back to where it started but how the golfer's left glenohumeral joint is ahead of the hands, which are ahead of the club head, all in a straight line.

swing speed.[9,19] EMG muscle activity during the downswing indicates that the golf swing is indeed a balanced activity requiring equal net muscular output from both sides of the body. One study compared muscle firing activity during the golf swing to muscle activity during a manual muscle test (MMT). According to this original research, three prominent shoulder muscles on the right side (of a right-handed golfer) had marked activity (>60 percent MMT) during the forward swing and acceleration phases. The right shoulder muscles showing moderate to high activity during the forward swing were the subscapularis, pec-

toralis major, and latissimus dorsi. During the acceleration phase, these three muscles increased their activity by demonstrating more than 80 percent MMT activity. During the forward swing, the subscapularis and latissimus dorsi in the left shoulder fired at moderate levels (30 to 60 percent MMT) and were then joined by the pectoralis major to peak during acceleration, just before ball contact.[12] The authors note that the timing of these shoulder muscles' peak activity is very similar to that seen in overhead throwing and tennis serving. Although accurate in their data collection and methodology, the data concerning precise muscle firing patterns in golfers need to be considered thoughtfully secondary to the wide variation evident in swing technique and precision. This limitation is especially evident when applied to the action and activities of the upper extremities in the full golf swing.

The erector spinae muscles on the right side exhibited peak activity during the forward swing (75 percent MMT), whereas the left-side group peaked during acceleration (50 percent MMT).[22] The activity of the abdominal oblique muscles during the forward swing was 62 and 54 percent MMT for the right and left sides, respectively. During the acceleration phase, the right-side oblique remained high (64 percent MMT), whereas the left-side oblique diminished somewhat (42 percent MMT). The authors noted that the high level of right-side erector spinae activity during the forward swing was caused by a phenomenon called "a controlled fall." They concluded that since the subjects were falling forward while rotating from right to left, the right-side erector spinae muscles were trying to resist gravity and rotational forces in an effort to maintain body position.[22]

The same study demonstrated that the abdominal oblique muscle activity during the forward swing was high as a result of the trunk rotation movement, but the authors were unable to discern between internal and external oblique activity because of the limitations from using surface electrodes. The bilateral activity in the oblique muscles probably was due to nearby muscle overflow and the concept of contralateral muscles controlling rotation. During acceleration, the results indicated that there is a fairly consistent level of EMG activity bilaterally in both the abdominal oblique and erector spinae muscle groups. This is a logical assumption because rotation continues to occur throughout the swing and because the motion has centralized when contact is being made. When the club and force vectors come in line with the body, both erector spinae groups are needed to control vertical gravitational forces. These data support the notion that adequate strength, endurance, and control of the abdominal muscles are important for performance and injury prevention in chronic golfers. Again, caution needs to be taken concerning the EMG values for the trunk muscles because careful observation would reveal that the data can be influenced directly by the amount of lateral sway and spine angle maintenance present in individual golfers.

During the rapid time frame from pre- to postimpact, the trunk and spine undergo increased stresses as a result of simultaneous and multidirectional movements. At impact, the average amount of secondary spine angle was found to be 28 degrees (16 degrees at setup), whereas the primary spine angle averaged 34 degrees (45 degrees at setup) (see Fig. 7.10). These values actually have changed from their respective positions at setup (by about 10 to 12 degrees each), indicating a significant change in spine angle position. The spine angle changes that occur are actually opposite and equal reactionary movements that are produced by the forces created during the high-speed three-dimensional motion of the downswing. Although these changes really cannot be controlled, they are important to golfer health and swing success and occur as a result of the directional forces being created during the downswing.

The same data show that shoulder and hip rotation at impact averaged −27 and −43 degrees, respectively.[21] The negative numbers indicate that the hips and shoulders face left of the imaginary target line or open, whereas the difference in amount (approximately 16 degrees) represents a continued torsional stress to the trunk and spinal elements. Although prolonged torsion is usually not desired for the spinal elements, it is a necessary evil required to strike a golf ball successfully. Ironically, attempts to minimize the rotational separation of the spinal segments in golf can even lead to increased stress by eliminating the necessary time for transfer of energy and deceleration to occur smoothly and efficiently.

Although the knee joint forces generated during the golf swing are not considered large enough to be considered high risk for traumatic knee injuries, the downswing phase could place significant stresses on a lead knee that is considered vulnerable.[7] This dynamic work found that the back-side knee can sustain anterior shear forces of up to 10 percent of body weight at an approximate knee flexion angle of 33 degrees. This is of clinical significance for anterior cruciate ligament (ACL) patients when one considers the similarity of the peak forces in this position with those found in side-cutting and open kinetic chain movements and with the increasing quadriceps activity found with this flexion-extension moment. The authors also found the internal tibial rotation moments (1.41 percent BW • BH) and average flexion angles during these peak rotation moments (23 degrees) of the back-side knee to be similar to, and as detrimental to, a newly reconstructed knee or as troublesome for an ACL-deficient knee as a side-cut maneuver.[7]

Like the back-side knee, the forces in the lead knee are greatest during the downswing and, with the exception of peak posterior forces, are greater than the forces measured in the back-side knee. Although not significantly different from the back-side knee, the anterior, medial, and lateral forces were all greater in the downswing of the lead knee. With great speed, the left knee is simultaneously undergoing hyperextension, lateral rotation, and varus stresses that can place undue stress on the vulnerable knee. These multidirectional stresses are a result of the rapid lateral weight transfer and trunk rotation in a closed-chain position.[7] These stresses continue until the downswing is completed but reach their highest levels during the impact to postimpact time period.

Studies on vertical compression levels during the golf swing indicate that over 80 percent of the body weight is on the lead-side during impact, and this value can increase up to 85 percent into early follow-through.[1]

Barrentine et al.[1] found that the front foot applied maximum lateral shear and vertical compression forces (133 and 950 N, respectively) approximately 0.02 s after ball separation from the club face. Additionally, this same study found that the front foot applied a maximum torque of 23 N • m approximately 0.3 s after impact. These data simply indicate that the lead-knee is indeed exposed to significant forces during this phase of the swing. When compression and rotary torque forces are produced at high speeds, a great deal of stability and strength are required to withstand the potentially detrimental forces. Golfers with ligamentous and cartilage injuries are very cognizant of the stresses placed on the knee during an otherwise innocuous activity such as swinging a golf club. Golfers with total knee and hip replacements should be very wary of their respective levels of strength and stability, as well as the type of motion they will be attempting when returning to golf.

It has been reported that it takes approximately 0.82 s to complete the backswing phase but only 0.23 s to complete the downswing phase for a professional golfer.[4] From these data it can be surmised that the downswing is approximately 3½ times the speed of the backswing. When combining these data with EMG and angular velocity data, it is easy to see why the downswing phase produces the highest percentage of injury in both professional and amateur golfers.[2,6,16]

The Follow-Through Phase

Once the club head has made contact with the ball and the ball has been imparted on its flight, the golfer enters the follow-through phase.[12] During this phase, maximum effort has subsided, and the body attempts to decelerate its rotary motion with eccentric muscle contractions.[12,22] Herein lies the function of the follow-through phase. Following impact, the hands and wrists finish their release by following the right arm along the proper swing path (Fig. 7.11). The actions at the shoulder girdle and trunk are much the same as they were during the backswing, only reversed in an effort to decelerate and stabilize. The left shoulder and arm are now abducting and externally rotating, whereas the right shoulder and arm are adducting and inter-

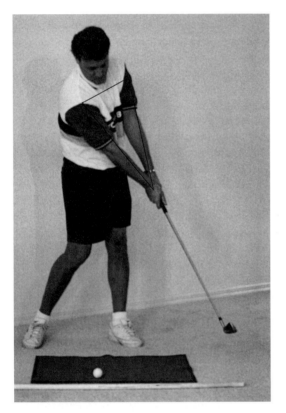

FIGURE 7.11

The postrelease phase of impact. Note how the golfer's head is still down and how the club and hands are extending down the target line. In the next instant, the right shoulder will come in contact with the chin and force the head to extend and rotate to the up position.

nally rotating toward a semi-impingement position. Proper rotator cuff function, scapulohumeral rhythm, and scapular stability are extremely important during the violent aspect of the downswing. When the arms reach about shoulder level, both elbows undergo flexion in an effort to decelerate arm speed and trunk rotation, minimize vertical translation, and maintain postural balance.[21]

Throughout early and late follow-through, the golfer's pelvic girdle and trunk continue to rotate to the left. The lumbar spine undergoes slight extension, continued rotation, and lateral bending as the golfer swings into the finish position[10] (Fig. 7.12). The left leg absorbs even more weight and inwardly rotates as the hip girdle rotates to the left. During this time, the left lower leg is outwardly rotating underneath the femur and is absorbing a posterior rotary varus stress, as described earlier. The left ankle is simultaneously being subjected to significant inversion and supination stresses. With this in mind, it is quite easy to see that golfers with instability and joint degeneration problems of the lead lower extremity do require special considerations for playing golf.

When the follow-through is finished, and hence the swing, the golfer should be balanced on the lead leg while his or her midsection faces the target.[9] Cooper's kinematic study of the golf swing revealed that weight (up to 85 percent) continues to be transferred (rotated) toward the front foot as the follow-through is completed.[5] At the finished position, the trunk should no longer be rotating but does assume a position of slight hyperextension and lateral flexion in an effort to counterbalance the golfer's center of gravity. Balance is also assisted by the finish position of the hands, since they should come to rest somewhat behind the left ear of a right-handed golfer.[9] The weight of the club also will act as a counterbalance if it is in the proper position. The golfer's head, which remained stationary throughout the first half of the swing, is finally pulled up and

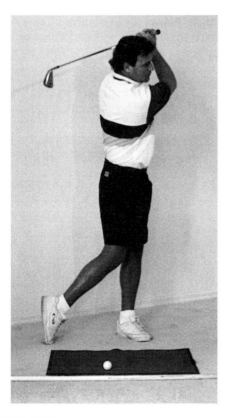

FIGURE 7.12

The finish position. Note how the golfer is vertically stacked, balanced, and on the left side with his weight.

rotated to the left by the turning trunk and swing momentum.[9]

EMG analysis of the follow-through phase reveals that selected shoulder muscles continue to be active bilaterally.[12] These data further indicate that golf is a bilateral activity. The erector spinae muscle activity diminishes during the early follow-through and stays at low levels throughout the late follow-through. The abdominal oblique muscles also diminish their activity but are considerably more active than the erector spinae groups.[22] Once the ball is hit, the trunk musculature continues to work, but the effort is now concen-

trated on deceleration and energy dissipation rather than on force production. As mentioned, it is important to maintain posture and balance throughout the follow-through phase, a skill that requires activity of the stabilizing muscles of the trunk.[22]

Injury Prevention

THE PHYSICAL NATURE OF GOLF

Recently, the physical demands and potential injuries associated with habitual golfing have received considerable attention from various forms of mass media. Recently, golf performance, fitness, and injuries have been the central theme of numerous articles, stories, and interviews in the various forms of media accessible to the golfing public. The increasing trend of professional tour players employing the services of personal physical therapists, athletic trainers, and personal fitness trainers to improve performance, prevent injury, and prolong careers has contributed heavily to this exposure. For the last several years, all three major professional tours have had full-time fitness and rehabilitation vans staffed with physical therapists, athletic trainers, and physicians offering a full range of medical, rehabilitative, and fitness services to the tour members.

As you will see in this chapter, there are many different causes and factors involved in the etiology and treatment of golf-related injuries and optimal performance. Some of the factors that will be addressed include full swing biomechanics, practice and play habits, gender differences, specific physical limitations, fitness, and exercise habits.

WARMING UP

Although use of a warm-up program is considered common practice among many athletes, there are still those who are not aware of the physical benefits associated with warming up. In addition, there are many athletes who warm up because they know it is "the thing to do" but are not quite aware of the physiologic and anatomic responses that come after warming up for physical activity. A proper warm-up program should be specific to the sport activity involved and should enhance flexibility, body temperature, blood flow, muscle and tendon suppleness, coordination, and nervous system readiness. It also should place progressive and functional demands on the body parts that are to be used for the upcoming activity and should include very specific sports skill drills or activities.

Many golfers, both recreational and competitive, fail to use a proper warm-up program prior to engaging in practice or playing sessions. Inadequate warm-up routines have been shown to cause a higher incidence of injury to the muscles and tendon units, while it is generally accepted that warming up prior to exercise can reduce this incidence of injury. Use of a warm-up program that includes a light form of exercise (jogging or muscle contractions), along with stretching exercises, is thought to increase muscular elasticity and help to reduce the rate of injury.

The following joints and muscles, along with some suggestions, should be exercised to gradually and progressively warm up before practice and play.

Stretching and Mobility

1. Thumb extensors with the Finklestein test (this should be done with the elbow fully extended) (This can be done in the car on the way to the course.)
2. Wrist extensors and flexors with the elbow fully extended (also can be done in the car on the way to the course)
3. Shoulder rotators and horizontal adduction (overlap stretches with club)
4. Spinal rotation in neutral and in golf setup position (be sure to include the spine angle principles while rotating)
5. Hip rotators and hamstrings (also can be done in the setup position with the hips rotated internally)
6. Feet and ankles via circumduction and inversion

Functional Exercises

1. Hammer thrusts (radial and ulnar deviation with club properly gripped in hand)
2. Figures 8's with the club and arm extended
3. Swing rotations with the club threaded behind back/between arms at slow speed
4. One-armed miniswings with pitching wedge for both arms
5. Two-armed miniswings with two clubs and feet together
6. Two-armed miniswings with feet apart and gradually increasing arc/length of swing
7. Full shots with pitching wedge
8. Build to full shots with each club in bag

GOLF-SPECIFIC EXERCISE

Since the golf swing requires the coordinated activity of practically all body parts interwoven into a very complicated kinesiologic pattern, the design of a golf-specific exercise program must be comprehensive and dynamic. Any effective sports-specific exercise program should focus on three fundamental issues: (1)the particular demands of the particular sport and/or position, (2) the physical limitations and deficiencies of the athlete, and (3) the sport- and fitness-related goals of the athlete. In simple terms, the goals and objectives of the exercise program for a basketball player should be different in scope and method from the program designed for an offensive lineman. Similarly, the exercise program of a retired 65-year-old golfer with a total hip replacement should be vastly different from that of a young professional golfer without any prior significant medical history.

Creating effective and functional exercise programs for golfers creates many challenges for the clinician. The golf swing has dynamic open- and closed-chain actions and uses both sides of the body in a very fast, complex, and three-dimensional fashion. The spine must rotate and yet be stable; both shoulder complexes must be strong, stable, and yet produce significant speed; the vulnerable hands and wrists must transfer a considerable amount of kinetic energy into the club and simultaneously absorb a significant amount of force from impact with the ground and the ball; and the knees and hips must continuously rotate and absorb close-chain torque from the ground and rotating upper links. To complicate matters even further, almost every muscle has a responsibility to stabilize, accelerate, or decelerate during a time span of less than 2 s.

Upper Extremity Exercises

Use of Theraband/tubing, pulley/cable systems, and free weights is strongly encouraged in order to promote and maintain functional flexibility and prevent muscle imbalance problems. Whenever possible, encourage full range of motion and incorporate diagonal and/or rotation patterns with all exercises. The following muscle groups should be addressed in order to improve golf fitness and minimize the risk of associated injury:

1. The wrist extensors and flexors (bilaterally)
2. The rotator cuff (particularly the lead side)
3. The latissimus dorsi and pectorals bilaterally (accelerate the club during the downswing)
4. The trapezii, rhomboids, and other scapulothoracic muscles bilaterally (Closed-chain scapular stability and open-chain training are needed.)
5. The upper traps and levator scapulae to stabilize the cervicoscapular regions

When called for, flexibility exercises should be incorporated for cervical rotation, scapular abduction and rotation, horizontal adduction (barring impingement conditions), wrist flexion and supination, and back-side shoulder external rotation (barring stability and/or rotator cuff problems).

Lower Extremity Exercises

Contrary to popular belief, the legs do not provide much power or club-head speed to the golf swing. Therefore, barring orthopedic or neurologic injury, the average person has adequate leg strength to play golf and to hit the ball a long way. Rather, clinicians and golfers alike should focus on general aerobic endurance of the lower extremities in an effort to promote better posture, balance, and support and to prevent fatigue to those golfers who walk during play. Low-stress cardiovascular exercise such as walking, biking, and Stairmaster are excellent for all golfers and will help delay postural muscle fatigue during the latter parts of a round and when golf is played in extreme environmental conditions. Closed-chain lower extremity exercises should be implemented when significant strength, endurance, or balance problems exist in order to minimize the associated stress of open-chain knee extension and to improve the functional aspects of the workout.

Flexibility exercises addressing the hip rotators and flexors, the hamstrings, and the gastronemius-soleus complex also should be incorporated. I favor a program consisting of equal parts static and dynamic stretching in order to better imitate the demands of the sport and prevent overelongation of collagen tissue.

Core Exercises

Golfers who wish to minimize their risk of low-back injury can start with basic abdominal strengthening exercises but should progress to functional lumbar stabilization exercises focusing on the transverse abdominis, internal and external obliques, and the lumbar mutifidi. Most important, they should progress to standing closed-chain abdominal exercises to promote a transfer effect to functional activity. See the section on functional rehabilitation for appropriate recommendations.

Mobility and flexibility exercises should only be incorporated if it is clinically prudent and with regard to the neutral pelvis position. Also, all rotary flexibility exercises should be done with consideration for the primary and secondary spine angle alignments. Of course, these exercises also should be monitored closely to prevent reaggravating the dysfunctional conditions and/or creating new ones. Again, it is suggested that the clinician focus more on slow, controlled, dynamic flexibility and mobility patterns and avoid chronic static stretching.

Etiology of Injuries

EXTRINSIC FACTORS

Setup Position

Failing to achieve a proper setup position is common among amateurs and accomplished players alike. Compromising the setup position can contribute significantly to poor performance and physical stress over time if left uncorrected. The most common characteristic of an improper setup position is failing to use a hip-hinge motion to obtain the primary spine angle. Many golfers employ spinal flexion rather than trunk flexion because it is more natural and less complicated (Fig. 7.4). Unfortunately, these golfers are not aware of the pathologic and mechanical consequences associated with prolonged lumbar flexion and posterior pelvic rotation. The stresses placed on the soft tissues and joints of the lumbar spine from excessive or prolonged spinal flexion activities are well known to

most medical professionals. However, most golfers are not aware of this relationship or of the negative influence poor posture can have a hip and shoulder rotation during the actual golf swing.

Use of spinal flexion during the setup phase will negatively affect the elements of the spine and swing efficiency in two primary ways: (1) shifting the golfer's center of gravity and (2) limiting the amount of rotation available in the spine. Proper use of hip-hinge motion, whereby neutral spine is maintained, will help to maintain the COG within the base of support or somewhere between the balls of the feet. In contrast, excessive spinal flexion will cause the COG to move posterior of the base of support, placing the golfer's weight more toward the heels. Because of the dynamic interaction between the various links in a kinetic chain, compromising posture early on in the kinetic sequence can have a significant effect on a golfer's dynamic motion, balance, and joint mobility during the latter firing links in the kinetic sequence.

A significant reduction in the amount of spinal rotation has been found in golfers who compromise their setup position and swing posture. Specifically, poor trunk posture can produce a sharp reduction in the amount of active hip and shoulder turn motion while simultaneously producing excessively high and abnormal spinal stresses. These findings can be demonstrated to the reader by attempting to rotate the thoracic cage in a seated position with the pelvis anteriorly rotated, in neutral, and posteriorly rotated. Then repeat the test with the spine in a neutral position and assess the difference in your rotation amount and comfort levels.

It is also very common for golfers to complain of increased discomfort and pain in the lumbar spine region when practicing their short game—putting and chipping. The postural requirements associated with putting and chipping combined with the need for excessive practice produces a significant strain on the posterior support structures of the lumbar and thoracic spines. Golfers with poor setup posture are even more prone to suffering from this type of positional strain.

Backswing Phase

The most common position seen at the top of the backswing is that in which the hip and legs move laterally, and the secondary spine angle is lost or even inverted—the aforementioned reverse weight shift. Rather than rotating the pelvis to the right in synchronization with the rotating shoulders, many novice golfers mistakenly attempt to use an excessive lateral weight shift of the lower body in an effort to increase their club-head speed. A lateral weight shift in the backswing causes the golfer to place his or her COG outside the base of support, thus compromising balance and dynamic sequencing of movement. When the lower body has shifted to the right, it now becomes impossible for the golfer to retain the secondary spine angle that he or she had at setup. If a golfer has shifted his or her hips to the right, the spine will then flex laterally to the left in a compensatory attempt to maintain balance. Ironically, the end result in this scenario is that the golfer places the majority of his or her weight on the front foot rather than on the back foot and loses the secondary spine angle—hence the term *reverse weight shift* or *reverse pivot.*

Regardless of ability, golfers who lose their secondary spine angle will be forced to attempt to get their upper torso behind the ball (reestablish their secondary spine angle) before impact in order to make contact with the ball. From this position, the golfer is forced to reverse his or her trunk inclination in the early part of the downswing by aggressively sliding the hips back laterally toward the target. In a chain reaction, this forces the spine to simultaneously flex laterally to the right in order to reestablish the original spine and torso inclination. Keep in mind that as this violent loss and reestablishment of the

spine angle are occurring, the spine is also undergoing significant rotary and shear forces. When this lateral movement and spine angle manipulation sequence is significant enough, the spine inevitably undergoes a tremendous hyperextension force during the latter stages of the swing (follow-through). The amount of hyperextension occurring is a direct result of the amount of movement required to reestablish the secondary spine angle. The nature and amount of forces created during the golf swing will be presented in more detail in the next section—the downswing.

Downswing Phase

The actions a golfer uses to make his or her move into the ball and the position the golfer achieves at impact are direct results of the previously achieved backswing. In general, golfers who maintain both spine angles, i.e., stay within their base of support while rotating through the ball and stay on plane throughout the swing, will have a high degree of proficiency and a lower level of physical stress. In contrast, golfers who lose their spinal angles and use excessive lateral weight transfers have trouble staying on plane, which leads to a lack of repeated swing success and higher injury rates.

Hosea et al.[10] evaluated the golf swings of amateur and professional players and the stresses placed on their L3–L4 motion segments while swinging a 5 iron. The authors found that professional golfers were generating 34 percent greater club-head speed, yet the amateurs were producing significantly greater spinal forces and 50 percent greater trunk muscle activity.[10] In comparison with professional golfers, amateurs produced 80 percent greater peak lateral bending and shear loads (560 versus 329 N), and 34 percent greater rotary torque forces. The authors also found that both groups of golfers generated compressive loads in the spine of up to eight times body weight, a value equating to other more vigorous activities that produce up to 4000 N of force. The authors offer a comparative analysis by pointing out that the loads produced in the lumbar spine of a golfer may predispose the golfer to muscle strains, a herniated nucleus pulposus, spondylolysis, and facet arthropathy with associated spinal stenosis.

Careful analysis of professional and amateur golfers has helped me to further pinpoint the reason for the discrepancy in force production between the two populations. Failure to maintain the secondary spinal angle during the backswing is the primary factor responsible for producing these dramatic levels of stress in the lumbar spine of amateur golfers. Remember, the more the secondary spine angle is lost, the more lateral movement is required to reestablish the position during the downswing. This chain reaction produces greater shear, lateral bending, and rotary torque forces and requires greater muscular effort to produce the movement. The work of Hosea et al.[10] supports the idea that professional golfers have more efficient swings and that amateurs produce higher forces that contribute to the development of injury and pathology. Arthrokinematically, the majority of these compensations occur in the thoracolumbar spine and consist of nonphysiologic spinal mechanics.

The moment of impact (ball and club face contact) only lasts for 0.0005 s. However, there is a great deal of energy being transferred through these joints and soft tissues and into the club during this very short time.[4] Based on this calculation, the total time period for full swing impact over 18 holes equates to approximately 0.018 s for a highly skilled player (based on a golfer shooting par golf by the book—36 full strokes and 36 putts—and excluding putts), and only 0.027 s for the typical 15 handicap amateur golfer (based on an average score of 90, taking 54 swings and 36 putts). The hand and wrist units are the last links in the kinetic chain and ultimately are responsible for transferring the speed and kinetic energy (which has been generated from other body segments and natural laws of physics) into the club. The demand placed on the small bones and soft tissues of the hand and wrist during this process and from contacting a semiyielding surface (grass, turf, dirt) at high speeds makes them very susceptible to injury.[5,11,12] Lateral epicondylitis ("golfer's elbow") of the left elbow is often the result of the "bowing" process of the left wrist during the preimpact phase, much like the action of the right elbow extensor muscle mass during the backhand swing in tennis.

Follow-Through Phase

Since the follow-through phase of a golf swing is merely a mirror image of the downswing,[6] one can learn a lot from both the actual follow-through and the resulting finish position. If a golfer does not maintain his or her center hub of rotation and ends up losing his or her balance, the finish position will not be balanced unless he or she uses some sort of compensatory move. Many "educated" amateur golfers fall victim to this scenario because they know what a proper finish position should look like but do not have the proper downswing mechanics required to achieve the "ideal" position. Hence they often compensate with their trunks to mimic the finish position and end up increasing the physical load placed on structures of the spine. Ironically, they often decrease the efficiency of their spine in the process.

Many teaching professionals and touring professionals alike used to teach and advocate a finish position that looked like a reverse-C (Fig. 7.13). It was thought that this position allowed the golfer to drive his or her body through the ball and increase the distance the ball was hit. As you can see, this position places an extreme hyperextension load on the lumbar spine, and the consequent development of increased low-back abnormali-

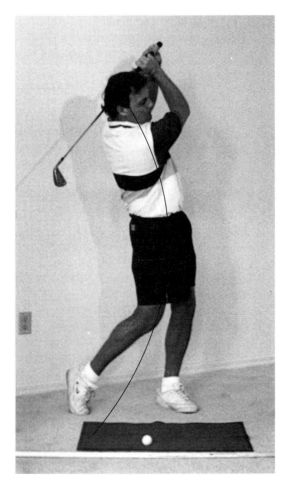

FIGURE 7.13

A *reverse-C* finish position. Produced by excessive lateral weight movement toward the target during the downswing, this position produces extreme hyperextension loads to the lumbar spine.

ties is the primary reason why most professionals have abandoned this technique.

INTRINSIC FACTORS

Playing the game of golf effectively and injury-free requires the golfer to possess certain attributes that traditionally have been assigned to other athletes. Swinging a golf club requires

coordination, balance, strength, timing, rhythm, endurance, flexibility, and mental stamina.[10] It has been established that there are significant injury rates for both professional and amateur golfers,[2,12] and professional golfers recently have begun to place an increased emphasis on the physical demands of the game by participating in conditioning and injury prevention programs. The PGA, Senior PGA, and LPGA tours now offer full-time fitness and rehabilitative vans that travel to tournament sites all over the country for the benefit of the touring professionals. The vans are staffed with physicians, physical therapists, and athletic trainers and offer on-site preventative exercise and physical therapy programs.

Posture and Physical Condition

The ability to achieve and maintain the primary spine angle and thus avoid a spinal flexion load depends on hamstring flexibility, postural habits, abdominal control, and leg endurance. Those with excessively tight hamstrings (>30 degrees shy of vertical in the supine position with the hip flexed 90 degrees) may have trouble getting comfortably into the hip hinge position. Golfers with a habitual slouched posture and those who sit at a desk consistently also have difficulty implementing a hip hinge posture into their setup positions. Out of postural habit, they tend to feel more comfortable in a slouched, kyphotic position as they set up over the ball. As with other lumbar pain patients, poor transversus abdominis control and tone also will influence the ability of a golfer to avoid a compromising posture at address. Finally, golfers with average to above-average leg endurance and cardiovascular endurance seem to be able to maintain their setup posture for longer periods of time (the back nine holes) than those who are otherwise unconditioned. Playing and walking in the heat seem to add to this problem for unconditioned golfers, and they tend to slouch more in the later rounds, thus increasing the pressures and forces on their lumbar spines and increasing their chance of injury.

Rotary Flexibility

The backswing phase of the golf swing is relatively nonstressful, but it requires significant flexibility of the thoracic cage, cervical and lumbar spines, shoulders and pelvic girdles, hip joints, and both hands and wrists. The left shoulder complex, and in particular the posterior rotator cuff musculature and capsule (on a right-handed golfer), is especially vulnerable at the top of the backswing. During this time, the left shoulder is being placed in an impingement position while it is simultaneously being stretched to significant lengths.[19] This functional demand is of particular importance for those with inherent shoulder dysfunction and for older golfers because of the rotator cuff degeneration that often occurs with age.[5]

A proper *body turn*, as it is termed in golfing circles, requires sufficient cervical and trunk rotary flexibility. If inadequate flexibility or dysfunctional joint mechanics exist in any of these areas, the golfer must compensate with other segmental involvement to achieve a full and proper backswing. Golfers with limited rotation or significant dysfunction in the cervical spine will have difficulty keeping the head still during the golf swing as they attempt to rotate back and through the swing. Severe rotational limits in the cervical spine can even cause golfers to lose their secondary spine angles as they attempt to keep their eyes on the ball. Ironically, this motion causes increased stress to the cervical, thoracic, and lumbar spines over time.

A golfer with limited mobility in the thoracic cage will need to have more rotation in the lumbar spine and hips to produce a full rotary backswing. This inevitably will place increased stress on both the hyper- and hypomobile segments of the thoracic and lumbar spine. Likewise, a golfer with excellent mobil-ity of the shoulders and very little rotary motion in the lumbar spine and pelvis will place greater demand on the upper torso and its motion segments. This common compensatory action of the upper and lower portions of the torso can cause an imbalance in the contributions of the two segments. This imbalance may create extreme rotary torques in the susceptible segment(s) and possibly can lead to injury and performance changes that are not advantageous to the golfer.

The majority of injuries in golfing occur as a direct result of repetitive swinging.[12] The downswing phase is responsible for generating club-head speed and therefore places the body under extreme loads. During the downswing, the torso undergoes a rapid rotational change of direction that involves sequential segmental rotation, linear movement, forward trunk flexion, and lateral bending all in one combined movement. The average golfer goes through this coiling-uncoiling process approximately 110 to 130 times during a typical day of golfing (warm-ups, practice, and match strokes). If sufficient endurance and control of the trunk musculature are not possessed, motor fatigue can occur, and subsequent compensatory movement patterns will take over.[16] When poor motor endurance and flexibility coexist with poor body and swing mechanics, the golfer is exposed to the possibility of injury.

Lead Shoulder Complex

The role of the lead arm in controlling the plane of the downswing, combined with the delay between hip and shoulder girdle rotation, places significant stress on the left rotator cuff musculature. As the body "uncoils" toward the target, it "pulls" on the elevated arm and rotator cuff muscles as they are working to outwardly rotate the arm.[19] Limitations in the amount of left shoulder motion possibly can place even greater loads on the posterior cuff musculature and eventually may lead to significant rotator cuff pathology with increased practice and play. Abnormal scapular mobility and stability can place even further stresses on the capsular and muscular restraints of the glenohumeral joint, particularly in the lead-side.

During the time from preimpact to postimpact, there are also significant stresses placed on the distal segments of the upper extremities. In this extremely short span of time, the tissues in these areas are going from elongated to shortened positions very rapidly and are also absorbing contact forces from the ground and ball during impact. Golfers with low strength and flexibility in the upper extremities should be made aware of these demands and possible risks.

Lower Kinetic Chain

Both the knee and patellofemoral joints are forced to withstand a considerable amount of multidirectional force as the golfer prepares to make impact with the ball.[8] Golfers with ligamentous instabilities, patellofemoral syndrome, or degenerative joint disease can be subjected to increased pain and decreased function while participating in practice and play. Functional rehabilitation, orthotic and bracing intervention, and mechanical adjustments should be considered when dealing with knee pathologies in the golfing population. Golfers with surgical anterior cruciate ligament reconstructions should be aware of certain criteria used for returning to play safely, especially when there is left (lead-side) knee involvement. Golfers with ankle and foot instabilities and pathologies will experience difficulties in transferring weight to the involved side and rotating in a closed-chain position. Adequate strength, stabilization, and proprioception should be present before allowing a full and unrestricted return to play.

The follow-through phase requires sufficient flexibility of both upper quarters and hips to reach the full finish position. Limitations in hip internal or external rotation or the shoulders will not allow the golfer to fully follow through and thus not allow sufficient time to safely decelerate the swing. Lumbar extension is also required to swing through the ball and finish in a high, balanced position. When physical limitations such as these are not addressed, increased stresses and compensatory actions inevitably can become a consistent component of the golf swing.

Many observers wrongly site trunk rotation as the primary cause of low-back stress in the golf swing when in reality injuries arise as a result of the combination of rotation and the need to maintain the primary and secondary spinal angles throughout each swing. Knowing that golfing requires this specific posture and rotary movement pattern and that golfers maintain, move in, and move out of this posture for approximately 5 hours during the course of a typical day of golf, one can understand the high volume of back injuries in the game. When this functional requirement of the game is understood, it is easy to see the role of adequate trunk and extremity flexibility, abdominal stabilization, and proper body mechanics in preventing and rehabilitating the injured golfer. Educating the golfer about these principles will allow for self-management and decreased reoccurrence rates, as well as increased performance.

Because the golf swing is not a natural activity for the human body, nor does it fit the model of sound body mechanics in many ways, golfers of all abilities and experience should be aware of the potential risks and harms involved with the game. It is important to remember that there are many anatomic differences among individuals and that there are many different and equally effective ways to swing a golf club. The combination of anatomy and the swing technique will dictate the relative levels of success and physical stresses produced in each individual golfer.

Common Injuries and Their Rehabilitation

Although overuse injuries occur more frequently than acute trauma in golfers, the golf swing does generate enough force to cause significant acute injury. Incorrect swing mechanics and poor physical conditioning usually combine to be the primary cause of acute injuries in the amateur golfing population, whereas chronic play and practice are responsible for the majority of injuries on the professional circuits. Regardless of skill level, however, it has been reported that most golf injuries occur at or near the moment of impact during the downswing.[16,17] McCarroll and Gioe[16] report that the follow-through phase of the golf swing accounted for nearly 30 percent of all swing-related injuries in professional golfers, the second highest incidence next to the impact phase (50 percent). As evidence of the potential for high physical stress, one needs to look no further than the golfer who sustained a fracture and dislocated patella during the impact phase of the golf swing.[8] Mishits (such as hitting a root or rock), hitting out of deep rough, and hitting off of uneven lies are common occurrences for all golfers and can produce significant trauma to the tendons, ligaments, joints, and muscles of the hands, wrists, shoulders, and back as well.[5,11,12]

PROFESSIONAL GOLFERS

Professional golfers play and/or practice at least 10 months per year and hit hundreds of golf balls on a daily basis, making themselves susceptible to chronic overuse injuries. One survey of professional golfers found that 190 of 226 respondents (85 percent) were injured as a direct result of their profession, with each of these players averaging two injuries during the course of their professional career.[16] In fact, 54 percent of professional golfers consider their injuries to be chronic. The left wrist was most commonly injured (24 percent), followed by the low back (23.7 percent), the left hand (7.1 percent), the left shoulder (7.1 percent), and the left knee (7 percent). When the statistics were broken down by gender, female golfers had more hand and wrist injuries than men (38.8 versus 22.9 percent), men had more back injuries than women (25 versus 22.4 percent), and men had more left shoulder injuries than professional women golfers (11 versus 3 percent). Right-handed golfers, which comprised the majority of subjects, generally sustained more injuries to the left wrist and hand.

AMATEUR GOLFERS

One study examining injury rates among amateur golfers found that 57 percent incurred at least one injury directly related to golfing, whereas another found that 62 percent of its respondents had sustained one or more golf injuries.[2,16] Batt[2] reported that 32 percent of all amateur respondents in his survey sustained injuries while actually playing golf. For clarity, the author termed these *actual injuries*. Forty-two percent of the respondents reported injuries that were not caused by golfing but ailments that noticeably affected their game. The author termed these previous injuries and pathologies that resurfaced secondary to the stress induced by playing golf *incidental injuries*.[2] Overall, the highest incidence was found to be the low back (33 percent), followed by the hand and wrist (27 percent), the elbow (13 percent), the shoulder (7 percent), and finally the knee (6.5 percent).[2] Together, these surveys of amateur, professional, and tour golfers suggest that the low back and the hand-wrist complex are the most vulnerable sites for injury. Individual differences between men and women in this study are broken down and reported in Fig. 7.14.

A later study on amateur golfing injuries found an equal incidence among men (62

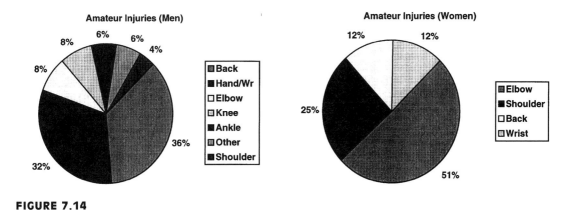

FIGURE 7.14

A. Golf injuries in men as reported by Batt.[2] *B.* Golf injuries in women as reported by Batt.[2]

percent) and women (61 percent), that back injuries prevailed as the most injured site across the whole group (35 percent), and that women sustained elbow injuries (36 percent) at an equivalent frequency to spinal injuries in the male subpopulation (36 percent).[17] As in other studies, the authors cited excessive play/practice and poor swing mechanics to be the most frequent causes of injury. The average respondent lost 5.2 weeks of playing time because of their injury, whereas 45 percent were still bothered by their injury at the time of the survey. Additionally, this study found that 65 percent of the golfers over the age of 50 years had been hurt playing golf.[17] This statistic is even more alarming when one considers that senior golfers (>50 years of age) make up 25 percent of the total golfing population (approximately 6.25 million golfers) and are responsible for 50 percent of the total rounds played every year (each played an average of 37 rounds in 1995).[20]

UPPER EXTREMITY

In many ways, the lead upper extremity is the most important element of a healthy golf swing. Unfortunately, it is also very commonly injured. After all, it forms the primary anatomic lever in the two-lever, one-hinge model. The anatomic lever pivots around the extremely mobile and susceptible glenohumeral joint and extends distally to the vulnerable and tenuous wrist-hand complex. DeQuervain's syndrome, hook of hamate fractures, golfer's elbow, and rotator cuff pathology have been associated with upper extremity requirements of the golf swing.[2,12,14,16,17,23,24,26]

Shoulders

In turn, glenohumeral joint function and health largely depend on the scapulothoracic joint's efficiency and health. Therefore, a healthy golfing shoulder requires adequate glenohumeral joint mobility and associated subacromial space, proper scapulohumeral rhythm, dynamic scapulothoracic stability, and a well-toned and well-trained rotator cuff.

Damage to the shoulder complex in golfers usually occurs in the lead (left in a right-handed golfer) shoulder and can include rotator cuff strains and tendinitis, impingement syndrome, bursitis, snapping scapula syndrome, and glenohumeral instabilities. Although most of these injuries are chronic in nature, acute damage can cause rotator cuff tears and glenohumeral subluxations to occur also. Typically, golfers will start out with a low-grade ache and discomfort in the shoulder after playing or practicing. Symptoms will increase during the backswing phase as the left arm adducts horizontally and rotates internally toward the end phase, placing the humeral head in close proximity with the acromion and restricting the subacromial space.

With continued swing stress, the low-grade inflammation can turn into more serious pathology and dysfunction if left untreated. Often, fatigue-related failures and/or abrupt tensile failures of the supraspinatus and infraspinatus can occur when the player executes a poor swing or hits a root or rock during the downswing. Taking an abnormally large divot (this can occur with an uneven lie in which the golf ball is above the golfer's feet on a hill and is also associated with an over-the-top downswing plane) also can cause full-thickness tears in the rotator cuff tendons or musculature.

Older golfers and those with years of stressful practice are candidates to develop multidirectional instabilities of the lead glenohumeral joint and present with signs and symptoms of secondary shoulder impingement syndrome. Greg Norman is a prime example, recently undergoing radiofrequency heat probe surgery to correct a long-standing instability in his left shoulder, which was caused by years of aggressive ball striking. Considerable care should be taken by the clinician to determine if the golfer with shoulder pain presents with primary or secondary shoulder impingement syndrome before implementing the plan of care.

Functional Rehabilitation. Golfers suffering from shoulder pain and/or dysfunction should be progressed similarly as overhead athletes with regard to reducing the inflammatory response, restoring glenohumeral mobility and scapulohumeral rhythm, enhancing scapular stability, and improving ro-

tator cuff firing and control. However, the clinician need not worry about strengthening the shoulder in the overhead position because the golf swing is an underarm pattern. A clinical paradox in treating the golfer's shoulder does exist, however. In order to perform full golf swings, the athlete must be able to fully horizontally adduct and internally rotate the lead arm. Obviously, this impingement creates a challenge for the clinician, especially if the patient presents with classic anatomic signs of primary impingement or a posterior glenohumeral instability.

Typically, these situations require the clinician and golfer to be more patient and progress with the rehabilitation schedule at slower rates. It is also advisable to work in conjunction with a professional golf instructor to modify the swing patterns of these golfers. This usually takes the form of shortening the backswing to more of a three-quarters position, letting the left elbow flex somewhat at the top of the backswing, and using more of a big muscle swing as opposed to an arm swing (use the trunk more and arms less).

Once the golfer reaches the functional restoration stage, the following exercises should help to return the golfer to play:

1. External rotation at neutral
2. Horizontal abduction without rotation in standing position with Theraband
3. Horizontal abduction with external rotation in golf swing posture (imitate the downswing) using The Golf Gym or a comparable device (Fig. 7.15)

Elbows

Again, the lead elbow is most commonly involved when injuries arise. The term *golfer's elbow* has been used to describe an inflammatory and degenerative condition of the extensor mass of the left elbow. Some references also have indicated that golfer's elbow occurs in the right elbow flexor mass. Indeed,

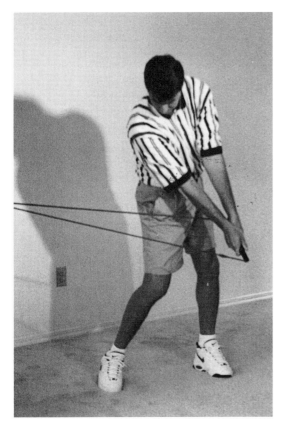 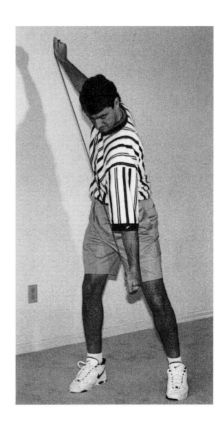

FIGURE 7.15

The golfer can perform this exercise with both hands in the early phases and then progress to using the lead arm only. Add internal rotation during the backswing and external rotation during the downswing only after the golfer can tolerate the movement.

both maladies are present in different populations. Skilled golfers who swing on plane and have good overall swing mechanics tend to overstretch the lead elbow extensor mass during the late downswing, whereas lower-skilled golfers who come over the top during the downswing tend to aggravate their medial flexor mass on the right elbow. Golfers suffering from this malady will present with identical symptoms to those athletes suffering from tennis elbow (extensor mass) or Little Leaguer's elbow (flexor mass). Weak shoulder musculature also has been found to contribute to the development of lateral epicondylitis in the lead arms of golfers.

There are also a significant number of golfers who are classified as being very "handsy" with their golf swings. They are termed such because of the large amount of pronation and supination present in the release phase of their downswings in order to square the club face during impact (see Lee Trevino and Corey Pavin). These golfers are also susceptible to elbow tendinitis and muscle strains due to the rolling-over effect of the muscles on the humeral epicondyles.

Functional Rehabilitation. Once the golfer reaches the functional restoration stage, the following exercises should help to return the golfer to play:

1. Radial deviation with a golf club using a proper grip position. This exercise can be progressed by adding Theraband to the distal end of the club.
2. Resisted pronation and supination (hammer/handle with Theraband).
3. Imitate the release motion of the downswing in a golf swing posture using The Golf Gym or a comparable device (Fig. 7-15).
4. Strengthen the external rotators, scapular stabilizers, and horizontal abductors as well.

Spine

Cervical Spine. Although acute cervical injuries are not very common in golf, golfers with preexisting conditions for cervical pathology and dysfunction can significantly irritate their condition if not careful. Golfers with poor cervicothoracic posture, limited rotational mobility, and degenerative conditions should be wary of the torque and stress placed on the cervical spine during a full swing. Attempting to keep the head still during the backswing without the proper rotational ability to do so will result in significant pain and dysfunction. Likewise, keeping the head down during the downswing will not allow the cervical and thoracic components of the spine to fully and efficiently rotate and will produce increased torque to the facet and vertebral joints. Diskogenic pain is rare in golfers less than 35 to 40 years of age, but radicular pain is somewhat common in the general golfing population and should be investigated thoroughly by the clinician.

Functional Rehabilitation. Once the clinician has reached the functional stage of rehabilitation with a golf patient presenting with cervical pain, reasonable attempts to restore cervical mobility and stability should be attempted. The clinician is somewhat limited as to what can be done here, and the major intervention in these patients lies with swing modifications, postural improvements, and pain control. Golfers with limited cervical rotation ability must

1. Use a proper hip hinge, primary spine angle setup position. Be sure to reduce or eliminate the amount of cervical flexion employed during the golf swing by teaching the golfer to look down at the ball during the setup out of the bottom of his or her eyes (as if reading from bifocal lenses). In effect, place the golfer in cervical neutral, and teach him or her to maintain it.
2. Maintain the secondary spine angles during the backswing.
3. Allow the head to move off the ball laterally, and avoid attempting to keep it perfectly still.
4. Teach the golfer to allow the head to rotate through and come up as the right shoulder moves through the impact zone and into the early follow-through phase. Keeping the head down throughout the follow-through reflects poor swing mechanics and significantly increases the forces applied to the cervical spine by limiting the ability to decelerate and finish its momentum.
5. Use adequate warm-up exercises to increase joint elasticity and mobility.

Thoracic Spine. Although not often injured in sports, the thoracic spine can present the opportunity for dysfunction and irritation in the golfing athlete. New evidence has demonstrated a high rate of costal stress fractures in the lead-side rib cage of beginning golfers, which had mostly gone misdiagnosed as "nonspecific back pain."[15] Vertebral and zygoapophyseal joint dysfunction is fairly common in the upper to middle thoracic spine as a result of the combination torque and shear forces that occur during the rotational aspects of the swing. Typically, golfers will present with pain and hypomobility in the lead (left) scapulothoracic area with associated soft tissue irritation in the paraspinal and vertebral scapular muscles. Visual and palpatory assessment of the orientation and mobility of the vertebral segments in question typically will reveal hypomobile and rotated segments and associated facet dysfunction at the corresponding vertebral levels. Lead-side facet dysfunction seems to be more prevalent in female golfers and males possessing less upper body strength (particularly in the rhomboid and trapezius muscle groups).

Functional Rehabilitation. Once normal spinal mechanics and mobility have been restored through appropriate manual and functional exercise, the clinician should focus on increasing the tone, strength, and endurance of the following muscle groups:

1. The external rotators (infraspinatus and teres minor)
2. The horizontal abductors (middle and posterior deltoid, long head of the triceps, latissimus dorsi)
3. The scapular adductors and downward rotators (lower and middle trapezius, rhomboids)

See the functional rehabilitation exercises for the shoulder for advanced, functional golf swing exercises.

Lumbar Spine. As evidenced in Fig. 7.14, Batt found that 48 percent of his respondents (both incidental and actual injuries) reported suffering from low-back injuries ranging from lumbosacral sprains to herniated disks. It has been speculated that between 90 and 100 percent of all touring professionals suffer from some degree of lumbar pain or dysfunction at some time in their career. As the literature reports, diskogenic pain is fairly com-

mon in golfers and should be investigated thoroughly and discriminately by the clinician. However, acute instances of disk pain and disruption are rare and, as in the general population, are usually associated with other contributing factors such as poor mechanics and posture, early injury, and poor lumbopelvic stability. As in the more proximal spinal segments, facet dysfunction and potential nerve root irritation are also possible in the lumbar spine and thus should be assessed in the clinical evaluation. Sacroiliac joint dysfunction and degeneration are also quite common in habitual golfers and therefore should be differentiated from lumbar diskogenic and/or radicular sources of pain.

Although not generally caused by golf per se, spondylolysis and spondylolisthesis can present significant problems in golfers with these conditions. Consider the level of shearing and rotary torque forces produced in skilled professional golfers who are able to maintain their spinal angles fairly well and the forces in lesser skilled players who do not maintain their spinal angles.[10] There is a fairly strong clinical relationship between those patients with poor swing mechanics and their respective chances for lumbar dysfunction. With these data in mind, it is recommended that patients presenting with symptomatic spondylolysis and spondylolisthesis should not be encouraged to partake in golf as a new hobby or recreational activity. Furthermore, it should be pointed out that individuals who have been playing golf for some time and those who wish to continue playing present formidable challenges for the clinician. Every attempt should be made to restore functional mobility and stability while simultaneously analyzing the golfer's swing mechanics and other potential sources of stress. This said, it is also the responsibility of the clinician to thoroughly inform such golfers of their physical and performance limits and of the associated risks of playing golf with such conditions.

Functional Rehabilitation. Golfers with lumbar spine dysfunction wishing to return to golf should be progressed gradually to seated and then standing closed-chain functional stability exercises that mimic the golf swing. After all, when is the last time a golfer had to swing a golf club lying supine on a table or in a "dead bug" position. Keep in mind that all exercises employed also should simultaneously address the neutral pelvic position, abdominal stabilization, and the golf swing postures and spinal angles. The following functional exercises should help ready the lumbar spine golfer to full activity:

1. Functionally and progressively strengthen the transverse abdominis, internal obliques, lumbar multifidi, and quadratus lumborum.
2. Hip hinge exercises with club, or T-bar, for visual and tactile feedback (Fig. 7.16).
3. Minibackswing rotations in a painfree range while maintaining spine angles (Fig. 7.17). You can perform this initially on the physioball and then in a standing position and can add tubing or weight resistance as the muscles respond. At first, perform only to the backswing side, and then add the downswing and follow-through motions as tolerated.
4. While seated on the physioball in pelvic neutral position:
   a. Neutral rotations with arms extended. Perform only half-rotations, from neutral to right and then back to neutral, etc., and then to the left side in the same manner. Progress to holding a Plyoball, Theraband/tubing, or cable pulley system for added resistance.
   b. Vertical chops between the legs and then overhead, avoiding lumbar hyperextension.
   c. Oblique rotations or seated wood chops to both sides using a diagonal pattern with slight forward flexion

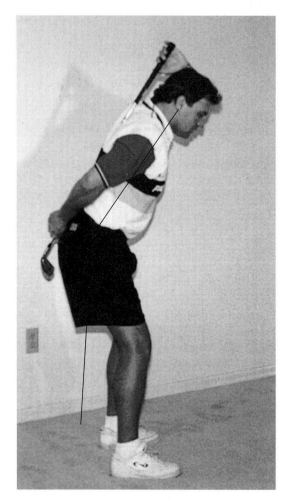

FIGURE 7.16

The hip hinge drill to promote a proper, spinal-neutral primary spine angle. Note how the club remains on the back throughout and how the knees automatically flex to support the body.

and extension movements of the upper spine.

5. Standing wood chops with a Plyoball keeping the hip hinge motion intact and synchronizing it with slight trunk rotation. Be sure to promote transverse abdominis stabilization, neutral pelvis position, and proper lower extremity flexion and extension throughout.

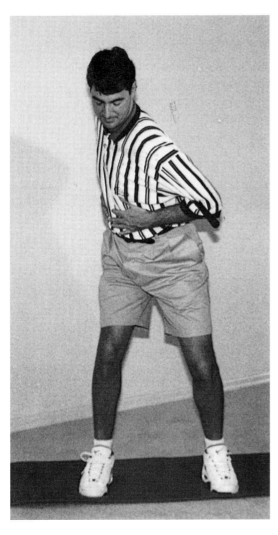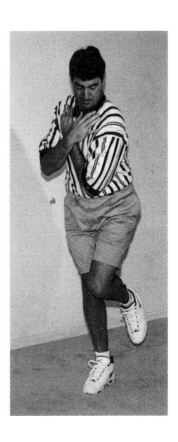

FIGURE 7.17

Miniswing rotations while maintaining both spine angles. The golfer should rotate within his or her painfree limits and work only on the backswing initially. Progress with quality and speed of motion as tolerated. Progress to one leg for an added emphasis on balance and proprioception

Return to Sport

As with any other sport or functional activity, considerable care should be taken when returning a golfer back to unrestricted play and practice. Also, follow the same general guidelines as other return-to-play programs by using alternating days at first, gradually increasing time before increasing intensity, and backing off whenever pain and discomfort arise secondary to a playing or practice session. Although it is impossible and would be considered imprudent to dictate the return-to-play criteria for all conditions and levels of play, the following criteria should be observed when returning your patient back to the links:

1. Begin with putting. Allow incremental bouts with a control on the amount of time spent in the putting posture. Be sure that your patient can tolerate practice putting sessions using a hip hinge to get in and out of the putting posture. Meanwhile, increase his or her ability to maintain pelvic neutral positioning and abdominal bracing throughout. *Do not* allow your golfer patient to stay in the putting posture for successive putts. Make the patient get in and out of the putting posture for each and every putt (this is critical). Depend-ing on the severity and nature of the injury, allow for the golfer to be capable of completing 3 to 5 successive days of putting practice (20 to 30 minutes each session) before progressing to the next level.

2. Progress to chipping with the same protocol as for putting. Back off to alternate days, begin with 10 to 15 minutes, and progress to 25 minutes on successive days. Keep in mind that the patient is still working on his or her functional stabilization programs at this point.

3. Now it is time to begin with miniswings and progress to the full swing. Back off to alternate days, and begin with a pitching wedge or sand wedge. Encourage the patient to practice half-swing pitch shots at 50 percent effort, and limit the initial practice session to 25 to 30 swings, again depending on the patient's level and condition. The golfer should be able to perform 50 swings on successive days before being allowed to progress to three-quarter swings at 50 percent effort.

4. This type of alternate-day, progressive volume routine should be used as the golfer moves up to a 7 iron, then 5 iron, then 3 iron, and finally a driver. Full-effort swings (100 percent speed) should not be encouraged until the golfer has been able to successively swing at three-quarter swing length and three-quarter effort on successive days without pain or residual discomfort. With pain and discomfort, gradually build up the endurance of the golfer to tolerate full-swing, full-speed stress before allowing him or her to return to play.

5. As the golfer is returned to play, allow 9 holes on alternate days, followed by 9 holes on successive days. As tolerated, gradually progress to 18 holes using the same pattern.

It is also suggested that the golfer use a golf tee during all functional rehabilitation sessions in an attempt to minimize the ground reaction forces associated with live ball striking. Also encourage the golfer to properly warm up and cool down prior to and following all ball-striking sessions. As always, commonsense pain guidelines and open, honest communication between the golfer patient and the clinician are critical to an effective and safe return to play.

References

1. Barrentine SW, Fleisig GS, Johnson H: Ground reaction forces and torques of professional and amateur golfers, in Cochran AJ, Farrally MR (eds): *Science and Golf II*. London: E & FN Spon, 1994.
2. Batt ME: A survey of golf injuries in amateur golfers. *Br J Sports Med* 26(1):63–65, 1992.
3. Bechler JR: Electromyographic analysis of the hip and knee during the golf swing. *Clin J Sports Med* 5(3):162–166, 1995.
4. Cochran A, Stobbs J: *The Search for the Perfect Swing*. Philadelphia: Lippincott, 1968.
5. Cooper JM, Glassow RB: *Kinesiology*. St. Louis: Mosby, 1976.

6. Duda M: Golf injuries: They really do happen. *Phys Sports Med* 15(7):191–196, 1987.

7. Gatt CJ, Pavol MJ, Parker RD, et al: Three-dimensional knee joint kinetics during a golf swing. *Am J Sports Med* 26(2):285–294, 1998.

8. Geisler PR: *The Kinesiology of Golf: Implications for Injury and Performance:* Self-published, 1996.

9. Hogan B, Wind WH: *The Modern Fundamentals of Golf.* New York: Simon & Schuster, 1957.

10. Hosea TM, Gatt CJ, Langrana NA, et al: Biomechanical analysis of the golfer's back, in Cochran AJ (ed): *Science and Golf.* London: Chapman and Hall, 1990.

11. Isaacs CL, Schreiber FC: Patellar osteochondral fracture: The unforeseen hazard of golf. *Am J Sports Med* 20(5):613–614, 1992.

12. Jobe FW, Moynes DR, Antonelli DJ: Rotator cuff function during a golf swing. *Am J Sports Med* 14(5):388–392, 1986.

13. Jobe FW, Schwab DR: *30 Exercises for Better Golf.* Inglewood, CA: Champion Press, 1986.

14. Knight B: DeQuervain's syndrome in golfers. *Sports Med Update* (Spring):12, 1990.

15. Lord MJ, Ha KI, Song KS: Stress fractures of the ribs in golfers. *Am J Sports Med* 24(1):118–122, 1996.

16. McCarroll JR, Gioe TJ: Professional golfers and the price they pay. *Phys Sports Med* 10(7):64–70, 1982.

17. McCarroll JR, Rettig AC, Shelbourne KD: Injuries in the amateur golfer. *Phys Sports Med* 18(3):122–126, 1990.

18. McTeague M, Anderson L: The science of the swing. *Golf Magazine,* December 1996.

19. Milburn PD: Summation of segmental velocities in the golf swing. *Med Sci Sports Exerc* 14(1):60–64, 1982.

20. National Golf Foundation: Latest golf participation study offers many encouraging signs. News release, National Golf Foundation, Jupiter, FL, April 28, 2000.

21. Personal communication: American Sports Medicine Institute, Birmingham, AL, 1994.

22. Pink M, Perry J, Jobe FW: Electromyographic analysis of the trunk in golfers. *Am J Sports Med* 21(3):385–388, 1993.

23. Stover CN, Wiren G, Topaz SR: The modern golf swing and stress syndromes. *Phys Sports Med* 4(9):42–47, 1976.

24. Torisu T: Fracture of the hook of the hamate by a golfswing. *Clin Orthop* 83:91–94, 1972.

25. Wiren G: *Golf: Building a Solid Game.* Englewood Cliffs, NJ, Prentice-Hall, 1987.

26. Yocum L, Mottram R: Rotator cuff surgery extends Morgan's career, in *On Tour* (A publication of the PGA). New York: McGraw-Hill, 1994.

CHAPTER 8

Dinghy Sailing

Kirsten Snellenburg

Sailing is one of the oldest modes of transportation for humans. It became a competitive sport when the Americas Cup Race started in England in the late 1800s. Since then, sailing has grown into a worldwide competitive sport. Sailing covers a wide range of disciplines from high-tech Americas Cup yacht racing, Olympic class dinghy racing, and regional or local events to the newest sport of windsurfing.

Even with technological advances, the small boat sailor has seen increases in related injuries within the sport. To date, little research has been done regarding injuries specific to the sport of dinghy sailing. The purpose of this chapter is to provide an overview of sailing and the sport-specific injuries that occur for a competitive dinghy sailor. The chapter will explore the fitness dinghy sailing requires, including the muscular strength and endurance, forces on the sailor, and the injuries common to the sport. The chapter will then aid the clinician in understanding the biomechanics of the sport and the appropriate treatment interventions that will allow the athlete to return to competition.

History of Sailing

Sailboats appeared more than 4000 years ago when the water was the only prudent mode of transportation and exploration. These vessels included Polynesian rafts that sailed from island to island in the Pacific and Indian Oceans. The Egyptians also used sailing in their civilization. The Egyptians developed sailing ships for cargo trade across the Mediterranean Sea, the Dead Sea, and the Red Sea.[1] Sailboats became invaluable vessels used in trading over the centuries. It was not until the nineteenth century, however, that sailboat racing gained international acclaim with the introduction of the Americas Cup. Most people around the world are familiar with Americas Cup racing. Yet, for the competitive athlete, the Olympics are considered by most the premiere sailing competition. In Sydney, Australia, for the 2000 Olympics, there were 10 classes of Olympic sailing. This included the men's and women's mistral windsurfing, women's Europe dinghy, men's fin class, men's laser class, men's and women's 470 double-handed, the 49er, and the Toronado class.

Biomechanics of Sailing

HIKING

In any type of sailing, there is *heeling,* a situation where the boat leans over or tips to one side because of pressure on the sails from the wind. In a small dinghy, the sailor counteracts this pressure by *hiking,* or leaning out over the side of the boat to counteract the heeling effect (Fig. 8.1). In light air, from 0 to 8 knots, the dinghy sailor does not need to hike out. Position is critical in light air to decrease surface area under the boat. The sailor balances his or her weight and allows the small amount of wind to play over the sails when racing. The position used in light air for the sailor is a forward trunk position over the center line of the boat, knees bent, and normally the upper body slightly twisted with the back hand close to the tiller.[2] In medium air, 8 to 16 knots, the sailor needs to work to keep the boat flat at all times. The best method of keeping the boat flat is simply by hiking.

There are two hiking methods: the bent-knee method and the straight-leg method. *Bent-knee hiking* occurs when the sailor has the legs in the hiking strap, the rear end is over the rail of the boat, and the knees, hips, and trunk are in flexion (Fig. 8.2).

Straight-leg hiking involves full knee extension and various amounts of hip and trunk extension (Fig. 8.3). It keeps the posterior part of the body from dragging in the water and slowing the boat down. Straight-leg hiking also allows the sailor to easily respond to changes in wind velocity simply by swinging the upper body in and out. This is accomplished by flexing the lumbar and thoracic spine.[2-5] In addition, straight-leg hiking helps the sailor move his or her weight further out over the water than the traditional bent-knee method. It is much more efficient than the "all or nothing" bent-leg hiking technique. However, straight-leg hiking requires an extreme amount of trunk and lower extremity strength to keep the legs perfectly straight and control the upper body.

SAILING

Light Air (0–8 mi/h)

In light air, the dinghy sailor keeps himself or herself close to the midline of the boat, as described earlier. This reduces drag (slowing of

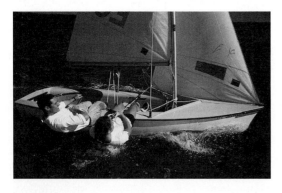

FIGURE 8.1

Hiking.

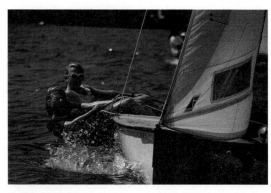

FIGURE 8.2

Bent-knee hiking.

The upper extremities in light-air sailing produce joint motions mainly of flexion and extension at the elbow and wrist, with the forearms usually in a pronated position. The elbow moves through 5° to 120° of flexion as the tiller or mainsheet line is manipulated. The axis of the force for the elbow is fixed, passing through the center of the trochlea of the humerus. The wrist is held in either a neutral or extended position while holding the tiller or the mainsheet line.

In light air, the movements must be slow and smooth to allow the boat to react with minimal water resistance. The head and upper torso are doing the majority of the movement while trimming and adjusting the dinghy's hull trim. In the neck, the anterior and posterior cervical muscles are active. The prime movers include the sternocleidomastoid (SCM), scalenes (anterior, middle, and posterior), upper trapezius, levator scapulae, splenius capitis and cervicis, semispinalis capitis and cervicis, and the suboccipitals. These muscles are going through isotonic and isometric contractions in light-air conditions. The thoracic and lumbar spines are also active in the light-air weight trim. The anterior and posterior muscles working include the rectus and transversus abdominis, internal and external obliques, psoas, quadratus lumborum, erector spinae, rotators, and multifidi.

The upper extremities are active in both steering the boat and trimming the sails. The muscles used during this activity include the triceps and biceps brachii, brachioradialis, coracobrachialis, and wrist flexors and extensors. Again, gentle and smooth movements are required throughout. Good proprioceptive feedback helps the sailor respond to the boat's reactions to the breeze, waves, and sail trim.

Medium Air (8–15 mi/h), Heavy Air (>15 mi/h)

In medium to heavy air, the dinghy sailor hikes out to counteract the forces in the sail. As described earlier, hiking acts as a lever

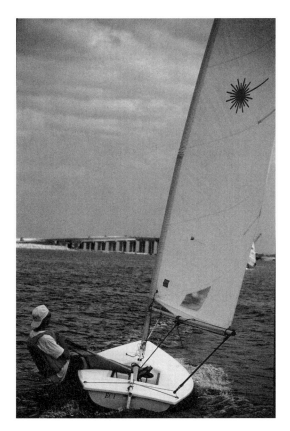

FIGURE 8.3

Straight-leg hiking.

the boat) by decreasing the surface area of the boat in contact with the water. This also allows for expert precision with sail trim and shape in the light-air breeze.

Joint motions in light-air sailing are small and smooth. The knees and hips are bent, with the knees up close to the midline of the boat. The knees are bent to 110° to 115°, and the hips to 100° to 150°. Most of the weight shifting occurs through the thoracic and lumbar spine. In this light-air position, the spine is not put into any end-range positions. Torsional forces are experienced with the coupling motions in the spine between T2 and L3.

arm against the center of effort in the sail. This maneuver keeps the boat flat, which reduces drag and maintains the maximum speed of the boat under these conditions.[2–4]

The movements and joint motions in medium and heavy air sailing are powerful and precise. The joints primarily used in medium and heavy air sailing are the ankle, knee, hip, and lumbar spine. The ankle is maintained at 0 to 5 degrees of dorsiflexion while the top of the foot is against the hiking strap. Posterior force is placed on the distal tibia and fibula and over the talocrural joint. The knee is kept in full extension. A majority of the sailing forces are translated to the knee and the low back.[5] It is estimated that during hiking, the dinghy sailor sustains forces up to 647 N. With pumping, the jerking movement increases forces up to levels of 843 N in the knee joints.[6]

The lumbar spine moves through a range of 160° of flexion to 20° of extension. The lumbar spine motion includes flexion, extension, side bending, rotation, torsion, and a small amount of shear. In lumbar extension while hiking, the posterior structures are subject to compression. This includes the disks, posterior ligaments, and zygapophyseal joints. Creep can occur during sustained loading over time, which leads to increased range of motion beyond normal limits. Many dinghy sailors with more than 5 years of experience will develop hypermobility in the lumbar spine. In lumbar flexion, the anterior structures are subject to compression, including the disks and anterior ligaments. Shear acts directly on the disk as each vertebra moves anterior to posterior.[7] Vertical force on the lumbar spine while wearing a 12-kg weight vest has been estimated at 4.5 N.[8] The torsional forces a sailor experiences are seen during axial rotation. The thoracolumbar junction from T7 to L2 takes a majority of the torsional forces. Axial rotation is considered a coupling motion specifically found with pumping the boat and working the boat through waves.

In the upper extremities, joint motion in medium to heavy air includes shoulder flexion, internal rotation, elbow flexion and extension, and a neutral wrist position. The force at the mainsheet is 111 N and increases to 289 N during pumping actions via shoulder and elbow flexion.[7,8]

The medium to heavy air movements for the dinghy sailor must be powerful. With winds greater than 15 knots, the boat maneuvers very rapidly, so the sailor's reactions must be of split-second timing and accuracy.

The lower extremity muscles absorb most of the forces and become the translation point of power from the sail into the sailor and then into the hull of the boat. In the ankle, the anterior tibialis muscle contracts isometrically against the hiking strap. In the knee, the quadriceps is contracting isometrically during straight-leg hiking. During bent-knee hiking, the quadriceps performs both isometric and eccentric contractions. The hamstrings, in both positions, assist in stabilizing the knee while hiking. The hip moves in flexion and extension, with the hip flexors and extensors working both isotonically and isometrically. The hip muscles include the psoas, rectus femoris, iliacus, sartorius, tensor fasciae latae, gluteus maximus, and hamstrings.[9,10]

The trunk moves in both flexion and extension, with some side bending and rotation. The muscles assisting with extension of the trunk include the erector spinae, quadratus lumborum, rotators, and multifidi. Trunk flexors include the transversus abdominis, internal and external oblique, rectus abdominis, and psoas major (Fig. 8.4).

The upper extremities are both steering the boat and trimming the sails. The muscles active during medium to heavy breezes include the rotator cuff, pectoralis major and minor, deltoid, triceps, biceps brachii, brachioradialis, coracobrachialis, and wrist flex-

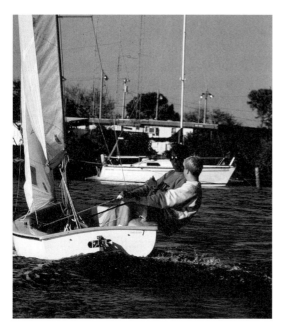

FIGURE 8.4

Trunk extensor musculature working in hiking.

ors and extensors. Rapid and powerful movements are required while the sailor adjusts the steering and trim of the sails.[9,10]

Injury Prevention

WARM-UP

On Land

Warming up is essential in the prevention of injuries when participating in athletic events. Sailing is no exception. Warm-up routines should include an aerobic component and stretching to increase circulation to target tissues. The aim of a warm-up routine is to raise the pulse rate by an aerobic activity such as walking, jogging, skipping rope, or cycling. The key joints to loosen up for the dingy sailor include the elbows, wrists, shoulders, low back, hips, knees, and ankles. Stretching for the dinghy sailor should include the lower back, upper extremities, shoulders, and lower extremities.[2,11,12]

On Water

Once sailors are on the water, there is often a long sail to the starting area or a waiting period on the water, which can result in muscles cooling down and stiffening up. The athlete should take at least 3 to 5 minutes prior to the start of the race for warming up. On the water, warm-ups should target the specific goals of increasing body temperature, increasing circulation, and stretching the muscles. Recommended exercises include arm circles, pedaling of the legs, sit-ups, general pumping action upwind, and stretching of the forearms and the rhomboids (upper back), as well as on-water drills of tacking and jibing repetitively and pumping upwind to raise the heart rate.[12,13]

STRETCHING

In the lower back, the target muscles to stretch are the erector spinae, quadratus lumborum, psoas major and minor, and abdominal muscles. Specific stretches include trunk flexion, extension, and rotation. (See Chap. 6 for illustrations.) Lower extremity muscles to stretch include the quadriceps, with attention to the rectus femoris, because this muscle crosses the hip joint. The hamstrings and the gluteus maximus also should be included. The shoulders and upper extremity muscles to specifically stretch should be the rotator cuff, pectoralis major and minor, latissimus dorsi, and teres major. The biceps brachii and brachioradialis also should be included at the elbow joint. These stretches include reaching behind the back in internal and external rotation and an anterior chest wall stretch using a wall. (See Chap. 5 for illustrations.)

The type of stretching initially performed by the dinghy sailor should be static with a hold of 30 s for each stretch. Next, the sailor should incorporate dynamic stretching drills that simulate the joint movements occurring on the water.

STRENGTHENING

In order to minimize and prevent injuries in dinghy sailing, the athlete should be on a regular exercise program to maintain and improve muscular fitness. Two elements are needed for muscular fitness in a dinghy sailor's exercise program. These include muscular strength and muscular endurance. Such muscular fitness can be accomplished through aerobic exercise, weight training, and/or circuit training.[5,13]

Aerobic training works well for laser sailors and dinghy sailors from the club level to the Olympic level (Table 8.1). Some type of cycling and/or StairMaster program is beneficial. The Norwegian laser sailors at the Savannah pre-Olympics in 1995 were training up to 3 hours per day 4 days per week road cycling. They stated that it increased their endurance for hiking and also gave them the ability to switch from aerobic to anaerobic levels without fatiguing. The other technique developed to work with aerobic exercise is the use of heart monitors. The majority of Olympic sailing coaches assert that heart monitors are important in regulating the aerobic and anaerobic threshold levels of their athletes.

Weight training can be performed with either free weights or weight machines. Weight training needs to have both an aerobic and anaerobic component, and any movement performed needs to have an isometric hold within it. For the lower extremities, closed-chain exercises are essential to train for the hiking position. These exercises include squats, leg press, lunges, and wall sits. Hiking benches are especially useful to assist with the sailor's overall training program because they increase hiking endurance (see "Special Equipment," below). A hiking-bench program for endurance should include approximately 20 to 40 minutes every other day.[3]

Upper extremity movements in dinghy sailing include trimming the sails and steering the boat. The upper extremity must produce powerful jerking movements for trimming the sails (pumping) or steering over waves. Strength training therefore should target the elbow flexors and extensors, including dumbbell curls, hammer curls, cable curls, triceps presses, triceps cable presses, and triceps dumbbell presses. For the anterior chest wall and pectoralis major and minor, exercises include the flat bench press, the inclined bench press, and inclined and flat flies. Address the forearm muscles with wrist curls.

For the lower and upper back, include chin-ups, rows, and lat pull-downs. Sailors should include upper abdominal curls, crunches, and hanging leg raises for strengthening abdominal muscles. Roman

TABLE 8.1

Recommended Aerobic Exercises

Cycling—approximately 1 hour, increasing time as well as speed.
StairMaster—30 to 50 minutes per day, 4 to 5 days per week.
Rowing machine (Concept II)—30 to 40 minutes per day, 4 to 5 days per week.

chair extensions to neutral will keep the trunk extensors strong. Rotational movements, with both crunches and trunk extension, should be included for stabilization of the lower back. Push-up activities with the lower extremities on the therapy ball (strengthening arms and developing trunk control) can be used for progressing the patient with trunk and abdominal dysfunctions. Closed-chain exercises will be used throughout the strengthening process because the tibia is in a fixed position in the hiking strap during hiking. Plyometric exercises can be added to increase eccentric strength and increase forces placed on the knee as in hiking.

SPECIAL EQUIPMENT

Hiking Bench

The hiking bench can be constructed out of wood using two by four's (Fig. 8.5). The length of the bench is 50 in., the width is 18 in., and the seat is 16 in. The edge of the seat to the hiking strap is 14 in., and the hiking strap is adjustable to the height of the seat. These are basic measurements for the bench; for more specific design, look for a laser racing book that can give specific directions on construction.[3]

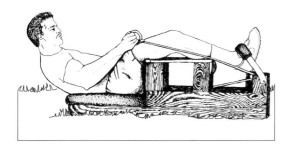

FIGURE 8.5

Hiking bench for off-water training.

Etiology of Sailing Injuries

In competitive sailing, the most common injuries include strains, sprains, and contusions. The three most common areas of injury include the lumbar spine, the knees, and the shoulders. Due to the lack of tracking in sailing, the actual incidence is not known. As with most sports, the specific etiology of sailing injuries can be attributed to intrinsic and extrinsic factors. Extrinsic factors that may contribute to injury include training errors, improper technique, and/or faulty equipment. Intrinsic factors may include impairments with range of motion (ROM), joint mobility, muscle dysfunction, and poor motor control.

EXTRINSIC FACTORS

Training Errors

Examples of training errors include overtraining and sailing in extremely windy conditions. Overtraining occurs over a period of time in which the sailor practices too many times in a week. Training errors also can take place under strong wind conditions in which the boat and sail can overpower the sailor. In these two examples, the sailor can develop strains, sprains, or more extensive pathologies.

Poor Technique

Good technique is essential while hiking with either the bent-knee technique or the straight-leg technique. Poor technique in hiking can be due to the sailor being out of physical shape, inexperienced, and having inappropriate or no coaching.

Equipment Failure

Equipment malfunctions occur too frequently in the sport of sailing. Most experienced sailors understand and live with the fact that equipment will fail during training and events. The most common equipment failures include the tiller extension breaking, hiking strap breaking, lines breaking, and sails ripping. These events usually take place when the sailor is in the hiking position, which will place abnormal stresses on the sailor. In such situations, the sailor can even fall out of the boat.

INTRINSIC FACTORS

Intrinsic factors include impairments with flexibility, joint mobility, muscle dysfunction, and poor motor control in the sailing athlete. Some of the common intrinsic factors are thoracic and lumber hypermobilities, tight hamstrings, and decreased lower extremity and trunk strength.

Etiology of Windsurfing Injuries

Windsurfing demands high levels of core strength, specifically the obliques. Common injuries occur to the shoulder and spine and are often the result of collisions with the boom. The risk of injury is 0.22 per 1000 participant hours, and most injuries are not major.[17,18]

Common Injuries and Their Rehabilitation

This section deals with the common injuries found in competitive dinghy sailing. It also addresses the potential causes of injury, methods of intervention, and sport-specific exercises for dinghy sailors.

LUMBAR SPINE

Sprains and Strains

Lumbar spine injuries typically include sprains of ligamentous tissue and strains of muscles. The common cause of lumbar spine injuries in sailing is excessive loading of the lumbar spine resulting from improper lumbar position and increases in wind velocities.

Disk Injury

With the repetitive movements in dingy sailing and the position of the lumbar spine during hiking, the disk is at risk. In addition, the repetitive compressive forces can increase the chance of disk injuries. Disk herniation and degeneration of the disk can lead to nerve root irritation.

Compression Fractures

Compression fractures in the lumbar spine can occur after a trauma such as a two-boat collision.

Treatment of Lumbar Spine Injuries

During the initial stage of rehabilitation, sprains and strains of the dinghy sailor should be handled in the same manner as for any individual. The goals include (1) establishing symptom relief for the athlete, (2) educating the athlete so that he or she can identify poor and/or at-risk positions and use modalities at home, (3) restoring the active range of motion for the athlete, (4) maintaining and developing balanced strength and stability of the injured area.

For the dinghy sailor, the final stage must include sport-specific training. The lumbar spine and trunk muscles need to be trained progressively using dynamic stabilization. Strengthening of the abdominal and extensor muscles should take place from 20° of extension to 160° of flexion, which will be used in hiking. Begin by isolating each of the groups and then progressively having the athlete use the trunk extensors and flexors together. The physiotherapy ball provides a good progression for the athlete. Exercises include seated ball exercises while using elastic resistance training to simulate trimming the sails and sit-ups on the ball with the legs straight and bent. Using a hiking bench is the best way to simulate hiking on the water and will help develop sport-specific strength.

KNEE INJURIES

Sprains and Strains

The knee is the focal point for the majority of forces during hiking. Common knee injuries in sailing include sprained ligaments, specifically the posterior cruciate ligament (PCL) and collateral ligaments.

Meniscal Tears

Meniscal injuries are also common when pivoting occurs on the fixed foot.

Tendinitis

Quadriceps tendinitis also can occur secondary to the repetitive eccentric activity of sailing.

Patellofemoral Syndrome

Sailors quite commonly present with patellofemoral syndrome, especially if they are training for long periods of time on the water. Frequently, chondromalacia develops. The undersurface of the patella shows degenerative changes of the articular cartilage as a result of the wear and tear. The patient may experience pain with hiking, ascending or descending stairs, and prolonged sitting.

Treatment of Knee Injuries

For the knee, sport-specific training needs to include appropriate strengthening goals. The therapist needs to know how much of the athlete's time is spent in a bent-knee hiking position or a straight-leg hiking position. This information can be gathered from the sailor. ROM needs to be incorporated with strength and endurance. Active stretching is important to have reflexive muscle relaxation. Once the athlete has begun active stretching, isometrics and eccentric exercises will assist with stability. As isolated strength and flexibility increase, exercises that improve core strength need to be incorporated. Squats, dead lifts, and bent-over rows will increase the core strength. Without proper strength and flexibility, though, these exercises can cause injuries. Plyometrics such as bounding and box jumping will prepare the athlete for the ballistic activities involved in sailing and windsurfing. Once there is adequate strength and stability, move to skill-specific activities such as the hiking bench. Progress slowly with time and intensity as muscle fatigue and soreness allow.

SHOULDER INJURIES

Rotator Cuff and Bicipital Tendinitis

The sailor uses the shoulder and upper extremity in sheeting and trimming the sail (adjusting of the sail) and steering the boat. Repetitive overuse of the shoulder muscles can create strain in muscle tissue, especially during eccentric contractions. Exercises should include shoulder and scapular dynamic stability. The athlete can use a 6-ft PVC pipe of one inch diameter to work on shoulder stability by holding the pipe in the middle and trying to vibrate it quickly back and forth. Different lengths and diameters will increase or decrease the challenge. Plyometric upper extremity exercises can include weighted ball throwing that incorporates trunk rotation, push-ups with a clap in between repetitions, hand stands against a wall with quick up and down movements, and using the hands on a StairMaster. These exercises incorporate strength and stability.

Return to Sport

No literature exists to support the best program for returning the sailor back to the water. If time permits, the sailor should return to the sport gradually. The general progression is to begin with light air first for 15 to 30 minutes for the first week and then slowly progress into medium and heavy air if the athlete remains symptom-free.

Develop plyometric sport-specific exercises, as well as practice on water. The athlete should be able to perform four 4-minute sessions on the hiking bench, and then he or she can start with light air on-water training blocks of 40 minutes. When the athlete can perform four 5-minute sessions, progress to six 8-minute sessions on the hiking bench. The athlete then can progress to moderate and heavy air in practice blocks, starting at 20- to 30-minute sessions. The athlete's tolerance should be used as a guide, along with the amount of inflammation and discomfort associated with the activity for the 24-hour period following the on-water practice session. Table 8.2 presents phase 3 of a lower extremity rehabilitation program for return to sport.

Definitions

Centerline of boat   The middle point of the boat that runs from the forward end to the back end.

Heavy air   Wind conditions greater than 15 mi/h.

Hiking   Leaning out over the side of the boat to counteract the heeling effect.

Jibing   To turn the stern of boat 180° in the opposite direction through the eye of the wind.

Laser   A 14-ft. fiberglass boat with a single mast and sail; this is designed as a one-person boat.

Light air   Wind conditions from 0 to 8 mi/h.

Mainsheet   A line that helps to pull the sail in and out to adjust to the wind.

Medium air   Wind conditions from 8 to 15 mi/h.

Pumping   To move the sail (rapidly) in such a manner that it creates more speed for the boat.

Tacking   To turn the bow of the boat 180° in the opposite direction through the eye of the wind.

Trim   A term used to describe adjusting the sail or sails.

Tiller   An extension (wood, aluminum, etc.) that is attached to the rudder that allows the sailor to steer the boat.

TABLE 8.2

Lower Extremity Rehabilitation for Return to Sport, Phase 3

Phase 3 (Advanced phase)
Therapeutic goals:
    Controlled mobility exercises and progression to plyometrics for sailing
    Continue ROM, muscular strength and endurance, proprioception
    Overall fitness and flexibility
    Restore athlete's confidence to resume sailing with full participation
Modalities:
    Cryotherapy and electrical stimulation (interferential, high voltage) after therapy, if
    inflammation arises
Therapeutic exercises:
    Stretching
    Open chain: Isokinetic quadriceps and hamstrings for concentrics and eccentrics
    Closed chain: Step up/down, band resistance in lungs, balance and proprioception exercises
    (single-leg balance), and trunk stabilization exercises with the physioball
    Hiking bench exercise: Start with two 3-minute sessions, and build on by minutes
Progression criteria: Return to practice when an 80 percent of strength, endurance, and
    proprioception is achieved

References

1. Allen JB: Sports medicine and sailing. *Phys Med Rehabil Clin Am* 10(1):49–65, 1999.
2. Bourke G, Rutherford M: *Championship Laser Racing.* New York: Fernhurst Books, 1998.
3. Tillman D: *Laser Sailing for the 1990s.* New York: International Marine Publishing, 1991.
4. Goff P: Biomecanique du rachis lombaire et navigation a voile. *Revue Du Rhumatisme* 55(5): 411–414, 1988.
5. Newton F: Dinghy sailing. *Practitioner* 233(1472):1032–1035,1989.
6. Mackie HW, Legg SJ: Preliminary assessment of force demands in laser racing. *J Sci Med Sport* 2(1):78–85, 1999.
7. Norkin C, Levangie P: *Joint Structure and Function, A Comprehensive Analysis.* 3d edition, Philadelphia: FA Davis, 2001.
8. Richert H: Sports medical aspects of sailing and windsurfing. *Dtsche Z Sports Med* 44: 301–303, 1993.
9. Kendall F, McCreary EK: *Muscles: Testing and Function,* 4th ed. Baltimore: William & Wilkins, 1993.
10. Netter F: *The CIBA Collection of Medical Illustrations,* Vol 1: *Nervous System, Anatomy and Physiology.* Paris: CIBA Foundation, 1986.
11. Vogiatzis I, Spurway NW, Boreham C: Assessment of aerobic and anaerobic demands of dingy sailing at different wind velocities. *J Sports Med Phys Fitness* 35(2):103–107, 1995.
12. Colby LA, Kisner C: *Therapeutic Exercise: Foundations and Techniques,* 3d ed. Philadelphia: FA Davis, 1996.
13. Spurway NC, Burns R: Comparison of dynamic and static fitness training programs for dinghy sailors—And some questions concerning that physiology of hiking. *Med Sci Res* 21: 865–867, 1993.
14. Shephard RJ: Biology and medicine of sailing: An update. *Sports Med* 23(6):350–356, 1997.
15. Cyriax J: Diagnosis of soft tissue lesions, in *Textbook of Orthopedic Medicine,* Vol1, 8th ed. London: Bailliere-Tindall, 1982.
16. O'Sullivan S, Schmitz T: *Physical Rehabilitation: Assessment and Treatment,* 3d ed. Philadelphia: FA Davis, 1994.
17. McCormick DP, Davis AL: Injuries in sailboard enthusiasts. *Br J Sports Med* 22(3): 95–97, 1988.
18. McLatchie GR, Lennox CM, Percy EC, Davies J: *The Soft Tissue Tissues, Trauma and Sports Injuries.* Oxford: Butterworth-Heinemann, 1993.

Additional References

Bennet G: Psychological breakdown at sea: hazards of single handed ocean sailing. *Br J Med Psychol* 47(3):189–210, 1974.

Bernardi M, Felici F, Marchettoni M, Marchettoni P: Cardiovascular load in off-shore sailing competition. *J Sports Med Phys Fitness* 30(2): 127–131, 1990.

Blackburn M: Physiological responses to 90 min of simulated dinghy sailing. *J Sports Sci* 12(4): 383–390, 1994.

Branth S, Hambraeus L, Westerterp K, et al: Energy turnover in a sailing crew during offshore racing around the world. *Med Sci Sports Exerc* 28(10):1272–1276, 1996.

Dunkelman NR, Collier F, Rook JL, et al: Pectoralis major muscle rupture in windsurfing. *Arch Phys Med Rehabil* 75(7):819–821, 1994.

Felici F, Rodio A, Madaffari A, et al: The cardiovascular work of competitive dinghy sailing. *J Sports Med Phys Fitness* 39(4):309–314, 1999.

Johns RJ: Sailing. *Trans Assoc Am Phys* 85:99–102, 1972.

Kemp R: The medical hazards of sailing. *Practitioner* 215(1286):188–196, 1975.

Legg SJ, Mackie HW, Slyfield DA: Changes in physical characteristics and performance of elite sailors following introduction of a sport science program prior to the 1996 Olympic games. *Appl Human Sci* 18(6): 211–217, 1999.

Legg S, Mackie H, Smith P. Temporal patterns of physical activity in Olympic dinghy racing. *J Sports Med Phys Fitness* 39(4):315–320, 1999.

Legg SJ, Miller AB, Slyfield D, et al: Physical performance of elite New Zealand Olympic class sailors. *J Sports Med Phys Fitness* 37(1):41–49, 1997.

Locke S, Allen GD: Etiology of low back pain in elite boardsailors. *Med Sci Sports Exerc* 24(9):964–966, 1992.

Mackie H, Sanders R, Legg S: The physical demands of Olympic yacht racing. *J Sci Med Sport* 2(4):375–388, 1999.

Marchetti M, Figura F, Ricci B: Biomechanics of two fundamental sailing postures. *J Sports Med Phys Fitness* 20(3):325–332, 1980.

Mitkova N, Raiceva V, Dimitrov M: Optimal nutrition and drinking diet of the crews in tropical conditions of sailing. *Biuletyn Inst Med Morskiej W Gdansku* 17(3):411–418, 1966.

Putnam CA: A mathematical model of hiking positions in a sailing dinghy. *Med Sci Sports* 11(3):288–292, 1979.

Saury J, Durand M: Practical knowledge in expert coaches: on-site study of coaching in sailing. *Res Q Exerc Sport* 69(3):254–266, 1998.

Schonle C: Traumatology of sailing injuries. *Aktuelle Traumatol* 19(3):116–120, 1989.

Shephard RJ: The biology and medicine of sailing. *Sports Med* 9(2):86–99, 1990.

Vogiatzis I, Spurway NC, Jennett S, et al: Changes in ventilation related to changes in electromyograph activity during repetitive bouts of isometric exercise in simulated sailing. *Eur J Appl Physiol* 72(3):195–203, 1996.

Walls J, Bertrand L, Gale T, Saunders N: Assessment of upwind dinghy sailing performance using a Virtual Reality Dinghy Sailing Simulator. *J Sci Med Sport* 1(2):61–72, 1998.

CHAPTER 9

Running

Brian R. Hoke

Running has for many years been the exercise of choice for thousands of individuals, whereas many others integrate running into their total fitness strategy. The popularity of running can be linked to a desire to achieve an aerobic and cardiovascular benefit, whereas other runners use running as a means to effectively control body weight and lean body mass. Running also can produce psychological benefits and can be a useful form of stress management. Finally, there are individuals who run to compete. A select few in top form aspire to "win the race," but many more simply work to better their own previous best effort and "personal record" (PR).

Recognizing the benefits derived from running aids the sports medicine practitioner in understanding why the injured runner may appear quite anxious and frustrated in seeking medical attention for his or her injury. The runner may be unable to derive the cardiovascular benefits to which he or she has become accustomed. Unless such runners modify their dietary caloric intake, a reduction in their running due to injury may be accompanied by weight gain, which actually may increase the forces that must be attenuated by the lower extremities during the running gait. Injured runners often feel an increase in their psychological stress levels that may be related to the absence of the endorphins released by the body during sustained exercise such as running. When injured, both recreational and competitive runners may notice that instead of setting new PRs, their race times are slowing. Adding to the frustration of the injured runner is a poor level of understanding by some medical practitioners, whose advice to any injured runner is simply, "If it hurts when you run, then just stop running." An appreciation for the biomechanics of running provides new insights into the mechanical basis underlying the etiology of many running injuries.

General Differences Between Running and Walking

To describe running as "fast walking" ignores critical differences in the biomechanics of walking versus running. The peak vertical forces in walking are approximately 110 percent of body weight, but these forces increase to 275 percent of body weight during running.[25] In walking gait, the stance phase lasts for 0.6 s and represents 62 percent of the gait cycle.[35] In running gait, the stance phase shortens to 0.2 s and represents only 31 percent of the gait cycle.[26] In walking, there is a transitional period termed *double-limb support* where both lower extremities are in contact with the ground at the same time. This overlap of the stance phase lasts for 12 percent of the early stance interval and again during the final 12 percent prior to toe-off, and in the period between, one limb remains in contact with the ground. Double-limb support does not occur in running; rather, the runner is in either single-limb support or a new phase termed *float* or *nonsupport* in which neither limb is in contact with the ground (Fig. 9.1). The base of gait narrows from 9 cm between the center of the heels during walking to 2 cm during running, and the center of the heel approximates the midline of the body in faster, more efficient runners.[9]

In walking, the loading of the stance limb typically begins at the lateral heel. In addition to narrowing the base of support, runners may load their foot differently during the gait cycle. It is not uncommon to see runners whose foot strike is in the midfoot or forefoot. In general terms, the faster the runner, the more is the tendency to increase the load on the forefoot, although runners who prefer to "run on their toes" can be found at every speed of running. The best way to study the point of impact and loading of the foot in running is with force-plate analysis and determination of impact point (*strike index*) and the path of loading (*center of pressure*), which have been described in detail by Cavanagh.[4]

Speed of forward locomotion for walking typically varies in a range from 2 to 4 mi/h (15–30 min/mi). Slower runners, often termed *joggers* in the literature but perhaps better described as *recreational runners*, typically run in a range from 5 to 9 mi/h (7 to 12 min/mi). Competitive runners often run 10 mi/h or faster (6 min/mi or less).[24]

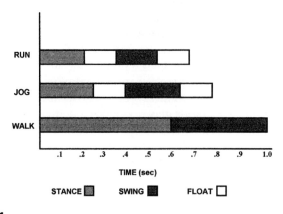

FIGURE 9.1

Cycle times for walking, jogging, and running.

The terminology used to describe the running gait cycle is different from the terminology classically used to describe walking gait. In walking, the *contact* period is from heel contact to foot flat, followed by the *midstance* period from foot flat to heel rise, *propulsion* from heel rise to toe-off, and *swing* phase from toe-off to heel contact. The description of the running gait cycle that follows is based on the classification by Slocum and James.[37] There are two phases, *support* and *swing*, and each phase has three functional periods. The support phase begins with *foot contact*, which is the period from initial ground contact to full weight acceptance. This is followed by *midsupport*, which is the period from full weight acceptance to the initiation of ankle plantarflexion. The final period within the support phase is *toe-off*, which is the period from the initiation of ankle plantarflexion to the time in which the foot leaves the supporting surface. The swing phase also encompasses three functional periods. The first is *follow-through*, which is from the time the

foot leaves the supporting surface to the point of maximal hip extension. This is followed by *forward swing*, which begins at the initiation of hip flexion and ends at maximal hip flexion. The swing phase ends with the period of *foot descent*, which lasts until foot contact (Fig. 9.2).

Biomechanics

ANALYSIS OF FORCES (KINETICS)

Running biomechanics involves both the study of forces (*kinetics*) and the study of motion (*kinematics*). The formal study of forces is usually conducted in gait biomechanics laboratories at universities or major hospital systems. Ground reaction force (GRF) can be quantified through the use of force plate platforms. GRF is the force reaction generated in response to the force transmitted to the ground by the foot or shoe. It is based on

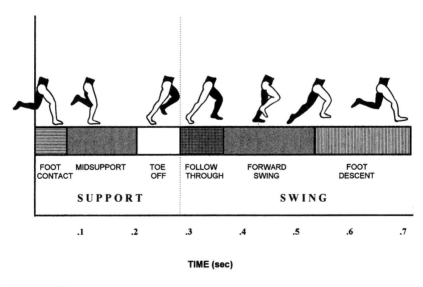

FIGURE 9.2

Phases and functional periods of the running gait cycle.

Newton's third law: For every action, there is an equal and opposite reaction. GRF represents the acceleration of the total body's center of gravity (more accurately termed the *center of mass*). There is considerable variability in the data between individuals and even between the right and left foot of the same individual.[4] Three components of GRF will be reviewed: vertical, mediolateral, and anteroposterior.

VERTICAL GROUND REACTION FORCE (VGRF)

Vertical ground reaction force (VGRF) in walking begins with an impact peak of less than body weight (BW) and then exceeds BW at the end of the contact period, dropping down during midstance and rising again to exceed BW, reaching its highest peak during the propulsive period. In the jogger (recreational runner), there is a VGRF impact peak of a magnitude of 1.5 to 2 times BW, followed a single propulsive peak at approximately 2 to 3 times BW. In the more efficient competitive runner, there is no VGRF impact peak, and there is a single propulsive peak approximately 2 to 3 times BW *but less than for jogging*[25] (Fig. 9.3).

MEDIOLATERAL SHEAR (MLS)

Mediolateral shear (MLS) in walking gait begins with an initial medial shear (occasionally lateral) after heel strike, followed by lateral shear for the remainder of the stance period. For the recreational runner, the MLS follows the same pattern as walking, but with a more pronounced medial shear at toe-off. For the competitive runner, the MLS again follows a pattern similar to jogging but with an appreciable decrease in the lateral shear and increasing amplitude of the propulsive medial shear[25] (Fig. 9.4).

Anteroposterior shear (APS) follows a similar pattern for walking and running. In the walking gait cycle, there is an anterior (braking) shear from foot strike to the end of the contact period and a posterior (propulsive) shear prior to toe-off. In the recreational runner, there is a brief anterior shear at impact, followed closely by an even longer anterior shear and then a posterior propulsive shear. In the faster competitive runner, there is a brief anterior shear, followed by a large posterior shear.[25] The greater magnitude in the APS is proportionate to the reduction in the VGRF for the faster runner (Fig. 9.5). One may observe this in watching a track workout where both

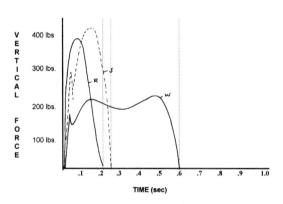

FIGURE 9.3

Vertical ground reaction forces.

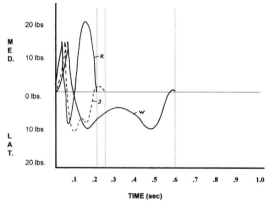

FIGURE 9.4

Mediolateral shear force.

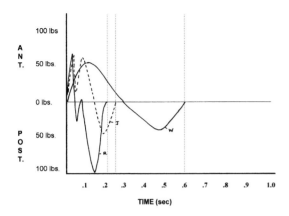

FIGURE 9.5

Anteroposterior shear forces.

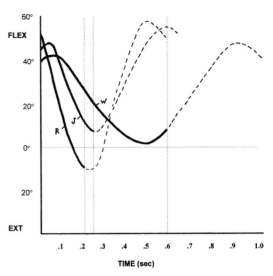

FIGURE 9.6

Hip flexion and extension walking, jogging, and running.

novice runners and competitive runners are present. The novice runner appears to have more "bounce" in his or her running gait, whereas the accomplished runner appears to "glide" around the track with less vertical displacement of his or her center of mass.

ANALYSIS OF SPECIFIC JOINT MOTION (KINEMATICS)

In contrasting the joint kinematic patterns for walking, jogging, and running, some general trends emerge: The total range of motion (ROM) increases, the duration of cycle decreases, and the resulting velocity of joint motion (degrees per second) dramatically increases.

Hip Joint Flexion and Extension (Fig. 9.6)

In walking, there is brief hip flexion after heel strike to aid in shock absorption, followed by hip extension as the pelvis moves over the femur, with maximal hip extension at heel-off. The hip then flexes through toe-off and into the swing, reaching a peak in the final 33 percent of the swing phase.

In jogging, the hip position at initial contact is slightly more flexed, and there is brief hip flexion after foot strike, followed by hip

extension throughout the remainder of stance. Peak hip extension occurs just after toe-off, with peak flexion occurring again in the final 33 percent of swing.[25]

In running, the hip is slightly more flexed at initial contact and then proceeds to extend throughout stance. Peak hip flexion and extension follow the same pattern as jogging but with significantly greater excursion.[25]

Hip Joint Adduction and Abduction (Fig. 9.7)

In walking, the hip is adducted 5 degrees at heel strike, adducting further until the end of contact phase. The hip then abducts from its adducted position throughout midstance and propulsion, reaching peak abduction shortly after toe-off. The hip then adducts through the final 66 percent of swing as the foot again approaches the ground.

In jogging, the hip is adducted 8° at foot contact, with peak adduction occurring at 40 percent of stance. The hip then abducts until

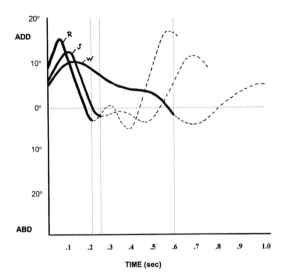

FIGURE 9.7

Hip abduction and adduction walking, jogging, and running.

early swing phase, when peak abduction occurs. During late swing, the hip again adducts, reaching peak adduction just before foot contact. As speed increases, the hip adduction at foot strike increases, narrowing the base of gait and placing the stance foot directly under the midline of the body.[25]

In the competitive runner, the hip is adducted 10 degrees or more at foot strike. The hip further adducts until 30 percent of stance and then abducts until 40 percent of swing phase. At this point the hip then adducts rapidly until just prior to foot strike.[25]

Lower Extremity Rotation (Fig. 9.8)

The pelvis, femur, and tibial segments all follow the same pattern of internal (medial) and external (lateral) rotation during human locomotion.[22] All internally rotate during the initial loading of the limb in early stance phase and then externally rotate until peak external rotation at toe-off. During the swing phase, all three internally rotate again. With regard

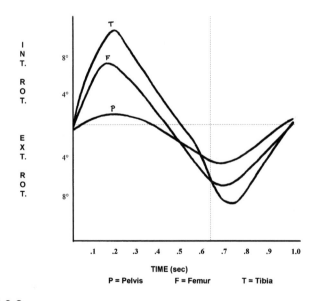

FIGURE 9.8

Rotational patterns of the lower extremity in gait.

to the magnitude of the motion, the femur rotates faster and farther than the pelvis, and the tibia rotates faster and farther than the femur. The velocity of lower extremity rotation is much greater as the speed of the gait cycle increases.

Knee Joint Flexion and Extension (Fig. 9.9)

In walking gait, the knee position at initial contact is near full extension, and the knee flexes to aid in shock attenuation until the end of the contact phase. Knee extension then occurs as the pelvis and femur advance forward over the slower-moving tibia, reaching a peak at heel-off. The knee flexes after heel-off, and this flexion continues through the swing phase. Knee flexion peaks early in the swing phase to aid in ground clearance and controlled acceleration of the advancing swing limb.

In jogging, the knee position at foot strike is appreciably more flexed, approximately 35°, and the knee flexes after the initial impact to a peak at 40 percent of stance. The knee then extends until just before toe-off, when the knee again flexes, reaching peak flexion (110°) halfway through the swing phase.[25]

In faster running, the knee is even more flexed at foot strike, approximately 45°, and the knee flexes further as the limb becomes fully weight receptive. The knee then extends until just prior to toe-off, which is followed by rapid swing-phase knee flexion to a peak of approximately 125° at 50 percent of the swing phase.[25]

Ankle Joint Dorsiflexion and Plantarflexion (Fig. 9.10)

In walking gait, the ankle is slightly dorsiflexed at heel strike. During the early contact period, the ankle plantarflexes in a controlled descent of the foot to the supporting surface, and then in late contact, dorsiflexion begins as the knee flexes, which requires forward ad-

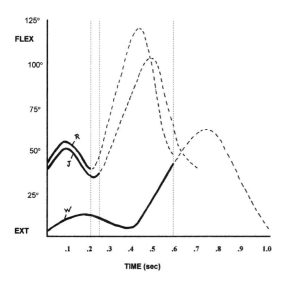

FIGURE 9.9

Knee flexion and extension walking, jogging, and running.

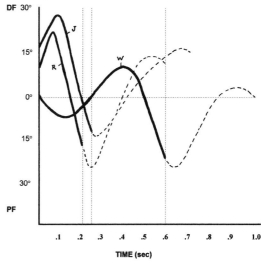

FIGURE 9.10

Ankle dorsiflexion and plantarflexion walking, jogging, and running.

vancement of the tibia over the talus. This forward advancement of the tibia over the foot continues the ankle dorsiflexion during midstance to reach a peak just prior to heel-off. During the propulsive period, the hip and knee flex, and the ankle joint plantarflexes until just after heel-off. Swing-phase clearance of the distal limb is accomplished by ankle dorsiflexion, which peaks at 66 percent of the swing phase.

In jogging, the ankle is dorsiflexed 15° at foot strike, but instead of initial plantarflexion, the ankle dorsiflexes further to a peak at 40 percent of the stance phase. This is followed by rapid plantarflexion until just after toe-off. During swing, the ankle dorsiflexes actively until just prior to foot strike.[25]

The faster runner begins the gait cycle at foot strike with the ankle 10° dorsiflexed, and there is further dorsiflexion until midway through the stance phase. Ankle plantarflexion then begins and continues through the remainder of stance, reaching a peak early in the swing phase.[25]

Subtalar Joint Motion (Fig. 9.11)

The subtalar joint in jogging and running follows the same general pattern of motion that has been described for walking. The foot is slightly supinated at foot contact, and pronation occurs during the initial loading of the foot. Peak pronation occurs near the transition from contact to early midstance. The foot remains in a pronated position throughout midstance, although supination begins following peak pronation and continues until just prior to toe-off. The subtalar joint achieves its maximally supinated position just prior to toe-off. During early swing, the subtalar joint pronates from its supinated position at toe-off to hover near neutral during midswing. In late swing, the subtalar joint again slightly supinates as the foot approaches the ground at terminal swing.

While the pattern of rear-foot (subtalar) motion appears very similar for walking and

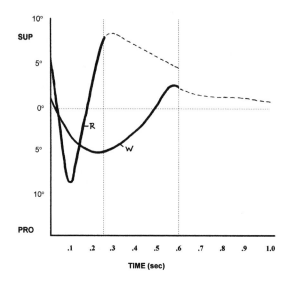

FIGURE 9.11

Comparison of rear-foot motion in walking versus running.

running, the magnitude and velocity of subtalar motion increase appreciably. Maximal pronation for walking is 6°,[36] and this increases to 9° to 10° for running.[6]

MUSCLE FUNCTION IN RUNNING

Typical muscle function during the running gait cycle involves a three-phase stretch-shortening cycle. The muscle activity begins with a deceleration of momentum during the stretch phase, followed by stabilization of the body segment during the amortization phase. The final phase is an acceleration of momentum accomplished through a concentric contraction of the muscle. Muscle force production is enhanced during the amortization and shortening phases by virtue of the preload delivered to the muscle fibers through the stretch phase.[3] Several authors have provided a comprehensive analysis of muscle function for various speeds of running that is summarized in Fig. 9.12.[1,24–26,28] The hip flexors' peak electromyographic (EMG) activity occurs dur-

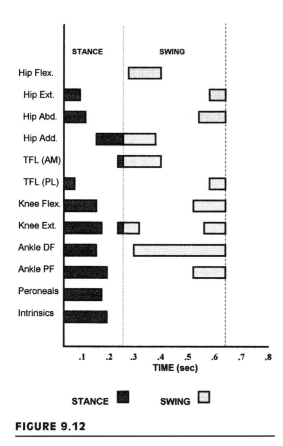

EMG activity during the running gait cycle.

ing forward swing. The primary function of this muscle group is to accelerate the forward momentum of the swing limb. The hip flexors appear to be the main muscle group that increases the speed of running gait.[24]

Hip/Thigh

The hip extensors show maximal activity beginning in foot descent, with activity continuing into foot contact and midsupport. The functions of the hip extensors are to decelerate the thigh at the end of swing, stabilize the hip and pelvis at foot contact, and accelerate hip extension in midsupport.

The hip abductor group functions in concert with the hip extensors, showing a similar period of peak activity. The hip abductor

muscle activation begins during foot descent and continues into foot contact. The function of this activity is to control the hip adduction occurring just prior to foot strike to bring the foot to the supporting surface closer to the midline of the body. Foot placement closer to midline places the foot more directly under the center of mass. The hip abductor group has a very important role in stabilizing the hip and pelvis in the frontal plane during the support phase. In the late support phase, the hip abductor functions concentrically as the hip undergoes abduction.

The tensor fasciae latae are composed of two functionally distinct parts: the anteromedial portion and the posterolateral portion.[32] The anteromedial fibers reach peak activity at toe-off and during early swing, assisting the hip flexors in accelerating the momentum of the thigh. The posterolateral fibers function in concert with the hip extensors and abductors, reaching peak electrical activity in late swing and early support phase. In doing so, the posterolateral fibers assist in preparing the swing limb for stance and, on foot contact, stabilizing the hip and pelvis.

The hip adductors show electrical activity throughout the entire running gait cycle.[26] Their function is to stabilize the pelvis to the thigh in stance and stabilize the position of the thigh to the pelvis in swing. Peak activity in the adductor longus occurs just prior to toe-off. It is hypothesized that this activity is to increase the stability of the support limb and ensure a smooth transition of weight to the contralateral limb.[23]

Knee

The knee extensors show the greatest activity in late swing and in the early support phase. They play a critical role for the lower extremity in controlling late swing-phase flexion of the knee and decelerating knee flexion at impact. This eccentric knee extensor activity provides "cushioning flexion" of the knee joint, which is a key mechanism for shock attenuation during the running gait. There is also a brief peak in knee extensor activity in follow-through and forward swing representing activity of the rectus femoris and vastus intermedius.[24,26,28]

The knee flexors are active primarily in the final 25 to 40 percent of the swing phase, and this activity continues briefly into the support phase.[24,28] Their function is to act eccentrically in decelerating forward flexion of hip and controlling late swing-phase knee extension. The early support-phase activity represents a cocontraction with the powerful knee extensors in providing stabilization of the knee joint as the support limb accepts weight.

Ankle

The anterior group, also known as the *ankle dorsiflexors,* is active throughout swing, with activity continuing into the early support phase. The function of this group is to accelerate and maintain dorsiflexion of the ankle, hallux, and lesser digits to aid foot clearance during swing. While there is some activity of the anterior group after foot contact, this probably represents a stabilization role in concert with the superficial and deep posterior group because the ankle dorsiflexes on contact.[24]

The posterior group, also known as the *ankle plantarflexors,* reaches peak activity beginning in late swing and continuing through the first half of the support phase. The function of this group is to stabilize the ankle and foot and decelerate ankle dorsiflexion after foot strike. Muscle activity in the posterior group primarily assists in controlling the forward momentum of the tibia over the relatively stationary foot. There is also a brief period of activity in the proximity of toe-off as the ankle is plantarflexing at faster running speeds, representing a secondary acceleration function.

The peroneal group, also known as the *ankle evertors,* reaches peak activity during the early support phase. The peroneal muscula-

ture functions to assist in controlling the supinatory motion that follows peak pronation, and by virtue of its insertion into the plantar aspect of the first cuneiform and first metatarsal, it also has a role in stabilization of the medial forefoot, in particular the first ray.

Foot

The foot intrinsics show the greatest EMG activity from foot contact through midsupport. The role of the foot intrinsics is one of "dynamic stabilization." These muscles act as dynamic ligaments to restrain excessive mobility of the midfoot and forefoot during weight acceptance.

Muscle activity in the control of rear-foot (subtalar) motion is determined largely by the relative position and subsequent tendon pull of the lower leg musculature. Those muscles which pull from the medial aspect of the subtalar joint axis function to decelerate subtalar pronation and assist in accelerating subtalar supination. These muscles include the tibialis posterior, soleus, gastrocnemius, tibialis anterior, flexor hallucis longus, flexor hallucis brevis, flexor digitorum longus, and flexor digitorum brevis. The deceleration of subtalar supination is accomplished through the activity of muscles that have tendons pulling from the lateral aspect of the subtalar axis. These muscles also assist in the acceleration of subtalar pronation, and included within this group are the peroneus longus, peroneus brevis, extensor digitorum longus, and extensor digitorum brevis (Fig. 9.13).

Injury Prevention in Running Athletes

The prevention of running injuries is accomplished through proper attention to shoe selection, stretching, strengthening, and a logical and incrementally progressive schedule.

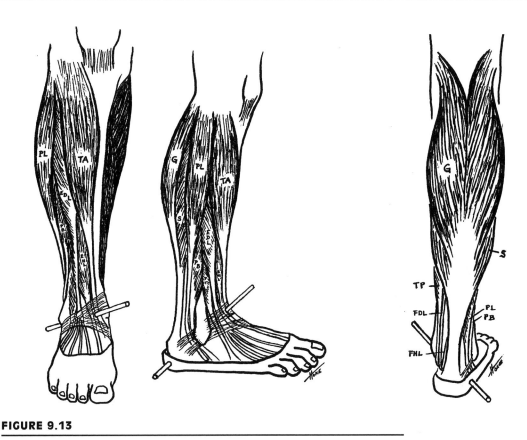

FIGURE 9.13

Relationships of lower leg musculature to the subtalar joint axis.

SHOE SELECTION

Shoe selection is critical in that the running athletes have very little protective equipment other than their footwear. The footwear industry has expanded exponentially in the past two decades, and a large number of appropriate running shoes are available from multiple manufacturers. Reviews of current footwear are available in popular national running periodicals such as *Runner's World* and *Running Times*. Running shoes are divided into three subclassifications: *Cushioned* shoes emphasize shock attenuation and are void of features that inhibit rear-foot motion; *stability* shoes are constructed to control the normal tendency toward pronation of the rear

foot on foot contact; and *motion-control* shoes are designed with additional support medially to aggressively inhibit excessive rear-foot pronation. Table 9.1 summarizes the features of these three categories of running shoes. The clinician may wish to have a ready reference "footwear prescription" to list desirable features for the runner's footwear based on the clinical examination and observed function. A sample form is provided in Fig. 9.14.

STRETCHING

Stretching programs, which emphasize a low-load prolonged stretch with active contraction of the antagonist, are recommended

TABLE 9.1

Recommended Shoe Features on Foot Biomechanics

	Supinated	*Neutral*	*Pronated*
Shoe classification	Cushioned	Stability	Motion control
Last shape	Curved	Semicurved	Straight
Construction	Central slip last or California slip last	California slip last	Combination last or board last
Midsole features	Single density EVA or PU with cushioning additions	Dual-density EVA	Dual-density EVA with plastic footbridge
Insole	Removable	Removable	Removable
Other notes	Often needs wide and/ or deep toe box; avoid pronation control features	Footframe	Reinforced heel counter and footframe

for the running athlete. The typical program includes attention to the hip flexors and quadriceps, hamstrings and lower back, posterior hip, lateral hip and iliotibial band, and gastrochemius soleus complex. It is recommended that runners stretch briefly prior to running in conjunction with a warm-up jog of several minutes at a pace approximately two-thirds of their typical training pace. An example of a common stretching program is presented in Fig. 9.15.

STRENGTHENING

Runners require a balance of strength throughout the lower extremities to avoid poorly controlled repetitive stresses that lead to injury. Particular attention should be placed on the lateral hip, the knee extensors, and the lower leg musculature. Simple programs requiring very little equipment enhance compliance and have proven to be the most successful. A sample program is included in Fig. 9.16. Alternatively, the running athlete may choose to use a well-equipped fitness center to accomplish these strength goals.

TRAINING SCHEDULE

The final component of injury prevention in runners is an incremental and progressive training schedule. Hoke's law states that "the body *responds* to small increments of change but will *react* to large increments of change."[17] The premise of this principle is that to effect a positive change, the stimulus must be beyond the present level of function but in doing so must not exceed this level by too great a margin. If the stimulus is too great, the body will react negatively, and further progression in the level of function actually will be delayed. An optimal training schedule incorporates a very gradual progression of increased time/ mileage, rest days, and cross-training with other activities such as cycling or swimming. A general rule for injury prevention is to keep the progression of time and/or mileage to no greater than 10 to 15 percent more than the previous week. All too often injuries are encountered simply because the individual had set a goal to be participating in a race, such as a marathon, without adequate forethought about the time necessary to safely and adequately prepare for the event.

PATIENT FOOTWEAR RECOMMENDATION

Type of Shoe (Activity):_____

Foot Structure (Shape):_____

Foot Function: o Over Pronation   o Neutral   o Under Pronation

Severity of Abnormal Function: o Mild   o Moderate   o Severe

SHOE FEATURES

Last (Shape):
   o Straight   o Semi-Curved   o Curved

Last (Construction):
   o Board   o Combination   o Central Slip   o California Slip

Midsole:
   o Polyurethane   o Compression Molded EVA
   o Firm Medial Midsole   o Rearfoot Cushioning
   o Single Density Midsole   o Forefoot Cushioning
   o Footframe

Uppers:
   o Low Cut   o Mid (3/4) Cut   o High Top
   o Reinforced/Extended Heel Counter
   o Deep Toe Box   o Wide Toe Box

Outsole:
   o High Density Rubber   o Blown Rubber
   o Rubber   o Polyurethane
   o Cleat   o Nubbed Sole

Insole:
   o Removable Insole for Orthotic

SPECIAL NEEDS:_____

_____

_____

_____

FIGURE 9.14

Shoe recommendation form.

Etiology of Running Injuries

SIX SOURCES OF SYMPTOMS

A number of factors are linked to the prevalence of injuries in running. I refer to the main areas of concern as the *six sources of symptoms*. The first source of problems is the runner's *schedule*. Training errors account for a significant proportion of running injuries. Common errors include rapid increases in weekly mileage, increasing the pace of workouts, and inadequate rest days. The second source of symptoms is *surfaces*. Included in this category are cambered roads, which have been linked to iliotibial band tendinitis of the downslope leg,[5] and hill running, which may increase stresses to the knee and achilles tendon.[11] The third source of injuries is the runner's *shoes*. While there are hundreds of models to choose from, it is still commonplace to encounter a runner who is trying to run in a shoe well beyond its useful life or a runner

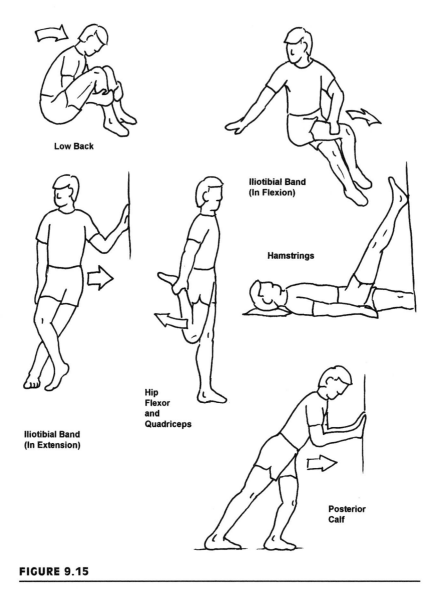

Low Back

Iliotibial Band
(In Flexion)

Hamstrings

Hip
Flexor
and
Quadriceps

Iliotibial Band
(In Extension)

Posterior
Calf

FIGURE 9.15

Flexibility exercises for runners.

whose running biomechanics and shoes are at odds. The fourth area of concern is *strength*. Runners may use running as their only form of regular exercise, and due to the cyclic nature of running gait, the same motor patterns are encountered thousands of times with each session. This can easily lead to imbalances that cannot be corrected simply by logging more miles. The fifth area of concern is *stretching*. While most runners understand that stretching can reduce the incidence and severity of injuries, stretching programs are often neglected or performed with improper technique. It is imperative that runners demonstrate their stretching methods when injured to make certain that the targeted

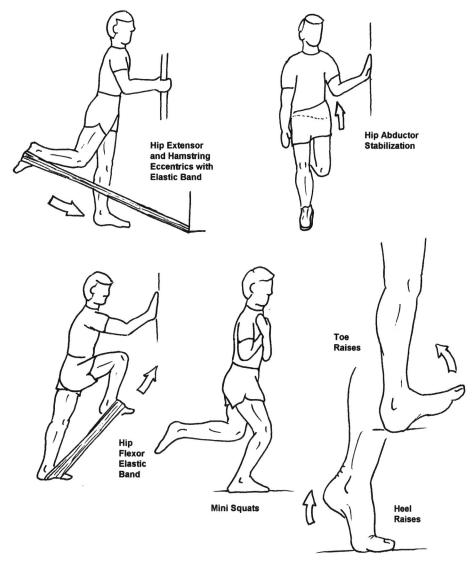

Hip Extensor
and Hamstring
Eccentrics with
Elastic Band

Hip Abductor
Stabilization

Hip
Flexor
Elastic
Band

Mini Squats

Toe
Raises

Heel
Raises

FIGURE 9.16

Strength training exercises for runners.

muscle group is indeed the recipient of the stretching exercise. The final area of concern is the runner's *structure*. The sports medicine practitioner who regularly deals with injuries to running athletes must develop clinical skills in evaluating lower extremity alignment and biomechanics. Running injuries are rarely due to trauma and generally fall into the classification of overuse injuries. The injuries commonly encountered by runners frequently are due to mechanical stresses imposed on tissues as the body seeks to compensate for intrinsic structural variations. There are many variations to this theme. Proximal factors such as internal femoral torsion and external tibial torsion result in a large Q-angle (valgus vector within the pull of the quadriceps). Over the course of many miles, these competing transverse plane factors may result in pain and dysfunction at the patellofemoral articulation. Distal factors also play a significant role, such as an excessive rear-foot and forefoot varus, which compensates through excessive subtalar pronation and midfoot hypermobility. The runner who encounters this compensatory mechanism over the thousands of repetitions in regular running may overload the tibialis posterior musculature. A more extensive discussion of the relationship between intrinsic factors and injury follows in the next section.

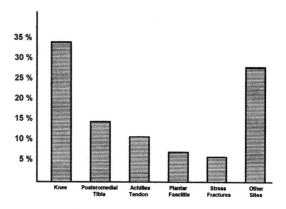

FIGURE 9.17

Running injury incidence.

Common Injuries and Their Rehabilitation

The cyclic and repetitive nature of running often leads to mechanical stresses that exceed the adaptation threshold of musculoskeletal tissues, resulting in injury. Numerous authors have described their experiences in the frequency of injuries to runners. Common sites include the knee, ankle, shin, hamstring, achilles tendon, calf, and plantar fascia. James and Jones[19] reported the following injury locations in a group of 180 runners presenting with 232 conditions: knee (34 percent), posteromedial tibia (13 percent), achilles tendon (11 percent), plantar fascia (7 percent), stress fractures (6 percent), and other sites (29 percent) (Fig. 9.17). An overview of each of these regions follows.

KNEE PAIN

Patellofemoral Joint Pain

Early investigators attributed patellofemoral pain to "chondromalacia patella," implicating the joint surface in pain production. While

this is without question a possibility in advancing osteoarthritis of the knee, many patients present with patellofemoral joint pain and no radiographic evidence of osteoarthritic changes and no crepitus on clinical examination. Investigators also have shown that regular participation in running did not coincide with premature osteoarthritis at the hip, knee, and ankle.[21] Dye et al. examined the sensitivity of various intraarticular structures of the knee by undergoing arthroscopy on his own knees without anesthesia. The synovium and infrapatellar fat pad were the most sensitive structures, whereas probing of a grade 3 chondral defect produced no acute pain.[8] It appears likely that the majority of running athletes who present to the sports medicine practitioner have pain related more to the synovial tissues and retinacular stresses than to degeneration of the patellofemoral joint. Clinical practice also has shown that many of these anterior knee pain patients achieve resolution of their symptoms within a few weeks following proper intervention, whereas it is well understood that cartilage defects at best require several months to heal with fibrocartilage.

As outlined previously, the knee extensor mechanism plays a crucial role in shock attenuation during weight acceptance following foot contact in running. This shock attenuation is accomplished through a smoothly controlled eccentric contraction of the knee extensors. The patellofemoral joint is a finely balanced system within the extensor mechanism that has multiple factors affecting its alignment and function. The runner frequently experiences pain in the patellar region when this system lacks the necessary "balance of power" between medial and lateral force vectors. Excessive pronation of the foot also has been cited by multiple authors as a contributory factor in the development of anterior knee pain.[15,17,19] The early peak in knee flexion following foot contact coincides with the peak in rearfoot pronation, and if the pronation of the rear foot becomes excessive, there will be adverse stresses on the knee in the sagittal (increased flexion), frontal (increased knee valgus), and transverse (increased tibial rotation) planes.

Treatment Treatment of patellofemoral pain in the runner focuses on changing the forces acting on the patella from the static and dynamic structures. Taping, using the techniques advocated by Grelsamer and McConnell,[15] frequently has resulted in symptomatic reduction and enabled injured runners to progress more quickly through their other rehabilitative interventions. A step-jump-hop program of weight-bearing concentric and eccentric loading is also helpful in developing fast-speed neuromuscular control of the knee extensor mechanism (Table 9.2). Particular attention must be given to the proximal and distal alignment of the lower limb during these exercises, avoiding excessive internal rotation of the femoral segment and maintaining the rear-foot function around its most congruent midrange (neutral) position. Strengthening of the hip extensors and external rotators in a closed kinetic chain environment will aid the control of femoral posi-

tion. In the presence of abnormal foot alignment, a properly posted (corrective) foot orthosis may prove extremely useful in the long-term management of the distal intrinsic factors.

Iliotibial Band Syndrome

The iliotibial band is a common site of injuries in runners, occasionally at the trochanteric region but more commonly at the knee. It is generally accepted that the irritation within the iliotibial band is created by friction as it passes over the bony prominence of the greater trochanter or the lateral femoral condyle. Magnetic resonance imaging (MRI) investigations have demonstrated thickening of the iliotibial band in symptomatic runners at the site where the band passes over the lateral femoral epicondyle.[10] The angle of knee flexion implicated in friction of the posterolateral fibers of the iliotibial band at the lateral femoral epicondylar eminence is 30° of knee flexion,[30] which in the running gait normally occurs just after foot contact.[31] Several factors increase the likelihood of injury to this structure in the running athlete. The first factor is that as the speed of forward ambulation increases, the base of gait narrows. Double-limb support no longer occurs, and the foot is placed much closer to midline to position the support limb directly beneath the center of mass. This narrowing of the base of gait is accomplished through increased adduction at the hip, placing the lateral hip musculature (including the iliotibial band) on increased tension. This may be even more stress to the female runner, who characteristically has a wider anatomic pelvic width than her male counterpart. An additional stress to the iliotibial band may be encountered if the hip abductor musculature fails to maintain a stable and level pelvis due to weakness or fatigue. As the contralateral hip drops inferiorly due to the weight of the swing limb, there is an effective increase in hip adduction

TABLE 9.2

Step-Jump-Hop Plyometric Progression

1. Step-ups	2. Step-downs
Level 1: 2-in. box	Level 1: 2-in. box
Level 2: 4-in. box	Level 2: 4-in. box
Level 3: 6-in. box	Level 3: 6-in. box
Level 4: 8-in. box	Level 4: 8-in. box
3. Jump-ups (two-legged)	4. Jump-downs (two-legged)
Level 1: 2-in. box	Level 1: 2-in. box
Level 2: 4-in. box	Level 2: 4-in. box
Level 3: 6-in. box	Level 3: 6-in. box
Level 4: 8-in. box	Level 4: 8-in. box
5. Hop-ups (one-legged)	6. Hop-downs (one-legged)
Level 1: 2-in. box	Level 1: 2-in. box
Level 2: 4-in. box	Level 2: 4-in. box
Level 3: 6-in. box	Level 3: 6-in. box
Level 4: 8-in. box	Level 4: 8-in. box
7. Hop-downs with repeat forward hop (single leg)	
Level 1: 2-in. box	
Level 2: 4-in. box	
Level 3: 6-in. box	
Level 4: 8-in. box	

to the support limb. Finally, the iliotibial band has a role in the transverse plane rotation at the hip and lower leg. The iliotibial band may come under greater tension when the runner exhibits excessive rear-foot pronation as the lower leg internally rotates. The increased tension produced through increased leg internal rotation can be compounded by external rotary influences at the hip, most notably femoral retroversion or tightness in the hip external rotators.

Rehabilitation Treatment of iliotibial band tendinitis in the runner must include stretching to the lateral hip musculature. It is suggested that these stretching exercises be performed in both extension and flexion of the hip to address both the anteromedial and posterolateral muscular attachments into the iliotibial band. Particular care must be taken to avoid lateral flexion of the lumbar spine when attempting to perform these stretches. Strengthening of the hip abductors is also an important component of treatment. It may be useful to use traditional side-lying leg lifts to create a foundation of strength in this group and then move to a weight-bearing environment to exercise this muscle group in single stance. In the weight-bearing exercise, the limb should be positioned in a manner similar to that encountered in running, with the stance foot positioned at midline through adduction of the hip. The stance-leg hip abductors may now be exercised by stabilizing the hip and pelvis and preventing a downward tilt of the contralateral pelvis.

Infrapatellar Tendinitis

As discussed previously, the runner uses eccentric contractions of the knee extensor mechanism to decelerate knee flexion that occurs at impact. Eccentric overloads have been implicated as a significant etiologic factor in the development of tendinitis in the athlete.[11,38] Anterior knee pain patients demonstrated significant knee extensor eccentric deficits that far exceeded the deficits in concentric strength.[2] The infrapatellar tendon typically becomes inflamed at its tenoperiosteal junction at the inferior pole of the patella, more posterior than anterior. The clinician may encounter difficulty in localizing the area of injury unless the patella is first tilted superiorly to increase exposure of the inferior pole, as described by Cyriax and Coldham.[7]

Treatment of this area may include the use of icing and/or deep transverse friction massage to the inferior pole using a simultaneous superior tilt to provide optimal exposure to the area of injury.[7] A knee extensor mechanism strengthening program emphasizing eccentric strength and control is recommended. This can begin by using open kinetic chain techniques designed to strengthen the knee extensors. A number of exercise modes can be used in this manner, such as cuff weights, formal weight-stack units, or sophisticated computer-controlled isokinetic machines. It is critical to emphasize control during the lowering or eccentric phase of the exercise. To integrate this into a functional environment, the step-jump-hop progression is suggested (see Table 9.2).

SHIN PAIN

Shin pain in the runner has three main subclassifications: stress fractures and stress reactions, exertional compartment syndromes, and musculoskeletal "shin splints." The runner may assist the practitioner with the differential diagnosis, since each of these subclassifications typically has a different clinical presentation.

Stress fractures can affect a variety of sites in the runner but are most common in the tibia (34 percent), fibula (24 percent), metatarsals (20 percent), and femur (20 percent).[21] With 58 percent of the stress fractures occurring in the shin, the sports medicine practitioner must be suspicious of any pain along the bony contours of the leg that worsens during each run but decreases following the run. Ultrasound may cause pain in the presence of a stress fracture.[14] Early radiographs may prove unremarkable, and a bone scan may be required to rule out increased metabolic activity within the osseous system.

Exertional compartment syndromes in the shin area typically present as a feeling of pain and "tightness" or "cramping" in the shin brought on by exercise. Continued exercise frequently results in distal paresthesias and motor weakness. Suspicions of compartment syndrome are investigated through dynamic pressure testing using an indwelling intracompartmental catheter during an exercise protocol. In the presence of compartment syndrome, the intracompartmental pressure frequently rises above typical values, and when exercise is stopped, there is a delay in the time to return to resting pressure values.[16,33,39,40]

Musculoskeletal "shin splints" include the remaining disorders of the muscle-tendon unit that are brought on by sustained exercise such as running. A knowledge of muscle function in the control of the rear foot and midfoot is necessary to discern which mechanical stresses have exceeded the capacity of the muscle-tendon unit. The anterior compartment is responsible for dorsiflexion of the ankle and foot to provide adequate clearance of the swing limb. The anterior compartment also has an eccentric function in controlling ankle and digital plantarflexion. By virtue of the medial pull of the tibialis anterior, the anterior compartment also has a secondary role in the deceleration of rear-foot pronation. The lateral compartment controls rear-foot supination and provides balance for the strong inverter pull from the anterior and posterior compartments. The peroneus longus also plays a significant role in stabilization of the first ray in the late support phase. The posterior compartments include both the superficial and deep compartments. The deep posterior group, and particularly the tibialis posterior, provide control of rear-foot pronation and prevent midfoot collapse during weight acceptance. The soleus fibers[27] and the flexor hallucis longus[13] also have been implicated in symptom production in cases of posteromedial shin splints symptoms.

Rehabilitation

Treatment of shin splints begins with classifying the source of the problem correctly. When shin splints are due to stress fracture or stress reaction, training must be suspended to allow the injury to heal. This typically requires a 4- to 6-week interval. During this period, the runner is encouraged to maintain their conditioning and fitness through alternative nonimpact training such as cycling, deep water running, or exercise using recently developed elliptical trainers. The return to running can be based on an absence of clinical findings, radiographic evidence of healing, or a lack of symptom reproduction with ultrasound over the site of the injury.

In the case of compartment syndrome, acute episodes may resolve with an altered training schedule, foot orthotics, shoe modification, and attention to resolution of muscle imbalances.[35] In the case of chronic recurrent compartment syndrome symptoms, excellent results may be achieved through the judicious use of surgical release of the fascia. This frequently can be done through minimal-incision subcutaneous fasciotomy.[29,35]

In the treatment of musculoskeletal shin splints, the cause of the increased stress must be identified accurately through the biomechanical evaluation. The musculature, which is producing the symptoms, is strengthened through both open kinetic chain exercises such as elastic band exercises or a specifically designed weighted footplate (Ankle Isolator, Kelly Kinetics). As strength and endurance improve, closed kinetic chain (weight-bearing) exercises are used to integrate the progress in a functional manner. Many forms of exercise exist for this purpose, from single-leg stance balances to equipment-augmented exercises such as with the Biomechanical Ankle Platform System (BAPS, Camp International). When the runner has achieved an adequate level of healing and improved muscle performance, a gradual return to normal training is suggested. Foot orthoses with deep heel seats, high medial flanges, and medial posting in the rear foot and/or forefoot frequently are useful for posterior tibial tendinitis. Peroneal tendinitis frequently is improved with neutral rear-foot posting, lateral forefoot posting, and first-ray cutouts in the orthotic shell.

ACHILLES TENDINITIS

The achilles tendon is a frequent site of injury in the running athlete.[5,11,18,20,38] The distal fibers of the achilles tendon have an area of hypovascularity that extends approximately 5 to 6 cm above the insertion of the tendon into the posterior calcaneus. This hypovascularity can impede the reparative process in the presence of achilles tendinitis. In addition, as the fibers terminate at the calcaneus, the tendon undergoes a transition to a more fibro-cartilaginous structure, presumably to be better suited to the high concentration of forces at this area. Stresses through the achilles tendon are increased by the presence of intrinsic structural abnormalities such as ankle equinus, a tight gastrocnemius and/or soleus, and forefoot equinus (cavus foot). Excessive rearfoot pronation also places an increased stress across the fibers of the achilles tendon, and its insertion medial to the subtalar joint axis gives the achilles tendon a secondary role in the deceleration of subtalar pronation. Training also may play a role in excessive stresses to this area. Increasing pace, uphill training, and running with primary contact in the forefoot all increase the stresses through the achilles tendon.

Rehabilitation

Treatment of achilles tendinitis may incorporate the use of heel lifts to decrease stresses through the tendon. An eccentric exercise program beginning with non-weight-bearing exercise and progressing to weight-bearing heel raises is useful in restoring the strength to the calf group. When a stretching program is used for this muscle group, care must be taken to avoid compensatory motion at the oblique axis of the midtarsal joint. Both the talocrural joint and the oblique midtarsal joint share the same major components of motion.[17] For this reason, when a runner lacks soft tissue or articular mobility at the talocrural joint, he or she commonly compensates through hypermobility and collapse of the midtarsal joint through the oblique axis of motion. This common compensation must be avoided in stretching of the calf group and achilles tendon. This is accomplished by maintaining slight supination of the rear foot during stretching techniques.

Subtalar supination inhibits functional hypermobility of the midtarsal joint complex, and the resulting forces will be directed toward the talocrural articulation.

PLANTAR FASCIITIS

Medial heel pain is a common affliction within the running community. There are many causes of medial heel pain, but the most common diagnosis given to the injured runner is plantar fasciitis. The plantar fascia plays an integral role in stabilization of the midfoot and forefoot during running gait. As the heel begins to rise, the constant length of the plantar fascia places it under greater tension as it is "wound" around the metatarsal heads. This creates further stability for the late support phase, and this effect is commonly referred to as the *windlass mechanism*. When there is a loss of midfoot stability under the initial loading of the foot, the plantar fascia may come under tension prematurely. As the heel rises in the unstable foot, the added tension through metatarsophalangeal dorsiflexion may cause injury to the plantar fascia at its attachment to the medial calcaneal tuberosity. Midfoot and forefoot instability typically arises from one of two scenarios. The midfoot may have inherently poor static support through the plantar ligamentous structures, or there may be a secondary loss of midtarsal stability as the rear foot moves beyond the normal range of pronation.

Rehabilitation

Treatment of plantar fasciitis includes decreasing extrinsic stresses on the midtarsal joint from tight achilles tendons. A stretching program while maintaining a supinated rear foot can resolve this adverse influence. In recalcitrant cases, a night splint may be helpful in maintaining the calf group on stretch during sleep. If a night splint is used, it can be modified with a medial wedge under the heel and a 45-degree wedge under the hallux to maintain rear-foot supination in the splint and increase midfoot stability through the windlass mechanism. Taping the plantar aspect of the foot using a modified "low dye" method is also helpful in maintaining external support to the healing tissues during daily activities, and this typically is done sequentially for a 2-week period. A thorough evaluation of the intrinsic structure of the foot may reveal the need for external support through foot orthoses. In considering the influence of structural malalignment, the clinician must keep in mind the "rule of 3s": the support phase of running occurs three times faster, and the forces that must be attenuated are three times higher, so a mild structural fault will take on three times the significance that it would have for walking. In selecting an appropriate orthosis for a runner, the clinician must consider the weight of the runner, the foot type (cavus versus planus), soft tissue mobility ("rigid" hypomobility or "flexible" hypermobility), the speed of runner, the increased "functional limb varum" produced by narrowing of the base of gait, and the inherent control features of the runner's shoes.

Return to Running Progression

Typically, there are two runners who incur training errors in their training regimen. The best summary of the problem are the "three toos": *too much, too fast, too soon*. The first type of runner making frequent training errors is the novice runner. The second type of runner who frequently errs in his or her training schedule is the accomplished runner returning after an injury. In both these scenarios, the training errors encountered place the individual at high risk for the development of a new injury or aggravation of an existing one. When a running injury has been diagnosed properly, and treatment has brought about the desired reduction of symptoms, the runner typically will be very anxious to return to the road. It is suggested that the runner meet the following criteria for a progressive return to running: no joint effusion, no pain during daily activities for 2 weeks, and able to hop forward on the injured leg with good neuromuscular control. When these criteria have been followed, a gradual progression with rest/recovery days is suggested. A sample program is outlined in Table 9.3.

If at all possible, the sports medicine practitioner should follow the credo, "*Keep the runner running!*" It is important to remember all the positive effects of running for the individual. Complete rest is avoided, if possible, instead working with the runner to compromise by reducing mileage, frequency, and pace. The runner should be advised to integrate replacement sources of fitness training such as swimming, cycling, or other forms of aerobic exercise available using formal equipment such as motorized stairclimbers, elliptical trainers, or cross-country ski simulators. If a reduced training schedule is first attempted and it fails to provide resolution of the injury, the runner will be more willing to accept total rest in the management of his or her injury.

TABLE 9.3

Return-to-Running Program

The following is a training program for returning to running after injury. The runner should not attempt to resume a regular running schedule until he or she has gone 2 weeks without significant pain in daily activities. If pain should return on running, the runner may continue as long as

1. The character of the pain is not sharp.
2. The pain lessens or remains unchanged as the running session continues.
3. The presence of pain does not alter the runner's normal pattern of motion (no limping allowed!).

Begin each session with a brisk walk of 2 to 5 min to warm up, followed by stretching exercises for another 5 min. The following program is recommended, with a rest day between each step of the program:

Step 1: Walk 4 min.; jog 2 min. Repeat four times
Step 2: Walk 4 min.; jog 4 min. Repeat three times
Step 3: Walk 2 min.; jog 4 min. Repeat four times
Step 4: Walk 2 min.; jog 6 min. Repeat three times
Step 5: Walk 2 min.; jog 8 min. Repeat three times
Step 6: Walk 2 min.; jog 10 min. Repeat twice

On completing step 6, the runner may resume a gradual transition back to continuous running for 10 min. or more following a 2-min. warm-up walk. The runner may increase the running time by 2 to 4 min. per session, with at least 1 day of rest between runs for the first month.

TABLE 9.4

Flexibility Training Exercises for Runners

Low back: Sit down and bend both knees, placing feet flat about shoulder width apart. Drop both elbows between knees, and reach around outside the lower leg. Tense abdominal muscles, and pull body forward, assisting with arms. Stretch should be felt in lower part of back.

Iliotibial band in flexion: Sit down with one leg straight and knee bent. Place foot of bent leg over the straight leg, and turn trunk toward the side of the bent leg. Put opposite hand on upper thigh of bent leg, and pull bent leg across body and toward the side of the straight leg. Stretch should be felt in back of hip and outer thigh.

Iliotibial band in extension: Stand with hip you wish to stretch facing a wall. Shift outer hip toward the wall, keeping balance by placing hand on wall and crossing other leg over. Be careful not to bend sideways in your back. You should feel a stretch in the outer thigh of the side toward the wall.

TABLE 9.4   (cont.)

Flexibility Training Exercises for Runners (cont.)

Hip flexor and quadriceps: Stand on one leg. Bend the opposite leg at the knee, and grasp ankle of free leg. Use buttock muscle to pull hip backward, assisting with the arm holding the ankle. Do not arch your back. You should feel a stretch in the front of the hip and thigh of the side you are holding at the ankle.

Hamstrings: Lie on the floor in a doorway. Place one leg up against the door frame, keeping the knee straight. Gradually move buttock closer to the door frame, lifting foot higher in the doorway. Stretch should be felt in the back of the thigh and behind the knee.

Posterior calf: Stand facing a wall with one foot well ahead of the other. Keep heel of back foot on the ground, and keep knee straight. Bend forward at the hips and waist, and keep weight to the outside of the foot. Do not lift back heel off the ground, and do not let foot roll inward at ankle (pronate).

Note: Hold each stretch for 15 to 30 s, and repeat five times for each muscle group. Exercises can be performed several times a day and should be done regularly at completion of each running session.

TABLE 9.5

Strength Training Exercises for Runners

Hip extensor and hamstring eccentrics with elastic band: Stand facing a wall or door, and anchor elastic band low in doorway. Wrap or loop other end of elastic band around foot. Bend knee and pull foot and leg backward slowly to create tension in the elastic band. When hip reaches maximal extension, let tension off slowly, allowing hip to come forward and knee to straighten.

Hip abductor stabilization: Stand on one leg with foot directly under the middle of the body and opposite hip toward wall. Let hip of free leg drop down, and then lift it up using the muscles of the outer hip on the stance leg. Do not bend spine sideways.

Hip flexor elastic band: Stand facing a wall, and stand on one foot. Place one end of an elastic band under the foot of the stance leg. Wrap or loop other end of band around foot of free leg. Place hands on wall for balance, and lift hip and knee of free leg forward and upward against resistance of elastic band. Lower smoothly with control.

Mini squats: Stand on one leg and cross arms across chest. Lower body slightly by bending knee of stance leg. Hold this position briefly, and then straighten stance leg out, raising up in space. Keep hips and pelvis level as you do this, and try to maintain stance knee directly over stance foot.

Toe raises: Stand with weight evenly on both feet. Lift front of foot off the floor, pulling toes and forefoot up away from the supporting surface and keeping heels on the floor. Hold briefly, then return to flat-footed position.

TABLE 9.5 (cont.)

Strength Training Exercises for Runners (cont.)

Heel raises: Stand with weight evenly on both feet. Lift heels off the floor, bringing weight forward up onto the ball of the forefoot. Hold briefly, and then return to flat-footed position.

Note: Do three sets of each exercise to the point of muscular fatigue. Strength exercises should be done on alternating days to allow time for the body to respond to the increased demand.

References

1. Adelaar RS: The practical biomechanics of running. *Am J Sports Med* 14(2):497–500, 1986.

2. Bennett JG, Stauber WT: Evaluation and treatment of anterior knee pain using eccentric exercise. *Med Sci Sports Exerc* 18(5): 526–530, 1986.

3. Cavagna GA: Storage and utilization of elastic energy in skeletal muscle. *Exerc Sports Sci Rev* 5:89–129, 1977.

4. Cavanagh PR: The shoe ground interface in running, in Mack RP (ed): *AAOS Symposium on the Foot and Leg in Running Sports*. St. Louis: Mosby, 1982.

5. Clancy WG: Runners' injuries: Evaluation and treatment of specific injuries. *Am J Sports Med* 8(4):287–289, 1980.

6. Clarke TE, Frederick EC, Hamill CL: The study of rear-foot movement in running, in Frederick ED (ed): *Sport Shoes and Playing Surfaces: Biomechanical Properties*. Champaign, IL: Human Kinetics Publishers, 1984.

7. Cyriax JC, Coldham M: *Textbook of Orthopaedic Medicine*, Vol 2: *Treatment by Manipulation, Massage and Injection*, 11th ed. London: Balliere Tindall, 1984.

8. Dye SF, Staubli HU, Biedert RM, Vaupel GL: The mosaic of pathophysiology causing patellofemoral pain: Therapeutic implications. *Oper Tech Sports Med* 7(2):46–54, 1999.

9. Edington CH, Frederick EC, Cavanagh PR: Rear-foot motion in distance running, in Cavanagh PR (ed): *Biomechanics of Distance Running*. Champaign, IL: Human Kinetics Publishers, 1990.

10. Ekman EF, Pope T, Martin DF, Curl WW: Magnetic resonance imaging of iliotibial band syndrome. *Am J Sports Med* 22(6):851–854, 1994.

11. Fyfe I, Stanish WD: The use of eccentric training and stretching in the treatment and prevention of tendon injuries. *Clin Sports Med* 11(3):601–624, 1992.

12. Galloway MT, Jokl P, Dayton OW: Achilles tendon overuse injuries. *Clin Sports Med* 11(4):771–782, 1992.

13. Garth WP, Miller ST: Evaluation of claw toe deformity, weakness of the foot intrinsics, and posteromedial shin pain. *Am J Sports Med* 17(6):821–827, 1989.

14. Goodwin JS: Stress fractures diagnosed by ultrasound. *Mediguide Inflam Dis* 4:5, 1983.

15. Grelsamer RP, McConnell J: *The Patella: A Team Approach*. Gaithersburg, MD: Aspen Publishers, 1998.

16. Hargens AR, Ballard RE: Basic principles for measurement of intramuscular pressures. *Oper Tech Sports Med* 3(4):237–342, 1995.

17. Hoke BR, Lefever-Button SL: *When the Feet Hit the Ground, Everything Changes*, Level 2: *Take The Next Step*. Toledo, OH: American Physical Rehabilitation Network, 1994.

18. Jacobs SJ, Berson BL: Injuries to runners: A study of entrants to a 10,000 meter race. *Am J Sports Med* 14(2):151–155, 1986.

19. James SL, Jones DC: Biomechanical aspects of distance running injuries, in Cavanagh PR (ed): *Biomechanics of Distance Running*.

Champaign, IL: Human Kinetics Publishers, 1990.

20. Komi PV, Fukashiro S, Jarvinen M: Biomechanical loading of achilles tendon during normal locomotion. *Clin Sports Med* 11(3): 521–531, 1992.

21. Konradsen L, Berg Hansen E, Sondergaard L: Long distance running and osteoarthrosis. *Am J Sports Med* 18(4):379–381, 1990.

22. Levens AS, Inman VT, Blosser JA: Transverse rotations of the segments of the lower extremity in locomotion. *J Bone Joint Surg Am* 30A:859, 1948.

23. McBryde AM: Stress fractures in runners. *Clin Sports Med* 4(4):737–752, 1985.

24. Mann RA, Moran GT, Dougherty SE: Comparative electromyography of the lower extremity in jogging, running, and sprinting. *Am J Sports Med* 14(6):501–510, 1986.

25. Mann RA: Biomechanics of running, in Mack RP (ed) *AAOS Symposium on the Foot and Leg in Running Sports.* St Louis: Mosby, 1982.

26. Mann RA, Hagy JH: Biomechanics of walking, running, and sprinting. *Am J Sports Med* 8(5): 345–350, 1980.

27. Michael RH, Holder LE: The soleus syndrome: A cause of medial tibial stress (shin splints). *Am J Sports Med* 13(2):87–94, 1985.

28. Montgomery WH, Pink M, Perry J: Electromyograhic analysis of hip and knee musculature during running. *Am J Sports Med* 22(2): 272–278, 1994.

29. Mubarak SJ: Surgical management of chronic compartment syndromes of the leg. *Oper Tech Sports Med* 3(4):259–266, 1995.

30. Noble CA: Iliotibial band friction syndrome in runners. *Am J Sports Med* 8(4):232–234, 1980.

31. Orchard JW, Fricker PA, Abud AT, Mason BR: Biomechanics of iliotibial band syndrome in runners. *Am J Sports Med* 24(3):375–379, 1996.

32. Pare EB, Stern JT, Schwartz JM: Functional differentiation within the tensor fasciae latae. *J Bone Joint Surg Am* 63A(9):1457–1471, 1981.

33. Pedowitz RA, Gershuni DH: Pathophysiology and diagnosis of chronic compartment syndrome. *Oper Tech Sports Med* 3(4):230–236, 1995.

34. Pink M, Perry J, Houglum PA, Devine DJ: Lower extremity range of motion in the recreational sport runner. *Am J Sports Med* 22(4): 541–549, 1994.

35. Rampersand YR, Amendola A: The evaluation and treatment of exertional compartment syndrome. *Oper Tech Sports Med* 3(4):267–273, 1995.

36. Rodgers MM: Dynamic biomechanics of the normal foot and ankle during walking and running. *Phys Ther* 68(12):22–30, 1988.

37. Slocum DB, James SL: Biomechanics of running. *JAMA* 205:97–104, 1968.

38. Stanish WD, Curwin S, Rubinovich M: Tendinitis: The analysis and treatment for running. *Clin Sports Med* 4(4):593–609, 1985.

39. Styf JR: Diagnosis of exercise-induced leg pain in the anterior aspect of the lower leg. *Am J Sports Med* 16(2):165–169, 1988.

40. Styf JR: Intramuscular pressure measurements during exercise. *Oper Tech Sports Med* 3(4):243–249, 1995.

CHAPTER 10

Alpine Skiing

Michael R. Torry

J. Richard Steadman

The history of skiing dates as far back as 4000 B.C.[1] While these early skiers primarily used this mode of locomotion for warfare or hunting, it can be safely assumed that recreational aspects of skiing took place and that non-combat-related ski injuries most likely occurred in this population. The Norwegian Army held the first recorded organized skiing competition in 1767, and thereafter, the sport quickly grew in popularity in the European countries.[1] Skiing remained relatively unknown in North America until the 1932 Lake Placid Olympics. Advances in skiing techniques, skiing instruction, ski equipment design, automated lifts, easier ski destination access, international competitive events, and media exposure have increased the popularity of downhill skiing. Recreational participation has grown to approximately 4 million in the United States alone.[2] However, with these advances, new patterns of athletic injuries also have emerged.[2-15] Injury tracking and clinical database research have been instrumental in leading to the development of better equipment designs and have had a dramatic influence on the etiology and treatment of injuries incurred during alpine skiing. This chapter addresses the evolution of these advances, outlines the current trends in injuries and injury rates associated with alpine skiing, and discusses current biomechanical research and scientific developments governing the application of preventative injury training and postinjury rehabilitation in today's ski industry. As the reader will note, skiing injuries can encompass nearly every joint in the body. Thus, sections pertaining to mechanisms of injury, injury prevention, and rehabilitation will be associated with the most commonly injured joints among all skiers—the knee, shoulder, and hand.

Traditional professional and Olympic alpine ski racing venues consist of four major areas with varying levels of technical challenges. The slalom venue is often divided into two general events, the slalom and the giant slalom. The slalom is characterized by short-radius turns and requires technical skills to maintain carry speeds through a series of gates (the number of gates is variable but typically is between 45 to 75). Although it is considered a slower, more technical event, world-class alpine racers can ski a slalom course in 0:50:00 to 0:75:00 s and can attain speeds of 35 to 50 mi/h. The giant slalom is similar in that racers must use technical skills to navigate a series of gates (35 to 60); however, the turns generally are wider (larger radius), speeds average 40 to 60 mi/h, and the race can last for 0:50:00 s to 1:20:00 min. The "super G" race is a longer event, lasting from 0:75:00 s to 2:30:00 min, possesses fewer gates (20 to 35) allowing for greater-radius turns, and racers can achieve speeds ranging from 65 to 75 mi/h. The downhill event is characterized by 15 to 25 gates and lasts approximately 2:00:00 to 2:30:00 min. World-class downhillers can achieve speeds in excess of 80 mi/h through the course.

As skiing has become more popular, newer venues also have emerged. Competitions such as free aerial performance, small and large mogul racing (skiers navigate large, closely located snow mounds during a course), speed skiing (racers tuck and ski straight down the mountain often exceeding speeds of 100 mi/h), and extreme challenge skiing such as cliff jumping or skier cross are becoming more commonplace in both professional and recreational settings.

Biomechanics of Alpine Skiing

KINEMATICS OF SKI TURNS

Since the early 1980s, considerable research has been conducted regarding proper skiing mechanics, forces and loads on the human body during ski turns, and the proper muscle phasic relationships needed to smoothly accomplish these tasks. These important strides in research have allowed for the development of successful injury prevention and fitness training programs, injury mechanism identification, and surgical and rehabilitative treat-

ment of various skiing injuries as a whole. While there are many forms of alpine skiing, the information contained in this chapter will be confined mostly to alpine slalom recreational and elite skiing performance criteria.

Mastering alpine skiing is a tremendous neuromuscular effort. No two turns during a downhill race or casual ski day are ever the same because there is always something new to experience and unanticipated external forces to attend to. Thus, ski technique and equipment selection can vary widely according to terrain (steep slope versus subtle slope or "flats") and snow condition (fresh powder versus packed powder, ice, or slush). Nevertheless, in its simplest form, alpine skiing is sliding downhill on skis and making turns to control speed and avoid race gates, trees, rocks, and other skiers. For Olympic racers who compete in the four alpine disciplines of downhill, super G, giant slalom, and slalom, turning ability and carrying speed through the gates are the general skills that are emphasized in routine training regimes. To maximize turning ability and maintain sufficient speed through a turn or gate, a skier must maintain balance by controlling the center of gravity (COG) relative to the base of support (outside and inside ski edges). This is accomplished by a series of unweighting maneuvers and subtle anatomic position changes throughout the turn while the skier simultaneously adjusts for air friction, snow friction, ground–ski boot forces, and centrifugal and centripetal forces acting on the COG. The ski turn traditionally has been divided into four phases.

Phase 1 (Preparation Phase)

In preparation for a turn, the goal of the skier is to transfer his or her body weight from the outside ski of the previous turn to the outside ski of the upcoming turn. To accomplish this, the skier unweights his or her body by an upward extension of the arms and trunk and attempts to couple this motion with the energy return of the reverse camber of the skis initiated by the momentum of the previous turn. All these lower extremity motions are preceded and balanced by a downhill pole plant of the inside pole relative to the turn radius. While one may be able to ski successfully without a pole, the pole plant helps initiate the turning sequence by creating a body position that is able to unweight.

Phase 2 (Turn Initiation)

The skier initiates the turn by developing pressure on the medial edge of the outside ski. This is accomplished by levering the edge of that ski on the snow and by applying pressure to that edge using the medial aspect of the foot and quadriceps force. The force exerted by the skier bends the ski into a reverse camber. The skier leans into the turn, causing the outside ski to edge considerably. The greater the speed, the greater is the inward inclination of the body needed to increase the edge-to-snow angulation of the ski. This edging technique allows the skier to increase the pressure on the tip of the ski, driving it into the snow. This technique, coupled with the natural shape (camber) of the ski, makes the turn easier to accomplish.

Phase 3 (The Fall Line)

In this phase, the centripetal force is at a right angle to the line of gravity acting on the skier. Thus, the skier increases the outward pressure on the outside ski by increasing the uphill angulation of the knees and hips. Because a shorter-radius turn (slalom) possesses less centripetal force than a larger-radius turn (giant slalom), a skier either may change the magnitude of the inward lean of the trunk or increase the uphill angulation of the knees and hips to accomplish a shorter-radius turn without compromising downhill speed.

Phase 4 (Turn Completion)

At the end of phase 3, the momentum of the COG and centrifugal force are acting in the same direction, tending to pull the skier

down the hill. To complete the turn successfully, the skier must resist these forces by increasing the edging pressure on the outside ski. Kinematically, the ski turn is complete when the skis are parallel to the fall line and pointed in the direction of the next turn. By keeping the COG over the outside ski and by reducing angulation through knee extension, the skier is able to maintain speed into the next turn.

ELECTROMYOGRAPHY OF SKI TURNS

Human movement depends on neuromodulation of force output of the muscular system. The activity of muscles during athletic events can be assessed with electromyography (EMG). The use of EMG to understand which muscles create and absorb forces during skiing has become commonplace, and estimates of specific muscle onsets, durations, and amplitudes have been reported.[16–19] Keeping in mind that there are many techniques (mostly depending on skill level) to execute a ski turn successfully (e.g., wedge, parallel, and slalom), making direct comparisons between different ski turns and skiers becomes quite difficult.

Traditional ski instructors teach a progressive continuum of ski turns. The wedge or "snowplow" ski turn is often first taught to novice skiers. This turn is characterized by a wider base of support (feet wider then shoulder width) and an outward angulation at the rear of the skis and a toeing-in at the forefoot so that the skis form a triangle-wedge with the apex in front of the skier. This technique allows beginners greater control of their skis, greater control of speed, and thus greater stopping ability. Once this skill is mastered, novice skiers then advance to the parallel turn. This type of turn, as the name implies, constitutes keeping the feet shoulder-width apart or narrower and the skis parallel to each through all the phases of the ski turn. Lastly, skiers attempt to improve turning ability by establishing larger-radius, high-speed slalom turns.[20] Several laboratories have conducted research studies investigating the neuromuscular control of these ski turns. In general, the wedge turn typically expresses the least amount of muscular activity, whereas the faster slalom turn exhibits the greatest.[16–19] The dynamic nature of each turn may best be reflected by these EMG parameters. Wedge turns typically are slower, whereas slalom turns are much faster.[16–19] As mentioned previously, a skier attempts to maximize speed through a turn by a combination of increasing velocity and decreasing turn radius. These acts, however, create larger centrifugal forces that need to be controlled. Therefore, speed and/or a short turn radius can increase the muscular demand in skiing.[17,18]

Because so much emphasis is placed on the uphill or downhill legs in ski instruction and ski turn technique, it is no wonder that there is evidence that limb position, relative to the turn, influences muscular output.[21] A common observation from most EMG studies is that the uphill, or inside, limb during a turn exhibits considerably more EMG activity in the rectus femoris than the downhill limb at the same instance of a ski turn. Alternatively, others[16,17] found that the vastus medialis and vastus lateralis exhibit greater EMG output on the downhill limb compared with the uphill limb. Our own analysis of bilateral muscular output during slalom ski turns showed that the muscular outputs for most of the lower extremity muscles were consistent bilaterally at the beginning of a turn.[21] The exceptions were the medial gastrocnemius and the vastus lateralis, which demonstrated significantly greater activity in the outside limb. This was attributed to the slalom ski turn, which emphasizes medial pressure on the outside limb in the early portion of the turn. The remaining portion of the slalom turn allows the skier to remain relatively upright because he or she moves in a shorter

arc compared with the giant slalom turn. Thus, disparity between limb EMG activity was not apparent for most muscles. During the giant slalom, however, many more differences in bilateral muscular activity were identified at both phase 1 and phase 2 of the ski turn. It was observed that the vastus lateralis, biceps femoris, and gluteus medius were all dominant on the outside limb in nearly all phases of the turn. The most differences occurred in phases 2 and 3 of giant slalom turns. While these results are indicative of each turning style and provide considerable insight into potential complications when an elite skier returns to skiing after a unilateral limb injury, preseason conditioning should focus on double-limb training because turns are staggered in all alpine races.

High levels of co-contraction are evident in all ski turns that have been reported.[16–19] Additionally, there is evidence that skier ability can alter muscular output. Karlsson et al.[22] noted that novice skiers exhibit more constant levels of muscular output, whereas advanced skiers demonstrate distinct phases of EMG bursts and relaxation periods during a single turn. This finding suggests that advanced skiers achieve a higher level of motor efficiency throughout a race or ski day.

The EMG data that have been reported in the literature for several types of ski turns suggest that regardless of skier ability, preseason training and postinjury rehabilitation should focus on eccentric contractions of the hip adductors, gluteal muscles, quadriceps, hamstrings, lower back, and stomach muscles. Additionally, these exercises should be conducted in a manner that creates a heightened level of co-contraction about the hip and knee joints.

MECHANICAL LOADS DURING SKIING

Determining internal and external forces acting about a skier during a turn is technically challenging. To obtain accurate internal joint moments and joint reaction forces, the forces and moments between the ski and boot must be estimated. Additionally, the interaction of the skier and the ski-binding–boot system offers computational challenges as well. Thus it is not surprising that most early biomechanical data concerning skiing were derived from portable pressure sensors that could be implanted between the foot and boot.[23] These pressure patterns helped to reveal major differences between rear-entry boots and conventional boot designs. Later studies helped show that the pressures on the medial toe and instep are essential in initiating a ski turn.[24,25] Nonetheless, estimates of forces and moments about the lower extremity have been presented.[26–29] Peak internal forces and moments acting on a skier have been estimated at 270 N·m for hip extensors, 150 N·m for varus/valgus knee moments, 60 N·m for knee torsion moments and about 1300 N·m for anterior shear forces at the knee joint.[30–33] Hip joint contact forces can be in excess of 10 times body weight (BW) for large mogul skiing and between 5 and 7 times BW for small moguls. These forces are considerably higher than hip contact forces endured during walking or running. Ground reaction forces that occur in downhill skiing were evaluated and compared with forces of similar parameters that occur in cross-country skiing. The authors concluded that downhill skiing can produced forces of 6 kN per leg and are considerably higher when compared with the same forces encountered during cross-country skiing.[25]

Maxwell and Hull[32] measured the foot-boot ground reaction forces, joint moments, and thigh musculature EMG and the lower limb kinematic patterns of three individuals (rated as intermediate or advanced skiers) as they completed four ski turns (one wedge and three slaloms) on a beginner and an intermediate ski run. From these parameters, knee joint compressive loads were estimated at approximately 400 N for the snowplow and

300 N for the downhill limb during a parallel slalom turn. Posterior shear forces at the knee were roughly 60 percent less during the snowplow compared with the slalom turn for all participants.[32]

From these performance studies it can be concluded that low levels of skiing can be conducted with comparable stresses to lower extremity joints in relation to other forms of exercise (jogging and running). However, as with most sports, these forces can reach deleterious levels in extreme situations (large moguls). More important, these performance measures have been used as input to drive complex computer models designed to help researchers understand the internal loads that occur during skiing and investigate specific mechanisms of ski injuries and help improve equipment design. Herzog and Read[28] in 1993 employed resulting knee joint forces and moments from two World Cup downhill racers (one with good form and one with poor form) and incorporated this information into a complex model of the knee to estimate posterior cruciate ligament (PCL) and anterior cruciate ligament (ACL) stress. Their model predicted maximal quadriceps forces in excess of 8000 N·m. Surprisingly, maximal PCL force was estimated at nearly 3000 N·m, whereas ACL force was estimated at approximately 600 N·m. More complex modeling approaches are being developed, and great strides in understanding exact forces occurring in the inner aspects of the lower extremity joints will be forthcoming in the next decade.

Injury Prevention

Many of the studies cited in this chapter depend on many factors, and identifying a single most influential variable is very difficult. However, by possessing considerable knowledge of the injury rates, injury mechanics, and general performance and biomechanics of skiing, one can design specific off-season conditioning techniques to improve the safety of the recreational and professional skier. From the literature review, the following recommendations can be made to help reduce the probability of skier injuries[37,40]:

1. Skier ability has been associated with skiing injury rates. Advising beginning skiers to take supervised ski lessons can reduce the injury rate by one-half.
2. Proper equipment and equipment maintenance are essential for safe skiing. While biomechanical research has been focused on improving boot-binding and ski design, to date there is no foolproof equipment. Boots and boot-binding release systems have improved in the last 15 years and are most likely responsible for the continued decline of injury rates. Bindings should be evaluated and adjusted regularly by a trained ski mechanic. Boots should be fitted by skiing technicians who can make recommendations for specific manufacturers and boot designs to meet individual needs such as increased Q-angle, high arches, wide or narrow feet, and increased varus knee deformity. These small precautions and equipment adjustments can make dramatic improvements to the foot-boot-binding-ski system and allow for optimal skiing performance.
3. On-mountain skier safety such as knowing the terrain-rating scales at each individual resort and across resorts is also recommended. Ski mountains have a universal system for rating the difficulty of each run on the mountain. Each run is marked with a color code according to the steepness, length, and snow-covered terrain of the run. Green represents the lowest or easiest level to ski. Blue is termed intermediate and is for skiers who have mastered the basics in terms of ski turning and stopping. Black is for intermediate to advanced skiers, and double black diamonds are reserved for advanced skiers only. Unfortunately, many skiers attempt to ski outside their functional boundaries, stretching the limits of their skills and abilities. Additionally, these color rating scales are somewhat ambiguous and are not consistent across mountains or ski resort areas. For instance, a black run in the East of North America may not be the same as in the West or as in Swiss or Canadian ski resorts. Thus skiers always should inspect each course or send reliable scouts to test the rating scales for each new run or mountain prior to skiing unknown territory.
4. Skier fatigue is another factor often associated with skiing injuries. Skiing requires large, prolonged eccentric contractions of the lower back, abdominals, quadriceps, hamstrings, and gastrocnemius. Proper off-season conditioning of these muscles is required in preparation for skiing. The off-season conditioning section below outlines specific skiing exercises that all skiers can do to maximize their skiing potential.

Alpine skiing requires extensive eccentric power output from the leg musculature. Olympic skiing athletes have registered some of the largest isokinetic leg exercise scores compared with other Olympic athletes.[40,43] Traditional progressive resistance weight training is the typical training regime for these athletes. However, considerable emphasis is placed on eccentric work in all exercises. Both recreational and professional skiers use most of the lower extremity muscles and abdominal muscles and a large portion of the upper extremity muscles during pole planting. Thus, general strength training emphasizing upper and lower extremity muscles groups is recommended. While there are many stretches and strengthening exercises that can help a skier achieve greater potential, below are selected stretches and exercises that can be used by both professional and recreational skiers alike.

WARM-UP

Begin with a slow jog to increase your heart rate and body core temperature. Following the warm-up, the athlete needs to perform a stretching routine. Then begin skiing at lower levels while gradually increasing the speed and difficulty of the turns.

STRETCHES

Cross-Legged Stretch

This stretch loosens the iliotibial band, which is needed to keep the hips loose and allow the skier to get the skis out from under the COG while keeping the upper body aimed down the fall line during a turn.

Hamstring Stretch

This stretch loosens the three muscles in the back of the thigh and lower back. Flexible hamstrings allow for stronger skiing by allowing the skier to achieve a lower COG without bending at the waist. This is very important because skiing upright removes the mechanical advantage of the hamstrings to reduce anterior translation of the tibia relative to the femur. Begin statically and gradually progress to dynamic stretching.

Seated Squat Stretch

This stretch is conducted sitting in a chair with the feet 4 to 5 ft. apart and the forearms placed against the inner thighs. Bend at the waist, and attempt to touch the floor with the hands.

STRENGTHENING

Forward, Diagonal, and Lateral Lunges

This exercise works the quadriceps, abductors, adductors, and gluteals in an eccentric fashion. Use the shoulder barbell, handheld weights, or sports cords to add resistance.

Power Squats

This exercise uses traditional squatting techniques but with increasing and decreasing weights in a pyramid scheme to ensure fatigue training of the lower extremity musculature.

Abdominal Workout

Traditional crunches and sit-ups strengthen the torso, helping the skier to make effortless turns. It is important to work in diagonals to include the obliques. A physioball can be used to challenge the abdominals (Figs. 10.1 and 10.2).

Etiology of Skiing Injuries

ADVANCES IN EQUIPMENT DESIGN

Ski equipment design has had a major influence on injury types and injury severity over the past 25 years of North American skiing. For instance, in the middle to late 1960s, most recreational and professional skiers were skiing in leather boots that barely covered the ankle joint and were secured to the skis by metal, nonrelease bindings. Advances in plastics in the early 1970s allowed the introduction of plastic boots that provided more rigid ankle support. Thus, ankle injuries began to decline. It is believed that boot height also played an important role in reducing injuries to skiers. As plastic boots stiffened the ankle joint, they translated more stress up the limb, and greater incidences of tibial fractures and knee injuries were observed. From these early beginnings in

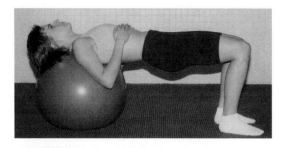

FIGURE 10.1

Abdominal exercise, bridging with physioball. *(Used with permission from Canavan PK: Rehabilitation in Sports Medicine. New York: Appleton and Lange, 19, Chap 8, Fig. 8-90, p 169.)*

ski boot design, continual improvements such as softer plastics, built-in canting, and superior boot fitting for differing ages and genders have all contributed to the etiology of injuries observed in the skiing population today. In today's ski industry, individuals with varus deformity, leg-length discrepancies, and forefoot and rear-foot abnormalities can seek professional guidance from boot manufacturers and professional ski shops that are capable of providing special moldings and boot-foot contouring to meet most needs. For instance, a simple heel pad or forefoot lift inside the boot

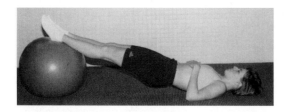

FIGURE 10.2

Trunk stabilization exercise with rolling the ball side to side and closer and further. *(Used with permission from PK Canavan: Rehabilitation in Sports Medicine. New York: Appleton and Lange, 19, Chap 8, Fig. 8-91, p 169.)*

can help skiers who have flat feet or high arches. Additionally, qualified ski technicians can provide built-in lifts in the boot or between the boot and the binding (canting) to help overcome outside ski edging problems due to varus deformity. These minor adjustments can help improve performance by increasing the skier's edging ability.

Not all aspects of ski injuries can be attributed to equipment, however. The style of skiing also has had an effect on injuries. The movement from the Alberg style of skiing to the high change of direction type of skiing pioneered by Claud Kelly has most likely contributed significantly to injury mechanisms as well.[1,23,34]

Advances in ski design also may play a role in reducing skiing injuries. The recent development of shaped skis offers anecdotal evidence of decreased energy needed to turn and thus decreases internal joint forces during a turn.[35] This fact, however, has not been scientifically justified. Novice skiers also may find that skiing with wider skis is easier, particularly in powder, because they tend to increase skier buoyancy, keeping the skier above the snow line.

Apart from skis and boots, bindings and release settings have garnered much attention in the last decade of skiing. Bindings secure the boot to the ski. There are many different types of bindings on the market. Nearly all bindings have an adjustable setting that allows a skier to tighten the binding according to his or her ability. The commercial purpose of this variable setting is to allow consumers to buy one binding and adjust the settings as they increase in their technical abilities. The technical purpose of the binding is to establish a safe zone of release for each skier. For example, when a skier falls and is tumbling down the hill, the bindings should release the skis. Thus, the torque is minimized about the lower extremity (especially the knee), decreasing the chance of injury. Moreover, the skier must only attend to stopping his or her momentum without worrying about his or her skis catching on snow, rocks, trees, or gates. In order for the bindings to release, they must sense a force threshold that has been set by the skier prior to competition. As one can see, if the release settings are too high, the bindings will not release during a fall, increasing the chances of severe injury. Conversely, if the release settings are set too low, they may release inappropriately when the skier is in a middle of a turn, jump, or landing when forces are high. The rule of thumb is to tighten the binding settings to match ability. Manufacturers provide a listing of these settings for their equipment, and they are based on the consumer's ability to rate his or her skiing ability. The higher the skier's ability, the higher or tighter is the setting. Ski technicians working at professional ski shops are trained to match skier ability to release settings for each brand of equipment.

Epidemiology of Skiing Injuries

A number of epidemiologic studies have been conducted to determine the injury rates and severity of these injuries in recreational and professional downhill skiers.[2-15] Because of these studies, tremendous strides in skier safety through improved training, teaching, and equipment design have emerged to greatly reduce the number of injuries incurred by skiers each year. Early in skiing history, the sport developed the reputation of being a relatively dangerous activity. The literature today, however, suggests that injury rates have enjoyed a steady decline since the early 1940s. One study estimated an average of 6.6 injuries per 1000 exposure hours in the 1950s and 1960s that has decreased to 2.8 injuries per 1000 exposure hours through the

1970s and 1980s.[3] Still other researchers have shown almost a 50 percent decrease in skier injuries in the past 15 years.[2,11] Consistent with this decline, there also has been a notable shift in the types of injuries occurring in the skiing population. Ankle and tibial fractures and nonknee sprains have all shown a significant decline over the past 15 years.[11] Results of our own database[14] show that 32 to 48 percent of all injuries are related to the knee, whereas the shoulder and back account for only 15 percent of all injuries recorded in 1998 (Fig. 10.3). Thus, while overall injuries have been declining, severe knee injuries such as ACL ruptures have increased 172 percent over the last 15 years and tripled over the last 22 ski seasons.[11] These trends are magnified when viewed as a percentage of all injuries or as a percentage of a particular injury group. For instance, in the past 15 years, third-degree knee sprains have increased from 3 to 16 percent of all reported injuries. As a percentage of knee sprains, they have increased from 16 to 66 percent in the last 15 years.[11] It has been the consensus of the literature that these trends can be attributed, in part, to specific improvements in equipment design.

Large epidemiologic studies have identified general trends in the skiing population at risk for injury. These studies suggest that smaller, younger, lighter, and less experienced skiers are at the highest risk for injury.[3] Within these categories, skier skill level seems to be the single most determining factor of risk of injury in that beginners are 33 percent more likely to be injured compared with 6.2 percent of skiers rated as intermediate or expert.[3] However, these factors also suggest that inexperienced skiers tend to have maladjusted equipment, also a significant factor.[3] It is interesting to note that the incidence of injury drops by one-half when beginners participate in supervised ski lessons.[3]

A considerable amount of clinical data suggest that one gender is more vulnerable to in-

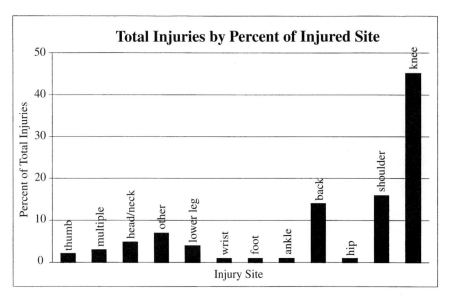

FIGURE 10.3

Total injuries by percent of injured site. Distribution of ski injuries as a percent of total injuries reported in an 8-year technical report to Vail Associates. *(Adapted from Briggs KK, Steadman JR: Pre-placement screening program for the ski resort industry: An 8-year study. Technical report 8. Vail, CO: Vail Resorts Association, 1998.)*

jury compared with the other gender, and several studies suggest that the injury patterns for each gender are drastically different from one another.[7–9] These studies report that females are two to five times more likely to injure their knees,[7,8] whereas males are more likely to injure their head and shoulders.[9] Other authors[5] reported that injury rates were similar between males and females, but females were 33 percent more likely to rupture their ACL. In a 1989 study, female ski racers were reported to be two to six times more likely to tear their ACL compared with their male counterparts.[4] A more recent study showed that among professional alpine skiers, the incidences of ACL rupture were 4.2 (males) and 4.4 (females) per 100,000 skier days, further suggesting that no significant difference exists between the genders with regard to ACL injury in the professional alpine skiing population.[10]

By closely screening individuals prior to the start of a ski season and by tracking these skiers throughout their employment and over multiple years of skiing, researchers have been able to identify several factors leading to injury potential within the professional skiing population. For instance, an 8-year preseason knee screening program (KT-1000 testing, Lachman and pivot shift examinations) conducted on employees of the Vail Valley Ski Resort area suggests that individuals who have had a previous knee injury are at greater risk for a more severe injury during a ski season.[14] Additionally, skiers who are ACL-deficient are three times more likely to reinjure their knee compared with those who have been reconstructed, and an ACL-reconstructed knee is twice as likely to rerupture compared with an uninjured knee.[10] Comparing reconstruction techniques, individuals reconstructed with the semitendinosus tendon technique are more likely to suffer a rerupture compared with those reconstructed with the bone-patellar-tendon-bone surgical technique.[10]

In a 1-year ski season, it was reported that shoulder injuries accounted for only 8 percent of all skier injuries.[36] Of these, acromioclavicular (AC) separations, anterior glenohumeral dislocations, rotator cuff injury, and shoulder contusions were most common. These rates are not uncommon or disproportionate to shoulder injury rates in other sports. Again, males are more at risk for a shoulder injury compared with females, and there appears to be no relationship of limb dominance to injury rate. Glenohumeral dislocations are closely associated with secondary injuries such as fracture (occurring in 10 percent of all anterior dislocations) and axillary nerve paralysis (3 percent). AC separations are reported to account for 18 percent of all shoulder injuries. Of these, 60 percent are usually first degree, 22 percent are second degree, and 18 percent are third degree. The occurrence of rotator cuff injuries has been estimated to be about 20 percent of all shoulder injuries, with most reported cases being either partial or complete tears. However, the probability of underdiagnosis is high compared with an AC separation or glenohumeral dislocation. Thus, there is a consensus among ski resort physicians that many smaller rotator cuff tears are unreported because medical attention is not sought immediately.

Injuries to the thumb constitute an estimated 40 percent of all injuries in the upper extremity, making it the most injured joint in the upper extremity. Of these, 85 percent are related to the ulnar collateral ligament (UCL) of the metacarpophalangeal (MCP) joint. Additionally, because the severity or pain of the UCL injury initially appears rather innocuous, it is speculated that this injury also goes unreported in many cases.

Common Skiing Injuries and Their Rehabilitation

KNEE

Determining what exact conditions contribute most significantly to injury is an arduous task given all the possible factors that can be accounted for in the sport of skiing. Nevertheless, several studies have identified various types of knee ligament injury mechanisms. In the *phantom foot mechanism*, the skier is falling backwards, the hips are below the level of the knee, and nearly all the skier's weight is on the downhill limb, which places a stress on the inside tail of the downhill ski. This stress causes a torque that points in the opposite direction of the foot, forcing the boot forward relative to the femur.[37]

In a *boot-induced ACL injury*, the mechanism is characterized by an off-balanced landing where an anterior drawer force is created by the tail of the ski that drives the boot forward, creating excessive anterior translation Other mechanisms include the downhill ski *sliding out* from the COG during phases 2 and 3 of the turn, the uphill ski *catching an edge or snow mound* during a turn, skier *collisions and falls* (especially collisions from behind), and *falls where the bindings do not release*, causing excessive knee torsional stress as the skier tumbles down the hill.[38]

After ACL rupture, skiers typically complain of instability. In the case of isolated ACL tears, many skiers may continue to ski until they notice this instability in turning or an increase in knee joint effusion. Conversely, some skiers may experience considerable pain and will need to be evacuated from the mountain by the ski patrol. Diagnosis of ACL injury is made routinely with clinical pivot shift and Lachman tests, followed by a magnetic resonance imaging (MRI) scan of the joint. Isolated ACL tears are common in skiing, but many tears are also associated with secondary restraint damages such as medial collateral and/or lateral collateral ligament injury. More common is an association with bone bruising or chondral defects of the articular surface of the femoral condyles and/or tibial plateau.

Rehabilitation   This section is concerned with the rehabilitation of the ACL-reconstructed athlete entrusted to the care of a physical therapist immediately following surgery. It should be noted that surgical technique and graft fixation should dictate the rehabilitation protocol. For this discussion, ACL reconstruction was conducted with a two-incision, 10-mm patellar tendon graft using interference screw fixation.[39,40]

After surgery, the patient is placed in a constant-passive-motion (CPM) device with a range set at approximately 30° to 70°. The CPM device prevents stiffness between therapy sessions and allows for earlier gains in ROM exercises. Furthermore, this passive ROM provides important physiologic effects that aid in the healing response of the newly placed graft and in articular cartilage nutrition. Most important, it also places essential (nondeformation) stresses on the graft to aid in collagen healing and the stimulation of collagen along the lines of the graft fibers.

Postoperatively, patients are placed in a protective brace, which is used for all ambulation during the first 6 weeks following surgery (Fig. 10.4*A*). A 90° knee flexion block is used to avoid excessive flexion angles that might rupture the patellar tendon graft site due to hyperflexion.

Immediately following surgery, the patient is taught effective patellar mobilization techniques to help in the avoidance of patellar tendon adhesions that may create flexion contractures or increase patellofemoral stress later in the rehabilitation process.

Strengthening is also begun immediately but is not emphasized to the extent of the ROM exercises. At this point, these exercises are aimed at preventing atrophy rather than providing strength gains. An emphasis is placed on well limb and upper body exercises and general aerobic conditioning.

At 2 weeks after surgery, unbraced bilateral limb bicycling is allowed, keeping the ROM of the knee within 10° to 90° and with little or no resistance. Deep-water running allows for aerobic exercise, ROM, and initiation of agonist and antagonist actions while eliminating the risk of impact loading.

At 6 weeks, forward and backward walking protocols are added, and resistance is increased on a stationary bicycle. Stair-stepper and inclined-treadmill walking is emphasized, and strengthening is now also emphasized. At this time, balance and proprioception exercises, and step-ups are performed when the patient has good muscular control.

Beginning at 12 weeks after surgery, patients are brought into light agility exercises, including side-to-side maneuvers with elastic resistance. Dynamic balance exercises should also increase in difficulty (Figs. 10.5 and 10.6). As strength and stability allow, a fitter can be used (Fig. 10.4 *B*). If strength and ROM are satisfactory at this time, open-chain exercises are also added.

From 16 to 24 weeks after surgery, the preceding activities are increased in both duration and intensity based on the individual's progression. At 6 months, patients start participating in a functional testing regime that includes resistance exercises with an elastic Sport Cord.[44] The Sport Cord test is designed to test the injured limb in a functional manner. It is comprised of four Sport Cord exercises that the patients have performed throughout their rehabilitation programs. The functional test is administered approximately 5 to 6 months postoperatively and by recommendation of the attending physician. The functional test includes:

1. *Single one-third knee bends* (Fig. 10.7*A*). With resistance provided by the Sport

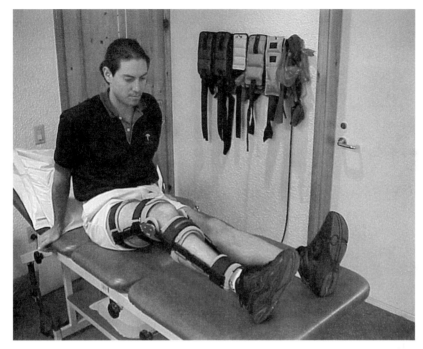

A

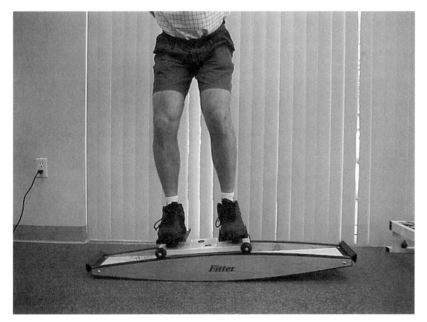

B

FIGURE 10.4

A. Postoperative, long-leg, hinged knee brace. *B.* Fitter.

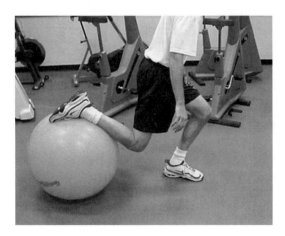 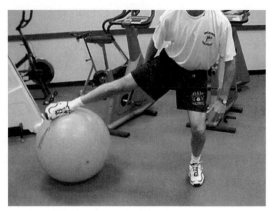

FIGURE 10.5

Physioball for dynamic balance.

Cord, the test requires the patient to perform single-limb knee bends (full extension to 35 degrees of flexion) for 3 minutes without stopping. The number of repetitions is counted, and the therapist ensures that the patient does not cheat on depth of the knee bends throughout the test. For each 30 s the

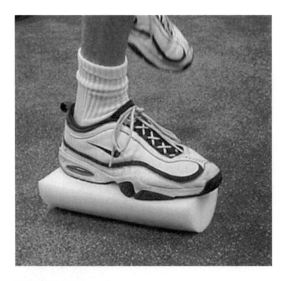

FIGURE 10.6

Half foam balance exercise.

patient successfully completes, a point is added. Thus, if the patient is able to complete the test with no pain or antalgic patterns, a score of 6 is given. If a patient is only able to complete 1 minute of knee bends, then a score of 2 is given; for 1.5 minutes, a score of 3; for 2 minutes, a score of 4; and so forth. If the patient complains of pain or if there is a noticeable shift in proper mechanics, a point for each fault is deducted from the final score.

   2. *Forward power running* (see Fig. 10.7B). A belt is worn, and the Sport Cord is attached to the waist of the patient. The patient first moves forward to a predetermined location marked with chalk on the floor. This location ensures that the Sport Cord will offer ample resistance. The patient begins by slowly jogging in place and then leans forward offering greater resistance to the Sport Cord. The therapist ensures that resistance is maintained, and a cadence monitor (set at a two-count repetition) may be used to help keep the patient at a constant pace. The patient runs in this manner for 3 minutes. A point is added for every 30 s that is completed. Thus, a maximum score of 6 is possible, and as with the knee-bend test, points are deducted if the therapist observes antalgic patterns or if the patient complains of pain.

3. *Backward power running* (see Fig. 10.7*C*). The technique and scoring for the backward-running test are similar to the forward test, only the patient jogs backward against Sport Cord resistance. As with forward running, a total of 6 points is allowed.

4. *Side-to-side jumping* (see Fig. 10.7*D*). This is similar to the forward and backward run, except that patients work on lateral movements. Standing with the Sport Cord attached to a clip on the lateral side of the waist, the patient jumps laterally, increasing the resistance in the Sport Cord. The patient is instructed to hold this position for a one count before allowing the tension of the Sport Cord to "pull" him or her back onto the opposite foot. Because considerable resistance is offered both in the jump away from the wall and in the return jump back to the wall, both limbs are exercised aggressively and in both a concentric and eccentric fashion. A cadence monitor will help the therapist keep the patient at a constant rhythm.

The scores for each test are summed, and a total score of 18 or higher is considered passing. Patients are then cleared for return to skiing. Generally, skiers are allowed to return to groomed skiing, starting with green runs and advancing on to more difficult groomed runs based on their self-determined confidence. Most skiers are back to aggressive skiing at 6 to 8 months after surgery. We have noted that recreational skiers are often 2 to 3 months behind in their rehabilitation compared with professional skiers and thus are not fully recovered until 8 to 9 months after surgery. We believe that this is due to precondition status and decreased time spent on rehabilitation. In addition, those who have had complications resulting in increased rehabilitation time take longer to return to ski-

ing. This includes individuals that did not attain full ROM early or did not achieve satisfactory strength in the 6- to 12-week period. In general, our approach to therapy of the ACL-reconstructed patient is based on establishing full ROM early because it is our belief that strength gains will come in time and with hard work, whereas stiffness requires surgical intervention.

Functional knee brace wear is controversial. While wearing a functional brace does not prevent all reinjuries, we encourage brace wear for up to 1 year after surgery to help prevent or limit the severity of injury due to unexpected slips or falls. It is our experience that skiers like the proprioceptive effects of the brace, and limited research has shown that brace wear can help the ACL-reconstructed patient achieve more normal eccentric, kinetic loading patterns.[41,42]

SHOULDER

Anterior Glenohumeral Dislocation

The most common mechanism of the anterior glenohumeral dislocation is a fall on an outstretched arm.[45] The arm abducts and externally rotates, forcing the humeral head anteriorly and inferiorly out of the glenoid fossa. The shoulder is painful on physical examination, palpation of the anterior humeral head is possible anteriorly, and movement is severely restricted. Treatment of glenohumeral joint dislocation is immediate reduction followed by immobilization for 3 to 4 weeks.

Rehabilitation Rehabilitation of the glenohumeral joint after anterior dislocation involves a three-phase treatment plan.[49] Recognizing that the surrounding tissues also will have experienced significant trauma, phase 1 emphasizes immobilization, rest, ice, and gentle isometrics for the wrist, elbow, and hand. Immobilization will depend on the attending physician's views but can last from 3 to 6 weeks. During the immobilization pe-

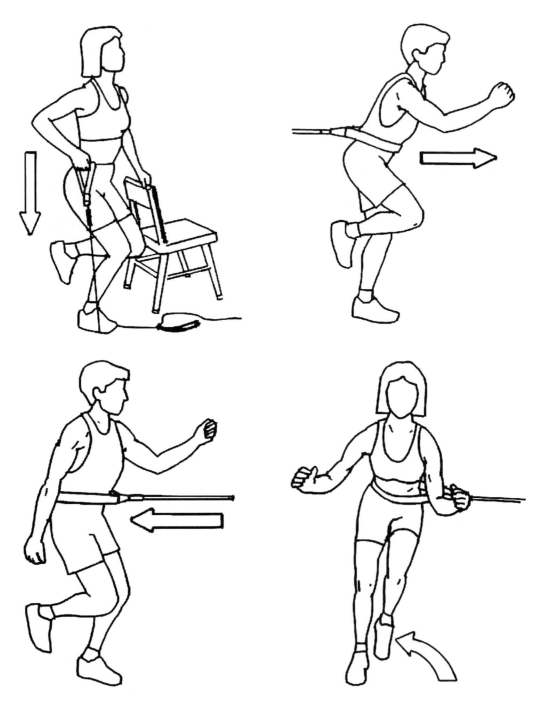

FIGURE 10.7

A. Single one-third knee bends. *B*. Forward power running. *C*. Backward power running. *D*. Side-to-side jumping.

riod, isometric contractions can be initiated at force levels tolerated by the patient. Through the exercises it is important that the therapist keep the arm anterior to the mid-coronal plane to discourage anterior humeral head migration.

Phase 2 starts at the completion of the immobilization period. This phase is characterized by passive and active posterior capsule stretching exercises with ROM limitations set for external rotation.[49] The goal of phase 2 is to provide the skier with painless internal rotation, elevation, and limited external rotation.

Phase 3 is initiated once the ROM criteria of phase 2 are met. This phase includes a strengthening regime beginning with exercises that keep the elbow below the horizontal plane of the shoulder (i.e., exercises with less then 90° of humeral elevation) to reduce capsular and other soft tissue irritation.[49] Strengthening exercises focus on the internal rotators because they provide considerable dynamic restraint against anterior instability at lower ranges of abduction. A variety of stabilization exercises should be performed in the closed kinetic chain. A hydraulic joystick can be used for sport-specific stabilization (Fig. 10.8). As strength gains are made, the patient progresses to isotonic exercises in cardinal planes and diagonal planes of motion (see Chap. 6 for illustrations). Return to full sports participation is allowed when full, painless ROM and plyometric exercises have been performed with sufficient strength as compared with the noninjured arm (see Chap. 12 for additional shoulder dislocation stabilization exercises). Full recovery from anterior dislocation can range from 6 weeks to 6 months depending on the involvement of secondary joint structures.[49]

Acromioclavicular Separation

Acromioclavicular (AC) separation mechanisms most often involve a direct blow to the shoulder driving the acromion down with re-

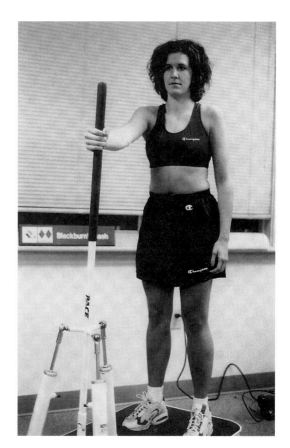

FIGURE 10.8

Joystick shoulder exercise. *(Used with permission from Canavan PK: Rehabilitation in Sports Medicine. New York: Appleton and Lange, 19, Chap 9, Fig. 9-48, p 201.)*

spect to the clavicle. Diagnosis is made by direct palpation and tenderness at the AC joint. In high-grade injuries, the clavicle may appear depressed or elevated with respect to the acromion. Treatment of acute AC separations is controversial, but most surgeons will attempt conservative treatment prior to initiating surgical intervention. Taping of the AC joint should be used in the return to function. (Refer to Chap. 14 for rehabilitation of AC joint injuries.)

HAND

Ulnar Collateral Ligament Thumb Injury

Ulnar collateral ligament (UCL) thumb injuries, "skier's thumb" or "game keeper's thumb," result from forced abduction and hyperextension.[44,46,47] During skiing, this often occurs as a result of a fall when holding onto the ski pole, which drives the thumb into the snow when the skier does not or cannot release the pole from the hand. Diagnosing UCL injuries begins with palpating for tenderness over the ulnar aspect of the thumb. Images may show bony avulsion from the phalanx. Functionally, the skier may have difficulty in grasping or an inability to pinch between the thumb and the index finger. Treatment depends on severity, and complete ruptures or avulsions may require surgical repair. Incomplete, grade 2 lesions may be treated with 4 to 5 weeks of cast immobilization followed by aggressive strengthening exercises. Grade 1 lesions may be treated with splint immobilization and followed by strengthening exercises when pain subsides.

Rehabilitation   Because the loss of thumb mobility or function can account for a 50 percent reduction in hand use, thumb injuries are quite serious. Incomplete UCL injuries can be treated conservatively as long as there is good residual stability.[48] Initial conservative treatment of UCL injuries involves immobilization with a thumb spica cast. The length of immobilization is determined by the severity of injury but should not exceed 3 weeks.[48] Rehabilitation is rapid, and return to sports also can be quick depending on the activity level. If chances of reinjury are high, patients respond well to removable splinting or molded-plastic protectors, which offer better protection than taping. Unfortunately, complete UCL injuries do not respond well to conservative treatment.[48] Such injuries typically require surgery to correct for major instability during pinching or grasping of ob-

jects. Rehabilitation should focus on restoration of both academic and functional hand movements. Academic recovery is the ability of the hand to regain temperature, pinprick, and touch sensations.[50] Functional recovery is aimed at restoring the patient's ability to use the hand for functional activities. Thumb injury rehabilitation should serve to allow the patient to use the hand to regain normal daily activities without compromising injured structures as early as possible. Hand therapy is not initiated with the intent to return to sporting competitions. This is secondary to normal function during daily activities.[50] Early rehabilitation is concerned with motion exercises. Strengthening is initiated with approval from the attending physician and is concentrated on the pinching motion.[48]

Return to Sport

Once athletes are able to complete the functional tests as outlined in the ACL rehabilitation section, skiers are allowed to return to groomed skiing. The skiers should start with green runs and advance to more difficult groomed runs when they can perform at each level with good biomechanics, strength, balance, proprioception, and endurance.

Summary

Epidemiologic studies have documented specific injuries and trends in injuries among recreational and professional skiers. The data suggest that while the incidence of all injuries declined dramatically over the last 15 years, it seems to have leveled off, and a new pattern of specific knee injuries has emerged. Collecting actual human performance data during a ski event poses particular environmental and physical challenges. Nonetheless, significant strides have been made in identifying weak links in both equipment design and the human interaction with that equipment during competitive situations. With constant advances in computer technology and mechanical testing apparatus, the future looks bright for compelling research to alter and improve the sport of alpine skiing for professional and recreational athletes alike.

To become an advanced-level skier requires many hours of practice and properly tuned equipment. Unfortunately, getting to these higher levels of performance predisposes a skier to documented risks and injuries. Most notably, ACL rupture continues to pervade the skiing industry. Technological, surgical, and rehabilitative advances to combat ACL injury have improved greatly in the last 10 years and have helped to minimize the lasting effects of a severe knee injury on the sport of skiing and the ski industry in general. Continued improvements in these key areas are needed, while more controlled, randomized studies investigating the effects of different therapeutic protocols are needed to further improve the treatment of injured skiers in the future.

Acknowledgments

We gratefully acknowledge the financial support of the NFL charities and Vail Associates in partial funding of some of the material presented in this chapter. We also acknowledge Karen Briggs of the Steadman-Hawkins Foundation Clinical Research Department for contributions in the epidemiology of skiing injuries, as well as Sean McKenroe and Gene "Topper" Hagerman of the Howard Head Sports Medicine and Rehabilitation Center for their contributions to the knee and shoulder rehabilitation sections of this chapter.

References

1. Rayner R: *The Story of Skiing*. London: David & Charles Newton Abbot, 1989, pp 9–15.
2. Johnson RJ, Pope MH: Epidemiology and prevention of skiing injuries. *Ann Chir Gynaecol* 80:110–115, 1991.
3. Shealy JE: Overall analysis of NSAA/ASTM data on skiing injuries for 1978 through 1981, in Johnson RJ, Mote CD (eds): *Skiing Trauma and Safety: 5th International Symposium* (ASTM STP-860). Philadelphia: American Society for Testing and Materials, 1985, pp 302–313.
4. Elleman B, Holmes E, Jordan J: Cruciate ligament injuries in female alpine ski racers, in Mote CD, Johnson RJ, Binet MH (eds): *Skiing Trauma and Safety: 7th International Symposium*. Philadelphia: American Society for Testing and Materials, 1989, pp 105–111.
5. Greenwald RM, Toelcke T: Gender differences in alpine skiing injuries, a profile of the knee injured skier, in Johnson RJ, Mote CD (eds): *Skiing Trauma and Safety: 11th International Symposium*. West Conshohochen, PA: American Society for Testing and Materials, 1997, pp 111–121.
6. Viola RW, Steadman JR, Mair SD, et al: Anterior cruciate ligament injury incidence among male and female professional alpine skiers. *Am J Sports Med* 27(6):792–795, 1999.
7. Cadman R, Macnab AJ: Age and gender: Two epidemiological factors in skiing and snowboarding injury, in Mote CD, Johnson RJ, Huaser W, Schaff S (eds): *Skiing Trauma and Safety: 10th International Symposium* (ASTM STP-1266). Philadelphia: American Society for Testing and Materials, 1996, pp 58–65.
8. Greenwald RM, France EP, Rosenberg TD, et al: Significant gender differences in alpine skiing injuries: A five-year study, in Mote CD, Johnson RJ, Huaser W, Schaff S (eds): *Skiing Trauma and Safety: 10th International Symposium* (ASTM STP-1266). Philadelphia: American Society for Testing and Materials, 1996, pp 34–44.
9. Shealy JE, Ettlinger CF: Gender related injury patterns in skiing, in Mote CD, Johnson RJ, Huaser W, Schaff S (eds): *Skiing Trauma and Safety: 10th International Symposium* (ASTM

STP-1266). Philadelphia: American Society for Testing and Materials, 1996, pp 45–57.

10. Oates KM, Van Eenanaam P, Briggs KK, et al: Comparative injury rates of uninjured, anterior cruciate ligament-deficient, and reconstructed knees in a skiing population. *Am J Sports Med* 27(5):606–610, 1999.

11. Johnson RJ, Ettlinger CF, Shealy JE: Skier injury trends—1972 to 1994, in John RJ, Mote CD, Ekeland A (eds): *Skiing Trauma and Safety: 11th International Symposium* (ASTM STP-1289). Philadelphia: American Society for Testing and Materials, 1997, pp 37–48.

12. Kocher MS, Feagin JA: Shoulder injuries during alpine skiing. *Am J Sports Med* 24(5): 665–670, 1996.

13. Johnson RJ, Ettlinger CF, Shealy JF, et al: Impact of super-side cut skis on the epidemiology of skiing injuries. *Sportverletz Sportschaden* 11(4):150–152, 1997.

14. Briggs KK, Steadman JR: *Pre-Placement Screening Program for the Ski Resort Industry: An 8-Year Study* (Technical Report 8). Vail, CO: Vail Resorts Association, 1998.

15. Mote CD: The forces of skiing and their implications to injuries. *Int J Sport Biomech* 3: 309–325, 1987.

16. Berg HE, Eiken O: Muscle control in elite alpine skiing. *Med Sci Sports Exerc* 31(7): 1065–1067, 1999.

17. Berg HE, Eiken O, Tesch PA: Involvement muscle actions in giant slalom racing. *Med Sci Sports Exerc* 27(12):1666–1670, 1995.

18. Hintermeister RA, O'Connor DD, Lange GW, et al: Muscle activity in wedge, parallel and giant slalom skiing. *Med Sci Sports Exerc* 29(4):548–553, 1997.

19. Hintermeister RA, O'Connor DD, Dillman CJ, et al: Muscle activity in slalom and giant slalom skiing. *Med Sci Sports Exerc* 27(3): 315–322, 1995.

20. Muller E: Analysis of the biomechanical characteristic of different swinging techniques in alpine skiing. *J Sports Sci* 12:261–278, 1994.

21. Hintermeister RA, Lange GW, O'Connor DD, et al: Muscle activity of the inside and outside leg in slalom and giant slalom skiing, in Muller E, Schwameder H, Kornexl E, Raschner C (eds): *Science and Skiing.* New York: Chapman and Hall, 1993, pp 142–149.

22. Karlsson JA, Eriksson A, Forsberg L, et al: *The Physiology of Alpine Skiing.* Park City, UT: US Ski Coaches Association, 1978, pp 30–41.

23. Rashner C, Muller E, Schwameder H: Kinematic and kinetic analysis of slalom turns as a basis for the development of specific training methods to improve strength and endurance, in Schwameder H, Kornexl E, Raschner C (eds): *Science and Skiing.* New York: Chapman and Hall, 1993, pp 252–261.

24. Schaff P, Senner V, Kaiser F: Pressure distribution measurement for the alpine skier from the biomechanical high tech measurement to its application as Swingdeep feedback system, in Muller E, Schwameder H, Kornexl E, Raschner C (eds): *Science and Skiing.* New York: Chapman and Hall, 1993, pp 160–172.

25. Babiel S, Hartmen, Spitzenpfeil P, Mester J: Ground-reaction forces in alpine skiing, cross country skiing and ski jumping, in Muller E, Schwameder H, Kornexl E, Raschner C (eds): *Science and Skiing.* New York: Chapman and Hall, 1993, pp 174–179.

26. Loui JK, Kuo CY, Guitierrez MD, Mote CD: Surface EMG and torsion measurements during snow skiing: Laboratory and field tests. *J Biomech* 17:713–724, 1984.

27. Nachbauer W, Schindelwig K, Mosner M, Kaps P: Forces and moments at the boot sole during carving. Abstract, XVII International Society of Biomechanics Congress, Calgary, Canada, August 8–13, 1999.

28. Herzog W, Read L: Anterior cruciate ligament forces in alpine skiing. *J Appl Biomech* 9(4): 260–278, 1993.

29. Antolic V, Kralj-iglic AI, Pavlovicic: Skiing technique in swing turns: Distribution of stress on the hip-joint articular surface, in Muller E, Schwameder H, Kornexl E, Raschner C (eds.): *Science and Skiing.* New York: Chapman and Hall, 1993, pp 174–179.

30. Hull M, Mote CD: Leg loading in snow skiing: Computer analysis. *J Biomech* 13:481–491, 1987.

31. Nigg BM, van den Bogart AJ, Read L, Reinschmidt C: Load on the locomotor system during skiing: A biomechanical approach, in Muller E, Schwameder H, Kornexl E, Raschner C (eds): *Science and Skiing.* New York: Chapman and Hall, 1993, pp 27–115.

32. Maxwell SM, Hull ML: Measurement of strength and loading variables on the knee during alpine skiing. *J Biomech* 22(6): 609–624, 1989.

33. Herzog W, Hasler E, Abrahamse SK: A comparison of knee extensor strength obtained theoretically and experimentally. *Med Sci Sports Exer* 23:108–114, 1991.

34. Feagin JA, Lambert KL, Cunningham RR, et al: Considerations of anterior cruciate ligament injury in skiing. *Clin Orthop* 216:13–18, 1987.

35. Kassat G: Turning skis without mechanisms of turning, in Muller E, Schwameder H, Kornexl E, Raschner C (eds): *Science and Skiing*. New York: Chapman and Hall, 1993, pp 132–140.

36. Weaver JK: Skiing-related injuries to the shoulder. *Clin Orthop* 216:24–28, 1987.

37. Ettlinger CF, Johnson RJ, Shealy JE: A method to help reduce the risk of serious knee sprains incurred in alpine skiing. *Am J Sports Med* 23(5):531–537, 1995.

38. McConkey JP: Anterior cruciate ligament rupture in skiing: A new mechanism of injury. *Am J Sports Med* 14(2):160–164, 1986.

39. Kursaka M: A biomechanical comparison of different surgical techniques of graft fixation in ACL reconstruction. *Am J Sports Med* 15: 225–229, 1987.

40. Steadman JR, Forster RS, Silferskiold, JP: Rehabilitation of the knee. *Clin Sports Med* 8(3): 605–627, 1989.

41. Decker MJ, Torry MR, Levene D, Steadman JR: Landing performance in ACL-deficient athletes with and without a functional knee brace. Paper presented at the American Academy of Orthopedic Surgeons, 67th Annual Meeting, Orlando, FL, March 15–19, 2000.

42. Decker MJ, Pecha FQ, Torry MR, Steadman JR: The effect of a functional knee brace on knee joint performance during drop landings. Paper presented at the American College of Sports Medicine, 46th Annual Meeting, Seattle WA, June 2–8, 1999.

43. Steadman JR, Swanson KR, Atkins JW, Hagerman GR: Training for alpine skiing. *Clin Orthop* 216:34–38, 1987.

44. Strickland JW, Retig AC: Collateral ligament injuries of the thumb, in *Hand Injuries in Athletes*. Philadelphia: Saunders, 1995, pp 101–103.

45. Mendoza FX, Nicholas JA, Sands A: Principles of rehabilitation of the shoulder, in Nicholas JA, Hershman EB (eds): *The Upper Extremity in Sports Medicine*. St Louis: Mosby, 1990, pp 253–263.

46. Mayer VA, McCue FC: Rehabilitation and protection of the hand and wrist, in Nicholas JA, Hershman EB (eds): *The Upper Extremity in Sports Medicine*. St Louis: Mosby, 1990, pp 619–639.

47. Primiano GA: Skier's thumb injuries associated with the flared ski pole handles. *Am J Sports Med* 13(6):425, 1985.

48. Mayer V, Gieck JH: Rehabilitation of hand injuries in athletes. *Clin Sports Med* 5(4):783, 1986.

49. Mendoza FX, Nicholas JA, Sands A: Principles of rehabilitation in the athlete, in Nicholas JA, Hershman EB (eds): *The Upper Extremity in Sports Medicine*. St Louis: Mosby, 1990, pp 251–264.

50. Strickland JW, Rettig AC: Collateral ligament injuries of the thumb, in Strickland JW, Rettig AC (eds): *Hand Injuries in Athletes*. Philadelphia: Saunders, 1995, pp 102–104.

CHAPTER 11

Ice Hockey

William J. Montelpare
Moira N. McPherson
Neil Purves

Ice hockey is often described as the fastest team game,[1-9] yet the speed and style of play have led to descriptions of ice hockey as a violent, aggressive sport[2] with a high risk for a myriad of injuries.[10] Ice hockey is a game played by two opposing teams, each consisting of six players (on the ice at any one time), made up of three forward players (a center and a right and a left winger), two defense players, and a goaltender. The objective of the game is for one team of players to place the puck into the opponents' goal by overcoming the defensive strategies and tactics of the opposition.

Ice hockey is played on an ice rink that is close to 200 ft in length and 100 ft in width. The playing surface, or rink, has rounded corners with a circular radius of 28 ft and is enclosed by 4-ft-high boards that can be made of wood, plastic, or fiberglass.

Independent ice hockey governing bodies organize and regulate rules concerning the use of certain types of equipment, protocols, and procedures. The ice hockey governing bodies are also responsible for adjudicating events that occur within the various leagues

and for enforcing punitive measures on individuals who break the rules. However, there are great differences in the rules across the various leagues as well as the consequences for infractions of the rules. For example, while all players participating in formal ice hockey leagues must wear ice hockey skates (not speed skates or figure skates), there is no unanimity concerning the use of dental protection or face shields. Likewise, while body checking is not tolerated in some leagues, it is encouraged in others. Such variability of rules and styles of play contributes to the difficulties in providing a comprehensive scientific description of the events within the sport and the techniques required to participate.

The purpose of this chapter is to outline the biomechanics of ice hockey beginning with a breakdown of the various skills that combine to enable an individual to participate. The skill breakdown is followed by a description of muscle actions required to perform the various skills. The section concludes with the kinematic and kinetic analyses of the motions required in the game of ice hockey. The second section is intended to discuss the etiology of ice hockey injuries and the importance of age, anthropometrics, and governance on injury risk. The third section covers the various ways that injuries can be prevented, especially warm-up exercises and stretching routines. The final section is a presentation of the specific rehabilitation techniques for injured ice hockey players. It is important to note that although ice hockey research has been reported in several languages, the information presented in this chapter is limited to previous research in English or French.

Biomechanics of Ice Hockey

Ice hockey is a complex sport that involves a combination of forward power skating, frequent starts and stops, lateral agility, and backward propulsion, as well as stick handling, passing, shooting, and body checking skills. Hockey players are constantly adapting, refining, and linking these skills as they respond to the dynamics of the game. The physiologic preparation of skaters, along with their perceptual motor abilities, confounds analyses of the techniques required to participate. The investigation of hockey skills is further complicated by the dynamics of the ice and skate interface. As a result, a comprehensive body of literature defining all ice hockey techniques is lacking. However, the muscle actions, movement patterns, and mechanics of the body during forward acceleration have received some scientific attention and are the focus of this section.

FORWARD POWER SKATING

The motion of each leg during forward power skating can be divided into three phases: *glide*, *push-off*, and *recovery* (Fig. 11.1).

Glide

The glide phase occurs when the body's weight is supported over one leg, which remains nearly constant in length and position until the push-off. The glide phase occurs during the recovery phase of the contralateral leg.[11] Ice skating is distinct from other forms of cyclic locomotion specifically in the mechanics of the push-off phase. In skating, the push-off leg must be externally rotated at the hip to establish an appropriate blade-ice surface angle. Ideally, the skate applies a force into the ice at an angle that is perpendicular to the direction of the opposite skate.[12] The body will accelerate forward in reaction to the propulsive forces generated from the push-off and will decelerate during any periods of glide as a result of the resistive forces of drag and friction.[13] The overall force of the lower extremity muscle contractions is summated during propulsion and can reach peaks values of up to 140 percent of body weight, magnitudes that may have a bearing on the frequency of observed hip muscle strains.

Push-Off

The beginning of the push-off phase is characterized by eccentric loading of the lower limbs by hip and knee flexion and ankle dorsiflexion. The push-off is initiated by extension, abduction, and external rotation of the hip and extension of the knee resulting from contraction of the quadriceps, gluteus maximus and gluteus medius, biceps femoris, and semimembranosus.[12,14] The ankle undergoes dorsiflexion and pronation followed by plantarflexion and supination. The powerful push-off of the hip and knee and forceful plantarflexion of the ankle finish the push-off phase. The phase is completed when the leg nears full extension and the skate blade loses contact with the ice surface.

Recovery

The recovery phase begins with completion of the push-off and finishes when the skate makes contact with the ice again, completing one cycle of the movement pattern. During

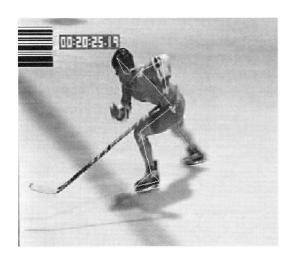
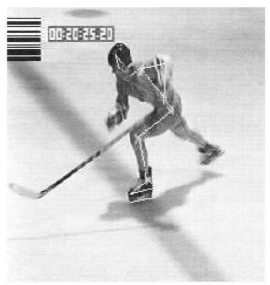
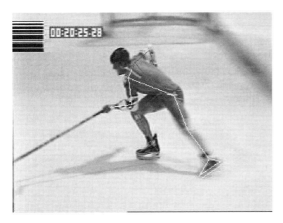
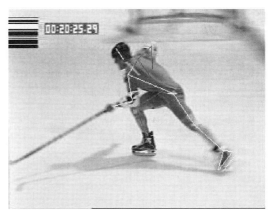

FIGURE 11.1

A. End of left-foot recovery, end of right-foot push-off. *B*. Start of left-foot push-off, start of right-foot recovery. *C*. End of right-foot recovery, end of left-foot push-off. *D*. Start of right-foot push-off, start of left-foot recovery.

the recovery phase, the hip and knee flex, the hip rotates internally to neutral, and the ankle is maximally dorsiflexed.[12]

Combined Leg Action

When examining the combined action of the legs, there are alternating periods of single support (one-skate in contact with the ice) and double support (both skates in contact with the ice).[12] The single-support period is often a glide phase, whereas propulsion or push-off occurs during the double-support period.[16] During acceleration, propulsion can occur during both double- and single-support periods. Often, after the first three strides, there may be no double-support phase.

PRIMARY MUSCLE GROUPS AND MUSCLE ACTIONS

Development of the lower body muscles is essential to the performance in the game of ice hockey.[48] The lower body, in particular the hip and knee flexors and extensors, play an important role in accelerating, turning, stopping and starting, shooting, and even body checking.[45,48] However, power generated by the lower body will be limited without adequate strength in the abdominal muscles, as well as the lower back and hip muscles. Development in the upper body musculature (shoulder, arm, and wrist muscle groups) contributes to shooting, puck control, and the control or warding off of opponents.[45,48]

Three forms of muscle action are prevalent in the sport of ice hockey: *concentric*, *eccentric*, and *isometric* contractions. The most common movements in the game of ice hockey involve primarily concentric contractions, whereby the muscle contracts, shortens in length, and produces force to generate movement.[48] Equally important in the game of ice hockey, however, are eccentric muscle contractions that occur during rapid stops, changes in direction, and when absorbing a body check.[48] Isometric contractions, while less frequent than both concentric and eccentric contractions, are involved primarily in stabilization of the body between the boards and opponents and when the player is fighting for the puck. In the case of an isometric contraction, the muscles are contracting, but there is no change in the muscle length.[49] It is essential that ice hockey players incorporate all three forms of muscle actions in training and practice.

KINEMATIC AND KINETIC VARIABLES ASSOCIATED WITH ACCELERATION

Researchers who have examined forward power skating have highlighted the important kinematic variables influencing skating performance and have developed regression equations to predict acceleration. Marino and Dillman[17] used regression analyses to determine the predictability of average acceleration over 20 ft, instantaneous skating velocity at the 20-ft mark, and the time to skate 20 ft. Using the means of the mechanical variables over the first three strides, the researchers found that toe to hip distance at touchdown, angle of takeoff, weight, stride rate, lean at touchdown, and leg length best predicted average acceleration. The total time taken to skate 20 ft was found to be a function of forward lean at touchdown, angle of takeoff, stride rate, and height. Further research found significant linear relationships between three variables and acceleration.[18] Single-support time and placement of the recovery leg at touchdown showed a significant negative relationship with acceleration. On the other hand, stride rate showed a significant positive relationship with acceleration. The propulsive angle of the skate and the body lean angle at touchdown also were related to acceleration.[19] These results suggested that a rapid acceleration was related to a rapid stride rate, which in turn was related to a large propulsive angle that reflected an outward rotation of the hip during push-off. It is proposed that the angle of body lean at touchdown is an indication of the optimization of propulsive forces in terms of magnitude and direction.[19]

An analysis of the 1983 U.S. National Hockey Team[20] showed that in order to maximize acceleration, the body should be in a position of greater forward lean, as indicated by the trunk and leg angle parameters. In addition, the skate should be placed close to the body, as indicated by a measurement of the toe to hip distance. An examination of the effects of fatigue on forward skating technique showed that as the quadriceps muscles began to fatigue, the skaters moved into a more upright position.

As a result of the complexity required to measure ice reaction forces, there have been few attempts to investigate the kinetic parameters associated with skating. Research using dynamometer recordings of the first three strides following three different starts from a force plate embedded into a synthetic skating surface demonstrated that the proper application of lateral or transverse force is characteristic of a good skating stride.

Etiology of Ice Hockey Injuries

Although several authors report ice hockey injuries, it is difficult to describe reliable and valid ice hockey injury trends. Research limitations may be attributed to such factors as poor compliance by the team designated to record injuries, the lack of an internationally accepted standard injury report form (including the inconsistency in using the previously reported definitions and classifications for injuries), differences in rules of play or differences in the enforcement of such rules across ice hockey leagues, and differences in rules regarding the use of protective equipment.

In a comprehensive review of the epidemiologic characteristics of ice hockey injuries, the most often reported mechanisms for injury were the stick, followed by the puck and then the skates.[1] Some authors also reported that the ice surface can be noted as a mechanism of injury, whereas the goal posts and boards were associated with collision injuries resulting from body checking.[1]

A summary of ice hockey injuries reported by several studies indicates that the head and face continue to be the most frequently involved body part.[5,21,22] However, the estimates of injuries by body part may be league-specific and influenced by rules about the mandatory use of face masks and helmets. Researchers reported from a study that all the injuries to the head resulted from direct blows to the face mask or to the top

of the helmet. Despite the use of helmets, a high rate of concussions resulted from head trauma (12 percent). Even more important is the consequence of the reported head trauma. The researchers indicated that blows to the head caused other symptoms such as double vision, blurred vision, and a loss of motor coordination.[21]

In studies that considered injury rates across all body parts, the knee was reported most often, followed by the shoulder, hands, and ankles. However, most of the reported injuries were soft tissue trauma resulting in contusions and lacerations.[23] Likewise, many of the injuries were accidental, with no penalty being administered.[23,24]

It is apparent from previous injury reports that the most prominent lower extremity injuries are reported for the thigh and the knee, followed by the ankle and foot. From studies of injuries across all body parts, the lower extremity injuries comprise approximately one-third of all injury reports.

EXTRINSIC FACTORS
Style of Play

Style of play is an important consideration in the prevention of injuries. It is essential that players, league administrators, and spectators recognize that injuries are not a necessary part of the game of ice hockey.[56] To this end, league administrators must continue to seek ways to reduce the rate, severity, and types of injuries.

Rules

The simplest mechanism for injury prevention is a change in the rules and enforcement of existing rules to prevent injurious behavior such as intentionally dangerous or violent contact by a player with a stick or near the boards.[56] In many ice hockey leagues, intentional collision (referred to as *body checking*) is not only within the rules, but exceedingly violent contact is often encouraged. Collisions and frequent illegal contact are precursors to injuries of varying severity.[1,10] In an attempt to reduce the prevalence of injuries that result from body checking, some leagues have eliminated even minimal body contact. However, risk of injury in even the most controlled environments during games and practices continues to exist.

Other equally notable considerations of rules that were designed to prevent injury include the mandatory use of specific types of equipment, especially helmets and face protection,[26,57] stricter enforcement of existing rules by league administrators and on-ice officials,[1,26,56,23] and the mandatory and continuous education of coaches, officials, and league administrators about injuries at all levels of hockey.[31,56]

Municipalities and ice hockey governing bodies must establish a formal, approved action plan to handle all forms of ice hockey–related emergencies, injuries, and accidents at all levels of play.[1] Furthermore, the municipalities and ice hockey governing bodies must establish a procedure for dissemination and compliance of the action plan for all individuals who assume responsibility in reserving the ice for an ice hockey event (practice or game).

Municipalities and ice hockey governing bodies must establish, approve, and enforce stricter penalties for infractions of rules that predispose individuals to injuries. The specific action to be taken with individuals who break the rules also should be incorporated into the plan and should be approved and enforced by a group external to the municipalities and ice hockey governing bodies.[60,61]

Municipalities and ice hockey governing bodies should establish rules of play for specific types of leagues at various levels and within various communities. These rules of play should include elimination of body checking and slap shots because these are noted as the primary causes of injuries. In specific leagues, and especially within certain levels, the no-contact, no-slap-shot rules should be enforced strongly.[1,29] Likewise, there must be an explicit move by the media, especially in specific television broadcasting of ice hockey games, to avoid sensationalizing the contact aspect of ice hockey. In addition, there should be a boycott on specific videos that display dangerous body checks. These activities promote injurious behavior.[56]

Equipment

It is recommended that in all leagues, including adult recreational pickup leagues, players must wear protective equipment at all times (i.e., while sitting on the bench or while participating in the game). The equipment includes helmets, face shields, and throat protectors that are approved by the Canadian Standards Association (CSA) and the American Society for Testing and Materials (ASTM).[5,26,58,59]

Among the most important changes in ice hockey related to equipment as a mechanism for injury prevention have been the CSA/ASTM-approved changes in helmet and face mask designs.[12] These design changes have led to greater protection of the head[56,58] and face.[5,26] Similarly, the redesign of skate blades has enhanced the safety of the game, resulting in a reduction in skate-to-player–related injuries.[12,59] The changes in skate design have been progressive. Significant design changes to the skate include adding a bumper or safety guard to the back end of the tube skate and the legislation of guidelines for plastic blade carriages that require that the plastic blade assembly portion extend 3 mm beyond the metal runner.[12,59]

INTRINSIC FACTORS

Age as a Factor in Ice Hockey Injuries

The age of introduction to a sport and the age at which high performance is achieved have dropped dramatically since the early 1960s.[42] Successful ice hockey players often enter professional hockey leagues as early as age 17. Although these players may be chronologically younger, it appears that most players are biologically mature.[42] For example, a review of data from representative hockey teams (such as the World Junior Championships) indicate that players who display superior size and strength characteristics, as well as an ability to initiate and receive violent collisions without interruption of play, are more likely to be recruited.[62]

In an attempt to reduce differences between players' sizes and the likelihood of an injury as a result of size differences, most ice hockey governing associations organize players according to a common age determination date and an age division strategy. The specific purpose of adopting an age determination date and an age division strategy is to reduce the potential discrepancies between players' relative to size and strength characteristics at various stages of growth and development.[62]

Size and strength developments are a function of maturation and are inconsistent across males and females. Maturation events, which include attainment of near-adult stature and developments of strength, occur during specific growth periods throughout the aging process but are most predominant during the years 9 through 13.[63,64] Therefore, given that the age categories of minor hockey players extend for a 12-month period, regardless of an individual's personal growth and development, there could be a 12-month chronological difference in ages between players in the same league age group. The chronological age difference that results from age grouping therefore can exacerbate any biological age difference that may exist between players in the same league. Such discrepancies are most noticeable in the representative leagues where the selection of players is commonly based on the anthropometric characteristics of stature and weight, as well as the strength developments.

In such leagues, the selection of players is biased by a single age determination date. The scientific research about physical growth and development indicates that there are distinct chronological age periods within which individuals mature. Specifically, the rate at which strength, stature, lean body mass, or emotional maturation occurs may differ across an age cohort, especially during the preadolescent and adolescent years.[62,64] Selecting players based on stature within an age group at or around the maturational years of age 9 through 13 is referred to as the *relative age effect*.[65] The relative age effect is characterized by physical and psychological growth differences between preadolescent and adolescent athletes in the same age cohort but with different birth dates throughout a specified calendar year.[62] The relative age effect is demonstrated by the following example. In Canada, the age determination date of December 31 favors players born earlier in the calendar year (January to April) and discriminates against players born in the latter part of the calendar year (September to December) secondary to a lack of physical and psychological development relative to other players within the same age cohort. The result of the relative age effect is a skewing of the distribution of ice hockey players relative to month of birth within any age division.

Anthropometric Differences among Players

Intrinsic injury risk factors include the physiologic events that occur during training and practice sessions or during the game of ice hockey.[23,50,51] Likewise, anthropometric differences between opposing players[52] can be considered as intrinsic risk factors. The studies by Roy et al.[36] and Bernard et al.[53] are of particular importance to studying ice hockey injuries and especially the role of body checking and aggressive play in amateur ice hockey. These studies reviewed differences in physical characteristics that could be attributed to the prevalence of injuries. The important findings in the two studies include that differences were observed for measures of weight, height, grip strength, and the force of impact generated by a body check of the smallest versus the largest players within each age group[36] and that statistically significant differences were observed between the shortest and tallest players (41 cm, 16.5 in), between the lightest and heaviest (47.7 kg, 105 lb), and between force of impact during body checking between the strongest and the weakest players (35.7 percent difference).[53]

Differences in the rate of development are thus expected to accentuate any relative age effects.[62] For example, the relative muscle mass for boys (defined as the amount of body weight attributed to the weight of muscle) can increase from 42 to 54 percent between the ages of 5 and 17 years. Similarly, the greatest increase in height gain is likely to occur between the ages of 12 and 14.5 years. Among other specific growth and development findings, it was reported that males achieved their greatest percentage of lean body mass (i.e., body mass without fat) between the ages of 16 and 17 years.[62]

A similar window for growth, development, and maturational changes was reported by the Saskatchewan Longitudinal Growth Study.[66] This study showed that the highest oxygen consumption capabilities occurred between the ages of 12.5 and 14.5 years, suggesting that the greatest potential for aerobic work was during the ages of 12 to 15 years. The results of the Saskatchewan Longitudinal Growth Study[66] were supported by others,[67] who showed that increases in the ratios of anaerobic power output related to aerobic power capacity were greatest between the ages of 8 and 14 years. These latter findings are of particular importance because they illustrate the period of growth when the individual is increasing his or her ability to perform anaerobically, which is extremely noteworthy for ice hockey performance.

Unfortunately, in striving for success at an early age, several growth and development considerations may be overlooked.[68,69] Increasing the training intensity at an early age without establishing a fundamental strength foundation that is developed from repeated regimens of low-intensity training may compromise the development of bone length and bone circumference.[42] Likewise, when a young athlete progresses well beyond the appropriate levels of training intensity, tendon and ligament development may be compromised and could result in injury or localized conditions such as tendinitis.[68] Torcolacci[68] noted that young athletes could experience a reduction in joint flexibility as a result of increases in regimens of high-intensity training, especially without adequate or proper stretching in the warm-up and cool-down phases.

Injury Prevention

WARM-UP

Several authors have suggested that the warm-up phase is a necessary part of the preparation for both practice sessions and events.[41-43] The primary effect of the warm-up is to initiate the early recruitment of the neuromuscular system, enhance blood flow, and raise temperature within the skeletal muscles and cardiovascular systems. The rise in temperature results from the production of heat generated by an increase in aerobic metabolism. This rise in cell temperature causes a further increase in the action potential of enzymes that catalyze metabolic functions. In addition, the rise in temperature caused by the warm-up leads to an increase in blood flow not only to the working muscles but also to the alveolar capillaries that ultimately enhances oxygen delivery to the working muscles and thereby supports continued aerobic metabolic functions. The warm-up increases neuromuscular facilitation, which leads to a decrease in reaction time and a decrease in muscle contraction time. Most important, by participating in a warm-up phase, the individual may reduce the risk of experiencing inadequate blood flow to the skeletal muscles and myocardium that results from partaking in an intense activity in a short time period.

The warm-up phase acts as the preanticipatory stage of the activity and thereby accounts for activation of the motor cortex and sympathetic neural system. This event causes an acceleration of heart rate, an increase in myocardial contractility, an increase in vasodilatation in the working muscles and a concomitant decrease in blood flow to the visceral organs, an increase in arterial blood pressure, and an initial recruitment of the muscle sense organs—the muscle spindles.

When an individual engages in an active warm-up, the initial recruitment of muscle fibers needed to perform the activity is detected by the muscle spindle (also called the *stretch receptor*). The muscle spindles monitor the amount of work required by the muscle and thereby moderate the stimulus-to-recruitment profile of the nerve-muscle system. Recruiting the muscle spindles in the warm-up stage has an indirect effect in injury prevention. During the warm-up stage, the monitoring function of the muscle spindle is effective in restricting muscle damage by preventing the rapid and complete recruitment of a muscle and only allowing necessary fiber utilization. Likewise, the muscle spindle monitors the economy of the muscle recruitment and preparation for activity by restricting unnecessary energy expenditure. Finally, the muscle spindles work in conjunction with the Golgi tendon organs, located at the muscle-tendon interface, to inhibit muscle contraction by accommodating the stress of muscle lengthening. The partnership between the Golgi tendon organs and the muscle spindles prevents damage to the nonelastic, noncontractile elements of the muscle.

In order to achieve the suggested sport benefits, which include optimizing the benefits gained during training and maximizing performance of an activity, and to achieve the physiologic benefits of a warm-up (i.e., raising core body temperature and stimulating the central nervous system), the initial warm-up activity for ice hockey should include a low-intensity activity such as a relaxed skate. In colder conditions, it is most important that the on-ice warm-up increases slowly and occurs over a longer period of time.[42,46] Since the comprehensive warm-up is expected to improve motor performance and reduce the risk of injury, the warm-up consist of two distinct parts: (1) the general warm-up and (2) the activity-specific warm-up.

During the relaxed skate (i.e., the general warm-up) players should progress through the range of motions typically used in the game. For example, a general warm-up should progress to short sprints, crossover striding in both directions, and intentional arm movements such as full arm circles. After the warm-up skate, it is recommended that players perform their stretching regimens, followed by sport-specific activities such as passing and shooting drills.

Some teams will use a pre-ice general warm-up that consists of low- to moderate-intensity activity such as jogging or cycling. These activities will recruit a large portion of the body's muscle mass.[42] Typically, the pre-ice general warm-up has a duration of 10 to 15 min; however, participants tend to customize the duration and intensity of the activities during this period to meet their particular needs.[42] It is therefore recommended that the pre-ice general warm-up should be followed by 5 to 10 min of general movement (e.g., a series of calisthenics such as leg swings and arm circles) to increase muscle, tendon, ligament, and joint mobility.[42] Research has shown that a passive warm-up using heat sources such as saunas, whirlpools, and heat pads can achieve increases in body temperature but may not provide the same benefits of an active warm-up.[42,44]

STRETCHING

The warm-up also should include a stretching phase, but it is important to recognize that the stretching phase is not the warm-up.[45] Often individuals stretch at the beginning of the warm-up when the muscle has not habituated to the ensuing stress of exercise. Ballistic loading of the unprepared muscles and tendons (i.e., a lack of neuromuscular facilitation) can lead to injuries that are further aggravated by continued activity.[46] It is recommended that the warm-up should be considered as a planned preparatory event that consists of four distinct activity protocols: (1) general warm-up (relaxed skate), (2) a static stretching phase, (3) a ballistic activity stage, and (4) a sport-specific stage.[43]

The static stretching phase should take place without bouncing or bursts of activity.[43,46] The static stretching phase should be initiated after a general warm-up involving low- to moderate-intensity activities.[42] The critical point of the stretching phase is that the athlete recruits those muscles which will be used during the activity. Therefore, the muscle groups of both the lower and upper extremities and midsection should be considered in the pre-event stretching routine. (See Chaps. 5 and 9 for illustrations.) In ice hockey, these muscle groups include the quadriceps, hamstrings, gluteals, and abdominals. The exercises of the pre-event stretch should include a slow progressive stretch and hold. It is generally recommended that the distance of the stretch for the muscle group be to the point of comfortable tension.[43] The amount of time to hold the stretch and the number of times to repeat the stretch maneuver depend on the type of stretch being performed. For example, a lower-back twist, in which the individual lies on his or her back and crosses one leg over the other while keep-

ing the knees straight and the back and shoulders flat (on the ice, floor, or mat), should be performed three times for each leg.[46] Each stretch should be held for a duration of 30 s. The lower-back twist is an excellent activity to stretch the rotators of the lower back and the hip abductors. Conversely, the shoulder towel stretch (recommended for internal and external rotators[45]), in which the individual begins by holding a towel overhead with arms outstretched and finishes with the towel held behind the back, is a range-of-motion (ROM) stretch activity that should be performed a total of 10 times in a slow-progressive manner.

STRENGTHENING EXERCISES

There are a number of widely accepted resistance exercises for hockey players.[45,72] A training program that includes such resistance exercises is recommended to reduce the risk of various types of ice hockey injuries. The specific protocols for each exercise are available in several published sources.[30,45,48,73] These exercises can be grouped according to the number of joints involved in the movement and/or the muscle groups recruited for the movement. Likewise, the order of prioritizing the exercises can be arranged according to the importance of the movement to the sport and the skill level required to complete the movement. For example, movements requiring a high level of skill should be presented at the start of the exercise training session.[73]

All strength exercise programs should begin with exercises that are being taught or practiced. Introducing exercises that require a level of learning above that which would be common to the sport at the beginning of the exercise session reduces the inhibitive effects of fatigue on the performance of the exercise.

The multijoint exercises, such as the power clean, which are designed to recruit multiple muscle groups in series, are among those exercise types which require higher levels of skill to perform appropriately and therefore should be scheduled at the start of an exercise/training session.[73] In such complex exercises, a potential problem exists in that the exercise must first be learned before it can be used effectively. The exercises are not necessarily isolated as training regimens for ice hockey but have been shown to be effective in strength and conditioning programs for ice hockey.

A multijoint, multimuscle exercise stimulates a number of muscle groups around more than one joint. In ice hockey, the multijoint, multimuscle movements focus on the rapid drive of the body to develop the propulsion phases of skating. Examples of multijoint exercises include power cleans, power snatches, hang cleans, hang snatches, and high pulls. Other exercises that provide benefits to the propulsion phase of skating include the lateral squat and the crossover step-up. The lateral squat is a multijoint exercise that aids in developing strength in the muscles around the knee and hip joint. The crossover step-up is intended to strengthen the muscles of the lower body and is most like the motor pattern a player experiences during the crossover for power strides in skating. The athlete can train on a slide board.

Exercises for the lower body can be divided into single-leg versus double-leg movements. The importance of training unilaterally is that single-leg exercise enables the player to develop neuromuscular recruitment patterns that are consistent with the events in the game. (See Chap. 10 for illustrations.) By loading the single limb in training, the participant is replicating the typical load experienced during skating, since skating is a biphasic skill.

Exercises that strengthen the muscles of the lower body and thereby reduce the risk of injuries include single-leg squats, lateral squats, crossover step-ups, split squats, and single-leg presses. Double-leg exercises such as squats (back squats, front squats), double-leg presses, and dead lifts (power lifting technique) are important for developing the stabilizing strength that is required by players to initiate and receive a body check and to maintain position during play. Furthermore, it is recommended that single-leg exercises be performed before double-leg exercises.

Exercises for specific muscles of the lower body such as the muscles around the hip joint, knee joint, and thigh include but are not limited to quadriceps extensions, hamstring curls, and exercises that require abduction and adduction of the hip joint, as well as hip flexion and extension. Hamstring curls and calf raises are examples of single-joint exercises that focus the stress around a single joint (Fig. 11.2). Exercises that strengthen the muscles around the ankle include inversion, eversion, dorsiflexion, plantarflexion.

The lower back and abdominal musculature are collectively known as the midsection and is an area requiring emphasis in strength training. Exercises that enhance the strength of the lower back include back extensions using a standard exercise apparatus, reverse

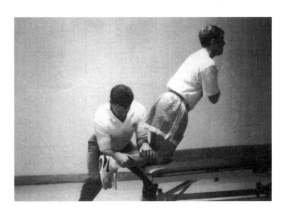

FIGURE 11.2

Kneeling leans for eccentric and concentric hamstrings. *(From Prentice W: Rehabilitation Techniques in Sports Medicine, 3d ed. New York: McGraw-Hill, 1999, Chap. 22, Fig. 22-4, p 419.)*

back extensions, and lying back extensions (a.k.a. "superman extensions"). Rotation of the upper body can be added to any of these extension exercises to facilitate strengthening of the rotators and multifidi. The abdominal exercises should be performed in sequence from lower abdominal muscles (knees to the chest) and oblique abdominal muscles (any twisting motion) to middle upper abdominal muscles (chest to knees). Lower abdominal exercises include abdominal sits and leg raises. Exercises for the oblique abdominal muscles include Russian twists, seated or standing bar twists, plate twists, or medicine ball twists; middle upper abdominal muscle exercises include all crunch-type exercises. (Additional midsection stabilization exercises are pictured in Chapters 6 and 10).

Exercises for the upper body should consider muscle balance around the joint. The notion is that the activity of pressing along one plane should be followed by the action of pulling in the same plane. For example, a bench-press activity should be balanced by using seated rowing or one-arm rowing afterward. Likewise, inclined-bench-press exercises using dumb-bells or barbells are counterbalanced with t-bar rowing. Shoulder presses, either wide or close, are countered with lateral pull-downs and chin-ups. Examples of single-joint exercises for the upper body include biceps curls, triceps extensions, shoulder lateral raises, and upright rowing, as well as flies and pullovers for the chest.

Pressing exercises (e.g., bench and shoulder presses) that involve the muscle groups around the shoulder and elbow joints are examples of multijoint exercises for the upper body.

ANAEROBIC AND AEROBIC TRAINING

Ice hockey can be classified as an intermittent exercise requiring bursts of activity in shifts lasting between 30 and 90 s.[54] Participation requires large volumes of ATP produced by recruiting fast oxidative glycolytic muscle fibers. For most players, the rest bouts, which range between approximately 0.5 and 3 min (depending on the level of play and personal ability), provide the opportunity to vent off lactate as carbon dioxide through the events of aerobic metabolism. However, for many participants, the rest period is simply not long enough to allow sufficient aerobic metabolic compensation.[55] An individual's aerobic and anaerobic capacity will limit his or her performance. That is, in order for an individual to meet the energy demands of the game, the individual must have an exceptional anaerobic capacity to deliver energy without oxygen.[2] Likewise, the participant must have an efficient aerobic power and aerobic endurance to mobilize the metabolic end products of anaerobic metabolism to carbon dioxide, energy, and water. However, although a well-developed aerobic system is essential to the recovery of anaerobic energy production pathways, development of the aerobic system cannot be achieved merely by regular participation in game situations.[2] Rather, even in elite players who may receive as much as 35 min of playing time in a game, there is a need to add at least two to three aerobic training sessions per week. This notion is supported by other researchers who found it possible to maintain specific endurance by performing two to four high-power interval sessions per week according to the competitive schedule and relative importance of the games being played.[48]

Adding aerobically based training sessions can prevent detraining, which occurs during the season and is especially important during the recovery stages needed between training sessions and/or games.[2,48,54] In ice hockey, the need to enhance the ability of the aerobic system to provide a recuperative pathway for intense anaerobic activity is most important when one considers the inhibiting action of accumulations of muscle cell metabolite concentrations on performance.[41]

During the off-season, general aerobic endurance training programs should comprise the largest proportion of training and must continue at a reduced frequency throughout the playing season.[2,42] The development of aerobic endurance training requires a high volume of continuous steady-state activity of moderate to medium intensity at least 5 days per week throughout the off-season. The main objective of a regimen of aerobic endurance is to increase the participant's ability to tolerate the end products of anaerobic metabolism that result from participation. As such, throughout the training sessions, the aerobic endurance program should include activities that are similar to those encountered during a game situation. In particular, the training program should include continuous activities such as stationary cycling[2] and interval-type activity (where the frequency of rest is less than or equal to the time in activity). The intermittent activity of the training session should reflect the participation profile. That is, ice hockey is an intermittent activity in which a player may be required to accelerate for 20 to 30 s and rest for 5 to 10 s. High-power intervals (20–85 s), performed at a 1:1 work-to-rest ratio over a long duration (20–45 min), will be most effective in habituating the individual to the work typically experienced during a game.[42]

Common Injuries and Their Rehabilitation

INJURIES TO THE HEAD AND FACE

Despite the specific rule changes about checking from behind and high sticking, as well as the mandatory use of helmets and face masks, reports of varying severity of trauma to the head and facial areas continue to be amassed across different leagues.[1,10,25–28] For example, an investigation of ice hockey injuries in the Finnish National League and Division 1 League (Finland) indicated that 18 percent of injuries were to the head or face.[10] Similar studies of elite Swedish ice hockey players showed that the risk of concussion injuries during a career is about 20 percent.[25] Yet epidemiologic reports of head and facial injuries are not restricted to elite ice hockey players. Adult male recreational and old-timer players demonstrated similar proportional risks of injuries to the head/neck and face of 32 and 25 percent, respectively.[29]

Although injuries to the head/neck and face are important, a mere review of injury report forms within any given league is an inappropriate method for analysis or evaluation of the true prevalence of such injuries. A compilation of injury report forms indicating injuries to the head and facial areas can lead to overreporting because these injuries typically require immediate treatment, and therefore, the more severe the injury, the more likely it is to be reported and recorded.[26,27]

UPPER EXTREMITY INJURIES

The organization of injuries by body part includes the following upper extremities: the neck, shoulder, clavicle, chest/rib, arm, and hand. Upper extremity injuries typically are caused by collisions with an opponent as the result of either a legal or an illegal check.[30] For example, recent research of a single National Hockey League (NHL) season[12] showed that body contact caused a fourfold increase in injuries over a 12-week period. Nevertheless, contact with an opponent's stick, collisions involving players and the boards, being hit by the puck, and colliding with the goal posts are also major causes of upper extremity injuries.[28,31–35]

It is important to note that the severity of upper extremity injuries ranges from severe cervical spinal trauma (C1–C7),[27] to fractures, separations, and dislocations,[12] to contusions of soft tissue.[34–37] In addition, research also has reported that injuries to the upper extremity may be age-related.[32] For example, a study of emergency departments in a city in northeastern Ontario, Canada, demonstrated that for reported injuries (i.e., the player sought medical treatment), most occurred to individuals over the age of 16 years and that 30 percent of injuries in this older cohort were to the head, neck, and facial areas.

LOWER EXTREMITY INJURIES

The prevalence of injuries reported for the lower extremities is illustrated in Table 11.1. Typically, injuries to the knee and ankle are caused by trauma to the ligament or meniscus. Often these injuries result from collisions with other players or from collisions with the boards or the net. However, in some cases, knee and ankle injuries have been associated with extreme joint torque caused by a player catching an edge of the skate blade on the ice. The hockey ankle sprain[38] results from a severe dorsiflexion, eversion, and external rotation of the ankle, again as a result of catching the skate blade in an ice rut. However, such an injury can result from being involved in a forward fall over the ankle while the ankle is caught in external rotation and dorsiflexion.

TABLE 11.1

Injuries Reported by Body Part

Prospective study over 15 years at a retina clinic (N = 1600): 33 cases, or 13.2 percent of all injuries related to hockey, with 2 percent of retinal detachments related to hockey (Antaki et al., 1977).

Retrospective study from patient records from emergency room treatments (N = 38): 9 ocular lacerations, 4 fractures to eye skeleton, 13 hyphemas, 7 angle recessions, 12 cases of traumatic iritis, 9 corneal abrasions, 5 cases of retinal edema (Vinger, 1976).

Retrospective study from British Columbia Amateur Hockey Association (1972–1973 season) (N = 35,435): 41 percent dental injuries, 59 percent head and face not dental injuries (Kropp et al., 1975).

Retrospective study part 1: Finnish amateurs (N = 108,921) and four professional Finnish teams (N = 100): 6885 injuries reported, 11.5 percent maxillofacial and dental injuries.

Retrospective study part 2: All registered Finnish players (1984–1985) (N = 62,185): 2989 injuries reported, 10.7 percent to head and face (Sane et al., 1988).

Experimental design of U.S. college intramural hockey, 1968 control year (69 teams), 1969 experimental year (73 teams): 8.2 injuries per 1000 athlete exposures, 8.3 percent head injuries in control year versus 3.8 percent in experimental year (Kraus et al., 1980).

Cross-sectional survey of members of Minnesota Committee on Ophthalmology (1974): 47 cases of eye injury due to ice hockey (Horns, 1976).

Cross-sectional survey of injuries in amateur, intercollegiate, and professional players: facial bone fractures, dental loss, and lacerations (Wilson et al., 1977).

Cross-sectional survey of youth, adult, and semiprofessional teams: facial lacerations, facial bone fractures, and dental loss (Daffner, 1977).

Cross-sectional survey of head injuries among college and junior players in Canada and the United States based on injury report forms for 22 teams (1465 injuries): 79 percent facial injuries, 12 percent cerebral trauma, 8 percent scalp, 1 percent skull fracture (Bolitho, 1970).

TABLE 11.1 (CONTINUED)

Injuries Reported by Body Part

Review of literature and reports by physicians and ophthalmologists: Over 800 intraocular and extraocular injuries (Pashby, 1979).

Prospective study for 3 years of one elite Swedish ice hockey team ($N = 25$): Game injury rate = 78.4 per 1000 athlete exposures, practice injury rate of 1.4 per 1000 athlete exposures. Injuries were distributed as 7.4 percent shoulder, 17 percent arm/hand, 4.2 percent chest, 11.6 percent spine, 10.5 percent groin, 9.5 percent thigh, 22 percent knee, and 11.6 percent foot/ankle (Lorentzon et al., 1988).

Prospective study of a Junior B team for the 1977–1978 season, age 15 to 19 years ($N = 20$): 83 injuries recorded (1.57 injuries per game, 78.3 injuries per 1000 athlete exposures), distributed as 5 percent hand/wrist, 7 percent forearm/arm, 5 percent shoulder, 5 percent elbow, 6 percent chest/ribs/back, 8.4 percent hip/pelvis/abdomen, 10.8 percent groin/celiac plexus (Park and Castaldi, 1980).

Retrospective study of a professional team over three seasons; 20 players reported 233 injuries for 234 games (50 injuries per 1000 athlete exposures): 19 percent of injuries were major, 6.5 percent fractures to hand/wrist, 1.3 shoulder-related (Rovere et al., 1978).

Retrospective review of x-rays of amateurs and professionals with previous shoulder injury ($N = 87$: 10 amateurs, 24 active professional players, 53 retired professional players): All injuries were related to the clavicle (Norfray et al., 1977).

Retrospective review of 12 secondary schools during the (1982–1983) season; coaches and players were surveyed ($N = 263$): 45 injuries to the shoulder, 38 percent acromioclavicular joint injuries, 4 percent sternoclavicular joint injuries, 4 percent fractures, 40 percent muscle strains/contusions, 14 percent other (Finke et al., 1988).

Cross-sectional survey based on 210 respondents from 266 players: 4.7 injuries per 1000 athlete exposures, 19 percent of injuries attributed to upper extremity, 4 percent foot/ankle, 13 percent knee, 9.5 percent groin/leg (Jorgensen and Schmidt-Olsen, 1986).

Cross-sectional survey of Swedish ice hockey players from two leagues ($N = 300$): 63 injury reports where 48 respondents indicated three or more dislocations, 32 respondents indicated that they had received corrective surgery as a result of participating in ice hockey (Hovelius, 1978).

Cross-sectional survey using a questionnaire forwarded to neurosurgeons, orthopedic surgeons, and physical medicine and rehabilitation specialists in Canada (1966–1991) ($N = 1000$): 182 spinal injuries reported with the following distribution: 75.8 percent cervical C1–C7/T1, 1.6 percent thoracic T1–T11, 4.4 percent thoracolumbar T11/12–L1/2, 3.8 percent lumbosacral L2–S5 (Tator et al., 1993).

A biomechanical approach to examining the type and severity of joint ligament injuries during such trauma was conducted by Nordin.[39] The results showed that the risk of injuries to ligaments, such as that experienced in the hockey ankle sprain, depended not only on the size and the shape of the liga- ment but also on the speed at which the liga- ment was loaded and the position of the joint in relation to the externally applied load.

The condition of *myositis ossificans trau- matica* was described as a sequelae that arises from a severe contusion, hematoma, or fracture.[40] This condition is common among hockey players who suffer injuries from trauma such as a blow by a hockey stick or a severe body check. In such cases, the players usually return to play following a regimen of treatment and therapy.

Knee Rehabilitation

Consider that a player has incurred medial collateral and anterior cruciate ligament injuries and has undergone an anterior cruciate ligament reconstruction. Although the rehabilitation time can vary with the accelerated approach, the athlete can see a return to sport in 4 to 6 months. With a more conservative approach, the athlete can see a return to sport in 7 to 12 months.[74] A basic 16-week regimen would include the following specific events:

1. For the first 6 weeks, the leg is placed in a long-leg brace, and the athlete is encouraged to perform upper body exercises. In the first week, the leg is moved passively through the range of 0 to 90 degrees. Similarly, the athlete may be allowed limited weight bearing with some quadriceps isometric exercises and straight-leg raises. By the end of the first week, the patella can be mobilized.

2. In weeks 2 and 3, the athlete is encouraged to move the leg actively and passively through the range of 0 to 110 degrees. Full knee extension is desired at this time. Hamstring and calf stretching is initiated. There is a gradual increase in weight bearing, and closed-chain strengthening exercises are initiated (e.g., gait retraining, toe raises, wall sits, minisquats).

3. In weeks 4 through 6, the athlete is progressed to full weight bearing in the brace. Active and passive movements are advanced through the range of 0 to 120 degrees. Stationary cycling can begin at this time. The rehabilitation program includes a regimen of unilateral leg strengthening (e.g., knee bends, calf raises, step-ups), leg pressing, a swim-

ming/aquatics program, stairclimber, and most important, active assisted knee flexion.

4. In weeks 7 to 10, the athlete discontinues the use of the long-leg brace, but wears a functional brace during an on-ice skate. The trainer observes the motion to ensure that muscle tone and strength are sufficient. During these weeks, the athlete continues full passive and active movements through the range of 0 to 130 degrees. Exercises include knee flexion hamstring curls (90 degrees), hip abduction/adduction (painfree), walking, ski machine, and balance and proprioceptive training (e.g., weight shifting, minitrampoline). The trainer conducts isokinetic evaluations to ensure that strength in the involved knee has attained 70 percent of the unaffected knee. Following this assessment, the trainer may begin lateral movements (e.g., shuffles, kariocas, slide board, fitter, agility drills), jogging, and light plyometrics.

5. Finally in weeks 11 to 16, the athlete should be capable of moving the leg through the full ROM, increasing the intensity and volume of linear (forward/backward) and lateral (agility) activity. At this time, rotational movements are introduced to the program. The exercise program includes strength training exercises, isokinetic evaluation at two speeds (180 and 300 degrees per second are commonly used), and sport-specific activities with a gradual increase in intensity. At this time the athlete is allowed to begin on-ice training.

6. Over the next 5 to 12 months, the athlete should be able to enjoy a complete return to hockey at full participation but with monitoring to ensure that the leg can move through the full ROM with no effusion while maintaining good knee stability. The trainer monitors pain and edema, ensuring that the athlete continues stretching all muscle groups around the injured region and using caution on the gradual increase in intensity of effort.

Return to Sport

Preseason preparation and postinjury rehabilitation generally involve activities that improve anaerobic power and anaerobic capacity such as interval-type training. Weight-bearing exercises such as running, inline skating, and slide-board training, combined with hill work or intermittent cycling, may be used to develop and maintain the participant's anaerobic fitness. Plyometrics need to be performed for power and explosive movements (Figs. 11.3 and 11.4). Examples of these are box and depth jumps and single-

and double-leg bounding (see Chap. 13 for additional examples of plyometric exercises). A fitter also can be used to simulate the side-to-side movement.

Recovery from injuries and return to participation require a staging sequence similar to the preseason preparatory regimen for cardiovascular and strength conditioning. That is, following an injury, the athlete should consider first the development of general strength rehabilitation followed by sport-specific exercises.

Complex training involves the combination of strength training with plyometrics, sprint and/or sport-specific training to maxi-

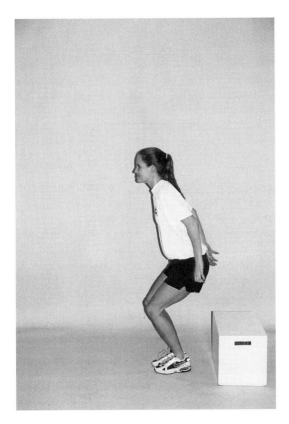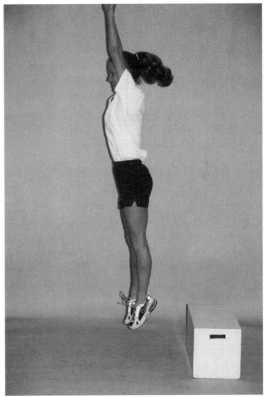

FIGURE 11.3

Box jumps. *(From Prentice W: Rehabilitation Techniques in Sports Medicine, 3d ed. New York: McGraw-Hill, 1999, Chap. 23, Fig. 23-19, p 453.)*

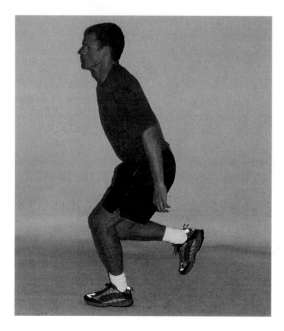 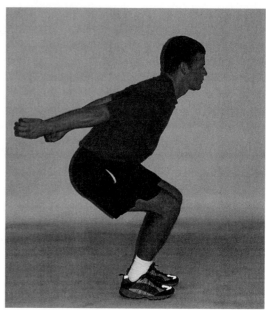

FIGURE 11.4

Single- and double-leg bounding. *(From Prentice W: Rehabilitation Techniques in Sports Medicine, 3d ed. New York: McGraw-Hill, 1999, Chap. 23, Fig. 23-19, p 453.)*

mize the development of muscular power, and central nervous system (CNS) activation.[70] While the use of strength training or plyometrics alone will increase power, some researchers[68,70] have indicated that the greatest improvements in muscular power result from combining these two forms of training, which is accomplished through a regimen of complex training. Complex training therefore is recommended for ice hockey players because it can develop strength and speed in such essential events as production of explosive leg power during skating or upper body strength required during initiating or avoiding a body check.

Speed is a crucial element of an ice hockey player's performance. However, because the playing surface is limited, players are unable to maintain top speeds for prolonged episodes. Yet speed is not limited to

skating. Speed is required to perform such skills as moving the puck, evading opponents, and invoking game strategies. As a result, a player must rely on agility and the ability to accelerate rapidly.[19,48] Activities that develop speed and increase agility are essential to the participant's training regimen, particularly those activities which improve movements and skill performance. Skills that incorporate speed and agility may be practiced during the warm-up and cool-down at a slow to moderate pace. However, once the skill is learned, it should be performed at maximal speed during the training session. In this way, speed will be developed as a consequence of CNS habituation and the development of appropriate motor unit firing patterns.[48,68]

Injuries may occur during speed training when the participant is experiencing muscular fatigue, since the compensatory mechanisms to overcome fatigue can change the dynamics and recruitment of the motor pattern.[48,68,71] As with the maintenance of strength,[48] it is recommended that speed and agility drills be performed two to four times per week throughout the competitive season to avoid detraining.

References

1. Montelpare WJ, Pelletier R, Stark R: Ice hockey injuries, in Caine D, Caine C, Lindner K (eds): *Epidemiology of Sports Injuries.* Champaign, IL: Human Kinetics Publishing, 1996, Chap 15.

2. Cox M, Miles DS, Verde TJ, Rhodes EC: Applied physiology of ice hockey. *Sports Med* 19(3):184–201, 1995.

3. Pelletier R, Montelpare W, Stark R: Intercollegiate ice hockey injuries: A case for uniform definitions and reports. *Am J Sports Med* 21(1):78–82, 1993.

4. Daly P, Sim F, Simonet W: Ice hockey injuries: A review. *Sports Med* 10(3):122–131, 1990.

5. Lorentzon R, Werden H, Pietila T, Gustavsson B: Injuries in international ice hockey: A prospective, comparative study of injury incidence and injury types in international and Swedish elite ice hockey. *Am J Sports Med* 16(4):389–391, 1988.

6. Pforringer W, Smasal V: Aspects of traumatology in ice hockey. *J Sport Sci* 5(3):327–336, 1987.

7. Bull C: Hockey injuries, in Schneider R, Kennedy J, Plant M (eds): *Sports Injuries: Mechanisms, Prevention, and Treatment.* Baltimore: Williams & Wilkins, 1985, pp 90–113.

8. Mack R: Ice hockey injuries. *Sportsmed Dig* 3(1):1–2, 1981.

9. Sutherland G: Fire on ice. *Am J Sports Med* 4(6):264–269, 1976.

10. Molsa J, Airaksinen O, Nasman O, Torstila I: Ice hockey injuries in Finland: A prospective epidemiologic study. *Am J Sports Med* 25(4): 495–499, 1997.

11. Allinger TL, Van den Bogert AJ: Skating technique for the straights, based on the optimization of a simulation model. *Med Sci Sports Exerc* 29(2):279–286, 1977.

12. Minkoff J, Varlotta GP, Simonson BG: in Fu FH, Stone DA (eds.): *Sports Injuries, Mechanisms, Prevention and Treatment.* Baltimore: Williams & Wilkins, 1994, pp 397–444.

13. Marino GW, Weese R: Kinematic analysis of the ice skating stride, in Terauds J, et al (eds): *Science in Skiing, Skating and Hockey.* Del Mar, CA: Academic Press, 1978.

14. Kahn J: Hockey. *Phys Med Rehabil Clin North Am* 10(1):1–17, 1999.

15. Marino GW: Biomechanics of power skating: Past research, future trends, in *Proceedings of the 13th International Symposium on Biomechanics in Sport.* 1995, pp 246–252.

16. Marino GW: Acceleration-time relationships in an ice skating start. *Res Q* 50(1):55–59, 1979.

17. Marino GW, Dillman C: Multiple regression models of the mechanics of the acceleration phase in ice skating, in Landry F, Orban WM (eds): *Biomechanics of Sports and Kinanthropometry.* Miami: Symposia Specialists, 1978.

18. Marino GW: Kinematics of ice skating at different velocities. *Res Q* 48(1):93–97, 1977.

19. Marino GW: Selected mechanical factors associated with acceleration in ice skating. *Res Q* 54(3): 1983.

20. Greer N: Application of biomechanics to ice hockey. *American Hockey Magazine* 5(7): 21–23, 1998.

21. Goodwin-Gerberich S, Finke R, Madden M, et al: An epidemiological study of high school ice hockey injuries. *Childs Nerv Syst* 3:59–64, 1987.

22. Daly P, Foster T, Zarins B: Injuries in ice hockey, in Renstrom P (ed): *Clinical Practice of Sports Injury Prevention and Care.* London: Blackwell Scientific, 1994, pp 375–391.

23. Hayes D: Hockey injuries: How, why, where, and when? *Phys Sports Med* 3(1):61–65, 1975.

24. Benton J: Hockey: Optimizing performance and safety, a round table. *Phys Sports Med* 11(12):73–83, 1983.

25. Tegner Y, Lorentzon R: Concussion among Swedish elite ice hockey players. *Br J Sports Med* 30(3):251–255, 1996.

26. Pashby T: Eye injuries in sports. *J Opthalm Nurs Technol* 8(3):99–101, 1989.

27. Tator C, Edmonds V: National survey of spinal injuries in hockey players. *CMA J* 130(7):875–880, 1984.

28. Tator C: Neck injuries in ice hockey: A recent, unsolved problem with many contributing factors. *Clin Sports Med* 6(1):101–114, 1987.

29. Voaklander DC, Saunders LD, Quinney HA, Macnab RB: Epidemiology of recreational and old-timer ice hockey injuries. *Clin J Sport Med* 6(1):15–21, 1996.

30. Wolynksi D, Brubaker D, Radulovic P: The use of specific exercises in preventing hockey injuries. *Strength Condit* 12:62–66, 1998.

31. Roberts WO, Brust JD, Leonard B: Youth ice hockey tournament injuries: Rates and patterns compared to season play. *Med Sci Sports Exerc* 31(1):46–51, 1999.

32. Rampton J, Leach T, Therrien SA, et al: Head, neck, and facial injuries in ice hockey: The effect of protective equipment. *Clin J Sport Med* 7(3):162–167, 1997.

33. Finke R, Goodwin-Gerberich S, Madden M, et al: Shoulder injuries in ice hockey. *J Orthop Sports Phys Ther* 10(2):54–58, 1988.

34. Rielly M: The nature and causes of hockey injuries: A five-year study. *Athletic Training* 17(2):88–90, 1982.

35. Hastings D, Cameron J, Parker S, Evans J: A study of hockey injuries in Ontario. *Ont Med Rev* 41:686–692, 1974.

36. Roy A, Bernard D, Roy B, Marcotte G: Body checking in pee-wee hockey. *Phys Sports Med* 17(3):119–126, 1989.

37. Rovere G, Gristina A, Nicastro J: Medical problems of a professional hockey team: A three-season experience. *Phys Sports Med* 6(1):58–63, 1978.

38. Hunter R: Hockey, in Reider B (ed): *Sports Medicine: The School-Age Athlete.* Philadelphia: Saunders, 1991, pp 590–600.

39. Nordin M: Biomechanics of ligaments, in Törnquist C (ed): *Proceedings of the 3rd International Conference on the Coaching Aspects of Ice Hockey.* Gothenburg, Sweden: The Swedish Ice Hockey Association, 1981.

40. Tredget T, Godberson C, Bose B: Myositis ossificans due to hockey injury. *CMA J* 116(1):65–66, 1977.

41. Fox E, Bowers R, Foss M: *The Physiological Basis for Exercise and Sport,* 5th ed. Toronto: Brown and Benchmark, 1993.

42. Bompa TO: *Theory and Methodology of Training,* 3d ed. Dubuque, IA: Kendall/Hunt Publishing Company, 1994.

43. Sleamaker R: *Serious Training for Serious Athletes.* Champaign, IL: Leisure Press, 1989.

44. DeVries HA: *Physiology of Exercise for Physical Education and Athletics* Dubuque, IA: William C Brown, 1966.

45. Stone WJ, Kroll WA: *Sports Conditioning and Weight Training Programs for Athletic Competition,* 2d ed. Boston: Allyn and Bacon, 1987.

46. Prentice W: *Fitness for College and Life,* 3d ed. St Louis: Mosby, 1990.

47. Williams WH: *Lifetime Fitness and Wellness,* 4th ed. Toronto: Brown and Benchmark, 1990.

48. Twist P: *Complete Conditioning for Ice hockey.* Champaign, IL: Human Kinetics, 1997.

49. Zatsiorsky VM: *Science and Practice of Strength Training.* Champaign, IL: Human Kinetics, 1995.

50. Houston M, Green H: Physiological and anthropometric characteristics of elite Canadian ice hockey players. *J Sports Med* 16:123–128, 1976.

51. Green H, Bishop P, Houston M, et al: Time-motion and physiological assessments of ice hockey performance. *J Appl Physiol* 40(2):159–163, 1976.

52. Bouchard C, Landry F, Leblanc C, Mondor JC: Quelques-unes des caracteristiques physiques et physiologiques des jouers de hockey et leurs relations avec la performance. *Mouvement* 9(1):95–110, 1974.

53. Bernard D, Trudel P, Marcotte G, Boileau R: The incidence, types and circumstances of injuries to ice hockey players at the bantam level (14 to 15 years old), in Castaldi C, Bishop PJ, Hoerner EF (eds): *Safety in Ice Hockey,* Vol 2 (ASTM STP-1212). Philadelphia: American Society for Testing and Materials, 1993, pp 45–55.

54. Twist P, Rhodes T: A physiological analysis of ice hockey positions. *NSCA J* 15(6):44–46, 1993.

55. Green HJ: Bioenergetics of ice hockey: considerations for fatigue. *J Sports Sci* 5:305–317, 1987.

56. Murray TM, Livingston LA: Hockey helmets, face masks, and injurious behavior. *Pediatrics* 3:419–421, 1995.

57. Pashby T, Pashby R, Chisholm L, Crawford J: Eye injuries in Canadian hockey. *CMA J* 113: 663–666, 1975.

58. Bishop P, Norman R, Pierrynowski M, Kozey J: The ice hockey helmet: How effective is it? *Phys Sports Med* 7(2):97–106, 1979.

59. Castaldi C: Ice hockey, in Adams S, Adrian M, Bayless MA (eds): *Catastrophic Injuries in Sports: Avoidance Strategies*, 2d ed. Indianapolis: Benchmark Press, 1987, pp 81–99.

60. Watson R, Singer C, Sproule JR: Checking from behind in ice hockey: A study of injury and penalty data in the Ontario University Athletic Association Hockey League. *Clin J Sports Med* 6:108–111, 1996.

61. Sullivan P: Sports MDs seek CMA support in bid to make hockey safer. *Can Med Assoc J* 142(2):157–159, 1990.

62. Montelpare WJ, Scott D, Pelino M: Tracking the relative age effect across minor amateur and professional ice hockey leagues, in *Safety in Ice Hockey*, Vol 3 (ASTM STP-1341). Philadelphia: American Society for Testing and Materials, in press.

63. Stalheim-Smith A, Fitch GK: *Understanding Human Anatomy and Physiology*. New York: West Publishing Company, 1993.

64. Gallahue DL, Ozmun JC: *Understanding Motor Development: Infants, Children, Adolescents, Adults*, 4th ed. New York: McGraw-Hill, 1997.

65. Daniel TE, Janssen CT: More on the relative age effect. *CAHPER J* 21–24, 1987.

66. Cameron N, Mirwald RL, Bailey DA: Standards for the assessment of normal absolute maximal aerobic power, in *Proceedings of the International Seminar on Kinanthropometry, Leuven, Belgium, Kinanthropometry II*. Baltimore: University Park Press, 1979.

67. Blimkie CJ, Bar-Or O: Trainability of muscle strength, power and endurance during childhood, in *Encyclopedia of Sports Medicine*, Vol 4: Bar-Or O (ed): *The Child and Adolescent Athlete*. London: Blackwell Scientific Publications, 1995, pp 113–129.

68. Torcolacci M: Personal communication (PHED 301/401), Advanced Weight Training Seminar Notes, Queen's University, Kingston, Ontario, 1997.

69. MacAdam D, Reynolds G: *Hockey Fitness: Year-Round Conditioning On and Off the Ice*. Champaign, IL: Leisure Press, 1988.

70. Chu DA: *Explosive Power and Strength*. Champaign, IL: Human Kinetics, 1996.

71. Marion A: Designing an annual training and competition plan: A step-by-step approach, in *Pro Pulses Plan: Training Program Management Software User Manual*. Montreal: Coaching Association of Canada, 1998.

72. Mikhailov VV: Recovery following hockey injuries. *Sov Sci Rev* 190–194, 1990.

73. Fleck SJ, Kraemer W: *Designing Resistance Training Programs*. Champaign, IL: Hardcourt Publishers, 1997.

74. Shelbourne DK, Nitz P: Accelerated rehabilitation after anterior cruciate ligament reconstruction. *Am J Sports Med* 18:292–299, 1990.

References for Table 11.1

Antaki S, Labelle P, Dumas J: Retinal detachment following hockey injury. *CMA J* 117(3): 245–246, 1977.

Bolitho N: Head injuries in ice hockey at the amateur level. *CAHPER J* 37(2):29–34, 1970.

Finke R, Goodwin-Gerberich S, Madden M, et al: Shoulder injuries in ice hockey. *J Orthop Sports Phys Ther* 10(2):54–58, 1988.

Horns R: Blinding hockey injuries. *Minn Med* 59(4):255–258, 1976.

Hovelius L: Shoulder dislocation in Swedish ice hockey players. *Am J Sports Med* 6(6):373–377, 1978.

Jorgensen U, Schmidt-Olsen S: The epidemiology of ice hockey injuries. *Br J Sports Med* 20(1): 7–9, 1986.

Kraus J, Anderson B, Meuller C: The effectiveness of a special ice hockey helmet to reduce head injuries in college intramural hockey. *Med Sci Sports* 2(3):162–164, 1979.

Kropp D, Marchant L, Warshawski J: An analysis of head injuries in hockey and lacrosse, Sport Safety Research Report, Fitness and Amateur

Sport Branch, Department of National Health and Welfare, 1974–1975.

Lorentzon R, Werden H, Pietila T, Gustavsson B: Injuries in international ice hockey: A prospective, comparative study of injury incidence and injury types in international and Swedish elite ice hockey. *Am J Sports Med* 16(4):389–391, 1988.

Norfray J, Tremaine M, Homer C, et al: The clavicle in hockey. *Am J Sports Med* 5(6):275–280, 1977.

Park R, Castaldi C: Injuries in junior ice hockey. *Phys Sports Med* 8(2):81–90, 1980.

Pashby T: Eye injuries in Canadian amateur hockey. *Am J Sports Med* 7(4):254–257, 1979.

Rovere G, Gristina A, Nicastro J: Medical problems of a professional hockey team: A three-season experience. *Phys Sports Med* 6(1):58–63, 1978.

Sane J, Ylipaavalniemi P, Leppanen H: Maxillofacial and dental ice hockey injuries. *Med Sci Sports Exerc* 20(2):202–207, 1988.

Tator C, Edmonds V, Lapczak L: Spinal injuries in ice hockey: Review of 182 North American cases and analysis of etiological factors, in Castaldi C, Bishop PJ, Hoerner EF (eds): *Safety in Ice Hockey,* Vol 2 (ASTM STP-1212). Philadelphia: American Society for Testing and Materials, 1993, pp 11–20.

Vinger P: Ocular injuries in hockey. *Arch Ophthalmol* 94(1):74–76, 1976.

Wilson K, Cram B, Rontal E, Rontal M: Facial injuries in hockey players. *Minn Med* 60:13–19, 1977.

CHAPTER 12

Football

Ryan P. Vermillion

History relates that the origin of football dates back many centuries. The ancient Greeks playcd a type of football, which was referred to as *harpaston*. The early Romans are said to have adopted a similar game, which was called *calcio*. This game was brought to Britain by invading Romans.[1]

In North America, the term *football* refers to the game that we know as American football, whereas in the rest of the world the term *football* refers to soccer. It is certainly one of the most commonly played sports on the North American continent at all age levels and at both amateur and professional levels.[1]

Football has evolved from the brutal game of the 1800s that was almost outlawed to the million-dollar marketing marvel that it is today. Initially, American football was played without the use of any or very little protective equipment. Over the years, rules have been changed, and equipment has been introduced to the game. Even with the addition of equip-

ment, the game is still brutal and can take its toll on the human body.

With the introduction of synthetic turf in North America, a large number of professional and university football games are being played on this artificial surface. This probably has resulted in an increased injury rate as a result of minor injuries due to abrasions and impact on this less resilient surface. The artificial surface has an added disadvantage that it becomes extremely warm on hot days, adding the risk of heat exhaustion. Opinions vary as to whether this artificial surface is responsible for more frequent and more serious injuries than those that result from playing on a natural surface. Most athletes certainly would prefer to play on natural turf.[1] This chapter will deal with many of these injuries, their rehabilitation, and return to the game. Understanding the athletes who play football will help the clinicians treating them. Certainly the game is not for the physically meek, and athletes with a higher tolerance for pain seem to perform better.[2]

Biomechanics of the Football Field Goal Kick

The field goal or extra point kick in professional football is a complex event. A snapper snaps the football back to a holder who has to control the football and place it down on the ground so that the kicker is able to kick the football through the goalposts with an oncoming rush from the defense. All this must be accomplished in less than 1½ s. The kick has evolved over the years from a straight-on kicking style to the soccer-style kick that professional kickers use today. The thought behind the soccer-style kick is that more strength is generated with adding rotation of the lower extremities and upper body. When looking at the soccer kicking style in detail, it can be broken down into six different components. For ease of explanation, the description of the field goal kick will be one for a right-footed kicker.

STANCE

The place kicker stands 3 to 3½ yards behind and 1 yd to the left of the football. The upper body is relaxed with a slight forward lean to help with the initiation of forward movement. The right leg is positioned behind the left, with the knee and hip extended

FIRST STEP

The first step is taken with the left foot and is described as a "jab step." It is a 6-in step that initiates forward movement of the body. This is a controlled but powerful step. The upper body is still relaxed with a forward lean.

SECOND STEP

The right leg then steps in front of the left leg with a comfortable slight overstep. The upper body begins a slight rotation to help begin the forceful rotation of the body through the ball.

THIRD STEP

With the third step, the left leg is placed next to the football. This step is the longest of all the steps. It is an aggressive overstep that will help the right leg generate enough force to propel the football. The path of the football depends on this step and the left foot position. The kicker is able to direct the football left, right, or straight depending on the position of the left foot.

SWING

The right leg swings to make contact with the football, and the kinetic energy of the right leg is transferred to the ball. The upper body rotates left to help with forward momentum. The left shoulder is horizontally adducted across the body, which keeps the body centered and the core strength under control. The swing limb follows through, propelling the kicker off his feet and into the air.

LANDING

The landing is described as a "skip landing" onto the left leg. The force that is generated through the right lower extremity lifts the left leg off the ground, and the left leg is the first to contact the ground as the kicker lands.

Biomechanics of the Long Snap

The long snap is a critical component of the punt. Without a quick and accurate snap, the punter will not have time to punt the ball. There are four main phases: stance position, acceleration, release and follow-through, and contact-ready position.[16]

STANCE POSITION

The stance position of the long snap is similar to the position for a snap to a quarterback, whether the quarterback is under center or in a shotgun position, or a snap for a field goal. The snapper's ankles are dorsiflexed, knees flexed, hips flexed and slightly abducted, spine flexed, shoulders flexed to 90 degrees and adducted, elbows slightly flexed, and the wrists in a neutral position.[16] The other three components of the stance position can be varied: eye contact, stance, and grip. The snapper can look at the punter until the punter catches the ball, or the snapper can use the nonvisual method and look at the defense. The snapper can stand in an even or offset stance. The offset stance may assist in blocking the oncoming rush of the defense to block the punt. The third variable component is the grip on the football. The snapper can use one hand, which is not usually recommended in wet weather. The football also can be easily deflected at the line of scrimmage. The second grip is both hands gripping the football on opposite quarters of the front half of the football. In the third grip type the snapper holds the football with the dominant hand, as if he were throwing a pass. The opposite hand is placed near the middle or top half of the football with the fingers extended toward the front tip of the football to guide the football. An equal amount of pressure from both hands provides the increased velocity.[16,18,19]

ACCELERATION PHASE

The acceleration phase begins with movement of the ball. The shoulders and elbows extend and adduct while the wrist flexes and ulnarly deviates to elevate the ball off the ground toward the punter. The ankles are plantarflexing, knees extending, and the hips and trunk flexing in unison to drive the ball between the legs.[16]

RELEASE AND FOLLOW-THROUGH PHASE

In this phase, the ball is passed between the legs. The joint motions are a continuation of the acceleration phase along with shoulder internal rotation and forearm pronation to create a clockwise rotation for the right-handed snapper. Once the ball is released, follow-through occurs to eccentrically slow all the joint movements of the body to prepare for the contact position.[16]

CONTACT POSITION

Following the release of the ball, the snapper needs to be prepared to block the oncoming rush of the defense. The ankles dorsiflex, knees flex, and the hips and trunk extend to a semiupright position. The shoulders and elbows are flexed upward to begin to block. It is important that the snapper get into a balanced position.[16]

Injury Prevention

One of the major differences from the conception of football to now is the preparation for the football season. Gone are the days of working yourself into condition during training camps. The game today is a full-time job. Players maintain excellent physical condition the entire year. Many of the top university teams are adopting the same year-round regimen. The off-season conditioning programs begin shortly after the last game has finished and continue until the new season begins. Within the off-season, there are many training camps that focus on football skills as well as enhancing the conditioning program. The philosophy of many of the best conditioning programs is to make the athletes better football players.

The exercises both in the weight room and on the field are football-specific and are performed to help train each athlete in a manner that will prepare him to play his certain position. The conditioning program for an offensive lineman is not the same as the conditioning program for a wide receiver.

Their demands on the football field are different, so their conditioning programs need to be different. For example, an offensive lineman needs power and strength within a short period of time and distance. Most linemen run between 2 and 10 yards per offensive play. On the other hand, a wide receiver will run from 2 to 60 yards depending on the play and his certain objective during that play. The tailored conditioning program needs to address strength, power, flexibility, speed, and agility and then combine all these together to perform a certain skill.

STRENGTH TRAINING

Strength is a must for all football players. Any movement on the football field requires strength, whether it is running, jumping, blocking, tackling, or throwing. All these movements require force—without force there would be no movement. *Power*, as described by many, is force times velocity, or the rate at which you can apply your strength. In football, this is referred to as *explosiveness*. With a football-specific conditioning program, a better football player can be developed who is less likely to be injured.

Explosiveness is more important than absolute strength because football players have only a short time to apply force during a play. A conditioning program must address plyometrics and explosive drills to prepare the player for the game. Box jumps are an excellent form of explosive exercise for the lower extremities, whereas the medicine ball toss and catching are excellent forms of upper extremity exercise.

FLEXIBILITY

Flexibility is an often-overlooked part of a conditioning program. Rarely is it an overlooked portion of a rehabilitation program. Possibly, if more flexibility drills were performed prior to games and practices, there would be fewer injuries. Despite the large size of many football players, they must have good flexibility. Decreases in range of motion (ROM) secondary to tight muscles will lead to less coordinated movements. The athlete has to fight against his own internal resistance while moving. A good flexibility program can keep football players out of the training room or the therapist's office. Flexibility needs to be multidimensional and performed in more then one plane (Fig. 12.1). Stretching the upper body in the frontal plane and the lower body in the sagittal plane is a good example of multiplane stretching (Fig. 12.2). After static stretching, dynamic stretching should be performed. The dynamic movements used will vary for each player.

SPEED

Speed can be defined as the ability of an athlete to move his body or specific limbs at a high rate of velocity. Many people believe that in professional football, speed is the most important physical component needed. Agility is the ability to move in multiple directions, includ-

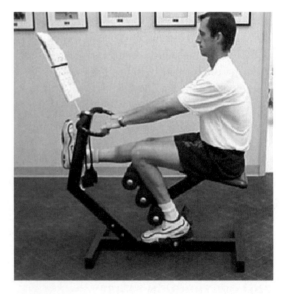

FIGURE 12.1

Multi-position stretch machine.

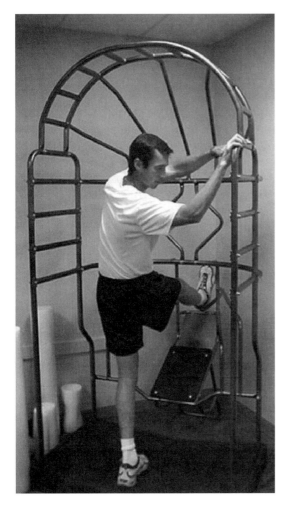

FIGURE 12.2

Multi-plane stretching.

ing stopping and starting, cutting and changing directions, moving the joints in all the planes of motion. This is an important part of the conditioning program. Each drill must address and prepare the athlete to compete in the game. The conditioning program must address all the planes of motion, not just the sagittal plane. We can never predict what movement will occur to an athlete's joints. The athlete must be able to handle all movements. This is accomplished by addressing the frontal, trans-verse, sagittal, and triplanar movements.[7] Triplanar movement is movement of a joint in all three planes. A complete and tailored program for each position is the athlete's greatest ally.

PROTECTIVE EQUIPMENT

The game of American football involves many collisions, and there is just so much that a health care practitioner can do to help prevent injury. Protective equipment has evolved from skin and shirts to the body armor of today's game. Protective equipment can be used to protect an athlete from injury or protect an injury from additional trauma.[9] The National Football Association (NFL) and the National Collegiate Athletic Association (NCAA) have rules about what a football player must wear during a game. An example of this would be the NCAA's Rule Section 4, Article 4, which states, "All players shall wear head protectors which carry the manufacturer's or reconditioner's certification indicating satisfaction of National Operating Committee on Standards for Athletic Equipment (NOCSAE) test standards."[8]

Face Masks and Mouth Guards

Before face masks were added to football helmets, 50 percent of football injuries were in or around the mouth. After the addition of face masks, mouth injuries fell to 25 percent of the total. The face mask, however, offers little protection against blows under the chin from forearm blocking, from knees, and from kicks. It also does not block blows to the top of the head that snap the jaw shut.[8] Today's combination of the face mask and mouth guard has made mouth injuries very rare. Mouth guards not only have reduced injuries to the mouth, such as split lips and broken teeth, but also have helped decrease concussions. They do this by absorbing the energy from blows, thus damping the transmission of forces to the brain.[6] This equipment must be fitted to an individual and maintained properly for the athlete to receive the greatest benefit.

Helmet

The football helmet has evolved from a leather shell to the suspension helmet to air-cell pads. Different shells of helmets have been studied regarding the reduction of head injuries.[23] Air-cell pads offer protection without adding weight. These helmets must be fitted properly for each individual. The steps below must be followed when fitting a football helmet to ensure its proper sizing.

1. The player's haircut should be the style and length that will be worn during the competitive season, and the player should wet the hair to simulate game conditions. The helmet should fit snugly on the player's head with the cheek pads snug against the sides of the face. The front straps of the chinstrap should be applied first, followed by the back straps. The chin pad should be an equal distance from each side of the helmet.
2. The helmet should be 1 inch (one or two finger widths) above the player's eyebrows. The face mask should extend two or three finger widths away from the player's nose.
3. The face mask should allow for a complete field of vision.
4. The back of the helmet should cover the base of the skull, and the ear holes should match up with the external auditory ear canal. With the chinstrap secured, the helmet should not move when you pull the face guard up and down or side to side.[10]

Maintenance of the football helmet is also very important in the overall care of the athlete. If the helmet is not maintained properly, the athlete can be predisposed to head and cervical spine injuries. Weekly helmet maintenance should include[11]:

1. Visual inspection to rule out any stress defects.
2. Check of the padding for wear and deterioration.
3. Check of the air cells for leaks and proper inflation levels.
4. Check of the face mask for bends and cracks. Screws and grommets that secure the mask to the helmet also should be checked for deterioration and looseness.
5. Helmets should be reconditioned on an annual basis.

Cleats

With different playing surfaces and different weather conditions such as rain and snow, different types of football shoes are worn. There are five main types of shoes: a flat-soled basketball-style turf shoe, a natural-grass soccer-style shoe, and three different mulitstudded (star studded, square studded, and conical studded) turf shoes. The length of the studs is an additional variable.[24-29] The dilemma that players face is that with better traction, there is an increase in the fixation of the foot to the ground surface and, consequently, an increase in the risk of injury.[25] Laboratory tests correlate foot fixation with cleat length.[24,26,27] The frictional release depends not only on the length of the cleat but also on the type of turf and the temperature of the turf. The largest area of concern is on artificial turf. An increase in artificial turf temperature increases the interface friction. The lowest friction occurs when the turf is less than 60°F and the highest when the turf reaches temperatures of 110°F. As far as shoes are concerned, the flat-soled basketball-style shoe had the lowest friction interface, with the soccer-style cleat having the highest friction. When an athlete wears a soft rubber-soled shoe on hot artificial turf, he is exposed to significantly higher friction levels, which can increase his risk of injury.[24]

TAPING IN FOOTBALL

The use of adhesive substances in the care of external lesions goes back to ancient times. The Greek civilization is credited with formulating a healing paste composed of lead oxide, olive oil, and water that was used for a variety of skin conditions. This composition was changed only recently by the addition of resin and yellow beeswax and, even more recently, rubber. Since its inception, adhesive tape has developed into a vital therapeutic adjunct.[12]

Uses of Tape for Injury Care

When used in sports, adhesive tape offers a number of possibilities for the care of injuries:

1. Retention of wound dressings
2. Stabilization of compression-type bandages that are used to control external and internal hemorrhaging of acute injuries
3. Support of recent injuries to prevent additional insult that might result from the activities of the athlete
4. Preventive support to protect against possible injury

Uses of Tape for Injury Protection

Protecting against acute injuries is an extremely important function of athletic tape. Protection often can be achieved in one of the following two ways:

1. Limitation of joint movements by using a predesigned taping
2. Stabilization by securing protective devices[12]

Etiology of Injuries

Another constant in the game of football is the unfortunate occurrence of injuries. Although football is called a contact sport, it would be more accurate to call it a collision sport. One play is made up of many different and separate collisions. The professional game is made up of approximately 130 plays when you combine offensive, defensive, and special team plays. The number of collisions that occur during these 130 plays is far too many to count. On the field at one time, there are 11 offensive players and 11 defensive players. Their goal is to score a touchdown on offense or prevent a touchdown on defense. The collisions will add up throughout the game, and no position is absolved from the possibility of traumatic or overuse injuries. The National Sports Injury Surveillance System collected data during the 1986 and 1987 playing seasons from a national sample of 6229 college football players. The overall injury rate for the two seasons was 6.32 per 1000 athlete exposures, or 45.27 injuries per 100 athletes. In a 1997 NCAA study, the injury rate for practice was 3.8 per 1000 athlete exposures in practice and 34.1 per 1000 athlete exposures in games.[22] Offensive players incurred more injuries than defensive players did. The knee and ankle were the most common injury sites, and sprains were the most common injury. Injuries during games occurred most frequently in the third quarter and least often in the first quarter. This finding suggests that players might benefit from warming up and stretching during halftime rather than resting and cooling off.[3] Inadequate conditioning could also be a factor.

The clinician's knowledge of the game of football will help his or her understanding of the injuries in football when they occur. Fortunately, all professional sports and Division 1 athletic programs have full-time certified athletic trainers on staff, and many high school programs are adopting the same thoughts and hiring full-time certified athletic trainers to care for their athletes. A study conducted by the National Athletic Trainers Association of high school football demonstrates that 62 percent of all reported injuries at the high school level occur during practice.[6] This fact leads to the importance of having certified athletic trainers at all high school athletic football practices and games. One of the most significant findings in high school football is that 36 percent of the athletes sustain at least one time-loss injury. This finding was consistent for both the 1986 and 1987 seasons. Additionally, the high school football data from three seasons demonstrates the following findings:

1. Seventy-three percent of the reportable injuries were minor, or caused the athlete to miss less than 7 days of participation.
2. Sixteen percent fell into the moderate group, causing the athlete to miss 8 to 21 days of participation.
3. Eleven percent were major injuries that caused the athlete to be restricted for more than 21 days.

It is important to note that the findings reported for the three seasons are consistent within each season, even though the number of reporting schools varied from year to year and included over 195 schools from 44 states.[6] The implementation of a solid strength and conditioning program should help reduce injuries for high school football athletes.

Many positions have a higher incidence of predictable injuries. In football, those being tackled are the most likely to be injured. The next highest incidence of injury occurs while performing a tackle or while blocking. Considering all players collectively, the most frequently injured body site is the lower extremity, with 20 percent of all injuries occurring to the knee.[3] Because football is a heavy contact sport, ligamentous injuries to the knee are extremely common.[1] Classically, the player will be supporting the body weight on a flexed knee, which is then struck from the lateral aspect, or on which the athlete pivots with the foot fixed on the ground, resulting

very often in an audible pop or snap and intense pain in the joint. There may be an associated torn medial or lateral meniscus in a very high percentage of such injuries involving the anterior cruciate ligament, and there may be involvement of the medial or, less commonly, the lateral collateral ligament.[4]

Fortunately, the most severe injury in American football, that of trauma to the spine, is relatively rare. The medical profession has helped considerably in minimizing this injury by having football management alter the rules and equipment.[1] The single greatest advancement was a 1976 rules change, coupled with a responsive change in coaching technique and strict enforcement by officials. Eliminating the spearing tackle has reduced the incidence of catastrophic injury to the cervical spine. The defensive player should no longer initiate contact with another player by striking him with the top of the head/helmet.[2] Changes in rules, improved tacking and blocking techniques, and better-conditioned athletes with improved protective equipment have helped lower the incidence of catastrophic injuries. Despite these measures, a total of 105 catastrophic permanent cervical and spinal cord injuries occurred in the United States from 1977 to 1989.[5] Football injuries to the head and cervical spine have been related to 97.7 percent of the total number of fall sports catastrophic injuries.[6]

Common Injuries

HEAT EXHAUSTION

A common injury that can affect all players on a football team is heat exhaustion. Football is the organized sport where heat illness is most pronounced because heavy equipment preventing heat loss is worn. The individual who is highly competitive and overenthusiastic should be watched carefully during periods of heat stress. He is often the one doing more than the rest of the team. An athlete may be participating in a practice or game and is unable to replace the lost fluids as rapidly as those fluids are lost. The sensation of thirst is not a reliable indicator of when to hydrate. It usually occurs too late and does not occur until the athlete has lost 2 percent of his body weight.[13] Therefore, pre-event hydration is very important in football. The classifications of heat disorders are circulatory instability, water and electrolyte balance disorders, and heatstroke or heat hyperpyrexia.

Circulatory instability is often characterized by heat syncope or fainting. Since football players are constantly changing postural movements, they are particularly susceptible to heat syncope, a form of exercise-induced heat exhaustion. In circulatory instability, peripheral vasodilatation takes place with a tendency toward venous pooling and hypertension. There is an immediate drop in blood pressure with a rise in pulse rate. Recovery is rapid if the athlete spends a few minutes in a reclining position.

Effects of Dehydration

- Decreased anaerobic capacity
- Decreased aerobic capacity
- Decreased gastric emptying
- Decreased sweat rate
- Decreased skin blood flow
- Decreased renal blood flow
- Decreased blood volume
- Increased heart rate
- Increased body temperature at which sweating begins
- Increased core temperature
- Increased incidence of gastric distress

Heat affects the performance of the football players, and there is a direct correlation between heat and minor injuries, illness, and irritability. Heat seems to decrease a person's willingness to work rather than his or her capacity to work.[13] (See the hydration section under "Injury Prevention" in Chap. 13 for more information.)

BRACHIAL PLEXUS INJURIES ("BURNERS" OR "STINGERS")

Another common injury that all football players can suffer is an injury to the brachial plexus. Commonly called a "burner" or a "stinger," this injury can become a chronic and debilitating injury. It has been reported that more than 50 percent of collegiate football players have sustained such injuries in the course of their playing careers.[14] The usual presentation is transient, burning upper limb pain and paresthesias following a block or tackle. Most brachial plexus injuries appear to be neuropraxias. There is temporary disruption of nerve function, with full recovery in a matter of minutes and with no subsequent signs of axonal degeneration. In some cases, however, weakness persists for weeks, and electromyography (EMG) is consistent with axonal degeneration. As a rule, substantial recovery occurs by 6 weeks, which indicates that these injuries are probably mixed neuropraxias and axonotmeses. Very rarely, there is no recovery of nerve function even after 6 or more months, indicating that there is neurotmesis, or complete axonal disruption.[14] Any of the nerve roots, trunks, divisions, or cords or peripheral nerves that make up the brachial plexus may be injured. Most commonly, the upper trunk is injured. Clinical and EMG examinations of athletes with persistent weakness characteristically reveal involvement of the upper trunk–supplied muscles: deltoid, supraspinatus, infraspinatus, and biceps.

Although isolated, spinal accessory, suprascapular, axillary, and long thoracic peripheral nerve injuries do occur. They are produced typically by different mechanisms of injury.[14] When evaluating an athlete with nerve injury, care should be taken by the medical staff not to allow the athlete to return to competition too soon. With upper extremity weakness, not only can the football player further damage the brachial plexus, but he also places himself in a compromised position secondary to the weakness. Another part of the body can be injured, in particular the cervical spine. Shoulder pads and extra padding can channel and help protect the football player and dissipate any forces from hits that might occur. The most important aspect of rehabilitation following a brachial plexus injury is rest and avoiding aggravating the injury.

CONCUSSIONS

Another debilitating injury that has received a great deal of attention over the past few years is concussions. Football at any level has certain risks that players must assume. Through improved medical coverage and medical advancements, concussions will decline steadily, as did most of the other catastrophic injuries that once plagued the game of football. The first hurdle that the medical staff must cross is the actual diagnosis and grading of the concussion. Not all players will divulge that they have been injured, and, to their defense, they might not understand how to communicate their injury to medical personnel.

Grading of Concussions

Grading a concussion is confusing because of the many different scales. This confusion can lead to misdiagnosis of a head injury. It is important for the medical staff to have set grades and guidelines that can be used when necessary.

An example of grades as stated by the Colorado Medical Society would be:

Grade 1 (mild): Confusion without amnesia and no loss of consciousness

Grade 2 (moderate): Confusion with amnesia and no loss of consciousness

Grade 3 (severe): Loss of consciousness

Once the head injury has occurred, the guidelines for return to competition are then implemented:

Grade 1 (mild): The athlete might state that he had "his bell rung" or "his clock was cleaned." The athlete should be removed from competition and examined immediately on the sidelines and reexamined every 5 minutes for development of postconcussion symptoms. The athlete may return to competition if there is no amnesia or if no other symptoms appear after 15 minutes of rest.

Grade 2 (moderate): The athlete will be confused and may not remember the play in which he was injured or even who he is playing against. This athlete should be removed from competition and not allowed to return during the game. The athlete should be examined and reexamined frequently on the sidelines for worsening symptoms. The athlete should be examined the following day, and if appropriate, the treating physician may then order special tests to be done (magnetic resonance imaging, computed tomographic scan). The athlete can return to competition after 1 week of being asymptotic at rest and with activity.

Grade 3 (severe): The athlete will have loss of consciousness. If the athlete is unconscious on the field for a prolonged time, he should be treated and transported as if he sustained a spinal cord injury. The athlete should be held out of competition for 1 month and be asymptotic at rest and with activity.

Sideline mental testing is an important factor in diagnosing a head injury. These tests help in assigning a grade and in deciding if the player can return to competition. Listed in Table 12.1 are sample questions and simple tests that medical personnel can use to test athletes during competition as prepared by the Colorado Medical Society.

Minor head injuries are more common than severe head injuries in sports. When a player does suffer a concussion, he is more likely to sustain another concussion if he is not evaluated and treated properly. Medical staffs must be able to deal with athletes properly once the injury has occurred. Diagnos-

ing, grading, and special tests are all tools that the medical staff can use to help them determine when a player can return to competition safely.

Risk by Position

Under game conditions, the running play is repeatedly shown to be associated with the highest risk of injury. The running play is a more aggressive play. There is forward confrontational movement of the offensive linemen toward the defensive linemen during the

TABLE 12.1
___

Simple Tests and Questions to Ask in a Sideline Mental Examination

Orientation: Is the player oriented to time, place, person, and situation?
    What is your name?
    Where are you?
    Against what team are you playing?
    What time is it?
Concentration: Is the player able to concentrate and solve problems?
    Recite numbers.
    Recite those same numbers backwards.
    Tell me the months of the year in reverse order.
Memory: Is the player able to remember the names of famous people or recent events?
    Who is the President?
    Who is the mayor of the city?
    What is your responsibility on a certain play?
Exertion provocative test (physical testing): Is the player able to do exercises without his symptoms getting worse?
    Sideline running.
    Push-ups.
    Sit-ups.
    Squats.
    Monitor for any signs of headaches, dizziness, nausea, and blurred or double vision.
Neurologic testing: Is the player responsive? Does he show signs of neurologic damage?
    Pupil symmetry and pupil reaction: As the athlete opens and closes his eyes, watch for pupil symmetry and reactions to light.
    Coordination: finger to nose test: Watch for coordinated movements.
    Sensation: With the athlete's eyes closed, examine his sensation to sharp and dull objects.

play. During a passing play, the offensive linemen are not allowed to move aggressively across the line of scrimmage past a specific distance until the pass is thrown, and the receivers generally are trying to avoid contact with a defender until a reception is made. Defensive players almost always try to react to the movement of the ball and move toward it. Defensive players are at relatively high risk on plays run inside and outside the tackles, whereas offensive players are at greatest risk on plays run outside the offensive tackles. Confrontation with the defensive players who may initiate contact with the head can provide enough force to cause a concussion injury.[15]

When determining who is at greatest risk for concussion injuries during a game, the specific play must be considered. The offensive and defensive linemen are at their highest risk during running plays. The running backs are at greatest risk during running plays in between the tackles. This is secondary to the small area to which they are confined with the defensive lineman and linebackers all trying to stop them. The tackle is violent and forceful. The hits are usually head to head or head to knee, both of which potentially can cause a concussion.

The quarterback is also at relatively high risk when he is being tackled while throwing. He often does not see the defensive player coming and consequently cannot prepare for the hit. Quarterbacks are not accustomed to hitting and try to avoid contact as much as possible.

Wide receivers are at risk when being tackled secondary to vulnerable positions into which they must put themselves to catch the football. The receiver is frequently airborne when he is tackled, increasing the force of impact when he hits the ground.

The defensive secondary is usually made up of smaller players who generate speed from their positions when coming in for a tackle. Their speed, coupled with the offensive player's running force, can generate

enough force to cause a concussion for either the defensive or the offensive player.[15]

Position-Specific Injuries and Their Rehabilitation

All the rehabilitation programs discussed in this chapter will follow four distinct phases: *early phase*, *intermediate phase*, *advanced phase*, and *return-to-activity phase*. This will allow the reader to see the advancement through each phase. All the programs are tailored; no concrete timetables must be followed without deviation. Movement from one phase to another will follow tissue healing and functional outcomes of the athlete's progress. To prepare the athlete to return to competition with the most success and the least chance of reinjury, rehabilitation must be functional. We cannot rehabilitate them one way and then ask them to perform in the functional arena in another way.

QUARTERBACKS

The quarterback is susceptible to many different types of injuries. Oncoming defensive linemen can hit him, or blitzing linebackers and defensive backs can run full speed into him. The defensive players can outweigh the quarterback by as much as 100 lb, and the quarterback usually wears lighter shoulder pads.[21] The common injuries for quarterbacks are acromioclavicular (AC) separations of the throwing shoulder, tears of the medial collateral ligament (MCL) of the throwing elbow, rotator cuff strains of the throwing shoulder, nondominant anterior cruciate ligament (ACL) sprains/tears, and achilles tendon injuries

Achilles Tendon Rupture

Probably the most common injury that has plagued many of the greatest quarterbacks is an overuse and repetition injury. The repetition of dropping back to throw the football typically has resulted in a rupture of the Achilles tendon. A quarterback may throw the football up to 50 times in a game and a few hundred times during practice. This repetition of dropping back, decelerating, and planting the right foot for a right-handed quarterback can lead to Achilles tendinitis that can slowly cause degeneration of the tendon. The tendinitis weakens the tendon and makes it susceptible to tearing. The tendon also can tear from the trauma of a one-time violent deceleration and planting motion without any previous problems with the tendon.

The diagnosis of an Achilles tendon rupture is fairly easy with the Thompson test. In addition, a defect in the tendon can be detected with palpation in many cases. Surgery usually is performed rather quickly after a rupture, and an open repair typically is the surgery of choice.

Rehabilitation Early Phase: Following surgery, a cast is placed on the involved leg in slight plantarflexion. The gait status for the first week following surgery is non-weight-bearing. After the first week, the surgeon will reevaluate the repair, and the surgical site is inspected for signs of infection. The patient is recasted, remaining in slight plantarflexion for another week. At 2 weeks after surgery, the cast is removed, and the involved lower extremity is placed in a walking boot, with the foot again in a slightly plantarflexed position. The athlete begins to ambulate partial bearing his weight with crutches. Rehabilitation should include active ROM for inversion and eversion, seated subtalar joint supination and pronation, and dorsiflexion from the plantarflexed position into neutral. The most important aspect of early rehabilitation intervention is soft tissue healing and wound care. Isometric exercises are initiated in all planes except for plantarflexion. Joint and scar mobilization also can be started at this time.

Strengthening exercises to the proximal joints of the lower extremity in a non-weight-bearing position will help prepare the lower extremity for an increase in the weight-bearing status.

Intermediate Phase: During this phase, frontal plane exercises are started, progressing to sagittal plane exercises in the weight-bearing position. The weight-bearing status should be progressed from partial to full weight bearing in a walking boot.

Crutches can be discontinued once the athlete's gait is normalized. Stationary bike riding is a great form of aerobic exercise that can be initiated at this time. As healing continues, the walking boot can be removed in favor of an athletic shoe with a graduated heel lift. Bilateral minisquats and wall sits can be added to the program. A treadmill-walking program needs to be started with side stepping (shuffles) and progressing to forward and backward walking. Bilateral proprioception stance exercises should be performed, progressing to unilateral exercises. The BAPS board is an excellent exercise for ROM, balance, and proprioception. Scar and joint mobilization should continue if indicated.

Advanced Phase: Starting in the frontal plane and progressing to the sagittal plane, the preceding exercises should be continued with the addition of surgical tubing or dumbbells to the minisquats. Progress to lunges in all planes while adding resistance with dumbbells, a weight vest (Fig. 12.3), or surgical tubing. Changing the surface to a foam (Fig. 12.4) or wobble board will increase the difficulty of the exercise. The stairstepper with changing foot positions from neutral to toe-in and toe-out will increase the aerobic demands and is a good closed-chain exercise for the lower extremity. A slide-board program can begin with changing board lengths and speed modification. Resisted walking with sport cords forward, backward, lateral, cariocas, and shuffles is used to help with leg strength and is a good form of concentric and eccentric exercise. Calf raises can be per-

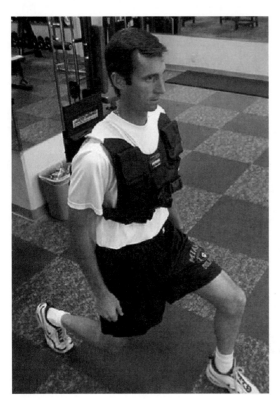

FIGURE 12.3

Weight vest with lunges.

the needs of the position will prepare the athlete for specific position demands. A resisted running program using chutes, weight vests, or tubing resistance is a fun and a progressive alternative to straight-ahead running for the athlete. The plyometric jumping program should be started to increase the explosive speed and strength of the lower extremities. See the sport-specific quarterback running program in Table 12.2.

RUNNING BACKS

The next highest profile player on the football field is the running back. There have been many high profiled running backs over the years. NFL records held by running backs are

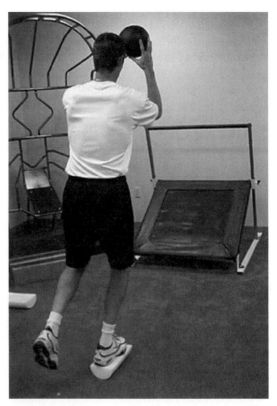

FIGURE 12.4

Single-leg ball throwing on foam roll.

formed bilaterally at first, followed by bilateral concentric–unilateral eccentric raises and then unilateral raises. Weights can be used, and both the soleus and the gastrocnemius need to be trained.

Return-to-Activity Phase: The athlete must have full strength and ROM before entering the return-to-activity phase. Following the functional progression will allow you to know when the athlete is ready to enter this phase. Tests that can be performed to determine when an athlete is ready to enter this phase include the single-leg hop test, single-leg jump test, unilateral timed-balance test, and single-leg box jump test. Sport- and position-specific running programs tailored to

TABLE 12.2

Quarterback Running Program

Performed with a football in the throwing position when dropping back.

20-yd sprint, jog/walk back
3-step drop, jog/walk back
5-step drop, jog/walk back
7-step drop, jog/walk back
5-step drop roll left, jog/walk back
5-step drop roll right, jog/walk back
20-yd zigzag every 5 yards, jog/walk back
40-yd sprint, jog/walk back
7-step drop shuffle left, jog/walk back
7-step drop shuffle right, jog/walk back

spoken about with reverence and awe. Their records of running show both strength and stamina over a long period of time. The common injuries are contusions, ankle sprains, hamstring strains, and ACL sprains/tears. One of the most common knee injuries experienced by running backs is the MCL sprain. With the demands that running backs place on their knees in addition to the constant hits they take on their knees, the MCL takes its share of stress.

MCL Sprain

This injury can be diagnosed with a physical examination of the knee. During the valgus overload examination of the knee, the practitioner will see an increase in laxity of the medial structures of the knee. This laxity is then evaluated and graded from less severe to more severe using a grading system of 1 to 3. A grade 1 injury indicates minor damage with no instability. A grade 2 injury indicates more significant damage with some degree of laxity perceived. However, there is enough integrity left to prevent full opening of the joint. A grade 3 injury indicates total rupture with

loss of restraint and ensuing instability. The immediate care of the athlete will be based on the degree of injury. A grade 1 MCL sprain is treated differently than a grade 3 sprain.

Grade 1 sprain. There is no immobilization of the knee. Crutches can be used if the athlete is unable to ambulate without a limp. A Zumi unloader can be used for gait training to decrease weight bearing (Fig. 12.5). Exercises are initiated immediately in a protected ROM. The goal is to prevent stress on the ligament during the rehabilitation process until it has had enough time to heal properly. Maintaining a good quadriceps contraction through quadriceps isometrics and functional electrical stimulation or biofeedback will help decrease any swelling and also maintain good muscle tone.

Grade 2 sprain. Early immobilization can be helpful to help control swelling, protect the ligament from further disruption, and assist with early healing. Crutches should be used until the gait pattern is

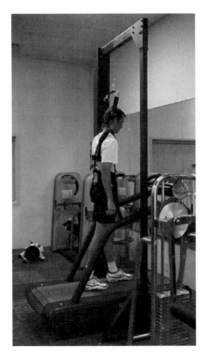

FIGURE 12.5

Zumi unloader.

normalized. A protective brace, such as a short, hinged knee brace, should be used even after the crutches have been discontinued to help prevent any unnecessary ligament stress. Progression from sagittal plane exercises to frontal plane exercises should be slower than for grade 1 sprains.

Grade 3 sprain. Early immobilization is imperative to prevent further injury and eliminate unnecessary force to the ACL and PCL. Many physicians prescribe a long-leg, hinged brace. Using this knee brace during the first phase of rehabilitation also can help prevent any unnecessary strain to the MCL during exercise. Progression through the phases will be slower, and precautions should be taken to limit the stress placed on the ligament during rehabilitation.

Rehabilitation Early Phase: The early phase begins with work in the sagittal plane but not allowing for excessive flexion of the knee. End-range flexion of the knee places unnecessary stress on the MCL. EMG biofeedback in conjunction with quadriceps isometrics will help decrease swelling through muscle pumping action as well as help retard muscle atrophy. Straight-leg raises can be performed in all planes, with the precaution of hip adduction because this movement can increase stress on the MCL. Multiangle proprioceptive neuromuscular facilitation (PNF) exercises and multiangle isometric wall sits are exercises that will work leg strength and not aggravate the ligament. Balance exercises with changing knee and foot positions can be performed with equipment such as the Airex, DynaDisc, foam rolls, and Kat Balance systems.

Intermediate Phase: The stationary bike will challenge aerobic demands and increase lower extremity strength. The stairstepper, starting with a small range and increasing the range as healing continues, also will challenge aerobic demands and increase lower extremity strength. In the intermediate phase, begin to work into frontal plane exercises. As the athlete progresses, begin with standing balance and reaching exercises in all planes including box step-ups and step-downs forward, backward, and laterally. Resisted walking especially side-stepping, will appropriately stress the MCL. Manual resistance squats with changing hand and force positions also will challenge strength and proprioception.

Advanced Phase: The athlete should continue with isotonic leg extensions and leg curls to build leg strength and power. During this phase, the athlete should work into the transverse plane with the exercises. Squats with changing foot positions, multiplane lunges, and multiplane box step-ups with rotation will increase the demand on the lower extremity. Standing multitouch drills in all planes will challenge the joint in all planes with a combination of hip, knee, and ankle movement. The slide board will challenge the muscular system anaerobically and aerobically. Using resistance weight belts or vests also will increase the challenge. Standing single-leg rotation exercises can be progressed with added resistance using balls, tubing, and hand weights. Resisted tubing frontal plane shuffles, slides, and cariocas are recommended. The athlete also needs to have a high level of balance and proprioception and can use a dynamic roller board to achieve this (Fig. 12.6).

Return-to-Activity Phase: The athlete must have full strength and ROM before entering this phase. Performing a functional progression of exercises and functional tests will tell you if the athlete is ready to return to activity. Sport- and position-specific running drills need to be added at this time to prepare the athlete to return to competition. Plyometrics will challenge the explosive properties of the lower extremities, as will a resisted running program using chutes, a weight vest, and surgical tubing. See the specific running back running program in Table 12.3.

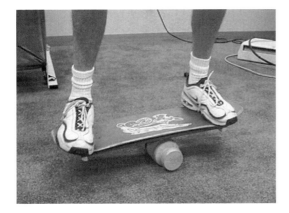

FIGURE 12.6

Dynamic roller board for dynamic balance.

OFFENSIVE LINEMEN

The offensive line is made up of the largest players on the field. Frequently, these were the boys who were bigger than all the rest growing up and were placed on the offensive line simply because of size. These five players can dictate the outcome of many games. Television commentator and offensive line enthusiast John Madden says, "The game is won and lost up front with the offensive line." Blocking and protecting the superstar quarterbacks and running backs is their job. Blocking without holding the opposition is challenging, especially when working against players who are faster and quicker than they are. Back problems are common in both offensive and defensive linemen. The mechanics of repetitively hitting blocking sleds are a major cause of lumbar injuries.[20] Many knee ligament and shoulder problems can arise from the continual blocking. The shoulder is especially vulnerable when blocks are made with the arms stretched out. Also, these players must work out hard in the weight room. Shoulder problems frequently begin with or are exacerbated by improper technique or the lack of proper muscle balance.

Posterior Shoulder Instability/Dislocation

Posterior shoulder instability can become a detrimental and chronic condition for offensive linemen if it is not diagnosed and rehabilitated early. The player will present with complaints of pain and weakness of the shoulder. Internal rotation and forward flexion movements are the most painful. The rotator cuff musculature (supraspinatus and infraspinatus) normally are the weakest. A posterior apprehension test can be performed by transmitting a posterior force to the humeral head. The push-pull test is also popular. Often these athletes do very well with conservative care and proper weight lifting.

Rehabilitation Early Phase: Shoulder passive ROM and pendulum exercises can help restore proper movement to the joints

TABLE 12.3

Running Back Running Program

Performed with a football and starting from a three-point stance

40-yd sprint, jog/walk back
10-yd square in right, jog/walk back
10-yd square in left, jog/walk back
6-yd post right, jog/walk back
6-yd post left, jog/walk back
30-yd zigzag every 5 yd, jog/walk back
15-yd swing pass right, jog/walk back
15-yd swing pass left, jog/walk back
10-yd come back right, jog/walk back
10-yd come back left, jog/walk back

after a dislocation. T-bar ROM exercises along with grade 1 and 2 joint mobilizations can help decrease pain and inflammation. Care should be taken not to stress internal rotation and horizontal adduction. Isometric strengthening exercises are beneficial.

Before moving into the next phase, the athlete must have full active and passive ROM. A core strengthening program should be started. Core strength will help with the return to activity and help decrease some of the stress on the shoulder during contact with other players.

Intermediate Phase: The intermediate phase progresses with shoulder girdle muscle strengthening with an emphasis on the rotator cuff and scapular muscles using manual techniques, surgical tubing, and dumbbells. The upper body ergometer can be used with a shortened ROM to limit stress to the posterior capsule.

Quadruped weight-shifting exercises, wall weight shifting, and quadruped cufflink exercises are closed-chain exercises for the upper body. The Body Blade exerciser and supine rhythmic stabilization exercises are good open-chain exercises. Starting in the neutral position so as not to stress the posterior cap-

sule, PNF resistance exercises should be incorporated in the supine and standing positions, starting with manual resistance and progressing to external resistance with tubing or cuff weights. A progressive resistance dumbbell program with an emphasis on the posterior shoulder and rotator cuff musculature is a good open-chain exercise approach.

Advanced Phase: The stairstepper can be used for the upper body (starting in the quadruped position and progressing to the push-up position), and wall push-ups using manual resistance or a weight vest can be added to challenge shoulder strength and stability during closed-chain exercises (Fig. 12.7). Push-ups can be progressed from the floor to a medicine ball with varying sizes of balls and hand positions (Fig. 12.8). Push-ups with the arms in a horizontally adducted position maximally stress the posterior capsule and should be performed with caution. Other closed-chain exercises include quadruped upper extremity slide board excursions in all planes.

Return-to-Activity Phase: This phase should be monitored very closely to determine if the player can return to full contact football without surgical intervention. The

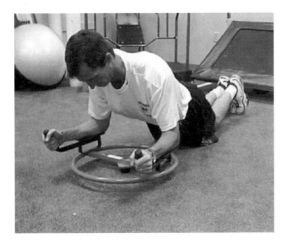

FIGURE 12.7

Upper extremity balance ring.

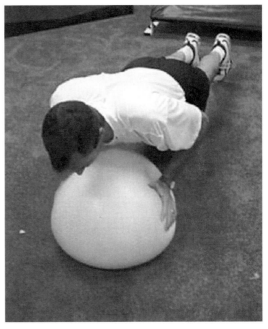

athlete must have full strength and a negative posterior apprehension sign.

Functional exercises must be introduced at this stage, but close supervision should be provided. Blocking drills with a Studman (Fig. 12.9) or blocking sleds along with upper extremity plyometrics will challenge the upper extremity and prepare the athlete for

FIGURE 12.8

Push-ups with physioball for increased proprioception.

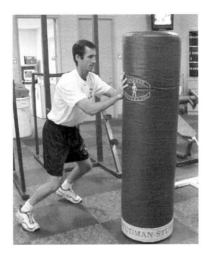

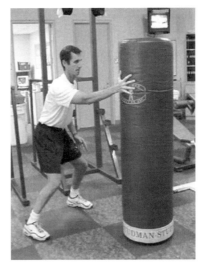

FIGURE 12.9

A. Studman blocking forward. *B.* Studman cross-blocking sideways.

ballistic upper extremity activities. Ballistic wall push-ups, medicine ball catches and tosses, and physioball bounce push-ups will continue to challenge the posterior musculature and capsule and help the rehabilitation professional determine if the athlete is ready to enter into full competition. See the sport-specific offensive and defensive linemen running program in Fig. 12.10.

WIDE RECEIVERS

With all the sprinting and cutting required of receivers during a game, it is no wonder there are numerous hamstring strains and ACL tears. Often a receiver will plant and turn to run a pass route, and his cleat will become caught in the turf or he can receive a direct blow to the knee. To prevent noncontact ACL injuries, there may be a benefit to retro-running drills to increase the proprioception and motor training of the hamstrings. See the sport-specific wide receiver running program in Fig. 12.11.

DEFENSIVE BACKS

Defensive backs often have upper extremity injuries when defending or blocking the offensive player. Finger dislocations and hand and wrist sprains are seen when the upper extremity gets caught in a face mask or jersey. Neck and shoulder sprains are also seen during tackling, especially when the athlete tackles or collides with someone who outweighs him by up to a hundred pounds.

KICKERS

Both field goal kickers and punters develop overuse injuries. The field goal kicker most often has responsibilities for extra point kicks and kick-offs. The most common injury is a hip flexor strain in the proximal muscle belly. This occurs during the eccentric contraction when the muscle is overstretched just prior to the forward swing phase of the kick. This can occur in punters, but hamstring strains are more common. They occur during the eccentric elongation of the hamstrings during the follow-through phase of the kick. Low-back strains are also common as a result of the rotation accompanied by hyperflexion movements.[21]

Return to Sport

SPORT-SPECIFIC RUNNING PROGRAMS

The rehabilitative running program should mimic and simulate what the football player will be doing on the field. As stated previously, the different football positions place different demands on the muscular systems of players as well as their cardiovascular systems. When they are performing their running program, this should be kept in mind. The running program should stimulate the joints in all the planes of movement. When possible, receivers and running backs should carry the football and have someone throw the football to them. Defensive backs and linebackers should do more than half their running backwards to simulate covering the receiver and their position-specific demands. These drills can be performed at different speeds, depending on what your goals as the rehabilitation specialist are: full speed with a jog back, half speed with a walk back. The variations depend on the individual's certain recovery status.

The programs are made up of 10 different runs. The order of the runs can be changed to fit what the rehabilitation specialist is trying to accomplish. See the quarterback running program (Table 12.2), the running back running program (Table 12.3), the defensive back running program (Table 12.4), the offensive lineman running program (Fig. 12.10A), the defensive lineman running program (Fig. 12.10B), and the wide receiver running program (Fig. 12.11).

OFFENSIVE LINE- METABOLIC WORKOUT

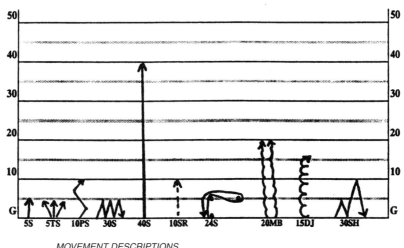

MOVEMENT DESCRIPTIONS

5S	5 yard sprint
5TS	5 yard triangle shuttle
10PS	10 yard pass shuffle at 30 degree angle backward (w/45lb)
30S	30 yard shuttle
40S	40 yard sprint
10SR	10 yard set-reset, etc. (facing sideline)
245	24 shuttle drill
20MB	20 yard Medicine Ball repels
15DJ	15 yard double leg jumps
30SH	30 yard shuttle

SET 1	SET 2	SET 3	SET 4	SET 5
5TS	5S	5S	10SR	40S
10PS	24S	10SR	24S	5S
40S	5TS	15DJ	5TS	5TS
10SR	5S	40S	10PS	20MB
5S	10PS	5S	30S	30S
24S	30SH	20MB	5S	24S
30S	20MB	30S	40S	5S
15DJ	10SR	10PS	20MB	15DJ
5S	40S	5S	30SH	30SH
30SH REST	5S REST	5TS REST	5S REST	5S

FIGURE 12.10

A. Offensive lineman running program.

Conclusion

The sport of football means many different things to different people. It can bring back memories of childhood games or time-honored family traditions of attending games with fathers or grandfathers. Some say that football has a certain smell—cool fall air, grass, and sweat. Whatever your individual thoughts and feelings are, just about everyone has a special relationship with the great game of football.

DEFENSIVE LINE- METABOLIC WORKOUT

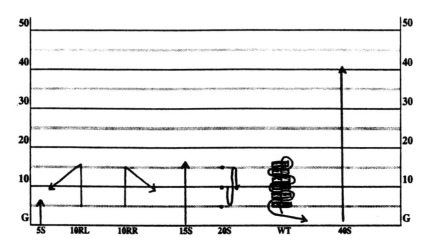

MOVEMENT DESCRIPTIONS

5S	5 yard sprint
10RL	10 yard rush, retreat left at 45 degrees to sideline
10RR	10 yard rush, retreat right at 45 degrees to sideline
15S	15 yard sprint
20S	20 yard shuttle (3 cone)
WT	Weave & Trash Drill w/5 yard sprint out
40S	40 yard sprint

SET 1	SET 2	SET 3	SET 4	SET 5
10RL	15S	5S	10RR	20S
WT	5S	WT	5S	15S
40S	20S	40S	WT	5S
5S	40S	10RR	40S	10RL
15S	10RL	15S	40S	5S
5S	WT	5S	5S	40S
10RR	5S	40S	15S	5S
20S	5S	10RL	20S	WT
5S	15S	20S	5S	10RR
40S REST	10RR REST	5S REST	10RL REST	15S

FIGURE 12.10 (CONTINUED)

B. Defensive lineman running program.

WIDE RECEIVERS- METABOLIC WORKOUT

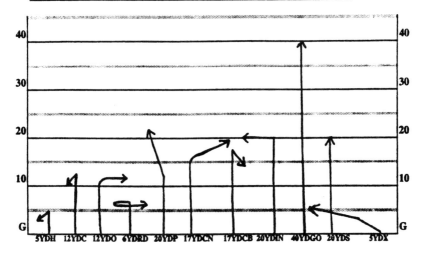

MOVEMENT DESCRIPTIONS
5YD H	5 yard hitch (1 route)
12 YD C	12 yard curl (6 route)
12 YD O	12 yard out (3 route)
6 YD RD	6 yard reverse delay 2 route)
20-21 YD P	20-21 yard post, break at 12 yards (8 route)
17 YD CN	17 yard corner (7 route)
17 YD CB	17 yard comeback (5 route)
20 YD IN	20 yard In (4 route)
40 YD GO	40 yard to (9 route) can pump like 5 route
20 YD S	20 yard sprint
5 YD X	5 yard cross (0 route)

Note: If possible, have someone throw you the ball during this workout.

SET 1	*SET 2*	*SET 3*	*SET 4*	*SET 5*
17 YD CN	12 YD O	40 YD GO	5 YD H	6 YD RD
20 YD P	20 YD IN	20 YD P	12 YD O	40 YD GO
40 YD GO	17 YD CB	6 YD RD	17 YD CB	17 YD CN
5 YD H	40 YD GO	20YD S	40 YD GO	20 YD P
12 YD O	12 YD C	20 YD IN	17 YD CN	12 YD C
20YD S	5 YD H	12 YD C	6 YD RD	20YD S
5 YD X	6 YD RD	5 YD X	20YD S	20 YD IN
17 YD CB	17 YD CN	12 YD O	5 YD X	40 YD GO
6 YD RD	20 YD P	17 YD CB	12 YD C	5 YD H
20YDIN (R	20YD S (R)	5 YD H (R)	40 YD GO(R)	17YD CB (R)

FIGURE 12.11

Wide receiver running program.

TABLE 12.4

Defensive Back Running Program

Performed as if covering a wide receiver or with someone throwing the player the ball.

20-yd sprint, jog/walk back
5-yd backpedal turn, sprint 10 yd, jog/walk back
20-yd backpedal, jog/walk back
10-yd backpedal, stop, and break right, jog/walk back
10-yd backpedal, stop, and break left, jog/walk back
40-yd sprint, jog/walk back
15-yd backpedal, turn, and sprint right at 45-degree angle, jog/walk back
15-yd backpedal, turn, and sprint left at 45-degree angle, jog/walk back
10-yd backpedaling W's, jog/walk back
5-yd sprint, jog/walk back

Acknowledgments

I would like to thank John Gamble and Mike Woicik for the running examples.

References

1. McLatchie GR, Lennox CM: *The Soft Tissue: Trauma and Sports Injuries*. Oxford, England: Butterworth-Heinehann, 1993.
2. Porter CD: Football injuries. *Phys Med Rehabil Clin North Am* 10(1):95–115, 1999.
3. Zemper ED: Injury rates in a national sample of college football teams: A 2-year retrospective study. *Phys Sports Med* 17(11):100–113, 1989.
4. DeHaven KE: Diagnosis of acute knee injuries with hemarthrosis. *Am J Sports Med* 8(1): 9–14, 1980.
5. Mueller FO, Blyth CS, Canter R: Catastrophic spine injuries in football. *Phys Sports Med* 17:51–53, 1989.
6. Frederick O: *Prevention of Athletic Injuries: The Role of the Sports Medicine Team*. Philadelphia: FA Davis, 1991.
7. Gray G: *Chain Reaction Plus*. Wynn Marketing Course Seminar, Fort Lauderdale, FL: 1994.
8. Roy S, Irvin R: *Sports Medicine: Prevention, Evaluation, Management, and Rehabilitation*. Englewood, Cliffs, NJ: Prentice Hall, 1983, pp 45–51.
9. O'Donoghue D: *Treatment of Injuries to Athletes*, 4th ed. Philadelphia: Saunders, 1984, pp 16–24.
10. Anderson MK, Hall SJ, Hitchings C: *Fundamentals of Sports Injury Management*. Baltimore: Williams & Wilkins, 1997, pp 184–185.
11. Ellison A: *Athletic Training and Sports Medicine*. Chicago: American Academy of Orthopeadic Surgeons, 1985, pp 101–106.
12. Klafs C, Arnheim D: *Modern Principles of Athletic Training*, 5th ed. St Louis: Mosby, 1981.
13. Perrin D: *The Injured Athlete*, 3d ed. Philadelphia: Lippincott-Raven, 1999, pp 204–238.
14. Garrick J, Webb D: *Sports Injuries: Diagnosis and Management*, 2d ed. Philadelphia: Saunders, 1999, pp 198–202.
15. Buckley WE: Concussions in college football: A multivariate analysis. *Am J Sports Med* 16(1):51–56, 1988.

16. Ohton D: A kinesiological look at the long snap in football. *NSCA J* 10(1):4–13, 1988.

17. Hay JG: *The Biomechanics of Sports Techniques*. Englewood Cliffs, NJ: Prentice-Hall, 1978.

18. Henrici RC: A cinemgraphical analysis of the center snap in the punt formation. MS thesis, University of Wisconsin, 1967.

19. Rubican CA: A comparison of the differences in speed and accuracy between two methods of spiral center pass to the punter in football. MS thesis, Springfield College, Springfield, MA, 1965.

20. Gatt CJ Jr, Hosea TM, Palumbo RC, Zawadsky JP: Impact loading of the lumbar spine during football blocking. *Am J Sports Med* 25(3):317–321, 1997.

21. Dorson J: Football injuries reflect position specific demands. *Biomechanics* 5(8):65–70, 1998.

22. National Collegiate Athletic Association's Injury Surveillance System, 1997. Health and Safety Education Outreach, P.O. Box 6222, Indianapolis, IN 46206.

23. Torg, JS, Harris, SM, Rogers, K, Stilwell, GJ: Retrospective report on the effectiveness of a polyurethane football helmet cover on the repeated occurrence of cerebral concussions. *Am J Orthop* 28(2):128–132, 1999.

24. Torg J, Stilwell G, Rogers K: The effect of ambient temperature on the shoe-surface interface release coefficient. *Am J Sports Med* 24(1):79–82, 1996.

25. Levy IM, Skovoron ML, Agel J: Living with artificial grass: A knowledge update, part 1: Basic sciences. *Am J Sports Med* 18:406–412, 1990.

26. Stanitski CL, McMaster JH, Ferguson RJ: Synthetic turf and grass: A comparative study. *J Sports Med* 2:22–26,1974.

27. Torg JS, Quedenfeld TC: Effect of shoe type and cleat length in incidence and severity of knee injuries among high school football players. *Res Q* 42:203–211, 1971.

28. Torg JS, Quedenfeld TC, Landau S: The shoe surface interface and its relationship to football knee injuries. *J Sports Med* 2:261–269, 1974.

29. Valiant GA: Friction, slipping, traction. *Sportverlez Sportschaden* 7:171–178,1993.

Additional References

Arciero RA: Adolescent football injuries and sexual maturity. *Clin J Sport Med* 6(1):69, 1996.

Bernhardt DT: Football: A case-based approach to mild traumatic brain injury. *Pediatr Ann* 29(3): 172–176, 2000.

Blivin SJ, Martire JR, McFarland EG: Bilateral midfibular stress fractures in a collegiate football player. *Clin J Sport Med* 9(2):95–97, 1999.

Collins MA, Millard-Stafford ML, Sparling PB, et al: Evaluation of the BOD POD for assessing body fat in collegiate football players. *Med Sci Sports Exerc* 31(9):1350–1356, 1999.

Collins MW, Grindel SH, Lovell MR, et al: Relationship between concussion and neuropsychological performance in college football players. *JAMA* 282(10):964–970, 1999.

Cooper ME, Wolin PM: Os trigonum syndrome with flexor hallucis longus tenosynovitis in a professional football referee. *Med Sci Sports Exer* 31(suppl 7):493–496, 1999.

Delaney JS, Lacroix VJ, Leclerc S, Johnston KM: Concussions during the 1997 Canadian Football League season. *Clin J Sport Med* 10(1): 9–14, 2000.

Gomez JE, Ross SK, Calmbach WL, et al: Body fatness and increased injury rates in high school football linemen. *Clin J Sport Med* 8(2): 115–120, 1998.

Fukuoka Y, Shigematsu M, Itoh M, et al: Effects of football training on ventilatory and gas exchange kinetics to sinusoidal workload. *J Sports Med Phys Fitness* 37(3):161–167, 1997.

Jones DM, Tearse DS, el-Khoury GY, et al: Radiographic abnormalities of the lumbar spine in college football players: A comparative analysis. *Am J Sports Med* 27(3):335–338, 1999.

Kennedy MA, Sama AE, Sigman M: Tibiofibular syndesmosis and ossification. Case report: Sequelae of ankle sprain in an adolescent football player. *J Emerg Med* 18(2):233–240, 2000.

Kenter K, Behr CT, Warren RF, et al: Acute elbow injuries in the National Football League. *J Shoulder Elbow Surg* 9(1):1–5, 2000.

Lovell MR, Collins MW: Neuropsychological assessment of the college football player. *J Head Trauma Rehabil* 13(2):9–26, 1998.

Maddali S, Rodeo SA, Barnes R, et al: Postexercise increase in nitric oxide in football players with muscle cramps. *Am J Sports Med* 26(6): 820–824, 1998.

McCarthy P: Artificial turf: does it cause more injuries? *Phys Sports Med* 17:159–164, 1989.

Meese MA, Sebastianelli WJ: Pulmonary contusion secondary to blunt trauma in a collegiate football player. *Clin J Sport Med* 7(4):309–310, 1997.

Metzl JD: Sports-specific concerns in the young athlete: Football. *Pediatr Emerg Care* 15(5): 363–367, 1999.

Naunheim RS, Standeven J, Richter C, Lewis LM: Comparison of impact data in hockey, football, and soccer. *J Trauma* 48(5):938–941, 2000.

Paulos LE, Drawbert JP, France P, et al: Lateral knee braces in football: Do they prevent injury? *Phys Sports Med* 14:108–119, 1986.

Palumbo MA, Hulstyn MJ, Fadale PD, et al: The effect of protective football equipment on alignment of the injured cervical spine: Radiographic analysis in a cadaveric model. *Am J Sports Med* 24(4):446–453, 1996.

Ross DS, Swain R: Acute atraumatic quadriparesis in a college football player. *Med Sci Sports Exerc* 30(12):1663–1665, 1998.

Schlegel TF, Boublik M, Ho CP, Hawkins RJ: Role of MR imaging in the management of injuries in professional football players. *Magn Reson Imag Clin North Am* 7(1):175–190, 1999.

Shaffer B, Wiesel S, Lauerman W: Spondylolisthesis in the elite football player: An epidemiologic study in the NCAA and NFL. *J Spinal Disord* 10(5):365–370, 1997.

Smith RS, Guilleminault C, Efron B: Circadian rhythms and enhanced athletic performance in the National Football League. *Sleep* 20(5): 362–365, 1997.

Stilger VG, Yesalis CE: Anabolic-androgenic steroid use among high school football players. *J Commun Health* 24(2):131–145, 1999.

Stocker BD, Nyland JA, Caborn DN, et al: Results of the Kentucky high school football knee injury survey. *J Ky Med Assoc* 95(11):458–464, 1997.

Stone MH, Sanborn K, Smith LL, et al: Effects of in-season (5 weeks) creatine and pyruvate supplementation on anaerobic performance and body composition in American football players. *Int J Sport Nutr* 9(2):146–165, 1999.

Strong LR, Titlow L: Sagittal back motion of college football athletes and nonathletes. *Spine* 22(15):1755–1759, 1997.

Thomas BE, McCullen GM, Yuan HA: Cervical spine injuries in football players. *J Am Acad Orthop Surg* 7(5):338–347, 1999.

Thompson N, Halpren B, Curl WW, et al: High school football injuries, evaluation. *Am J Sports Med* 15(2):117–124, 1987 [published erratum appears in *Am J Sports Med* 15(3): 257,1987].

Waicus KM, Smith BW: Renal fracture secondary to blunt trauma in a football player. *Clin J Sport Med* 9(4):236–238, 1999.

Weinberg J, McFarland EG: Posterior capsular avulsion in a college football player. *Am J Sports Med* 27(2):235–237, 1999.

CHAPTER 13

Basketball

Eric Shamus
William Kelleher
Bill Foran

Basketball is a sport that requires strength, power, and agility. Athletes of all ages and skill levels play the game. It can be played as an organized sport or recreationally, such as pickup games. Basketball dates back to 1891, when Dr. James Naismith created an indoor recreational game to be played in the winter. The game originated with a leather soccer ball that was thrown into two peach baskets. Women formally began playing the sport at Smith College, and the first rules for women were adopted in 1903.[1] Basketball was played for the first time as an Olympic sport in 1936. One of the most significant changes in the game of basketball over the years involves the jump shot. Prior to 1950, all shots were taken with one foot on the ground.

In the traditional game of basketball, there are five players. The positions are the center, power forward, small forward, shooting guard, and point guard. The athletes play both offense and defense. Depending on the players' athleticism, they may play more than one position. It is common to see recreational games of one on one, two on two, three on three, four on four, or five on five in both half- and full-court formats.

The overall dimensions of the basketball court are different for secondary schools (high schools) as compared with collegiate and professional levels. In secondary schools, the court is 50 ft by 84 ft, whereas college and professional courts are 50 ft by 94 ft. The backboard is usually rectangular. The rectangular backboards are 72 in wide by 48 in high.[1] The basketball rim has a diameter of 18 in and is positioned 10 ft above the ground. The ball varies in size and weight for both men and women. For men, the circumference of the ball is between 29 and 30 in, and it is inflated with 7 to 9 lb of air and weighs between 20 and 22 oz. For women, the circumference of the ball is between 27 and 29 in, and it is inflated with 6 to 8 lb of air and weighs between 18 and 20 oz. The ball and height of the rim may be smaller for ages 12 and under. The game can be played both indoors and outdoors. A leather composite ball is usually used indoors, and a rubber-based ball is used outdoors. The court construction can vary from suspended wood floors indoors to concrete and asphalt surfaces outdoors.[2]

The sport of basketball exposes the athlete to injury as a result of the running, jumping, cutting, pivoting, and explosive movements that occur during acceleration and deceleration.[3] This chapter will review the biomechanics of the sport, injury prevention, etiology of injuries, and common injuries and their treatment. Applying sport-specific knowledge to training and rehabilitation should result in decreased injuries and fewer games missed.

Biomechanics of Basketball

The game begins with a jump ball, where two players jump vertically to tip a tossed basketball toward a teammate for possession. Players on offense need to dribble, handle, pass, and shoot the ball while maneuvering themselves for an offensive rebound. Players on defense need to be quick and powerful in order to jump and block a shot or elevate for a rebound and guard their opponents. A breakdown of the fundamentals of each skill will be presented. There is little research regarding the biomechanics of the skills used in the game of basketball.

VERTICAL JUMP

The vertical jump is important in rebounding, playing defense, and shooting and passing the ball. The takeoff in a vertical jump can be from one or two feet.

Running Vertical Jump

The running vertical jump is performed by taking off of one foot during a layup or a shot block attempt. The initial phase of a single-foot takeoff is performed by running or stepping forward with the plant foot. The foot

plants hard on the ground while the opposite knee and hip flex to bring the lower extremity into the air. There is a rapid eccentric moment throughout the planted lower extremity, with the ankle dorsiflexing and the knee and hip flexing to prestretch and load the muscles to gain elastic energy. The rapid eccentric moment evokes the stretch reflex, or the stretch-shortening cycle, which results in greater concentric contraction of the same muscle. During the stretch-shortening cycle, the muscles and tendons elongate to gain elastic energy. Elastic energy is the force absorbed by muscle fibers as a result of elongation of the muscle and tendon.[4] The mechanics of the plant lower extremity are similar to the initial contact through midstance phases of running.

Once the plant leg is eccentrically preloaded, the concentric or push-off phase begins. Concentric plantarflexion knee, hip, and trunk extension elevates the player off the ground. The hip and knee extend to neutral (0 degrees), while the foot supinates and the ankle plantarflexes to 20 degrees. Between 15 and 25 percent of the force is generated from the ankle plantarflexors, between 32 and 49 percent from the knee extensors, and between 28 and 38 percent from the hip extensors. The contralateral hip and knee continue to forcefully drive upward.

Once the athlete becomes airborne, the contralateral, nonplant lower extremity extends rapidly. The last phase of the jump is the eccentric landing component, which is similar to the preload phase. As the player lands, the lower extremity musculature eccentrically contracts to absorb the shock. The anterior and posterior tibialis, gastrocnemius, and soleus eccentrically control pronation and dorsiflexion of the ankles. Knee flexion is eccentrically controlled by the quadriceps, and hip flexion is eccentrically controlled by the gluteals. Often an overload force is absorbed by the pelvis and lumbar spine, leading to injuries of the joints and intervertebral disks.

There have been many studies on the amortization phase of the vertical jump. This is the time between the eccentric preload and the concentric push-off phase of the jump. It has been found that a shorter amortization phase results in higher jumps. As the amortization phase increases, there is a loss of elastic energy and jumping height.[4-6]

In the running vertical jump, the player can jump higher because of momentum but risks loss of control in the air. If a player is off balance, he or she is more likely to sustain foot and ankle injuries on landing. The ankle plantarflexors are also at risk of injury because they are one of the largest energy generators and absorbers for both vertical jumps. The resulting joint movement and power patterns of the lower extremity are similar to those for the standing vertical jump.[7]

Vertical Jump from Two Feet

The primary difference between taking off from two feet rather than one foot is that there is no leg driving upward; both legs are planted and eccentrically loading. This explains why one-legged jumps only achieve 58.5 percent of the height reached by two-legged jumps. There is also higher muscle activation of the hip and knee extensors and ankle plantarflexors in the two-legged jumps. To achieve maximum performance in the two-legged vertical jump, each lower extremity should be trained individually and then trained in unison.[8]

The upper extremities play a role in the vertical jump from two feet. Arm swing can increase knee extensor torque by 28 percent. Arm swing also assists hip extensor torque by slowing the rate of trunk extension. This facilitates better muscle length tension ratios in the hip extensors.[8]

SHOOTING

The jump shot, free throw, hook shot, and layup are the four basic basketball shots. With all shots, it is important to hold the ball by the fingers and not the palm. Some players with very large hands may have a tendency to allow the ball to contact the palm, which decreases the amount of control of the ball. To be accurate with all the shots, practice is mandatory. A routine that allows for relaxation and concentration will increase accuracy.

Free Throw

When shooting a free throw from the foul line, a set shot is used. The foot on the side of the shooting hand is 10 to 12 inches in front of the opposite foot. The feet should be shoulder width apart, and the knees should be bent slightly. The center of gravity is slightly forward toward the front foot. The shooting elbow, wrist, and hand are all in the same plane as the lead foot.

The ball is held with both hands by the face, with one hand on the side of the ball for control. When beginning the shot, the knees extend, and the shoulders flex. The elbow is pointed toward the basket and moves from a flexed position into extension. The ball should be released at approximately 50 to 60 degrees of elbow flexion and from the index and middle fingers of the shooting hand.[1,9,10] The finger thrust and wrist snap into flexion[2] at ball release produce backspin on the ball. In the follow-through, the shooting arm should extend fully along with full forearm pronation and wrist flexion. Speed of 7.3 m/s with a spin of –2 to +2 m/s have been shown to be the most accurate for free throws.[11]

Free-throw percentages have declined to 73 percent for the NBA, a 25-year low.[12] Centers have the lowest percentage (67 percent in 1994), and point guards have the highest (79 percent in 1994).[13] Weight training and aerobic conditioning do not appear to have any detrimental or beneficial effect on the accuracy of free-throw shooting.[14]

Balance, elbow position, and follow-through[2] are some of the common areas that can affect the accuracy of free-throw shooting. Lack of knee flexion when beginning the shot and poor position of the feet (not aimed toward the basket) are also contributing factors. Research has determined that visual attention also can play a role in free-throw success. One study compared elite basketball players who shot above 75 percent and below 65 percent. The basketball players who shot above 75 percent located the target earlier, selected a single location (front of the rim), and maintained quiet eye fixation for almost a full second before initiating the shot (1400 ms). The players who shot under 65 percent demonstrated increased head movements, higher frequency of gaze shift, and shorter fixation during the preparatory phase (950 ms).[15,16] The results of this study demonstrate that shooting practice alone may not be enough to improve free-throw percentage. Players may need drills to help them focus and train their visual system.[15–17]

Hook Shot

The player begins the hook shot with the ball in both hands, centered at chin height, with the back to the basket. For a right-handed hook shot, the left foot steps toward the direction of the shot and is placed on the ground parallel to the baseline. The body and left upper extremity rotate toward the left foot. The ball is transferred to the right hand. The left lower extremity eccentrically loads, and the right lower extremity extends and then drives into the air. The ball is brought above the head with shoulder elevation in the scapular plane with the elbow and wrist in extension. As the ball is being released, the wrist flexes and the forearm pronates.[2]

Layup

The layup shot can be taken with or without a dribble. A skilled player can lay the ball up with either hand. The layup shot can be taken from various angles and from either side of the court. When taking a layup shot with the right hand, the ball is held with both hands on the outside of the right hip. The player will step and jump off the left foot and use the right hand to softly lay the ball off the backboard about 12 to 15 inches above the goal.[1] The greatest challenge is elevating less horizontally and more vertically. This will decrease forward momentum, allow for a softer shot, and decrease charging calls.

Jump Shot

The shooting motion of the upper extremity and foot placement in the jump shot are similar to those of the foul shot. The difference is simply the vertical jump into the air. It is important to square the shoulders to the basket before initiating the shot, take a comfortable jump, and maintain a normal rhythm. If a maximal jump is attempted every time, fatigue eventually will set in and alter the height of the jump, causing the shot to be short. Players who are off balance are often unable to control the shot.

As the distance of the shot increases, so does the ball release speed. However, the release angle of the elbow does not significantly change: 52 to 55 degrees for closer distances and 48 to 50 degrees for further distances.[9] The increased ball speed is mainly created by an increase in angular velocity of the elbow joint of the shooting arm. There is also a notable increase in the velocity of the center of mass of the body toward the direction of the basket at ball release. The forward center of mass is influenced greatest by the ankle joint.[10] As the distance increases, players also demonstrate an earlier timing of release, which causes an earlier rotation of the shoulder axis and an increase in angular velocity of shoulder flexion.[9,10]

SKILLS

Positioning

Positioning is critical for the athlete to allow for quick movements and changes in direction. Two common positions are the *offset stance* and the *parallel stance*. The offset stance is used for forward and backward balance and changes in direction. The feet are placed one in front of the other and are shoulder width apart. On offense, this is considered the triple-threat position: The player is able to pass, dribble, and shoot. This position also can be used for playing defense. In the parallel stance, the feet are side by side and shoulder width apart. The parallel stance is used for lateral movements.

In both positions, the feet are slightly toed out. The body weight should be distributed evenly from side to side and front to back. The player should be in a semisquat position with the ball held at a level even with the axilla. The ankles are normally in 5 to 15 degrees of dorsiflexion, the knees are flexed between 60 and 90 degrees, the hips are in 100 to 110 degrees of flexion, and the trunk is slightly flexed. For a defender, the ready position includes looking forward, the shoulders abducted to 90 degrees, and the elbows extended to block the pass or shot. The arms can easily be drawn close to the side from this position for quick movements. The entire foot should be in contact with the ground, with the weight on the balls of the feet. When initiating movements, weight shifting should be performed toward the direction of movement. It is important to maintain a low center of gravity for balance and quickness.

Pivoting

A player with the ball is allowed to move one foot to turn or rotate the body, but the other (pivot) foot must not move. Players need to pivot on the ball of the foot, keep the head level, and the feet shoulder width apart. Pivoting on the heel is illegal. Pivoting places a great deal of stress on the knees and can lead to injuries secondary to the rotational forces incurred.

Passing

There are basically four types of passes: the *chest pass*, the *bounce pass*, and the *overhead pass* with one or two hands. In the chest pass,

the ball should begin close to the chest, with the hands in a neutral position (the thumbs pointing up). When passing the ball, the shoulders flex and internally rotate, the elbows extend, and the forearms pronate. In the bounce pass, the ball is in the same starting position, but the ball is directed downward at an angle, and the thumbs are used to create a backspin. To pass the ball overhead, one or two hands can be used. The single-hand pass is used for longer distances and is similar to the mechanics of a baseball throw. The two-handed overhead pass is used for shorter distances. With this pass, the ball begins over the head, with the elbows slightly flexed and the thumbs pointing backward. As the ball is brought forward, the shoulders and elbows extend, and the forearms pronate. Variations of both passes can be performed depending on the situation.

Steps

There are three fundamental steps: the *slide step*, the *running step*, and the *forward/backward step*. In the slide step, the stance position can be offset or parallel. The feet are at least shoulder width apart. The first step is taken by the lead foot in the direction of movement, while the opposite foot pushes off. The lead foot continues to be positioned toward the direction of movement, while the back foot slides toward the direction of movement. Short shuffle steps continue to be taken in this manner without the feet crossing over. Players need to slide side to side and diagonally. These steps maintain the center of mass between the feet to allow for quick movements.

In a running step, the weight is shifted in the direction of movement. This is a controlled fall in the direction of movement to initiate momentum. In the forward/backward step, the player should shift his or her weight and push off with the back foot. The forward/backward step makes it difficult for the opposition to anticipate the player's direction of movement. An example of this is cutting.

Ball Handling and Dribbling

The basketball should be held by the fingers of both hands. The fingers should be spread out as far as possible, and the palms should not touch the ball. Players dribble without looking at their hands, so good tactile sense is important. The ball is controlled by the fingertips of either hand and by wrist and elbow movements. The downward pushing motion is initiated with finger and wrist flexion and elbow extension. The eyes should be looking forward, scanning the court. A lower dribble is used for control, whereas a higher dribble is used for increased speed.

Rebounding

The most important components of rebounding are positioning, anticipation, and athleticism. Once a player is in the proper position and anticipates the direction of the ball for a rebound, a vertical jump must be performed. This requires balance, strength, power, and overhead reaching. When possible, rebounding should be performed with two feet and two hands to increase control.

Ball Approach Angle

When shooting, the arc of flight of the ball is very important. A shot that is more like a line drive or has a flat arc has a poor angle of entrance into the basket. A shot with a larger arc enters the basket closer to a vertical position and is less likely to hit the rim and bounce out. The angle of release on a medium-arc shot is approximately 60 degrees of elbow flexion.[2]

Injury Prevention

The National Basketball Association (NBA) regular season lasts for 6 months and involves 82 games. If a team makes it into the playoffs, the season can extend an additional 2 months. With such a long season, it is imperative that players maintain a high level of fitness to stay injury-free. This can be challenging secondary to the unique combination of strength, speed, and power over various time intervals that basketball requires. Sport-specific year-round training is essential not only for performance enhancement but also for the prevention of injury.[18] This section will cover the various aspects of a comprehensive conditioning program. Many factors need to be assessed for injury prevention, including warm-up, stretching, strengthening, periodization and conditioning, prophylactic devices, shoe wear, psychology, and nutrition.

WARM-UP

Prior to playing in a game or practice, players need to warm up. An adequate warm-up consists of 5 to 10 min of jogging or stationary cycling.[4] The athlete should begin to perspire. This can decrease injuries as a result of

- Increased blood flow and muscle temperature
- Increased oxyhemoglobin breakdown and released oxygen from myoglobin
- Increased sensitivity of nerve receptors and speed of nerve impulses
- Decreased activity of alpha fibers and sensitivity of muscles to stretch
- Increased cardiovascular responses to sudden strenuous exercise
- Increased relaxation and concentration[19]

This will help prepare the muscles for the demands of basketball.

STRETCHING

In basketball, as well as other sports, stretching should be performed following the warm-up and again during the cool-down period. Stretching can assist with injury prevention and warm-up.[4,20,21] Stretching during the cool-down can decrease muscle soreness,[22] facilitate range of motion (ROM),[23] and increase muscle relaxation.[4] Stretching that causes pain will not increase flexibility but may cause muscle or connective tissue damage.[4] Table 13.1 lists the key muscles to target.

Stretching can be performed actively or passively. A *passive* stretch occurs when an outside force provides the stretching force. Examples are the use of a device (strap or belt) or a partner. *Active* stretching occurs when the athlete supplies the force of the stretch with the antagonist (opposite) muscle. This can be performed statically, dynamically, or ballistically.

A *static* stretch can be performed passively or actively and is held in one position. The static stretch includes passive relaxation and elongation of the muscle and connective tissue. Static stretching needs to be performed at a level that does not elicit the stretch reflex.[24] The stretch reflex is elicited when a quick stretching movement activates a muscle spindle. A sensory neuron from the muscle spindle innervates a motor neuron in the spinal cord that facilitates a muscle contraction of the muscle being stretched. This reflex acts as a stretching monitor to prevent injury.[4]

Proprioceptive neuromuscular facilitation (PNF) stretching techniques incorporate alternating contraction and relaxation of the agonist and antagonist muscles to cause neural responses that reflexively inhibit muscular contraction and facilitate muscular relaxation of the muscle being stretched.[4] The relaxation of the agonist during a maximal isometric contraction is called *autogenic inhibition*.[23] A submaximal isometric contraction of the agonist produces increased tension that stimulates the Golgi tendon organ (GTO) to reflexively relax the agonist.[22] An example is if the athlete contracts the hamstrings, the hamstrings will relax reflexively, allowing them to be stretched further.

A contraction of the agonist will reflexively relax the antagonist muscle. This is called *reciprocal inhibition* or *inverse stretch reflex inhibition*.[24] An example is if the athlete contracts the quadriceps, the hamstrings will relax reflexively, and the hamstrings can then be stretched further.

The three basic types of PNF stretching are hold-relax, contract-relax, and slow-reversal-hold-relax.[4] A benefit of the PNF techniques of stretching is the increased muscle length and the possible increase in motor learning within the new ROM.

PNF stretching provides reflexive relaxation of the muscle being stretched through reciprocal and autogenic inhibition. Before athletic competition, this is preferable to a

TABLE 13.1

Key Muscles to Target in Stretching

Lower Extremities	Trunk	Upper Extremities
Hamstrings	Low back	Pectoralis
Quadriceps	Obliques	Posterior shoulder musculature
Groin, adductors	Lattisimus dorsi	
Gluteals		
Calves		
Piriformis, hip rotators		

passive stretch, where a partner or a device provides the force of the stretch.[25] After active stretching, dynamic stretching should be performed.[4]

Dynamic stretching incorporates flexibility during sport-specific movements.[26] A good way to incorporate dynamic stretching is to start at one end of the basketball court and perform different drills for the length of the court. Each drill should be performed for at least one court length. The following progression of sport-specific movements with increasing intensity is recommended[4,27,28]:

- Forward/retro jogging
- Lateral shuffles and cariocas
- High-knee skips
- Bounding
- Butt-kick runs
- Angle cuts
- High-knee runs

Ballistic stretching involves bouncing movements at the end range of motion. A ballistic movement creates an end-range stretch but may cause muscle or tissue damage and is not usually recommended.[24]

STRENGTHENING

It is important to develop a good strength base with basketball players. This is developed through a weight training program with an emphasis first on the hips and legs, then core strength (including the abdominals, obliques, and back extensors), and finally, the upper body. The entire body needs to be strong, yet flexible.

The key to developing the lower body and midsection is with compound movements. A *compound movement* includes multiple joints in multiple planes. Compound exercises that focus on the lower extremities are listed in Table 13.2. [27,28] Compound exercises that focus on the midsection are listed in Table 13.3. Compound exercises that focus on the upper body are listed in Table 13.4.

POWER

The two ways to develop power are Olympic lifts and plyometrics. These are typically performed with the greatest volume and intensity in the off-season. Weight room power exercises include power and hang cleans, snatches, and power pulls. The reader is referred to the book by Baechle[4] for proper technique with Olympic lifts. A progression for high-intensity jumping plyometrics to be performed on the court is described in the conditioning section.

Plyometric exercise enables a muscle to reach maximal strength in as short a time as possible.[4] Plyometric exercises use gravitational forces to store potential energy in muscles. The energy, if used immediately in an opposite direction, will produce kinetic energy.[29] Plyometric exercises develop *speed strength*, which is the ability to exert maximal force during high-speed activities.[4,30] Plyometric exercises provide an overload with speed.

The three components of a plyometric exercise are the eccentric, amortization, and concentric phases. Greater power and speed are produced when the eccentric preloading is short and rapid. The rate of stretch is more important than the load.[4] Caution needs to be taken with plyometrics because if the athlete does not have excellent strength, flexibility, balance, and proprioception, injuries can occur. It is important to progress plyometric exercises from basic to difficult and from low to high intensity. Frequency, volume, and intensity need to be considered.

Frequency is the number of workouts (sessions) per week. The range for plyometric workouts is one to three times per week with 2 to 4 days of rest between.[4] With higher volume and intensity, the frequency needs to decrease.

TABLE 13.2

Lower Extremity Compound Exercises

Two-Legged	One-Legged
Squats with the bar positioned in the front or rear	Lunges, multidirectional
	Step-ups
Leg presses	

Volume for plyometrics is usually described in the number of foot contacts per total workout. Volume for the off-season should be 80 to 100 foot contacts per session for beginners, 100 to 120 foot contacts per session for intermediate-level athletes, and 120 to 200 foot contacts per session for advanced/elite athletes. During the preseason, the total number of foot contacts of a trained athlete can increase up to 50 percent. With higher intensity, volume needs to be decreased.[4,5,29,31]

Intensity is the amount of force or stress applied to the body. Intensity can be increased by the type of activity, whether one or two feet contact the surface at the same time, the speed of the activity, if an external weight is used, or by the number of foot contacts per set. There should be a 2- to 3-min rest period between sets. The athlete's body type needs to be taken into consideration when choosing a plyometric exercise.[4,5,29] See Tables 13.5 and 13.6 for upper and lower extremity plyometric drills.

CONDITIONING

The conditioning program for any sport must take into account the demands of the position, age of the players, and time available to condition. Basketball consists of high-intensity anaerobic bouts throughout each 12-min period. Prolonged rest only occurs during 20-s or 1-min time-outs, between periods, or if the player is substituted and leaves the game. Consequently, the player must have an excellent aerobic base to aid in quick recovery. This should be developed in the off-season. The anaerobic training takes place in the last phase of the off-season and preseason. This is accomplished with interval training runs of 400, 200, and 100 m on a track or football or soccer

TABLE 13.3

Midsection Compound Exercises

Back Extensors	Abdominals	Obliques
Roman chair	Crunches	Rotational sit-ups
Reverse hypers	Leg lifts	Medicine ball tosses
Dead lifts	Double-leg lifts	Side sit-ups
One-leg dead lifts	Medicine ball crunches	

TABLE 13.4

Upper Body Compound Exercises

Pressing Movements	Pulling Movements
Bench presses	Lat pull-downs
Incline presses	Shrugs/upright rows
Military presses	Seated/bent-over rows
Dips	

TABLE 13.5

Upper Extremity Plyometric Drills

1. **Warm-up drills**
   Plyoball trunk rotation
   Plyoball side bends
   Plyoball wood chops
   ER/IR with tubing
   PNF D2 pattern with tubing

2. **Throwing movements—standing position**
   Two-hand chest pass
   Two-hand overhead soccer throw
   Two-hand side throw overhead
   Tubing ER/IR (both at side and 90 degrees
     of abduction)
   Tubing PNF D2 pattern
   One-hand baseball throw
   One-hand IR side throw
   One-hand ER side throw
   Plyo push-up (against wall)

3. **Throwing movements—seated position**
   Two-hand overhead soccer throw
   Two-hand side-to-side throw
   Two-hand chest pass
   One-hand baseball throw

4. **Trunk drills**
   Plyoball sit-ups
   Plyoball sit-up and throw
   Plyoball back extension
   Plyoball long sitting side throws

5. **Partner drills**
   Overhead soccer throws
   Plyobal back-to-back twists
   Overhead pullover throw
   Kneeling side throw
   Backward throw
   Chest pass throw

6. **Wall drills**
   Two-hand chest throw
   Two-hand overhead soccer throw
   Two-hand underhand side-to-side throw
   One-hand baseball throw
   One-hand wall dribble

7. **Endurance drills**
   One-hand wall dribble
   Around-the-back circles
   Figure eight through the legs
   Single-arm ball flips

Source: From Prentice W: *Rehabilitation Techniques in Sports Medicine,* 3rd ed. New York: WCB/ McGraw-Hill, 1999, Table 10-1, p. 164.

TABLE 13.6

Lower Extremity Plyometric Drills

1. **Warm-up drills**
   Double-leg squats
   Double-leg leg press
   Double-leg squat-jumps
   Jumping Jacks

2. **Entry-level drills—two-legged**
   Two-legged drills
   Side to side (floor/line)
   Diagonal jumps (floor/4 corners)
   Diagonal jumps (4 spots)
   Diagonal zigzag (6 spots)
   Plyo leg press
   Plyo leg press (4 corners)

3. **Intermediate-level drills**
   Two-legged box jumps
   One-box side jumps
   Two-box side jumps
   Two-box side jumps with foam
   Four-box diagonal jumps
   Two-box with rotation
   One/Two box with catch
   One/Two box with catch (foam)
   Single-leg movements
   Single-leg plyo leg press
   Single-leg side jumps (floor)

Single-leg side-to-side jumps (floor/4 corners)
Single-leg diagonal jumps (floor/4 corners)

4. **Advanced-level drills**
   Single-leg box jumps
   One-box side jumps
   Two-box side jumps
   Single-leg plyo leg press (4 corners)
   Two-box side jumps with foam
   Four-box diagonal jumps
   One-box side jumps with rotation
   Two-box side jumps with rotation
   One-box side jump with catch
   One-box side jump rotation with catch
   Two-box side jump with catch
   Two-box side jump rotation with catch

5. **Endurance/agility plyometrics**
   Side-to-side bounding (20 ft)
   Side jump lunges (cone)
   Side jump lunges (cone with foam)
   Altering rapid step-up (forward)
   Lateral step-overs
   High stepping (forward)
   High stepping (backwards)
   Depth jump with rebound jump
   Depth jump with catch
   Jump and catch (plyoball)

Source: From Prentice W: *Rehabilitation Techniques in Sports Medicine,* 3rd ed. New York: WCB/McGraw-Hill, 1999, Table 10-2, p. 165.

field. This training is specifically designed to develop the phosphagen, glycolytic, and oxidative energy systems, which are used primarily in power sports lasting 1 to 10 s.[32,33]

For adolescent players, skill acquisition and overall conditioning should be emphasized more than sport-specific conditioning.[34] Sport-specific conditioning drills are appropriate for high school, college, and professional basketball players. Consequently, drills help develop a quick first step to move in any direction at any time, good jump height, and quick reaction times. These drills include on-court drills with and without a basketball, quick-feet plyometrics, agility drills, jumping plyometrics, and medicine ball drills. On-court conditioning drills also can incorporate dribbling.

On-Court Conditioning Drills with and without a Basketball

On-court conditioning drills with and without a basketball are performed to develop anaerobic power. As such, a rest period of 2 to 2½ times the running time should be provided after each drill. For example, if an athlete runs a 5½ in 32 s, the rest is 64 to 80 s before the next 5½ is run.

5½s The athlete runs 5½ lengths of the court (baseline to baseline five times and then finish at half court) as fast as possible.

Line Drills ("Suicides") The athlete starts at one baseline, runs to the closest free-throw line, then back to the baseline, then to half court, then back to the baseline, then to the opposite free-throw line, then back to the baseline, and then the full court, finishing back at the baseline.

17s The athlete runs sideline to sideline 17 times as fast as possible.

Lateral Resistance Training

Lateral resistance training drills focus on lateral movement and body control. The athlete holds or wears rubber tubing or bands. Against resistance, the athlete moves laterally to the right for three quick steps and returns back to the starting position under control. This is repeated 5 to 10 times or for a period of 10 to 20 s without pausing. The movement is repeated to the left after a 30- to 90-s rest.

Conditioning Drills with Shooting

Sideline-Touch Corner Jump Shots The athlete shoots a jump shot at the right corner of the free-throw line and then sprints to the opposite sideline and back to the left corner of the free-throw line for a jump shot. The athlete then sprints to the other sideline and back to the right corner of the free-throw line for a jump shot. This is continued for 30 s to 2 min or for a certain number of baskets made. *Variation:* The athlete shuffles laterally to the sideline and sprints back.

Endline Touch, Top-of-the-Key Jump Shots The athlete shoots a top-of-the-key jump shot and then sprints to the opposite baseline and back to the top of the key for another jump shot. This is repeated for a certain amount of time or for a certain number of baskets made.

Corner-Touch Perimeter Jump Shots The athlete shoots a perimeter jump shot and then sprints to one of the court's four corners and back for another perimeter jump shot. The athlete then sprints to a different corner and back for a jump shot. This is repeated for a certain amount of time or for a certain number of baskets made.

Quick-Feet Plyometrics

To develop quick feet, the athlete needs to practice moving his or her feet as fast as possible. Quick-feet plyometrics will improve foot quickness. One drill involves marking four spots 12 to 18 in apart on a shock-absorbing surface such as wood (not cement). The spots are numbered 1 to 4 like the sample below:

```
3              2
4              1
```

With these four spots, a number of different patterns can be executed. The drills can be performed with two feet or with one foot. When performed with two feet, the drills can last for 10 to 20 s, and the one-foot drills last for 10 s. Each drill must be performed as quickly as possible, minimizing the amount of time the feet spend on the ground. The following movement patterns are used:

Two-Number Patterns	Three-Number Patterns	Four-Number Patterns
1-2	1-2-3	1-2-3-4
1-4	1-3-2	1-4-3-2
1-3	1-4-3	1-3-2-4
4-2	1-3-4	4-2-3-1

The number of times the athlete lands on the starting spot during the allotted time should be counted. Adequate rest time for a good recovery between drills is 20 to 90 s depending on the fitness level of the athlete. Four to six jumping drills and four to six hopping drills per lower extremity should be performed for each workout.

Agility Drills

Agility drills should last 10 to 20 s with maximum effort. They can involve quick starts and stops, changes of direction, and movements in all directions.

Lane Shuffles The athlete starts on one side of the free-throw lane and then moves laterally as quickly as possible to the other side of the lane and back. The back-and-forth movement continues for 20 s. The number of times the athlete crosses the lane is counted.

Around the Lane This drill incorporates forward, lateral, and backward movements. The athlete starts at the baseline where the lane and sideline intersect. The athlete sprints up the line to the free-throw line, moves laterally across the free-throw line to the opposite lane line, backpedals to the endline, and moves laterally back to the starting position. The athlete immediately repeats the movements in the opposite direction.

Jumping Plyometrics

Box Jumps The athlete stands 0.6 m in front of one to eight boxes located 1 to 2 m apart. The athlete jumps onto a box, lands softly on the box, and explodes again as high and far forward as possible (if more than one box is used, the sequence is continued to the next box). Repeat for 5 to 10 jumps. The starting height can range from 0.4 to 1.1 m, with 0.75 m being the norm.[4,6] After the athlete can perform four sets of 10 jumps (intermediate level), he or she is ready for weighted box jumps. In weighted box jumps, the athlete can wear a weighted vest or ankle cuff weights. This drill develops power and quickness.[4,27,28]

In-Depth Jump The athlete starts on top of a 0.4- to 1.1-m box, steps off the box onto the floor with the feet 20 to 30 cm apart, and as quickly as possible jumps onto another box or in a vertical or horizontal position. The athlete swings his or her arms in the direction of the jump. This drill also develops power and quickness.

Single-Leg Box Jumps The athlete stands in front of a 0.4- to 1.1-m box on one foot. The athlete jumps with one leg up on the box and jumps down to the starting point on the same leg. The athlete jumps for up to 10 times without the use of the other leg. It is then repeated with the other leg. This drill develops balance, stability, and one-legged power. An increase in the amortization phase with this exercise will decrease elastic energy. It is important to have the shortest amortization phase as season training begins for proper motor learning.

With box jumps, the athlete should not flex the knees greater than 45 degrees on landing. If he or she does, the box is too high. Jump training programs can be effective in decreasing landing forces, decreasing abduction and adduction movements at the hip, increasing hamstring strength, and increasing jump height. Plyometric training also significantly enhances the rate of eccentric lower body force production.[35]

Medicine Ball Drills

Medicine ball drills develop core strength, power, and quickness. Listed below are three medicine ball drills. The first two drills develop core strength, and the third teaches the athletes to sit deep and to stay low on defense.

Side Toss Two athletes face each other about 10 to 12 ft apart. One is holding the medicine ball with both hands next to his or her right hip. He or she fully rotates the midsection to the right and then tosses the ball as he or she rotates back to a neutral position. The ball should be tossed to the partner's right side, and the partner rotates to the right as well and then tosses it back. After 10 tosses each, the drill is repeated to the left side. For the drill to be plyometric, the ball's momentum should not be stopped.

Over-Under/Under-Over   Two athletes are back to back about 1 ft apart. The athlete holding the medicine ball lifts it over his or her head, handing it to the partner, who hands it back between his or her legs. After 10 repetitions, they reverse the direction for 10 more repetitions. The athletes should stabilize the spine throughout the drill with appropriate muscular activation.

Deep-Squat Overhead Passes   Two athletes face each other about 10 to 12 ft apart. They both get in a deep-squat position (heels on the floor, knees over the feet not the toes, head up, shoulders back, and hips as low as the knees). The partners play catch with overhead passes for 20 passes.

PERIODIZATION

Seasons

For high school on, basketball's year-round training program has four distinct seasons: *preseason, in-season, postseason,* and *off-season.* The difference is the length of each season.

Preseason

The preseason is the 2- to 4-week time period from the start of practice until the first game. The first week to 10 days may include two practices per day. There is a drop in the volume of strength training with a maintenance of load. Endurance and plyometric sessions are also reduced to one to two times per week. Exercise selection should be as sport-specific as possible, including basketball drills.[4,28]

In-Season

The basketball season is the time to use the strength, power, quickness, speed, agility, and conditioning that was developed in the off-season. A solid in-season program will maintain the improvements developed in the off-season. Intense, quality basketball practices will eliminate the need for additional conditioning, jumping plyometrics, and agility drills. The players who are not getting playing time in the games may need extra conditioning to maintain their fitness level.

For basketball players to maintain their strength and power throughout the season, they need to be involved in an in-season weight-training program. In-season weight training should be performed twice a week. It needs to be a total-body program that includes multiple joint activities in order to be time-efficient.

NBA Year-Round Schedule

Jan.	Feb.	March	April	May	June	July	Aug.	Sept.	Oct.	Nov.	Dec.

----In-season---------------------|----Post----|-----------Off-season-----------|--Pre--|---------------

College Year-Round Schedule

Jan.	Feb.	March	April	May	June	July	Aug.	Sept.	Oct.	Nov.	Dec.

------In-season----|--Post--|--------------Off-season----------------------|-Pre-|--------------------

High School Year-Round Schedule

Jan.	Feb.	March	April	May	June	July	Aug.	Sept.	Oct.	Nov.	Dec.

---In-season------|-Post-|-----------------Off-season----------------------|-Pre-|--------------------

The program listed below is set up with five minicircuits of three to four exercises in each circuit. For example, the first minicircuit of a pushing movement (bench press), a pulling movement (lat pull), and a leg exercise (squats) is performed in succession, and then a 2-min rest is taken before repeating the circuit at a higher weight. After two or three sets of 8 to 10 repetitions of the first minicircuit, the athlete moves to the next circuit. A total-body program can be performed in a short period of time with minicircuits. Circuit training can cause delayed-onset muscle soreness (DOMS) because of the increase in blood lactate.[36]

Minicircuit 1: Bench press, lat pulls, squats
Minicircuit 2: Military press, shrugs, lunges, step-ups/downs
Minicircuit 3: Triceps pressdowns, arm curls, leg extensions, leg curls
Minicircuit 4: Calf raises, rotator cuff, wrist curls
Minicircuit 5: Abdominals, low back/trunk

After a game, any player with minimal playing time should perform aerobic and anaerobic activities to simulate game demands. This will maintain the fitness level of substitute and bench players.

Postseason

The postseason is a 2- to 4-week period of active rest. The athletes recover from a long season and prepare for a productive off-season. Fitness activities such as swimming, jogging, circuit training at a low volume and intensity, racquetball, and volleyball are encouraged. Even a little recreational basketball is permitted.[4,27]

Off-Season

The first few weeks of the off-season focus on basic weight training and general conditioning. Players start the process of building a new strength base and conditioning base. The athlete's 5- to 10-repetition maximum is often recalculated at this time. The last 12 to 16 weeks of an off-season training program focus on functional training.

The off-season is the time for basketball players to become better players. They can improve their skill, speed, agility, jumping ability, strength, power, quickness, flexibility, and conditioning. To develop all these components, the athletes need a well-rounded program that incorporates skill development, weight training, agility drills, conditioning, stretching, jumping plyometrics, quick-feet plyometrics, and medicine ball work. Table 13.7 shows a 1-week off-season training schedule that includes all the components of an off-season program.

Each workout starts with some aspect of skill development. Shooting, dribbling, ball handling, passing, and other basketball skills are all improved on at this time. The Monday and Thursday workouts include upper body weight training, agility drills, sport-specific conditioning, and flexibility. The Tuesday and Friday workouts include lower body weight training, jumping plyometrics, quick-feet plyometrics, and flexibility. Wednesday is the recovery day, with just medicine ball work and flexibility after skill development.

Weight training is the key to developing a solid strength base. Athletes with a solid strength base get the most out of plyometrics and agility drills. Table 13.8 shows a total-body split-routine weight-training program.

It is important that the upper body is strong and balanced. This program has four pressing movements and four pulling movements. For time efficiency, each pressing movement is followed by a pulling movement and then a rest period. A beginner's program could start with three pressing movements and three pulling movements, eliminating the incline press and seated row. The abdominal work should be three to five sets of a variety of crunches, leg raises, and twisting crunches.

TABLE 13.7

Off-Season Training Schedule: One-Week Sample

Monday	Tuesday	Wednesday	Thursday	Friday
Skill dev.	Skill dev.	Skill dev.	Skill dev.	Skill dev.
Wt. training, upper body	Wt. training, lower body	Med. ball	Wt. training, upper body	Wt. training, lower body
Agility drills	Quick-ft. plyos		Agility drills	Quick-ft. plyos
Conditioning	Jumping plyos	Conditioning		Jumping plyos
Stretching	Stretching		Stretching	Stretching

PROPHYLACTIC DEVICES/SHOE WEAR

Many basketball players wear ankle braces or have their ankles taped for practice or games. Ankle taping and bracing have been found to decrease the rate of injury.[37,38] This may be secondary to the fact that taping has been shown to improve the muscle reaction time of the peroneus brevis of unstable ankles.[39] The proprioceptive role of bracing and taping seems to be greater than its ability to limit the overall ROM of the ankle joint.

TABLE 13.8

Sample of a Total-Body Split-Routine Weight-Training Program

Upper body day:	
Bench press	2 to 4 sets
Lat pull	2 to 4 sets
Military press	2 to 4 sets
Shrugs	2 to 4 sets
Incline press	2 to 4 sets
Seated row	2 to 4 sets
Tricep pressdown	2 to 3 sets
Arm curl	2 to 3 sets
Ab work	3 to 5 sets
Rotator cuff work	1 to 2 sets
Wrist curls	1 to 2 sets

In comparing injury rates, basketball players wearing no tape and low-top shoes had the highest incidence of injury, i.e., 33.4 ankle sprains per 1000 player games. In comparing low- and high-top basketball sneakers, the incidence of injury decreased to 30.4 ankle sprains per 1000 player hours. High-top basketball shoes increase resistance to an inversion force. The basketball shoes studied increased the maximal resistance to an inversion moment by 29 percent for a neutral ankle and 20 percent for the ankle in 16 degrees of plantarflexion. The basketball shoe inversion resistance averaged 28 N·m of force. Neither the high- nor the low-top basketball shoe shows resistance to an eversion moment.[38,40] When players wore the high-top sneakers and had their ankles taped, the incidence of injury decreased to 6.5 ankle sprains per 1000 player hours. Based on this information, it is recommended that basketball players wear high-top sneakers and use ankle taping or bracing.[38,41,42]

Although one author determined that wearing athletic tape or a brace does not impede muscle performance,[43] several studies have shown that the use of external ankle supports by basketball players does adversely affect basketball-related performance tests. Vertical jump height is less with the ankles taped as compared with no tape, whereas jump-shot accuracy is better with tape as compared with the Swede-O Universal lace-up brace. Oxygen consumption and energy expenditure are higher with the Aircast brace as compared with tape.[44] The Active Ankle brace impairs performance the least out of the support devices tested. The prophylactic benefit of bracing needs to be weighed against the impairment of performance.

OVERTRAINING AND PSYCHOLOGY

The physiologic requirements of basketball are high, placing considerable demands on the cardiovascular and metabolic capacities of players.[45] It is not difficult to experience the effects of overtraining. Overtraining aerobically can cause a parasympathetic response. These symptoms include a decreased resting heart rate, early fatigue, decreased performance, increased sleep, demented counterregulatory capacity against hypoglycemia, and depression. Mood changes also can accompany the changes in performance.[46]

Overtraining anaerobically can cause a sympathetic response. These symptoms include a plateau followed by a decrease in strength gains, increased resting heart rate by 5 to 10 beats per minute, decreased lean body mass, decreased performance, decreased appetite, decreased sleep, decreased recovery after exercise, increased resting diastolic blood pressure, increased irritability, a cold that just will not go away, and decreased maximal plasma lactate level during exercise.[46,47] Both the sympathetic and parasympathetic systems have large effects on the psychology of a basketball player.

Psychology

Sports injuries happen to individuals who are much more than a combination of muscles, tendons, ligaments, bones, and/or joints that are injured. Even though the discipline is relatively young, sport and exercise psychology has already provided some solid support for the importance of addressing the prevention and rehabilitation of athletic injuries *holistically*. This includes consideration of such factors as the person's emotions, thoughts, habits, social network, life stressors, and coping skills as well as the actual physically damaged structures. It would be wise and ethically responsible, therefore, for the health care professional involved with athletes to be aware of how these factors can play a part in an athlete's increased vulnerability to injury and the more or less successful recovery from it.

Injury Vulnerability Some of the initial injury vulnerability research was designed to investigate the possible relationship of life stressors (major life changes or unwanted events) to the incidence of injuries in a variety of sports. The overall results from this research have been equivocal.[48] A few studies have found athletic injury to be positively related to life stressors[49,50]; other studies found no such relationship.[51] This is reminiscent of the results from the large body of stress-response research in clinical psychology and other disciplines that have found that it is *not simply* what events happen to a person that determine how stressed he or she will become. How that person perceives the life event and what coping skills he or she brings to bear on the experience will have more of an impact on the degree of the person's stress response.[52]

Building from this finding, sport psychologists have proposed and researched a multicomponent model for better understanding the role of stress and psychological factors in affecting an athlete's vulnerability to injury.[53] In this model, an athlete can be facing a potentially stressful situation in playing his or her sport (such as having to defend the opposing team's best scorer in a division championship basketball game), but the degree of stress the athlete experiences will depend on how much the person perceives the situation as a threat, in addition to how well the person uses coping skills. The coping skills could include confidently believing he or she has the ability for the task (also known as self-efficacy), relaxing at appropriate times to keep down excessive physical arousal, striving for his or her best effort rather than demanding constant perfection, managing anger at a referee's "bad" call, or recovering emotionally from a mistake in preventing the opponent from scoring. In the worst-case scenario, where the athlete perceives the responsibility of guarding this player as a serious threat and does not use any of the coping skills mentioned, the model proposes that the athlete will experience considerable "state" (situational) anxiety, excessive muscle tension, and impaired ability to attend to the play of the game. Excessive muscle tension can be associated with sympathetic nervous system over-arousal, a negative impact on smoothness of coordination, more impulsive movement, and an increase in the potential for physical injury.[54] Vulnerability for injury is further increased by the anxiety and stress response, having a negative influence on peripheral attention and the scope of the person's peripheral vision.[55] In our example, the stressed basketball player is more at risk to miss seeing a screen that is set up to his or her side and then run into the opponent setting the screen. The resulting fall or collision increases the risk of injury.

A study of basketball players, wrestlers, and gymnasts supported the multicomponent model as well as consideration of an additional factor, namely, degree of social support, in explaining vulnerability to injury.[56] In this study, life stress was found to be associated with athletic injuries only in the group of athletes who had both low-level use of coping skills and decreased experience of social support. Other factors that have been observed to put athletes at increased risk for injury include attitudes such as "Act tough and always give 110 percent" and "If you're injured, you're worthless" held by some

coaches and adopted by their players.[57] These attitudes could well encourage an athlete to play while hurt and make him or her susceptible to even greater injuries.[58] An increased number of overuse injuries was found in children and adolescents who were on teams where winning was stressed more than learning and fun.[59] In addition, parental pressure to win was found to lead to fictitious injuries in some young athletes. This phenomenon is called *eager parent syndrome*. It has been suggested that some young athletes find injury their only escape from pressures imposed on them.[60]

Given these factors that have been found to contribute to an athlete's increased vulnerability to injury, it would seem very appropriate that professionals involved with the care, training, or coaching of athletes address these concerns in an injury prevention program. Such a program could include identifying at-risk individuals and teaching such coping skills. This would include having reasonable self-expectations, relaxing, having goals to do well without demanding constant perfection, and recovering quickly from mistakes. Other preventive efforts could be directed at fostering supportive relationships and encouraging parents and coaches to not prioritize winning over physical safety and/or personal enjoyment of the sport. The skill training for prevention of injury can be part of an overall psychological skills training (PST) program for performance enhancement. PST includes focus on increasing skills for goal setting, positive imagery, maintaining confidence, thought/attention control, arousal regulation, and emotional management.[58] Various studies have demonstrated the efficacy of PST for increased success in different aspects of playing basketball such as mental imagery training for improved free-throw shooting[61] and attentional training in focusing and centering for improvement in overall game performance statistics.[62] Thus PST serves not only an injury prevention purpose but also overall skill performance in the sport.

NUTRITION

Inadequate nutrition can compromise performance, and it also can increase the time needed for recovery following injury. Two important components to look at in the athlete's diet are the amounts of carbohydrates and proteins consumed. It is extremely important to have adequate muscle glycogen stores for sports participation. It is also necessary to replace these stores following exercise to aid in the recovery process. A high-carbohydrate diet with low saturated fat is an important part of an athlete's dietary regime. Glycogen stores need to be replenished within 2 hours of the exercise. The amount of carbohydrates required to achieve optimal rates of glycogen resynthesis is 0.7 to 3.0 g of glucose per kilogram of body weight.[19]

Adequate protein is important to prevent the breakdown of muscles. The recommended protein intake can be calculated based on a 12 percent total energy value from protein. For example, an athlete who weighs 70 kg and has a daily total intake of 5000 kcal should have a protein intake of 2.1 g/kg of body weight. Athletes should be cautious not to skip meals and to avoid diets that limit carbohydrate or protein intake.[19]

HYDRATION

Athletes need to drink a minimum of eight to ten 8-oz glasses of clear liquids per day. When outside in the sun, this should increase to 16 to 24 glasses per day. The fluids need to be colder than air temperature for quicker absorption. At a minimum, athletes need to drink at least 16 oz of clear fluids 2 hours before exercise and immediately prior to exercise. During exercise, they need to drink 8 oz for every 15 min of active participation to replace fluid loss. For prolonged activity, athletes need to add drinks with electrolytes and carbohydrates, up to 30 to 60 g/h of exercise. Athletes should weigh themselves before and after exercise and drink 16 oz of water for every pound lost.

Etiology of Injuries

The most common injuries in basketball are sprains, strains, and contusions. Fractures and dislocations are more rare.[63] In general, a sprain is an injury to a ligament, whereas a strain is an injury to a muscle or tendon.

INTRINSIC FACTORS

Muscle strength imbalances, joint laxity, proprioception deficits, decreased neuromuscular activation patterns, muscle fatigue, and bony alignment are all intrinsic risk factors that predispose the athlete to injury. All these factors can be addressed directly with an individualized, comprehensive strength and conditioning program that is periodized for the year. Preseason physicals and skill assessments are useful in identifying an athlete's deficiencies. Muscle and joint testing, vertical jump, body composition, aerobic capacity, pulmonary function, and agility testing all should be included in preseason screenings.[4,64]

Regardless of age, women are more likely to be injured. This is possibly secondary to poor preseason conditioning.[63,65] In high school basketball, the overall risk of injury for boys is 3.2 and for girls 3.6 per 1000 hours. Women are significantly more likely to injure their knees than men at the high school, college, and professional levels. Tears of the anterior cruciate ligament (ACL) are the most common.[66–73] In professional basketball, women are 1.6 times as likely to be injured as men. This also may be a result of women having an increased Q-angle and different muscle firing patterns.

EXTRINSIC FACTORS

Many extrinsic factors can increase an athlete's risk of injury. First is the shoe-surface interface. It is important that athletes wear shoes that are specifically designed for basketball. Such shoes and treads are specifically designed to withstand the multidirectional forces encountered during play. It is also important that the surface itself be clean, free of debris, and dry.[25,38]

The material of the playing surface can have a role in injuries. A raised, wooden floor is the best surface for shock absorption and can reduce stress on the body. Outdoor courts typically are made of concrete and can contribute to such injuries as stress fractures and shin splints.[25]

Athletes also need to be aware of the ambient temperature where they are playing. The higher the temperature, the more important fluid replacement becomes. Without adequate hydration, the athlete will fatigue more rapidly. Fatigued players are at a higher risk of injury.[25,74,75]

The game schedule also can influence susceptibility to injury. The greater the time between games, the better is an athlete's performance. Research has found that greater than 1 day between games increases the home team's score by 1.1 points and the visitor's score by 1.6 points. Peak performance occurs with 3 days between games.[76]

Training errors also can contribute to overuse injuries. Too much stress with too little time for healing and recovery leads to inflammation from repetitive microtrauma. Overtraining can be avoided with a periodized strength and conditioning program that takes the game schedule into account.[18,25,77]

Injury rates for basketball vary by the competitive level. Injuries in college occur more frequently during practices,[78] whereas injuries at the professional level occur more frequently during games.[79]

Finally, player-to-player contact can result in injuries. Basketball is not a collision sport like football, but it does involve contact. The majority of contact occurs when playing aggressive defense, when positioning for a rebound or when a flagrant foul is committed. Good officiating can reduce the amount of player-to-player contact and unnecessary injuries.[25]

Common Injuries and Their Rehabilitation

LOWER EXTREMITY

The majority of musculoskeletal injuries are to the lower extremity. The ankle is the most frequently injured area, followed by the knee and groin.[63,80,81] In a study of basketball players, 92 percent had suffered an ankle sprain at least once during their career. The injury frequency was 5.5 ankle injuries per 1000 activity hours.[82,83]

Foot and Ankle Injuries

Lateral ankle sprains involving the anterior talofibular ligament (ATFL), calcaneofibular ligament (CFL), and occasionally the posterior talofibular ligament (PTFL) are often the result of a player landing on the lateral border of one foot and rolling the foot inward.[72,84] This usually occurs when a player jumps and lands with the foot in a plantarflexed and inverted position or lands on someone else's foot. Lateral instability may occur depending on the grade of ligament sprain. Basketball players with a history of ankle sprains demonstrate a larger mean postural sway and have a larger sway area.[82,83]

A grade 1 sprain has tearing of some of the fibers with minimal pain and ecchymosis (swelling). A grade 2 sprain has partial tearing of the fibers with increased swelling and severe pain. A grade 3 sprain has complete rupture of the fibers, severe swelling, and instability. Depending on the severity of the swelling and pain, ROM may be limited. A muscle strain of the peroneals is also common and associated with eversion weakness. Special tests include an anterior draw test for the ATFL and the medial talar tilt for the CFL. The distal tibiofibular ligament also can be injured with a rotational mechanism of injury.

In the acute phase of rehabilitation, immobilization in slight eversion is recommended to allow for scar tissue to be laid down around the torn ligament. This should be accompanied by rest, ice, compression, and elevation (RICE). Other modalities such as contrast baths, electrical stimulation, and neuromuscular electrical stimulation (NMES) can be helpful to decrease the swelling. Immobilization is often accomplished with bracing, but casting is used in more severe sprains. Once the swelling and pain are decreased, active ROM is initiated along with submaximal isometric training in midrange. This can be accomplished with manual resistance or resistance against a fixed object. Caution should be taken with allowing end-range plantarflexion and inversion secondary to the stress placed on the ATFL. This includes avoiding early calf raises. Soft tissue mobilization is used to align collagen fibers. Strength training is progressed gradually to eccentric resistance. Theraband or a cuff weight around the foot is helpful to isolate muscles in an open-chain environment.

A progressive water resistance and isokinetic program also can assist in building strength. While performing these exercises, the inversion motion should be limited. As stability and strength increase, controlled mobility exercises can be initiated with balance/proprioception exercises in the midrange. Useful exercise include single-leg squats and single-leg stance while the patient maintains a subtalar-neutral position. When static balance is at least 30 s, dynamic balance exercises such as with a BAPS board can be added. The motion should be pain-free, and the athlete should not watch his or her foot when performing the activity. Balance and proprioception are extremely important for all basketball players. Following ankle sprains, athletes have demonstrated shorter myotatic reflexes in the triceps surae muscle, increased area covered for center of foot pressure displacements, and difficulty maintaining postural control.[85]

A proprioception program for the lower extremities should include:

- Double-/single-leg stance (eyes open to closed)
- Balance/rocker board (two feet to one foot)
- Minitrampoline (hopping, jumping forward/backward/diagonal) progressing from two feet to one foot

As the patient progresses to jogging, the focus shifts to sport-specific rehabilitation. This includes advancing the athlete to jumping, cutting, and pivoting. Table 13.9 shows a step-hop-jump plyometric program for the lower extremities.

The rehabilitation is the same for peroneal injuries. If there is peroneus longus involvement, first metatarsal stabilization exercises should be included. Soft tissue mobilization is also important. This can be performed with cross-friction massage over the area of injury to assist in realigning scar tissue. Ruptures of the lateral retinaculum can occur. This can lead to snapping of the peroneus longus tendon over the lateral malleolus. Testing for this involves resisting eversion throughout the ROM. The snapping can be minimized by modifying the ankle position and limiting the ROM as exercise is performed.

Medial ankle sprains are less common but also can occur from landing improperly or by pushing off the outside foot, causing the ankle to evert excessively.[72] The deltoid ligament is very strong, and consequently, an avulsion fracture of the medial malleolus can occur. Occasionally, there is tearing of the interosseous membrane as well. A lateral talar tilt/eversion stress test can screen for medial instability. The rehabilitation principles would be the same as for the lateral ankle sprain. However, excessive eversion is limited in the early phases. Eccentric strengthening, proprioception training, and sport-specific drills remain important. Sprains also occur of the distal tibiofibular ligament. Athletes with such sprains will have pain with excessive dorsiflexion as a result of the wider anterior portion of the talus spreading the tibia and fibula. They also will complain of pain with rotational movement.

Tarsal tunnel injuries also occur in basketball players. The symptoms are pain on the anteromedial side of the ankle and numbness and tingling along the medial column of the foot. Treatment involves promoting good bony alignment through intrinsic and extrinsic strengthening. Orthotics often are prescribed to correct the faulty biomechanics.

Achilles Tendinitis

Achilles tendinitis is common in basketball players because of the repetitive eccentric loading of the tendon. The forces that need to be attenuated during the contact phase of running and jumping are approximately eight times body weight.[86] A 2 to 4 percent elongation strain causes initial deformation of the tendon's structure, where the collagen fibrils tighten. At 8 to 10 percent of elongation, there is breaking of the collagen crosslinks, and mechanical failure occurs. The most common region for failure is 2 to 6 cm proximal to the insertion of the tendon. This is a region of poor circulation.[86]

Treatment in the acute stage includes RICE and modalities. Once the inflammation is decreased, eccentric training needs to be the main focus, beginning with manual resistance or Theraband and progressive weight bearing. The athlete should ideally have 15

degrees of active dorsiflexion while in subtalar neutral before ambulating full weight bear in a sneaker.[72] Heel lifts can be used to decrease stress on the achilles tendon, and orthotics are often used to control excessive rear-foot motion.[87] Once strength is 85 percent, box jumping and sports drills should be incorporated. Extreme caution should be taken with cortisone injections because of secondary tissue deterioration. If proper care is not given, an Achilles tendon rupture can occur. It is also important to inspect the sneakers. Extra padding in the back lip of the shoes can cause a friction rub where the tendon inserts into the calcaneus.

Achilles tendon ruptures can occur with forceful eccentric loading into ankle dorsiflexion. Athletes will state subjectively that they felt like they were hit with a baseball bat or kicked in the back of the calf. A special test for a completely torn Achilles tendon is the Thompson test. To perform this test, the athlete lies prone, and the calf muscle is squeezed. With an intact Achilles tendon, the foot will plantarflex. Most tears and complete ruptures require surgery for return to sport. When reattaching the tendons, surgeons often reinforce the repair with the plantaris tendon to assist with support and increase blood flow. (Refer to Chap. 12 for the rehabilitation approaches after an achilles tendon repair.)

Shin Splints

Medial shin splints are common in basketball players from the impact forces incurred during repetitive jumping and running. Players who excessively pronate can suffer from posterior tibialis tendinitis at the musculotendinous junction of the medial tibia. The posterior tibialis muscle concentrically supinates the foot and eccentrically controls pronation. Posterior tibialis tendinitis is usually associated with eccentric weakness of the posterior tibialis and weakness of the intrinsic foot muscles, flexor digitorum longus, and flexor

TABLE 13.9

Step-Jump-Hop Plyometric Progression

1. Step-ups
   Level 1: 2-in box
   Level 2: 4-in box
   Level 3: 6-in box
   Level 4: 8-in box
2. Jump-ups (two-legged)
   Level 1: 2-in box
   Level 2: 4-in box
   Level 3: 6-in box
   Level 4: 8-in box
3. Hop-ups (one-legged)
   Level 1: 2-in box
   Level 2: 4-in box
   Level 3: 6-in box
   Level 4: 8-in box
4. Hop-downs with repeat
   forward hop (one-legged)
   Level 1: 2-in box
   Level 2: 4-in box
   Level 3: 6-in box
   Level 4: 8-in box

2. Step-downs
   Level 1: 2-in box
   Level 2: 4-in box
   Level 3: 6-in box
   Level 4: 8-in box
4. Jump-downs (two-legged)
   Level 1: 2-in box
   Level 2: 4-in box
   Level 3: 6-in box
   Level 4: 8-in box
6. Hop-downs (one-legged)
   Level 1: 2-in box
   Level 2: 4-in box
   Level 3: 6-in box
   Level 4: 8-in box

hallucis longus.[87,88] Treatment should include eccentric training by having the athlete begin in supination and control the lowering into pronation. The BAPS board with a weight in the posterior medial compartment also can be used to train the posterior tibialis. It is important to decrease excessive pronation through the use of orthotics or sneakers.

Knee Injuries

Knee injuries are the second most common injury, after ankle injuries.[63,89] Knee injuries are the most common cause of missed games (66 percent)[77] and can occur from contact, sudden changes in direction, or overuse. Overuse injuries are secondary to improper training or conditioning, excessive stress, or fatigue. Acute knee injuries can occur to the meniscus, ligaments, and patella.[90]

Meniscal Injuries Meniscal injuries often occur from jumping, pivoting, and cutting. The athlete may complain of a locking feeling, limited knee extension, joint-line tenderness, and a positive McMurray test.

Knee Ligament Injuries Ligament injuries can occur from tibial and femoral rotation during cutting, pivoting, deceleration, landing off balance, or another player falling into the lower extremity. A medial collateral ligament (MCL) injury is caused by a valgus stress, whereas a lateral collateral ligament (LCL) injury is caused by a varus stress, most often at 20 degrees of knee flexion. An ACL injury can be caused by a combination of any of these movements. ACL injuries usually occur with external or internal rotation of the tibia, with or without hyperextension. ACL injuries are not very common in professional basketball and frequently have a noncontact mechanism of injury.[91] Over six seasons of men's professional basketball (NBA), there were only 13 ACL injuries that required reconstruction. The injury rate was 1.4 percent per year. The breakdown by position is guards 0.8 percent per year, forwards 2.0 percent per year, and centers 1.7 percent per year.[92] (See Chaps. 11 and 12 for MCL and ACL rehabilitation.)

Patellar Tendinitis (Jumper's Knee) *Jumper's knee* usually refers to tendinitis of the patellar tendon at the insertion into the tibial tubercle. It is referred to as *quadriceps tendinitis* when it occurs at the insertion to the superior portion of the patella. The eccentric overload can cause a mineralization of the fibrocartilage.[93] With the repetitive stress of sprinting, deceleration, and jumping, microtears occur. The eccentric force of the quadriceps is usually much greater than the concentric force.[94,95] The goal of rehabilitation is to decrease the stress and inflammatory progression. Once the pain and inflammation have subsided, hamstring and quadriceps stretching and strengthening should be added. It is important to evaluate the playing surface and fitness level of the athlete. Hard surfaces, shoes with a lack of shock absorption, and deconditioning can be contributing factors to the injury. Often a Chopat strap–patellar tendon strap will assist in redistributing the forces along the patellar tendon. Strengthening often begins in the pool to decrease gravitational forces. Progression to minisquats and knee extensions will focus on the eccentric component and will assist in the rehabilitation progression. As the athlete moves to step-downs, a progression

to sport-specific activities is initiated. Jumping on a trampoline initially can help dissipate forces. Box jumps and other lower extremity plyometric exercises will help restore strength for a safe return to sport.

In adolescent athletes, it is often common to see Osgood-Schlatter's disease.[96] There will be tenderness to palpation over the tibial tubercle and an increase in bone growth at the tubercle. The initial focus of rehabilitation is relative rest, hamstring flexibility, patellar tendon strapping, and avoiding early quadriceps stretching. Hip strength should also be tested

Patellofemoral pain is also common from the continuous running and jumping. (See Chap. 9 for the rehabilitation of patellofemoral pain.)

Hamstring Strains

Hamstring strains can occur from large eccentric forces. They are often the result of training errors. The athlete may not have warmed up properly or stretched adequately (including dynamic stretching). In addition, excessive quadriceps training to increase vertical jump height and running speed can contribute to a quadriceps-hamstring strength imbalance. The recommended ratio is 3:2. Large concentric quadriceps forces can lead to hamstring strains.[63] Most often the strain occurs at the proximal origin, but it also can occur at the semimembranosus with discomfort along the posterior medial knee capsule.[97,98] Immediate treatment consists of RICE, after which strength, flexibility, and proprioception must be restored. It is important to check for lumbar spine involvement as well. Eccentric hamstring training and sciatic nerve mobilization should be part of the plan of care.

Upper Leg/Thigh Contusions

A contusion usually occurs from direct contact with an opposing player's elbow or knee.[63] As a result of this contact, blood vessels are damaged, and some hemorrhaging occurs. The severity of this injury is based on the depth and degree of damage. If a large hematoma forms, rest, ice, and compression are recommended. Deep massage is contraindicated secondary to the risk of developing myositis ossificans. Bone fractures and joint dislocations require emergency management.

Most injuries to the upper leg area are contusions from direct contact. Full recovery time can be estimated by the initial amount of ROM.[99] Treatments for contusions include RICE and progression to stretching and strengthening once the signs of acute inflammation are gone.

SPINE INJURIES

Most spine injuries in basketball occur in the lumbar spine. Lumbar spine injuries can be the result of repetitive trauma or a fall. Contusions, sprains, strains, and disk injuries do occur.[63,100] Most lumbar spine injuries are not serious, and they account for only 8.7 percent of the total reported injuries.[3,31,101] Most frequently, the athlete will complain of muscle spasms. Often muscle spasms occur as the body's protective mechanism from contusions, sprains, or strains. The basic treatment is rest, modalities, and a strengthening program to teach stabilization exercises for the trunk musculature.

With the repetitive extension movements during jumping and rebounding, basketball players may develop defects in the pars interarticularis.[100] These athletes will complain generally of unilateral pain and increased symptoms with hyperextension of the spine. A spondylolisthesis is a fracture of the pars interarticularis accompanied by vertebral instability. The symptoms usually are aggravated by lumbar extension and rotation. Education through lumbar spine exercises and trunk stabilization in neutral or slight flexion are important. Strengthening the multifidi has been found to be beneficial.[3] The athlete should be educated to minimize lumbar hyperextension.

The athlete can return to the sport after he or she demonstrates the ability to stabilize the spine during sport activities such as box jumping, running, and rebounding.

Sacral fractures are rare in basketball players unless they take a bad fall. Some basketball players use a jumping machine during training to increase their vertical jump height. This is basically a weighted squat machine. The repetitive axial loading can cause a sacral fracture. Caution must be taken with this type of exercise. Alternatives are weighted jump shoes and a weighted belt, which provide similar resistance without the axial loading.[102]

EYE INJURIES

Eye injuries can happen in basketball and are usually the result of being poked with a finger or elbow. Basketball accounts for 25 percent of all reported eye injuries sustained in sports.[103] Despite this statistic, it is reported that there are only 0.1 eye injuries per 1000 hours of practice and game situations.[104] These injuries generally need to be treated by a specialist.[105]

UPPER EXTREMITY
Wrist and Hand Injuries

Hand injuries such as sprains, contusions, and dislocations occur more frequently in basketball than in other sports.[80,106] Often, when deflecting a pass or with sudden changes in the direction of the ball, the fingers can become injured. This also can happen by getting a finger caught in the net or on another player's jersey. The fingers on both hands, especially the shooting hand, assist with ball trajectory and accuracy. When the return to sport is made too early, small injuries can cause long-term problems. These injuries often take a long time to heal. The small, permanent limitation in motion will cause lifelong problems, but these do not outweigh the desire of the athlete to play.[106,107]

Thumb Injuries

The metacarpophalangeal (MCP) joint is injured frequently. The metacarpal bone can become dislocated, and this is often difficult to detect.[106] Because of possible instability, the athlete is usually immobilized in a spica splint for 3 to 6 weeks and taped for protection following splinting. The collateral ligaments of the thumb also can be injured. The ulnar collateral ligament (UCL) is injured more commonly than the radial collateral ligament (RCL) and is referred to as *skier's thumb.* The injury is usually caused by excessive abduction of the thumb. For incomplete tears, a thumb spica cast is worn for 3 weeks with the MCP joint in 30 degrees of flexion. Once the cast is removed, isometrics and ROM need to be started on the MCP joint, avoiding end-range thumb abduction early on. Hand and thumb bracing or taping is important for protection against reinjury. (See Chap. 10 for rehabilitation of the skier's thumb.)

Carpometacarpal Joint Injuries

Injuries to the carpometacarpal (CMC) joints usually occur when the hand is in a fist.[111] There is often concern with the third and fifth fingers. A third CMC joint injury can damage the deep palmer arterial arch, and a fifth CMC joint injury can involve the ulnar nerve. Rehabilitation needs to begin with immobilization and modalities to decrease the swelling. Isometrics and wrist extension exercises are important. Tendon and nerve glides are also an important part of the rehabilitation. Instability can be a problem, for which splinting and taping can be useful.[108–110]

Proximal Interphalangeal Joint Injuries

Proximal interphalangeal (PIP) joint injuries can include damage to the capsule, ligaments, and tendons. Fractures also can occur.[111] A capsular/ligament injury is categorized into three grades. A grade 1 injury is stable with less than 20 degrees of angulation with varus or valgus stress. A grade 2 injury will have instability with varus or valgus stress with greater than 20 degrees of angulation. A grade 3 injury will be unstable. There is deformity with active ROM. Surgical repair is required for a grade 3 injury, whereas a grade 2 injury requires splinting for 2 to 4 weeks and "buddy taping" for 6 to 8 weeks. A grade 1 injury requires buddy taping or protective splinting.

A boutonniere deformity can occur with disruption of the central extensor tendon slip at its insertion into the middle phalanx. This is seen with forced flexion of the actively extended PIP joint.[109–111] With the extensor tendon being disrupted, the flexor tendons do not have an antagonist, and PIP joint flexion contractures can occur. Splinting the PIP joint in extension is required, but the patient is allowed to flex the distal interphalangeal joint.

Distal Interphalangeal Joint Injuries

The most common distal interphalangeal (DIP) joint injury is the mallet or baseball finger. This happens with a forced flexion of the DIP joint causing an avulsion of the terminal extensor tendon from the distal phalanx.[110] The athlete is splinted for 4 to 6 weeks with the DIP joint in extension, with movement allowed at the PIP joint. If an extension lag occurs over 35 degrees, surgery is usually indicated.[111]

Finger Fractures

Finger fractures that occur and are not displaced usually can be treated nonsurgically with splinting and buddy taping. Immobilization for 3 weeks is followed by an active ROM program. Passive ROM is initiated at 6 weeks with gentle strengthening. At 8 weeks, a full strength and conditioning program is permitted if there is no pain or swelling.[111]

Wrist Injuries

Wrist injuries usually occur as a result of falls. Fractures and ligament injuries can occur.

Wrist Fractures Scaphoid fractures are common and can be a serious injury. Pain is usually felt in the anatomic snuffbox and on the dorsal radial side of the wrist.[109–111] The concern is with nonunion scaphoid fractures because of possible necrosis of the bone. Healing depends on the blood supply, which is often damaged.

Wrist Ligament Injuries The ligament that stabilizes the scapholunate joint is often disrupted. A special test, the Watson test, can be performed to determine the stability of the joint.[111] The wrist is splinted to allow for protection, and wrist stabilization exercises are performed to increase stability around the joint. Early gripping exercises should be avoided because they cause spreading of the scaphoid and lunate and unnecessarily stress the ligament.

Shoulder Injuries

With repetitive overhead motion, basketball players can develop impingement syndromes and rotator cuff and biceps tendon degeneration. Repetitive shooting and rebounding drills can lead to this problem. (See Chaps. 2 and 6 for rotator cuff and impingement syndrome rehabilitation.)

Acromioclavicular (AC) injuries can occur from falling directly on the shoulder. This is usually associated with point tenderness and a possible step deformity between the clavicle and acromion. Early stabilization and attention to discomfort are very important. See the AC joint taping technique in Shamus and Shamus.[112] (See also Chap. 14 for rehabilitation approaches.)

HEAT EXHAUSTION

Basketball players, if not properly hydrated, can suffer from heat exhaustion. (See Chap. 12 for a discussion of the negative effects of heat exhaustion.) Heat exhaustion can be caused by a depletion of electrolytes and sodium. In normal, climatized individuals, rehydrating with water only can lead to heat exhaustion. It is important in athletes with high levels of activity to use replacement fluids that contain sodium and electrolytes. Athletes also can suffer from heat exhaustion simply as a result of the lack of water replacement.[63] See "Injury Prevention" above for proper rehydration procedures.

Return to Sport

PSYCHOLOGICAL ASPECTS

Sport and exercise psychology has made significant contributions to understanding the effective holistic response to the injured athlete, the rehabilitation process, and how to encourage the smoothest return to preinjury playing level and intensity. Athletes are vulnerable to having psychological reactions to injuries such that they can experience some degree of loss to identity as a skilled athlete, fear and anxiety regarding their future recovery, feelings of separation and loneliness from their teammates, a lack of confidence in their athletic and other skills, and performance decrements related to not properly pacing their return to playing status.[113] If an injured athlete is not approached and treated with an understanding of these potential responses, his or her rehabilitation and return to full function can, at the least, be delayed, stressful, or incomplete and, at the worst, result in continued reinjury, failure to resume playing, and/or serious emotional distress. Signs that an athlete is likely experiencing significant difficulties in adjusting to an injury include feelings of anger, depression, confusion, obsession with the question of when he or she can return to play, denial of the injury itself, dwelling on minor physical complaints, guilt about letting the team down, social withdrawal, substance abuse, eating disturbances, and/or repeated overly pessimistic statements about not being able to recover.

In light of these potential problematic reactions to injury, it is recommended that the professionals involved in the rehabilitation effort respond to the injured athlete by building rapport and showing sensitivity to what the injury means for the injured person, educating him or her about the injury and recovery process, teaching specific psychological coping skills, preparing for possible setbacks or plateaus in recovery, and fostering social support.[113] Of course, rapport building and coping skills training will likely proceed more smoothly if a sport psychologist had been involved with the athlete and his or her team in a preventive/educational role routinely prior to the injury. However, if this is not the case, as long as a referral is made to a sport psychologist in a sensitive manner as a regular member of the comprehensive rehabilitative team, the athlete will be less likely to misperceive the reasons for the referral, feel embarrassed or angry about it, and to refuse any such assistance. Similar to what was described previously, the psychological skills that have been found to be most helpful for rehabilitation include goal setting, positive self-talk, imagery and visualization, and relaxation training.[58,113–115] Appropriate sequencing of the rehabilitation process and the athlete's return to full playing status is critical, along with the importance of providing user-friendly skills instruction, practice with supervision and feedback, and graduated resumption of competitive play. These rehabilitation stages can be referred to as the *rapport-building phase, education phase, skills-development phase,* and finally, the *practice and evaluation phase.* Hopefully, the health care professional involved will develop and monitor the rehabilitation program in collaboration with the athlete's coaching personnel and supportive significant others (with the athlete's permission) to foster the least stressful and most successful recovery for the athlete.

LOWER EXTREMITY CONSIDERATIONS

If a player is recovering from a lower extremity injury, he or she usually can return to foul and set shooting prior to participating in a full practice session. Once the player can run without a limp, a gradual return to agility drills can be made. These drills include running forward, backward, sideways, diagonally, and in a zigzag fashion (Z course; Fig. 13.1), W sprints (Fig. 13.2), a box-run course (Fig. 13.3), and cariocas (crossovers). Cariocas are sideways running, crossing one leg over the other in front and then behind (Fig. 13.4). These drills should be progressed up to the full length of the basketball court (approximately 30 yd) for 10 repetitions. Next, dribbling around cones while catching and passing the basketball with another person should be added. Vertical jumping should be practiced at a 50 percent effort for 10 to 20 repetitions and progressed to 75 and 100 percent effort. This exercise can be transitioned to jumping while bouncing a basketball against the backboard. The goal per session is about 100 to 150 jumps. Players also need to practice layups, jump shots, set shots, and rebounding. Prior to returning to competitive play, the athlete must be able to perform plyometric exercises. Plyometric exercises can be found under "Injury Prevention" above.

After a proper warm-up and stretching, the athlete should participate in one-quarter, one-half, three-quarters, and then full practices. Following three full practices without pain or soreness, the athlete can return to competition.[90]

"Z" course (zigzag)

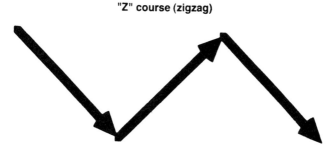

FIGURE 13.1

Zigzaging (Z course). *(Used with permission from Prentice W: Rehabilitation Techniques in Sports Medicine, 3d ed. New York: WCB/McGraw-Hill, 1999, Fig. 17-10, p 276.)*

CRITERIA FOR RETURN TO SPORT

Prior to returning an athlete to competition, the following criteria should be met:

- Time constraints for tissue healing have been observed.
- There is painfree full ROM of the joint.
- There is no persistent swelling.
- There is adequate muscle strength and endurance of at least 90 percent of the contralateral limb.
- Flexibility is equal bilaterally.

- Joint stability is maintained by muscle control and/or a brace or tape.
- There is good proprioception.
- Cardiovascular fitness is equal to or better than the requirements of competition.
- Skills have been regained.
- There is no biomechanical dysfunction.
- The athlete is ready psychologically.[19]

"W" sprint course

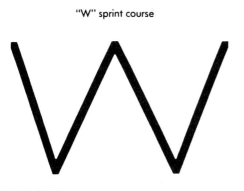

FIGURE 13.2

W sprints. *(Used with permission from Prentice W: Rehabilitation Techniques in Sports Medicine, 3d ed. New York: WCB/McGraw-Hill, 1999, Fig. 17-12, p 277.)*

Box run course

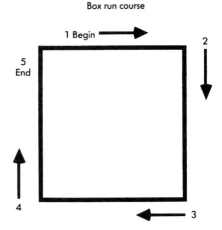

FIGURE 13.3

Box-run course. *(Used with permission from Prentice W: Rehabilitation Techniques in Sports Medicine, 3d ed. New York: WCB/McGraw-Hill, 1999, Fig. 17-13, p 277.)*

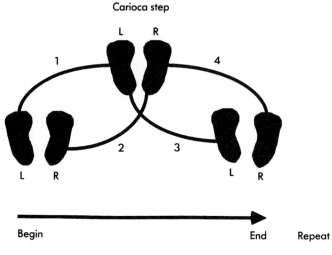

Carioca step

FIGURE 13.4

Carioca steps. *(Used with permission from Prentice W: Rehabilitation Techniques in Sports Medicine, 3d ed. New York: WCB/McGraw-Hill, 1999, Fig. 17-14, p 277.)*

References

1. Wilkes G: *Basketball: Sports and Fitness Series,* 7th ed. New York: McGraw-Hill, 1999.
2. Krause J: *Basketball: Winning Edge Series.* New York: McGraw-Hill, 1999.
3. Jackson D, Mannarino F: Lumbar spine in athletes, in Scott W, Nisonson B, Nicholas J (eds): *Principles of Sports Medicine.* Baltimore: Williams & Wilkins, 1984, pp 212–215.
4. Baechle TR: *Essentials of Strength Training and Conditioning.* Champaign, IL: Human Kinetics, 2000.
5. Chu D: Plyometrics, the link between strength and speed. *NSCA J* 5(2):20–21, 1983.
6. Aura O, Vitasalo JT: Biomechanical characteristics of jumping. *Int J Sport Biomech* 5(1): 89–97, 1989.
7. Stefanyshyn DJ, Nigg BM: Contribution of the lower extremity joints to mechanical energy in running vertical jumps and running long jumps. *J Sports Sci* 16(2):177–186, 1988.
8. van Soest AJ, Roebroeck ME, Bobbert MF, et al: A comparison of one-legged and two-legged counter movement jumps. *Med Sci Sports Exerc* 17(6):635–639, 1985.
9. Miller S, Bartlett R: The effects of increased shooting distance in the basketball jump shot. *J Sports Sci* 11(4):285–293, 1993.
10. Miller S, Bartlett R: The relationship between basketball shooting kinematics, distance and playing position. *J Sports Sci* 14(3):243–453, 1996.
11. Hamilton GR, Reinschmidt C: Optimal trajectory for the basketball free throw. *J Sports Sci* 15(5):491–504, 1997.
12. Taylor P: Clank! *Sports Illustrated* 81(19): 79–87, 1995.
13. Kingston G: Foul trouble. *The Vancouver Sun,* March 14, 1996, pp F1, F8.
14. Shoenfelt EL: Immediate effect of weight training as compared to aerobic exercise on free-throw shooting in collegiate basketball players. *Percept Motor Skills* 73(2):367–370, 1991.
15. Vickers JN: Control of visual attention during the basketball free throw. *Am J Sports Med* 24(suppl 6):93–100, 1996.
16. Vickers JN: Location of fixation, landing position of the ball and spatial visual attention

during the free throw. *Int J Sports Vis* 3(1): 54–60, 1996.

17. Posner M, Raichle M: *Images of Mind*. New York: Scientific American Library, 1991.

18. Stone WJ, Steingard PM: Year-round conditioning for basketball. *Clin Sports Med* 12(2): 173–192, 1993.

19. Brukner P, Khan K: *Clinical Sports Medicine*. Sydney, Australia: McGraw-Hill, 1993.

20. Beaulieu JE: *Stretching for All Sports*. Pasadena, CA: Athletic Press, 1980.

21. Walker SH: Delay of twitch relaxation induced by stress and stress relaxation. *J Appl Physiol* 16:801–806, 1961.

22. Prentice WE: A comparison of static stretching and PNF stretching for improving joint flexibility. *Athletic Training* 18(1):56–59, 1983.

23. Prentice WE: Flexibility, roundtable. *NSCA J* 6(4):10–22, 71–73, 1984.

24. Corbin CB, Dowell LJ, Lindsey R, Tolson H: *Concepts in Physical Education*. Dubuque, IA: William C Brown, 1978.

25. Bull RC: *Handbook of Sports Injuries*. New York: McGraw-Hill, 1999.

26. de Vries HA: *Physiology of Exercise for Physical Education and Athletics*. Dubuque, IA: William C Brown, 1974.

27. Foran W: *High Performance Sports Conditioning*. Champaign, IL: Human Kinetics, 2001.

28. Foran W, Pound R: *NBA Power Conditioning* (National Basketball Conditioning Coaches Association). Champaign, IL: Human Kinetics, 2000.

29. Chu D: Plyometric exercise. *NSCA J* 5(6): 56–64, 1984.

30. Lundin P: A review of plyometric training. *Track Field Q Rev* 89(4):37–40, 1989.

31. Ellison A: *Athletic Training and Sports Medicine*. Chicago: American Academy of Orthopeadic Surgeons, 1984, pp 409–411.

32. Fox EL: *Sports Physiology*. Philadelphia: Saunders, 1979.

33. Steingard SA: Special considerations in the medical management of professional basketball players. *Clin Sports Med* 12(2):239–246, 1993.

34. Sickles RT, Lombardo J: The adolescent basketball player. *Clin Sports Med* 12(2):207–220, 1993.

35. Hewett TE: Plyometric training in female athletes, decreased impact forces and increased hamstring torques. *Am J Sports Med* 24(6): 765–773, 1996.

36. Getchell B: *Physical Fitness, a Way of Life*. New York: Wiley, 1979.

37. Sitler M, Ryan J, Wheeler B, et al: The efficacy of a semirigid ankle stabilizer to reduce acute ankle injuries in basketball, a randomized clinical study at West Point. *Am J Sports Med* 22(4):454–461, 1994.

38. Ottaviani R, Ashton-Miller J, Kothari S, Wojtys E: Basketball shoe height and the maximal muscular resistance to applied ankle inversion and eversion moments. *Am J Sports Med* 23(4):418–429, 1995.

39. Karlsson J, Andreasson G: The effect of external ankle support in the chronic lateral joint instability. *Am J Sports Med* 20:257–261, 1992.

40. Shapiro M, Kabo J, Mitchell P, et al: Ankle sprain prophylaxis: An analysis of the stabilizing effects of braces and tape. *Am J Sports Med* 22:78–82, 1994.

41. Barrett JR, Tanji JL, Drake C, et al: High- versus low-top shoes for the prevention of ankle sprains in basketball players: A prospective randomized study. *Am J Sports Med* 21(4): 582–585, 1993.

42. Brizuela G, Llana S, Ferrandis R, Garcia-Belenguer AC: The influence of basketball shoes with increased ankle support on shock attenuation and performance in running and jumping. *J Sports Sci* 15(5):505–515, 1997.

43. Thacker SB: The prevention of ankle sprains in sports: A systematic review of the literature. *Am J Sports Med* 27(6):753–760, 1999.

44. MacKean LC, Bell G, Burnham RS: Prophylactic ankle bracing vs taping effects on functional performance in female basketball players. *J Orthop Sports Phys Ther* 22(2):77–81, 1995.

45. McInnes SE, Carlson JS, Jones CJ, McKenna MJ: The physiological load imposed on basketball players during competition. *J Sports Sci* 13(5):387–397, 1995.

46. Lehmann M, Dickhutn H, Gendrisch G, et al: Training overtraining: A prospective, experimental study with experienced middle and long-distance runners. *Int J Sports Med* 12: 444–452, 1991.

47. Fry AC: Resistance exercise overtraining and overreaching, neuroendocrine responses. *Sports Med* 23(2):106–129, 1997.

48. Brewer BW, Petrie TA: Psychopathology in sport and exercise, in Van Raalte JL, Brewer BW (eds): *Exploring Sport and Exercise Psychology*. Washington: American Psychological Association, 1996, pp 257–274.

49. Coddington RD, Troxell JR: The effect of emotional factors on football injury rates: A pilot study. *J Hum Stress* 6:3–5, 1980.

50. Cryan PD, Alles WF: The relationship between stress and college football injuries. *J Sports Med Phys Fitness* 23:52–58, 1983.

51. Williams JM, Tonyman P, Wadsworth WA: Relationship of life stress in injury in intercollegiate volleyball. *J Hum Stress* 12:38–43, 1986.

52. Lazarus RS, Folkman S: *Stress, Appraisal, and Coping*. New York: Springer, 1984.

53. Anderson MB, Williams JM: A model of stress and athletic injury: Prediction and prevention. *J Sport Exerc Psychol* 10:294–306, 1988.

54. Nideffer RM: The injured athlete: Psychological factors in treatment. *Orthop Clin North Am* 14:373–385, 1983.

55. Williams JM, Tonyman P, Anderson, MB: The effects of stressors and coping resources on anxiety and peripheral narrowing. *J Appl Sport Psychol* 3:126–141, 1991.

56. Smith RE, Smoll FL, Ptacek JT: Conjunctive moderator variables in vulnerability and resiliency research: Life stress, social support and coping skills and adolescent sport injuries. *J Person Soc Psychol* 58:360–369, 1990.

57. Rotella RJ, Heyman SR: Stress, injury, and the psychological rehabilitation of athletes, in Williams JM (ed): *Applied Sport Psychology: Personal Growth to Peak Performance*. Palo Alto, CA: Mayfield, 1986, pp 343–364.

58. Weinberg RS, Gould D: *Foundations of Sport and Exercise*. Champaign, IL: Human Kinetics, 1995.

59. Kozar B, Lord RM: Overuse injuries in the young athlete: Reasons for concern. *Phys Sports Med* 11:221–226, 1983.

60. Noakes TD, Schomer H: The eager parent syndrome and schoolboy injuries. *S Afr Med J* 63:956–968, 1983.

61. Savoy C, Beitel P: Mental imagery for basketball. *Int J Sport Psychol* 27:454–462, 1996.

62. Savoy C: Two individualized mental training programs for a team sport. *Int J Sport Psychol* 28:259–270, 1997.

63. Sonzogni JJ Jr, Gross ML: Assessment and treatment of basketball injuries. *Clin Sports Med* 12(2):221–237, 1993.

64. Scheller A, Rask B: A protocol for the health and fitness assessment of NBA players. *Clin Sports Med* 12(2):193–206, 1993.

65. Moretz JA III, Grana W: High school basketball injuries. *Phys Sports Med* 6(10):92–95, 1978.

66. Arendt E, Dick R: Knee injury patterns among men and women in collegiate basketball and soccer NCAA data and review of literature. *Am J Sports Med* 23(6):694–709, 1995.

67. Zillmer D, Powell J, Albright J: Gender-specific injury patterns in high school varsity basketball. *J Womens Health* 1(1):69–76, 1992.

68. Weesner C, Albohm M, Ritter M: A comparison of anterior and posterior cruciate ligament laxity between female and male basketball players. *Phys Sports Med* 14(5):149–154, 1986.

69. Gray J, Taunton J, McKenzie D, et al: A survey of injuries to the ACL of the knee in female basketball players. *Int J Sports Med* 6(6):314–316, 1985.

70. Ireland ML, Wall C: Epidemiology and comparison of knee injuries in elite male and female US basketball athletes. *Med Sci Sports Exerc* 22(S):82, 1990.

71. Micheli LJ, Metzl JD, Di Canzio J, Zurakowski D: Anterior cruciate ligament reconstructive surgery in adolescent soccer and basketball players. *Clin J Sport Med* 9(3):138–141, 1999.

72. Nicholas J, Hershman E: *The Lower Extremity and Spine in Sports Medicine*, Vol 1. St Louis: Mosby, 1986.

73. Rozzi SL, Lephart SM, Gear WS, Fu FH: Knee joint laxity and neuromuscular characteristics of male and female soccer and basketball players. *Am J Sports Med* 27(3):312–319, 1999.

74. Bolonchuk WW, Lukaski HC, Siders WA: The structural, functional, and nutritional adaptation of college basketball players over a season. *J Sports Med Phys Fitness* 31(2):165–172, 1991.

75. Hoffman JR, Stavsky H, Falk B: The effect of water restriction on anaerobic power and vertical jumping height in basketball players. *Int J Sports Med* 16(4):214–218, 1995.

76. Steenland K, Deddens JA: Effect of travel and rest on performance of professional basketball players. *Sleep* 20(5):366–369, 1997.

77. Molnar TJ, Fox JM: Overuse injuries of the knee in basketball. *Clin Sports Med* 12(2): 349–362, 1993.

78. Gomez E, DeLee J, Farney W: Incidence of injury in Texas girls' high school basketball. *Am J Sports Med* 24(5):684–692, 1996.

79. Zelisko JA, Noble HB, Porter M: A comparison of men's and women's professional basketball injuries. *Am J Sports Med* 10(5): 297–299, 1982.

80. Pfeifer JP, Gast W, Pforringer W: Traumatology and athletic injuries in basketball. *Sportverlezung Sportschaden* 6(3):91–100, 1992.

81. Engel J, Baharav U, Modan M: Epidemiology of basketball players. *Harefuah* 119(5–6): 121–124, 1990.

82. Leanderson J, Nemeth G, Eriksson E: Ankle injuries in basketball players. *Knee Surg Sports Traumatol Arthroscopy* 1(3–4):200–202, 1993.

83. Leanderson J, Wykman A, Eriksson E: Ankle sprain and postural sway in basketball players. *Knee Surg Sports Traumatol Arthroscopy* 1(3–4):203–205, 1993.

84. Blazina M, Fox JM, Carlson GJ: Basketball injuries, in Craig TT (ed): *The Medical Aspects of Sports*, Vol 15. Chicago: American Medical Association, 1974, pp 50–52.

85. Perrin P, Bene M, Perrin C, Durupt D: Ankle trauma significantly impairs posture control: A study in basketball players. *Int J Sports Med* 18(5):387–392, 1997.

86. Traina SM, Yonezuka NY, Zinis YC: Achilles tendon injury in a professional basketball player. *Orthopedics* 22(6):625–626, 1999.

87. McDermott EP: Basketball injuries of the foot and ankle. *Clin Sports Med* 12(2):373–393, 1993.

88. Hosea TM, Carey CC, Harrer MF: The gender issue: Epidemiology of ankle injuries in athletes who participate in basketball. *Clin Orthop* (372):45–49, 2000.

89. Chandy TA, Grana WA: Secondary school athletic injury in boys and girls: A three-year comparison. *Phys Sports Med* 13:106–111, 1985.

90. Peppard A: Knee rehabilitation, in Canavan P (ed): *Rehabilitation in Sports Medicine*. Stanford, CT: Appleton and Lange, 1998, pp 320–321.

91. Henry J, Lareau B, Neigut D: The injury rate in professional basketball. *Am J Sports Med* 10:16–18, 1982.

92. Starkey C: *National Basketball Association Injury Statistics*. New York: National Basketball Association, 1992.

93. Roels J, Martens M, Mulier J, et al: Patellar tendinitis (jumper's knee). *Am J Sports Med* 6: 363, 1978.

94. Bennet J, Stauber W: Evaluation and treatment of anterior knee pain using eccentric exercise. *Med Sci Sports Exerc* 18:526, 1986.

95. Pavone E, Moffat M: Isometric torque of the quadriceps femoris after concentric, eccentric and isometric training. *Arch Phys Med Rehabil* 66:168, 1985.

96. Mital M, Mitza R: Osgood-Schlatter's disease: The painful puzzler. *Phys Sports Med* 5:60, 1977.

97. Hunter S, Poole R: The chronically inflamed tendon. *Clin Sports* 6:371, 1987.

98. Ray J, Clancy, Lemon R: Semimembranosus tendinitis: An overlooked cause of medial knee pain. *Am J Sports Med* 16:347, 1988.

99. Jackson DW, Feagin JA: Quadriceps contusion in young athletes: Relationship of severity of injury to treatment and prognosis. *J Bone Joint Surg* 55A:95–101, 1973.

100. Herskowitz A, Selesnick H: Back injuries in basketball players. *Clin Sports Med* 12(2): 293–306, 1993.

101. National Basketball Trainers Association: *NBAT Injury Reporting System, 1990–1991 Season*. New York: National Basketball Association, 1991, pp 1–6.

102. Crockett H, Wright J, Madsen M, et al: Sacral stress fracture in an elite college basketball player after the use of a jump machine. *Am J Sports Med* 27(4):526–528, 1997.

103. Jones NP: Eye injury in sports. *Sports Med* 7:163–181, 1989.

104. National Collegiate Athletic Association Injury Surveillance System, Health and Safety Education Outreach, Indianapolis, 1989–1990.

105. Zagelbaum BM, Starkey C, Hersh PS, et al: The National Basketball Association eye injury study. *Arch Ophthalmol* 113(6):749–52, 1995.

106. Strickland J, Rettig A: *Hand Injuries in Athletes*. Philadelphia: Saunders, 1992.

107. McCue F, Baugher W, Kirlund D, et al: Hand and wrist injuries in the athlete. *Am J Sports Med* 7:275, 1979.

108. Amadio P: Epidemiology of hand and wrist injuries in sports. *Hand Clin* 6:379,1990.

109. Culver JE, Anderson TE: Fractures of the hand and wrist of the athlete. *Clin Sports Med* 9:85, 1990.

110. Doyle JR: Extensor tendons, acute injuries, in Green DP (ed): *Operative Hand Surgery*, 2d ed, Vol 3. New York: Churchill-Livingstone, 1988, p 2045.

111. Wilson RL, McGinty L: Common hand and wrist injuries in basketball players. *Clin Sports Med* 12(2):265–291,1993.

112. Shamus J, Shamus E: A taping technique for the treatment of acromioclavicular joint sprains: A case study. *JOSPT* 25:390–394, 1997.

113. Petitpas A, Danish S: Caring for injured athletes, in Murphy S (ed): *Sport Psychology Interventions*. Champaign, IL: Human Kinetics, 1995, pp 255–281.

114. Hardy CJ, Crace RK: Dealing with injury. *Sport Psychol Train Bull* 1:1–8, 1990.

115. Wiese DM, Weiss MR: Psychological rehabilitation and physical injury: Implications for the sportsmedicine team. *Sport Psychol* 1: 318–330, 1987.

Additional References

Applegate RA, Applegate RA: Set shot shooting performance and visual acuity in basketball. *Optom Vis Sci* 69(10):765–768, 1992.

Dendrinos G, Zisis G, Terzopoulos H: Recurrence of subtalar dislocation in a basketball player. *Am J Sports Med* 22(1):143–145, 1994.

Fernandez FM, Guillen J, Busto JM, Roura J: Fractures of the fifth metatarsal in basketball players. *Knee Surg Sports Traumatol Arthroscopy* 7(6):373–377, 1999.

Friedman SM: Optic nerve avulsion secondary to a basketball injury. *Ophthalmic Surg Lasers* 30(8): 676–677, 1999.

Goudas M, Theodorakis Y, Karamousalidis G: Psychological skills in basketball: Preliminary study for development of a Greek form of the Athletic Coping Skills Inventory-28. *Percept Motor Skills* 86(1):59–65, 1998.

Guyette R: Facial injuries in basketball players. *Clin Sports Med* 12(2):247–264, 1993.

Hakkinen K: Force production characteristics of leg extensor, trunk flexor and extensor muscles in male and female basketball players. *J Sports Med Phys Fitness* 31(3):325–331, 1991.

Hickey GJ, Fricker PA, McDonald WA: Injuries of young elite female basketball players over a six-year period. *Clin J Sport Med* 7(4):252–256, 1997.

Hoffman JR, Bar-Eli M, Tenenbaum G: An examination of mood changes and performance in a professional basketball team. *J Sports Med Phys Fitness* 39(1):74–79, 1999.

Johnson E, Markolf K: The contribution of the anterior talofibular ligament to ankle laxity. *J Bone Joint Surg* 65A:81–88, 1983.

Jukic I, Milanovic D, Vuleta D: Analysis of changes in indicators of functional and motor readiness of female basketball players within one-year training cycles. *Coll Antropol* 23(2): 691–706, 1999.

Khan KM, Cook JL, Kiss ZS, et al: Patellar tendon ultrasonography and jumper's knee in female basketball players: a longitudinal study. *Clin J Sport Med* 7(3):199–206, 1997.

Kioumourtzoglou E, Derri V, Tzetzis G, Theodorakis Y: Cognitive, perceptual, and motor abilities in skilled basketball performance. *Percept Motor Skills* 86(3 pt 1):771–786, 1998.

Kioumourtzoglou E, Kourtessis T, Michalopoulou M, Derri V: Differences in several perceptual abilities between experts and novices in basketball, volleyball and water polo. *Percept Motor Skills* 86(3 pt 1):899–912, 1998.

Lamirand M, Rainey D: Mental imagery, relaxation, and accuracy of basketball foul shooting. *Percept Motor Skills* 78(3 pt 2):1229–1230, 1994.

Landin DK, Hebert EP, Fairweather M: The effects of variable practice on the performance of a basketball skill. *Res Q Exerc Sport* 64(2): 232–237, 1993.

Liu S, Burton AW: Changes in basketball shooting patterns as a function of distance. *Percept Motor Skills* 89(3 pt 1):831–845, 1999.

Messina D, Farney W, DeLee J: The incidence of injury in Texas high school basketball. *Am J Sports Med* 27(3):294–306, 1999.

National Basketball Association, All-Star Break Team Physicians Meeting. Orlando, Florida, February 8, 1992.

Pynn BR, Bartkiw TP, Clarke HM: Ring avulsion injuries and the basketball player. *Br J Sports Med* 31(1):72–74, 1997.

Southard D, Miracle A: Rhythmicity, ritual, and motor performance: A study of free throw shooting in basketball. *Res Q Exerc Sport* 64(3):284–290, 1993.

Stephens DL: The effects of functional knee braces on speed in collegiate basketball players. *JOSPT* 22(6):259–262, 1995.

Trninic S, Perica A, Dizdar D: Set of criteria for the actual quality evaluation of the elite basketball players. *Coll Antropol* 23(2):707–721, 1999.

Tsur A, Shahin R: Suprascapular nerve entrapment in a basketball player. *Harefuah* 133(5–6):190–192, 247, 1997.

Whitehead R, Butz JW, Kozar B, Vaughn RE: Stress and performance: An application of Gray's three-factor arousal theory to basketball free throw shooting. *J Sports Sci* 14(5):393–401, 1996.

CHAPTER 14

Soccer

Suzanne Gassé

Each year thousands of new participants take to the soccer fields. Soccer is the most popular sport in the world, with an estimated 120 million participants worldwide.[1,2,37] In fact, the 1999 Women's World Cup final had the largest viewing audience of any women's sport in history. The explosion of participants can be attributed to several factors. The game is fairly easy to understand, relatively inexpensive to play, and easily accessible to children (and many parents encourage the participation in soccer over more so-called dangerous sports like football and hockey).[1] Because of this soccer craze, it is important for medical professionals working with these athletes to understand the demands of the sport and how to recognize and treat commonly seen injuries.

Outdoor soccer is played on a field 100 to 130 yd long and 50 to 100 yd wide, according to the governing body, the Federation International Football Association (FIFA). The goal is 8 yd wide by 8 ft high. A regulation game consists of two 45-min halves. The halftime does not exceed 15 min. In outdoor soccer, there are 11 players on the field at one time: 10 field players and 1 goalkeeper.

The soccer ball varies in circumference based on the player's age. A size 3, 4, or 5 ball is used. Size 3 is used for 6- to 9-year-olds. Size 4 is used for 10- to 13-year-olds. The size 5 ball is the regulation size for players aged 14 to adult and professional players.[3] It is 28 inches in circumference and weighs 14 to 16 oz. It is made of leather or a similar material. Uniforms consist of shorts, shirts, and cleats or turf shoes. The goalkeeper must wear a different color jersey from the rest of the team and the opponent's team. Shin guards are the only true protective equipment that a soccer player uses.

Indoor soccer varies slightly in field or court size, time of the match, and number of players on the field at one time. Indoor soccer is played on an artificial-turf field that is 27 to 46 yd long and 16 to 27 yd wide. Boards similar to that of an ice hockey arena surround the field. The boards keep the ball in play and allow for a faster pace of the game. The goal is 10 ft wide by 7 ft high. The game is divided into two 20-min halves with a half-time not to exceed 15 min. There are five players on the field, one being the goalkeeper.

Like outdoor soccer, the ball used for indoor play weighs 14 to 16 oz. The ball is also made of leather or similar material and is 24 to 25 inches in circumference. Uniforms are similar to outdoor soccer with the exception of the shoes. Because of the artificial playing turf, the players wear turf shoes or tennis shoes for improved traction.

The names of the positions vary based on the formations being used. Defenders are primarily responsible for preventing the opposition from attacking the goal and scoring. These positions include fullbacks, sweepers, and stoppers. Midfielders are the transitional line between the defense and forwards. They are responsible for both offense and defense. The "goal scorers" are the forwards or strikers. Their main role is to attack the opponent's goal and to score. The team with the most points at the end of the game is the winner. The goalkeeper is the only player allowed to use his or her hands in both indoor and outdoor soccer.

Skills of the sport include several types of kicking and passing. In most cases, the player may kick with the inside, outside, or instep of the foot depending on whether distance, accuracy, or a touch of chicanery is the objective. Other skills required include heading the ball, trapping or bringing the ball under control, and dribbling or progressing the ball with the feet while under control.

Biomechanics

KICKING

Kicking differs from walking and running because the main force is generated from the swing leg, not the stance limb. Another differ-ence is the speed of the limb. The speed of the swing leg is faster in kicking than in running or walking.[3] When studying the biomechanics of kicking, it is important to remember that it can vary greatly from one individual to the next as well as from one instance to the next in the same individual. A shot on the goal will have a different approach than a pass to another player making a run up the field. It is important to understand the key elements of a kick and the muscle groups involved. A basic knowledge of the muscles that are active at different moments of a kick will help the rehabilitation specialist prepare an athlete to return to the sport and also will help reduce injuries through proper preseason training and conditioning.

The most basic element of soccer is kicking.[3,5,38] There are three main factors that make a kick more or less successful. First is the development of velocity in the swing limb. Timing and the angle of approach of the kicker contribute to swing-limb velocity. Second is the placement of the foot on the ball. Third is the ability to maintain a rigid foot and ankle at ball contact.[3] There are six main components of kicking: the approach angle, plant-foot forces, swing-limb loading, hip flexion and knee extension, foot contact with the ball, and follow-through.[5] These components will now be discussed in detail.

Approach Angle

The approach angle dictates the path of the ball. Based on the kicking objective of the player, the angle at which he or she approaches the ball prior to foot contact will vary. In the straight approach, there is limited rotation around the vertical axis of the body. As the approach angle increases, the leg must rotate around the vertical axis to kick the ball straight. Also as the approach angle increases, the ground reaction force is reduced by the torque generated by the swing limb. At an angle of 45 to 60 degrees, a greater mechanical advantage is created by the swing limb that balances the resistance torque generated by body motion, thereby increasing leg and foot momentum on initial contact. Skilled players use this approach angle more frequently than their unskilled counterparts.[5]

A diagonal approach will increase swing-limb velocity and ball velocity. Peak ball velocity and peak angle velocity are greatest with a 45-degree angle of approach. However, peak velocity of the hip is greatest at a 15-degree angle of approach, and peak knee velocity is greatest at a 0-degree angle of approach. Two other factors that affect ball velocity are effective foot mass and foot velocity immediately prior to ball contact. Foot velocity before initial contact is similar in both straight and diagonal approaches; therefore, effective mass of the foot has the greatest effect on ball velocity in either a straight or angled approach.[5]

Plant-Foot Position

The position of the plant foot is important in determining the direction of the ball's path. Optimal plant-foot placement is 5 to 10 cm to the side of the ball. Placing the foot in a direct line perpendicular to the center of the ball allows for the most effective instep kick. (Fig. 14.1A). Skilled players are more likely to mimic this position versus their unskilled counterparts, who tend to place the plant foot further behind the ball.[5] If the plant foot is too far from the ball, the kicker will be off balance and therefore less efficient in the kick. Velocity subsequently will be compromised. In addition, the further behind the ball the plant foot is placed, the more likely it is that the ball will become airborne.

Skilled players also kick faster than do unskilled players. They can generate greater ground reaction forces vertically, anteriorly, posteriorly, and laterally. Both the plant-foot position and the approach path affect the ve-

locity of the ball. Greater efficiency in both these phases contribute to the greater kicking speeds of skilled players.[5]

Swing-Limb Loading

The backswing allows the hip flexors and knee extensors to be stretched in preparation for forward motion of the limb. Just prior to initiation of the forward motion, the kicking knee should be flexed, and the foot should be at hip height. As the plant foot contacts the ground next to the ball, the hip of the swing limb is extended, the knee is flexed, and the ankle is plantarflexed. The kicker's eyes are focused on the ball at least briefly. The position of the plant foot and the position of the hips at ball contact will dictate the path of the ball.[5]

Swing-Limb Acceleration

The hip flexors and knee extensors contract concentrically to initiate the forward motion of the swing limb. Just before ball contact, a large extension torque at the knee is produced to provide rapid knee extension (see Fig. 14.1B). The lower leg and foot internally rotate together from an externally rotated position. As the thigh decelerates, the lower leg and foot accelerate as the result of a momentum shift. This transfer of momentum from the thigh to the lower leg and foot plays a critical role in the kicking motion. There is also a subsequent shift in angular velocities from the upper to the lower leg. Swing-limb velocity is influenced by hip rotation, followed by hip flexion and knee extension prior to initial ball contact. Kicks with the least thigh deceleration showed the greatest knee extension velocity. This demonstrates the influence that one part of the kinetic chain has on the other. Skilled players demonstrate more efficient firing patterns during this phase than their unskilled counterparts, thus enhancing their performance.[5]

Foot Contact with the Ball

The kicker's plant-foot and contact-foot positions are critical to the outcome of a kick. At contact, the knee is flexed, and the foot is moving forward in an upward-sweeping direction. The hip of the kicking leg is flexing as contact occurs. Angular velocity of the thigh is minimal and contributes only minimally to the kick. Foot velocity at ball impact is not the primary factor that affects ball ve-

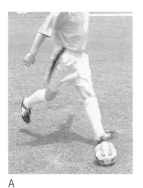 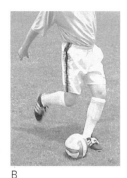

A   B

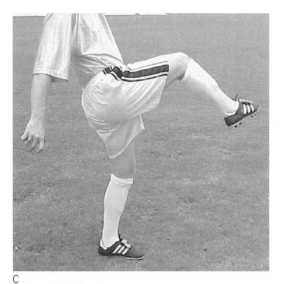

C

FIGURE 14.1

A. Kicking, plant-foot position. B. Kicking, acceleration. C. Kicking, follow-through.

locity. Rather, placement of the foot on the ball at contact has a greater impact on ball velocity. Skilled players contact the ball closer to the ankle and with a more rigid foot. Changing the angle of the ankle joint does not affect velocity as much as a change in the angle of the metatarsophalangeal joints. An increase in this angle correlates to a decrease in ball velocity.[5]

Follow-Through

The follow-through is an important phase in the kicking motion (see Fig. 14.1C). It allows for maximal contact between the body and the ball for the greatest time possible. The greater this period, the greater is momentum that can be achieved. Second, follow-through reduces injury to the swing limb. It allows forces in muscle, soft tissues, and joints to be dissipated. Immediately following ball contact, a large knee flexion moment is produced as the hamstrings eccentrically contract to control the rapid knee extension. If this flexor torque occurs too early, the kicker's foot will be slowed, which will decrease the ball's velocity. At the end of the follow-through, the hip extensors act eccentrically to slow the hip flexion moment.[5]

In kicking, only 15 percent of the swing limb's kinetic energy is transferred to the ball. The remainder of the energy must come from other mechanisms such as activation of the quadriceps. Stored energy in the muscles must have appropriate time to dissipate or injury can occur secondary to the large loads placed on the knee joint and surrounding soft tissues, which are already under stress immediately following the kick.[3,5]

When analyzing muscle activity during the kicking motion, the prevalence of eccentric activity is apparent. This pattern is described as the *soccer paradox*. This is so because knee flexor activity is dominant during knee extension and knee extensor activity dominates during knee flexion. The quadriceps are most active in the loading phase, when they are acting as antagonists. The maximum knee extensor moment therefore occurs very early in the kicking movement, during swing-limb loading. On the other hand, immediately prior to ball contact, there is no quadriceps activity. The hamstrings eccentrically dominate the last phase of the kicking motion. This reduces the angular velocity at the knee and aids in deceleration of the joint. Hyperextension at the knee is reduced, decreasing risk of injury and improving kick efficiency.[5]

Kicking is just one aspect of a soccer player's duties on the field. Heading and throw-in mechanics also will be examined for field players. Consideration also must be given to the difference in mechanics of the goalkeeper.

HEADING

Heading in soccer consists of three phases: preparation, contact, and recovery. These phases may vary based on the situation during play, but the basic technique remains constant. Using proper biomechanics when heading a soccer ball is important for both execution of the play and injury prevention. The most important initial element of heading is the player contacting the ball versus the ball hitting the player in the head.[3]

Preparation Phase

When jumping off the ground to head the ball, the legs should be slightly extended at the hips and flexed at the knees. Next, the player's trunk moves into extension with the head and body moving simultaneously. This initial extension moment provides for energy to be transferred via the trunk and hip flexors when striking the ball. The arms are extended in front of and away from the player's body to aid balance and serve as protection from opponents who are charging the ball.[3]

During the approach, the head and shoulders accelerate toward the ball by concentric contractions of the trunk and hip flexors. Eye contact needs to remain consistent throughout the heading motion to assist in controlling body motion as well as reducing velocity of the head after impact. The neck should remain isometrically contracted in a neutral position. The head should not lead the body in the forward movement. The arms are back and drawn in toward the body as the motion is completed. Momentum transfer from the player's body to the ball is controlled primarily by the trunk and hip flexors.[3]

The preparation phase is important for proper timing and form when heading the ball. The trunk musculature dominates the act of heading because it makes up the majority of total body weight. The trapezius and sternocleidomastoid muscles are active in the preparation phase, the latter being activated first in a jumping header.[3]

Contact Phase

The contact phase is characterized by initial impact with the ball at the player's hairline and recoil off the player's head. Total contact time is between 10 to 23 ms. Contact with the ball has three distinct phases. The first phase includes contact and deformation of the ball. Momentum is transferred from the player's head to the ball, causing the ball to change directions. The ball remains deformed during the second phase as it begins to travel in the same direction as the player's head. The third phase is characterized by the ball regaining its normal shape and breaking contact with the player's head.[3]

Recovery Phase

During the recovery phase of heading, the trapezius muscle remains active longer than the sternocleidomastoid. The trapezius assists in decelerating the player's head after ball contact. When heading the ball downward, the sternocleidomastoid becomes inactive faster than in any other heading situation in order to allow the head to get over the ball and direct the ball toward the ground.[3]

OVERHEAD THROWING

Field players use a two-hand overhead throw to bring the ball back into play when it goes out of bounds on the sidelines. The overhead throw includes cocking, acceleration to ball release, and follow-through. In the cocking phase, the player begins to dorsiflex the ankles, extend the hip and spine, flex the shoulders and elbows, and radially deviate the wrist.

As the player reaches the maximal cocking range, acceleration to ball release begins. If a player uses a split stance, the center of gravity begins to transfer forward. On ball release, the knees extend, the hips flex, the shoulders and elbows extend, and the wrists radially deviate. This forward-transferring motion is then controlled eccentrically through the follow-through.

GOALKEEPING

There are few studies analyzing the biomechanics of the goalkeeper. The demands of the game are very different for this player. The kicking motion of the goalkeeper involves punting the ball that is held in the hands, as opposed to a ball traveling on the ground. The phases of the kick are very similar, although the actual performance of the kick and the magnitude of the flexion and extension moments are very different. In addition, there are vertical and horizontal components in the follow-through when punting the ball.

A goalkeeper must jump both vertically and horizontally to save a ball. The drive of the arm and leg furthest from the ball, in the direction of the dive, is what actually helps the goalkeeper reach the ball. Research conducted on the biomechanics of a dive determined that a more experienced goalkeeper has more efficient synergistic movement of the muscles. This allows the goalkeeper to dive further than a less experienced counterpart. More research is still needed on goalkeeping to understand the different roles that muscles play at various stages of a dive. Increased knowledge of the position will further improve the progression of injured athletes back to competition and possibly will decrease injuries.

Injury Prevention

WARM-UP AND STRETCHING

Seventy-five percent of all injuries in soccer are avoidable.[6] For soccer players, the greatest form of prevention comes from proper warm-up and conditioning. An effective warm-up increases the temperature of tissues and increases range of motion (ROM).[7] Typical warm-up programs include running, calisthenics, dynamic stretching, and ball drills.[9]

Stretching is important for soccer players because they tend to be less flexible than their nonplaying counterparts of the same age.[7,9,10] Sixty-seven percent of the players studied had at least one tight muscle in the lower extremities.[7] There is a correlation between athletes with tight muscles and the incidence of muscle strains.[7,9] Muscle strains commonly affect soccer players and can end up sidelining them for weeks at a time. They are probably one of the most preventable injuries in the sport.

Static and contract relax stretching can be effective for increasing muscle length.[7,9] A combination of these techniques is important. The plantarflexor, hip adductor, knee extensor, knee flexor, and hip flexor muscle groups should be one focus of soccer players' stretching programs because they are the most frequently injured. (See Chap. 9 for illustrations of these stretches.) However, each joint in the lower extremity should be stretched in isolation and through dynamic movements. The soccer ball can be used to dynamically stretch these muscle groups. Figure 14.2 shows a dynamic hip adductor stretch. The back, neck, and upper extremities also need to be addressed prior to activity. These areas are often neglected because of the focus on the lower extremities in soccer players. After static stretching is completed, dynamic stretching to simulate sport activities should be incorporated.[13]

Shooting on the goal is one of the most common warm-up drills but is also related to quadriceps strains.[5] This can be a part of the warm-up routine if executed properly. It should only be allowed after stretching of the leg muscles is performed. Then shooting should begin with close, low-velocity shots and slowly increased to further distances with higher velocities. It is also important to remember the different demands of the different positions, namely, the goalkeeper. Prior to competition, more emphasis needs to be placed on upper body and trunk stretches for the goalkeeper than for field players.

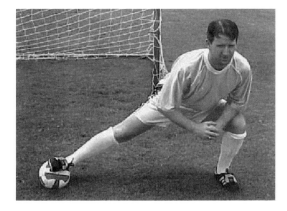

FIGURE 14.2

Stretching, adductors.

Other common practices can contribute to injury. First, players arriving late to practice or games rarely warm up appropriately. Second, during matches, players sitting on the bench are often thrust into action with little or no warm-up other than that in which they participated prior to the match. These common practices contribute to muscle injuries.

CONDITIONING

Conditioning, whether in-season or preseason, often has been the sole responsibility of the individual athlete. Frequently it is not until a player reaches the collegiate level of play that specific advice on how to condition for the sport becomes available. Even at this point, the program is general and not geared toward specific positional demands. With proper conditioning in the off-season, the player reduces the risk of many overuse injuries and injuries secondary to deconditioning.

As mentioned earlier, the running and sprinting demands of each position in soccer vary. Exclusive slow distance running is not necessarily the best method to prepare an athlete for the sport of soccer. It does not address the quick sustained bursts of energy needed to sprint to the goal on a breakaway or the goalkeeper's need to explode off his or her feet to make a diving save. Most runs in soccer vary in length from 5 to 30 yd.[12] Usually the player is running without the ball. Exercise intensity ranges from walking to sprinting for different time intervals.[12] This demand on various energy systems makes it important to train both aerobically and anaerobically. Interval training with jogging and sprinting may better prepare an athlete for the sport of soccer.

Each position also places different demands on the athlete. One research study calculated the total distance covered in a game as 10.8 km. Of this total distance, jogging comprises 36 percent of the distance, walking 24 percent, and actual distance with the ball only 2 percent. The player sprints an average of one time every 90 s for an average of 14 yd. Rest intervals are about every 2 min for approximately 3 s. By position, there are different conditioning demands for the athletes. Midfielders cover about 6.2 mi per game. Forwards and defenders cover a little less distance at 5.3 mi. Surprisingly, the goalkeeper, thought to be a stationary player, covers 2.2 mi per game.[4] Much of this distance includes the time moving around to stay ready while the play is away from the goalkeeper.

AEROBIC TRAINING

Aerobic training is necessary for athletes to compete in the 90-min matches throughout the season. *Aerobic training* refers to energy being derived when oxygen is used to metabolize substrates. This usually occurs when events are greater than 90 s in duration. For aerobic training, the activity should last 15 to 20 min at 70 to 85 percent of the maximum heart rate of the athlete.[13] Aerobic conditioning assists the athlete in performing for longer intervals at a higher intensity and allows for greater recovery between high-intensity exercise bouts. Since soccer uses a combination of the aerobic and anaerobic systems, there will be benefits both physiologically and psychologically to training in this fashion. With athletes conditioned to exercise for longer periods, they will be less likely to make mental errors as a result of fatigue.[12]

Aerobic conditioning should be both general and sport-specific. It should be performed from three to six times per week.[13] The general phase includes running at a slower pace. Then the specific phase follows, consisting of more runs that mimic the ones a soccer player makes during a match. The athlete alternates between walking, jogging, and sprinting. The pace is increased from the general phase and is performed at least four times a week, varying in intensity.[12]

ANAEROBIC TRAINING

Anaerobic exercise refers to activities that last less than 2 min. It involves the phosphagen and lactic acid energy sources. The phosphagen system is used almost exclusively in activities lasting under 6 s. Activities lasting 30 to 90 s rely on the lactic acid energy system. These systems are best developed using interval training methods.[13]

INTERVAL TRAINING

Interval training allows athletes to work at a higher intensity for longer periods than if they were to work continuously. This allows for greater intensity and duration of workouts. For an effective interval-training program, several goals must be met. First, the skills of the sport must be met. Second, all the energy systems must be enhanced by the training program. Lastly, the athlete must be able to manipulate the intensity and volume to meet specific needs of performance.[12]

PERIODIZATION TRAINING

A comprehensive conditioning program will incorporate a weight-training program along with a running program. In order for the athlete to peak at the optimal time, periodization of the training schedule should be employed. Periodization divides the athlete's year into phases of preseason, in-season, and off-season. These cycles are then used to train flexibility, strength, endurance, and sport-specific skills. The athlete spends 3 to 15 weeks per cycle, with an emphasis on strength, hypertrophy, or power. Within each cycle, the volume, intensity, and duration of the exercises are manipulated for the desired outcome. The athlete needs to perform exercises that are multijoint as well as train smaller muscle groups in different phases.[13]

A typical strength phase has moderate volume (three to five sets of 5 to 6 repetitions) and the intensity is 80 to 85 percent of the 1-repetition maximum. The hypertrophy phase has the largest volume (three to five sets of 10 to 15 repetitions) and the lowest intensity (50 to 75 percent of the 1-repetition maximum). The power phase has low volume consisting of five sets of 2 to 4 repetitions. Conversely, it has the highest intensity at 90 to 95 percent of the 1-repetition maximum. Generally speaking, the year is started with a hypertrophy phase lasting 3 to 4 weeks, followed by a strength phase lasting up to 4 weeks. The hypertrophy phase is probably the least important of all the phases for soccer players, and this is why it is shorter compared with other sports. The power phase is the last phase and lasts up to 3 weeks.[13] The length of each of these phases can be manipulated to obtain the desired results for a specific individual. These guidelines help to balance the athlete's training and prepare him or her for competition as well as to avoid overtraining.

In the off-season, the intensity of training can be greater than during competition. Plyometrics should be performed in the off-season more frequently than during the season because there is adequate recovery time. Performance in games can be compromised if plyometrics are used too heavily during the season. As the season nears, volume will be decreased in strength training, and exercises will be more sport-specific. During the competitive season, the volume of conditioning is at its lowest point, and plyometrics and weight training are alternated once a week.[13] There are transitional periods between the different phases to allow for the athlete to prepare his or her mind and body for the upcoming phases. Exceptions need to be made for players who do not receive game time.

These athletes should be trained following games at a level comparable with that of playing. This will assist in the conditioning and readiness of the players coming off the bench in future games.

STRENGTH TRAINING

Strength training that incorporates the stretch-shortening cycle of a muscle has been shown to enhance soccer performance. Concentric strengthening of the hip flexors and quadriceps, along with eccentric training of the hip extensors and hamstrings, is important to enhance soccer performance. However, it is not advisable to exclusively train a muscle either concentrically or eccentrically because that same muscle will play a different role in another instance. For example, although the quadriceps act eccentrically during phases of running, they act concentrically at ball contact during a kick. Designing a program that will effectively train muscles in both fashions will offer the greatest benefit to the athlete. Explosive muscle movements such as long and vertical jumps have been found to correlate with kick distance. Consequently, these exercises often are incorporated into a soccer player's training program for performance enhancement.[5]

Research has demonstrated that soccer players have good muscle symmetry between their dominant and nondominant lower extremities. Although most soccer players prefer to kick with one foot versus the other when shooting on the goal, most players use both feet somewhat evenly when dribbling and passing. On the other hand, peak knee extension torque is greater on the nondominant side than on the dominant side. This could be attributed to the role the nondominant leg plays in supporting the body's weight when kicking. The dominant leg, despite its lesser peak knee extension torque, was found to produce greater ball velocities.[5]

Weight-training exercises involving multijoint movements usually are performed prior to training individual muscle groups. Some multijoint exercises that are beneficial to soccer players include leg presses, squats, and lunges for the lower body. Squats are a demanding exercise because of the stress placed on the knees and therefore may be replaced by less stressful exercises if the athlete has a history of knee pain or injury. Many Olympic lifts such as the power clean and snatch are multijoint exercises but are not very sport-specific. These exercises also require a greater degree of skill to perform safely and may not be the best choice for soccer players. Single-joint lower body exercises should include seated leg extensions, hamstring curls, adductor and abductor exercises, and calf raises with both the legs straight and with the knees bent to train the gastrocnemius and soleus muscles, respectively.

Abdominal exercises are an integral part of the strengthening program. Maintaining core strength allows for all other segments of the body to be trained more efficiently. A program that targets both the obliques and the transversus abdominis is best suited for the athlete. These muscles can be trained by performing diagonal crunches. Using a physio ball can increase the difficulty level. It is also important to include exercises for the lumbar spine, including the paraspinals and multifidi.

Upper body exercises should include multijoint exercises such as the chest press as well as rowing, lateral pulls-downs, and front and lateral shoulder raises. Individual arm exercises for the biceps and triceps are of less importance than combined movements for soccer players. If the athlete chooses to exercise his or her arms, he or she should prioritize the other exercises first to optimize the time in the weight room.

Plyometrics

Plyometrics are a component of training programs for all athletes. These exercises have been found to increase performance and decrease injury risk.[14] Plyometrics are exercises that allow for a muscle to reach maximal strength in as short a time as possible.[13]

Plyometrics apply an overload to the muscle to strengthen it.[13] The three main components of a plyometric exercise are the eccentric, amortization, and concentric phases. The eccentric contraction elicits the stretch reflex, which allows for a greater concentric contraction to occur in the same muscle. This produces an increase in speed strength. The amortization phase is the period of time from the eccentric phase to the initiation of the concentric phase. The amortization phase should be kept brief in order to optimize the stretch reflex and therefore increase strength. The magnitude of the stretch is not as important as the rate of the stretch.[13] This method of training is very useful in soccer to train athletes to produce maximal force during high-speed movement.

When implementing a plyometrics program, it is important to keep a few things in mind. Make sure the athlete wears proper footwear for the surface. A nonslip supportive shoe is necessary. Grass is the best surface on which to perform these exercises because it is sport-specific, but elevated wooden floors are also acceptable. Trampolines and excessively padded surfaces will increase the amortization phase and thus decrease the benefits of plyometrics training. Consequently, they should be avoided.[13] Teaching the athlete how to land softly by toe-to-heel rocking is also important to reduce injuries. A high percentage of injuries occur from improper landings during sports.[14]

Most important, players must be at an appropriate skill and fitness level to perform these exercises to avoid injury. The basic features of the program that can be manipulated for the desired results are the volume, frequency, and intensity. *Volume* refers to the number of foot contacts per workout. The range should be between 80 and 100. *Frequency* is the number of times per week this training is performed. Usually, the athlete should perform one to three sessions based on the cycle of training he or she is in at the time (in-season versus off-season). *Intensity* is the amount of stress placed on the muscles, connective tissue, and joints. Different types of jumps place different amounts of stress on the joints. For example, skipping is a low-intensity activity, whereas in-depth jumps are high-stress activities.[13]

Plyometric exercises for the lower extremities include square jumps, box jumps, and depth jumps. To perform square jumps, make a cross on the floor using white athletic tape. The athlete stands in one of the four boxes and then hops forward, backward, sideways, diagonally, or any combination of these movements. The athlete also can be asked to hop clockwise or counterclockwise while being timed to advance the drill. Direction can be changed on the verbal command of the coach or therapist.

Box jumps are performed using a step from 0.4 to 1.1 m in height. Box heights of 0.75 to 0.80 m are used most frequently. At heights greater than 1.2 m, there is a great overload to the muscles, and many athletes are unable to maintain correct technique. The athlete stands about 0.6 m in front of the box. The feet are shoulder width apart. The knees and hips are slightly flexed. The athlete then jumps upward and forward to land on the box. As soon as the athlete lands on the box, he or she immediately jumps back down to the starting position and explodes back up. The less time spent in contact with the box, the more effective the drill. Proper landing technique is very important when performing this exercise to avoid injury. The shoulders should be over the knees on landing. Flexing

the ankles, knees, and hips will help to facilitate this.[13] This exercise can be performed for 10- to 30-s time intervals.

For field players, lower body plyometrics are the most useful. Depth jumps are used to increase leg power and strength. They are performed by stepping off a box and then immediately jumping up after landing on the ground.[13] A common plyometric exercise for the preparation of activity is side-to-side ball jumps. Field players and goalkeepers also may benefit from upper body and abdominal plyometrics for core stability. These exercises can be performed with weighted balls to increase the difficulty of the drill. (See Chap. 13 for a list of progressive upper and lower extremity plyometric drills.)

COOL-DOWN

Another aspect of injury prevention is the cool-down. This area has undergone very little research to date. Most players finish their practice and leave the field for the locker rooms. Few players take the time to actually cool down, whether stretching individually or with the team. A program allowing for 10 to 15 min of cool-down after training or games should be established to avoid muscle tightness. After vigorous exercise of the quadriceps and hamstrings, there is a decrease in ROM lasting 2 to 3 days.[7] When stretching follows the same vigorous exercises, no decrease in ROM is noted.[7] Muscle tightness may result from the accumulation of muscle stiffness after several days of practice or matches each week.[7] A cool-down program following practices or games that allows for muscles to be stretched adequately will be beneficial to athletic performance. Slow jogging over a short distance may be done at the end of practice, followed by 10 to 15 min of static stretching of the major muscle groups of the lower and upper extremities. Caution should be taken to avoid rushing through the cool-down because athletes are tired from the practice or match. Omitting this aspect of training can result in long-term effects that will be detrimental to the overall performance.

Hydration is an important issue for soccer players. Athletes compete for long periods of time. (Refer to Chaps. 12 and 13 for discussions of hydration.)

An injury prevention program that includes warm-up and cool-down using proprioceptive neuromuscular facilitation (PNF) stretching can result in a 75 percent decrease in injury occurrence, an 80 percent decline in medical costs, and a reduction in the time missed from play.[8] The education of coaches and athletes on the basics of warming up and cooling down could reduce the incidence of muscle strains and decreased flexibility among soccer players.

PROTECTIVE EQUIPMENT

As stated earlier, soccer players have very little protective equipment available to prevent injury. Shin guards are required at most levels of play. There are various types, from small plastic shin guards that are placed under the sock to larger shin guards that cover the malleoli and strap in place. Shin guards may reduce the incidence of contusions and bruises, but it is questionable if they dissipate forces enough to reduce the incidence of fractures.[15,36]

The uniform of the soccer player offers no protection to the body. Goalkeepers may wear jerseys with padding in the elbows, but this offers protection only against abrasions from the turf and not against contusions or possible fractures from falls on the elbow. Padding over the lateral thigh is also available in goalkeeper shorts, offering the same degree of protection against abrasions. Goalkeeper gloves are thought to offer protection to the hands. In fact, the gloves are worn to increase grip on the ball and are not used for protection.

HEADING

Some players may use mouth guards for protection of the mouth and prevention of mild concussions, but they are not mandatory. Dental injuries are not overly common in soccer but can occur when players go up to head a ball or when a goalkeeper and field player are both vying for an air ball. Concussions are incurred by the same mechanisms. There is also incidence of contact with the ground and goalposts, which can lead to concussions in soccer players, although these mechanisms of injury are not very common.

Some debate exists about the long-term effects of heading the ball. A study comparing Dutch professional soccer players with noncontact athletes showed through neuropsychological testing that some impairment occurs in memory, planning, and visuoperceptual processing.[16] However, in another study conducted on the U.S. National Team, no association was found between heading the ball and neurologic symptoms.[16] A soft protective helmet like one worn for boxing has been given some consideration as protective gear, but to date no mandates requiring its use have been implemented.

Heading should be minimized in practice to reduce possible injury from repetition. Reducing the weight of the ball during practice by using a lighter ball such as a beach ball also may reduce the risk of injury.[34] Education of athletes and coaches on neck strengthening exercises as well as proper form also could greatly reduce the risk of injuries in this category. Isometric and antigravity cervical spine exercises may be the easiest and safest method for training the spine stabilizers in preparation for heading. The ability to contract these muscles just prior to heading the ball will reduce the risk of injury due to a whiplash effect that may occur when a ball comes in contact with the athlete's head at high speeds.

The possibility that heading the ball may have long-term effects on the athlete has received considerable attention in recent years. A study using members of the U.S. National Team demonstrated an increased incidence of neurologic symptoms in these subjects.[1,3] These symptoms were thought to be related to the contact in the sport or repetitive heading.[1] A study using Dutch soccer players found that soccer players head the ball 8.5 times per game. A ball weighing 14 oz can travel at speeds of 50 to 80 mi/h.[34] Although these facts make it seem likely that repetitive forces at this weight and speed when applied to an athlete's head would have long-term effects, no conclusive evidence was found relating heading the ball to neurologic changes.[1] Most often soccer players complain of a headache with migraine-like symptoms initiated by heading the ball.[30]

GOALPOSTS

One other area of concern in injury prevention is the goalposts. Over a 13-year period, 18 individuals died from impacts with the goalposts. This is the most common cause of fatalities in soccer.[17] Some of these injuries occurred from the goalposts tipping over on people. In several instances, the person was performing a pull-up on the goalpost, and the goal collapsed, falling on the individual. One possible solution would be to make the goals stationary, but this actually may increase the number and severity of impact injuries. Research is being done on the use of different materials to pad the goalposts. The issue at hand is to find a material that will not change the play of the ball as it rebounds off the goalpost. Hopefully, some resolution to this issue can be found that will allow for similar play of the game while decreasing the risk of injury.

PROPHYLACTIC MEASURES

Prophylactic taping and bracing are used in the prevention of injuries. Since ankle sprains are the most common injury in soccer, great consideration has been given to preventative taping prior to practice and matches. This is very costly and time-consuming, and little research exists on the efficacy of prophylactic taping.[7] However, when a player has ankle instability or a history of ankle sprains, taping or bracing may be an effective means to prevent injury. Finding a brace that is appropriate should not be a decision that is left up to the player or the coach. Store-bought braces may not fit properly and can cause other problems for the athlete. Likewise, the athlete may pick out a brace that does not offer support for his or her particular injury. These factors may contribute to the ineffectiveness of prophylactic programs. Bracing should be the decision of the medical team, which includes the athletic trainer, physical therapist, and physician.

COACHING

Coaching players to use proper technique will help reduce the risk of injury. If a player heads the ball by stabilizing the neck first with active muscle contraction, then he or she is less likely to suffer an injury. Furthermore, a goalkeeper needs to be taught how to land properly when diving for the ball. By having the ball contact the ground first, followed by his or her hips, the ball can cushion the fall. This helps to decrease injury to the elbows and knees.

Coaches also need to understand the demand on the body as it relates to the appropriateness of progressing a player to a new skill.[7] This is especially true for coaches who are working with children. They need to recognize what prerequisite skills must be mastered in order to learn an advanced skill. Progressing a player too quickly can increase the risk of injury.

Etiology of Injuries

EPIDEMIOLOGY

Soccer is considered the most played sport in the world.[1,9] The number of people playing soccer and the number of associated injuries may be a reflection more of the popularity of the sport than of the inherent dangers from playing soccer.[9] Soccer has been the most popular sport in Europe since the 1800s.[1] It is not surprising to find that 50 to 60 percent of all sports injuries in Europe occur in soccer.[9] The number of injuries associated with soccer in the United States has clearly risen over the last two decades. This is most likely because of the sheer increase in numbers of people taking to the soccer fields.[1] Soccer is considered to be a relatively safe sport. Compared with American football, soccer has far fewer injuries.[18] A high school football player has an 85 percent risk of injury compared with a 30 percent risk of injury for soccer players.[1]

The rate of injury can be described in terms of incidence per 1000 hours of practice or games.[1,19] The definition of injury that a study uses may change the rate of injury. An *injury* can be defined as any incident reported to medical personnel. This allows for very minor injuries, such as abrasions, to fit into the definition of injury for the purpose of study.[1] Researchers studied 25,000 elite soccer players aged 11 to 18 years at a tournament in Norway. Males had a rate of injury of 14 per 1000 hours, and females had a rate of injury of 32 per 1000 hours.[1,19] Other studies with stricter definitions of injury, such as the loss of at least one game or practice, yielded lower injury exposure rates. These rates were 5 per 1000 hours for males and 12 per 1000 for females.[19] A Danish study found injury rates as low as 3.6 per 1000 practice hours and 14.3 per 1000 game hours for males.[10]

Injury exposure rates vary from practice to game settings. For males, the injury rate for practice is 7.6 per 1000 hours, and for games it is 16.9 per 1000 hours.[19] Injury rates for female soccer players are 7 per 1000 hours for practice and 24 per 1000 hours for game.[1] The rate of injury is at least two times as great in games than in practice.[1,9,18,19] Eighty-six percent of all injuries are said to occur in games.[2] This may be due to the fact that there is more physical contact in a game over a practice session.[18] In fact, college soccer players are nine times more likely to injure their anterior cruciate ligament (ACL) during a game versus a practice session.[1]

Most injuries in soccer are considered to be minor. This accounts for little to no loss of time from competition. Between 44 and 62 percent of all injuries are minor.[1,2,9,19] Moderate injuries account for 27 to 46 percent of all injuries.[2,9,19] Only 9 to 15 percent of all injuries are classified as severe, resulting in the loss of greater than 1 month of participation in practice or games.[2,9,19] Most of the serious injuries occur in 12- to 15-year-old females.[1,18] This is probably due to the high incidence of knee injuries found in females. These injuries often require a greater length of time away from the sport.[10]

Age Differences

Players older than 25 years of age have the highest injury rate at 18 percent.[2,18] This is partly due to the fact that this population contains former collegiate athletes with high skill levels and a more aggressive style of play.[18] Players in their thirties and forties who compensate for their lack of speed by a more physical play also fall into this group.[18] The increased physical contact may predispose these players to more injuries. The next age group, 18- to 25-year-olds, has a 17 percent incidence of injury.[2] Lowest injury rates are found in the younger populations, 15- to 18-year-olds.[2] The injuries to these players tend to be less severe, especially in school soccer.[2]

Gender Differences

Gender also plays a roll in injury rates. The risk of injury is greater in females than in males.[1] The incidence is almost two times as high in females versus their male counterparts. Furthermore, the severe injury rate is 60 percent for females and only 36 percent in males.[2] Several factors may contribute to this gender difference. First, females may lack the fitness levels necessary for safe participation. Females tend to train one-half the amount of time their male counterparts do.[19] Studies have shown that increased training can reduce injuries as a result of improved strength, coordination, and skill.[9] Part of the reason is also the definition of an injury. Female soccer players tend to miss more time due to injury. Male players are more likely to play hurt and do not miss time from the sport.[19]

The most common activity for a soccer player to be involved in at the time of injury is tackling.[18] *Tackling* is defined as a player attempting to gain control of the ball from another player who is in possession of the ball. Eighty percent of all injuries in soccer occur during physical contact between two players.[4,19,18] Contact includes being kicked by another player and colliding with another player.[18] Even though 80 percent of all first-time injuries are due to contact, most reinjuries actually happen while running.[10] At higher levels of play, more injuries involve running as the initial mechanism of injury.[10] These statistics hold true for both men and women. Higher levels of play have a higher rate of injury, probably due to increased skill levels and better competition with more physical contact between players. Fouls also occur more frequently at the higher levels of competition. Injuries that occur as a result of

a foul or a rule violation make up 15 to 30 percent of all injuries.[5,11,15]

There does not seem to be a significant difference in injury rates by position. One study found that goalkeepers were injured more frequently. Subsequent studies refuted this point and actually found an increased rate of injury in strikers. The differences by position lie in the mechanism of injury and body part injured rather than the frequency. Goalkeepers are more likely to be injured diving, tackling, or colliding with an object. They are more likely to injure their head, hands, fingers, and elbows. Field players are more likely to get injured kicking others, colliding with others, or running. These players exhibit more lower extremity injuries. Injuries rates do vary, however, by playing venue. Indoor soccer has an injury rate twice as high as outdoor soccer.[18]

Most injuries (69 percent) occur because of trauma, whereas 31 percent of injuries are due to overuse.[9] Between 84 and 88 percent of injuries in soccer occur in the lower extremities.[1,9,10,18] As mentioned previously, most of these injuries are minor and result in little to no loss of playing time. The rate of major injuries is 8 to 10 percent, mostly occurring in the lower extremities and including fractures, subluxations, and ligament injuries. Of all major injuries, ligament injuries to the knee are the most common. ACL injury is the number one knee injury in soccer, accounting for 50 percent of all severe injuries. It is seen more often in females than in males, 31 versus 13 percent, respectively.[1]

Many theories have been presented to explain why women injure their ACLs more often than men. These theories are broken down into intrinsic and extrinsic factors. Intrinsic factors include such variables as limb alignment, joint laxity, ligament size, notch dimensions, wider pelvis, increased genu valgum, and increased tibial torsion. Extrinsic factors include body movement, shoe-surface interface, muscle strength and coordination, level of skill and conditioning, and flexibility.[20,23,25]

Research indicates that a player's level of conditioning and skill are associated with ACL injury. The recent growth of women participating in soccer may mean that less skilled players are taking to the fields and are not trained and conditioned properly to participate safely at higher levels of play. Studies have found that with an increase in training, there was a subsequent decrease in the number of traumatic injuries. This could be due to improved coordination, better oxygen uptake, and greater strength and skill.[9] Since women spend less time training than men, this may contribute to increased injury rates of women.[19]

EXTRINSIC FACTORS

Body movement, playing surface, shoe type, shoe-surface interface, rule violations, muscular strength, and level of skill and conditioning are all factors that may contribute to injury rates. Specific body movements in soccer, including planting, cutting, landing from a jump, and decelerating, may have a role in the incidence of injury. Modifying the plant and cut maneuver to allow for more knee flexion and to keep the feet under the hips more when cutting and turning actually may decrease knee injuries. A flexed knee position also allows the hamstrings to have a greater contribution to knee stabilization by controlling rotation and anterior displacement, thus helping to reduce injury rates.[20]

Twenty-five percent of all injures in soccer can be attributed to poor field conditions. Irregularity in the playing surface and weather contribute to poor field conditions. To decrease the risk of injury, removing defects in the turf or repairing holes should be a priority. Since weather cannot be controlled, proper footwear selection for specific condi-

tions may be the most effective way to minimize the risk of injury. In general, screw-in cleats are associated with a higher risk of injury than molded cleats but are more popular for wet surfaces and grassy playing fields.[11] The benefits must outweigh the risks when the athlete chooses to play in these shoes.

A shoe-surface interface with a high coefficient of friction has been suggested to increase injury. Certain shoe types on artificial turf show a higher friction rate and correlate with an increased incidence of injury, particularly to the knee.[20] The player, coach, and training staff should carefully research shoes before making a final decision on footwear. The choice of a player's footwear is often based on appearance and fit but now is being recognized as an important part of injury prevention as well.

Rule violations also contribute to injury rates. As mentioned previously, 15 to 25 percent of all injuries are the result of a foul, and 30 percent of all traumatic injuries are sustained due to a foul.[11] Coincidentally, the player committing the foul is more likely to be the one seriously injured. Proper officiating and coaching are needed to protect athletes from these preventable injuries.

Conditioning and strengthening also can affect the incidence of injury. Teams with less than average training have a higher number of traumatic injuries. Increased training can affect skill and coordination, oxygen uptake, and strength positively. All these factors aid in decreasing injury.[13]

INTRINSIC FACTORS

Joint laxity, limb alignment, and notch dimensions are all intrinsic factors that can influence injury rates. These factors are important in understanding an athlete's predisposition to injury. Joint laxity and limb alignment are two factors thought to contribute to injury rates, but to date, limited data support these theories. Often, working on proprioception and using orthotics can help these athletes prevent injury. However, further research is needed on these topics to substantiate these claims.

Intercondylar notch size has been implicated as a reason for ACL failure in both newly injured and ACL-reconstructed knees.[20] *Notch width* is the ratio of the width of the intercondylar notch to the width of the distal femur at the level of the popliteal groove. Athletes with smaller notch widths are at higher risk for ACL injuries than those with notch widths considered in the normal range.[20]

Common Injuries and Their Rehabilitation

When looking at injuries in soccer, regardless of severity, the ankle sprain is the most common.[2,10,19] The knee is the second most commonly injured body part.[18] Skin lesions, contusions, muscle strains, and fractures make up a large percentage of the remainder of the lower extremity injuries.[2] Less common injuries include head and face injuries, shoulder dislocations, elbow fractures and dislocations, finger injuries, and groin and pubis injuries.[18]

LOWER EXTREMITY INJURIES

Ankle Injuries

Ankle Sprains With ankle sprains accounting for 36 percent of all injuries in soccer, it is important to understand the various mechanisms of these injuries. This will aid in determining proper rehabilitation techniques to return athletes back to competition as quickly and safely as possible. The mechanisms of injury are most often running or tackling. Eighty percent of first-time ankle injuries occur while tackling. In the cases where running was the mechanism of injury, there was a high incidence of previous ankle injury.[10] An ankle sprain in many instances can be worse than a fracture in terms of complete recovery.[21] Whereas fractures are immobilized and progressed gradually while they heal, quite often ankle sprains are rushed through the rehabilitation process, and the athlete returns to the sport before he or she has adequate strength and proprioception. This can lead to chronic swelling and instability of the ankle.[21] The athlete may be hampered by this ankle injury for an entire season if proper treatment is not received.

An inversion sprain is the most common type of sprain. One or two ligaments are commonly involved in inversion sprains. The most common ligament injured is the anterior talofibular ligament (ATFL). The second most commonly injured ligament is the calcaneofibular ligament (CFL). An eversion sprain is fairly uncommon due to the bony configuration of the ankle mortise. In addition, the foot would have to be forced outward for this injury to occur. This position would stress the strong deltoid ligament on the medial side of the ankle and often leads to an avulsion fracture of the tibia.[21]

The health care provider can grade ankle sprains based on the severity of injury. A grade 1 sprain is most common and usually involves the ATFL. There is minimal or no ecchymosis, minimal loss of function, mild pain and disability, and point tenderness over the ATFL. An anterior drawer test is negative on such an individual. A grade 2 sprain usually involves partial tearing of the ATFL and CFL. Pain is moderate, point tenderness is noted on palpation, ecchymosis appears 2 to 3 days after the injury, and the anterior drawer test elicits some excessive motion. A grade 3 sprain can involve the ATFL, CFL, and PTFL. Swelling is diffuse over the lateral aspect of the ankle, pain is moderate to severe, function is greatly limited, and anterior and posterior drawer tests are both positive.[21] Frequently, there is tenderness to palpation of the medial ligaments as well.

A grade 1 sprain may require immobilization for up to 5 days. A grade 2 sprain may require immobilization and the use of crutches for 5 to 10 days. A grade 3 sprain is typically casted for 2 to 4 weeks.[21] After the cast is removed, the same progression is followed with this athlete, usually at a much slower pace than for grade 1 and 2 ankle sprains because of the greater loss of motion and strength from casting. A grade 3 sprain occasionally requires surgical reconstruction.

The goals of ankle rehabilitation are to minimize stress to the healing ligament, decrease pain and swelling, restore motion in all planes, increase weight bearing, normalize gait, balance, and proprioception, increase strength, and initiate return-to-sport activities.[21] Initial treatment for ankle sprains includes rest, ice, compression, and elevation (RICE).[8,21] Rest allows the athlete to perform any activity that does not stress the injured body part. This allows the injury the time necessary to heal while avoiding overall deconditioning.[8] Ice is used to control swelling and inflammation after an injury. Compression is used to promote venous return and to decrease edema. Elevation is also used to promote venous return.[8] Many rehabilitation specialists recommend taping or bracing during this early phase to protect the ligament.

Based on the severity of the injury, ROM and stretching can be progressed as pain decreases. Some exercises that can be incorporated into the early rehabilitation process include towel crunches and picking up marbles with the toes to target the intrinsic muscles of the foot, ankle isometrics, and ROM of the toes. Ankle pumps and circles in the pain-free range can be useful to restore ankle ROM. As pain and swelling decrease, therapeutic tubing for inversion, eversion, plantarflexion, and dorsiflexion strengthening can be introduced.

These exercises, however, are initiated in the midrange to protect the ligament, and the range is increased as pain resolves. All these exercises can be performed in a non-weight-bearing position. Cross-friction massage to the ligament can assist with collagen fiber alignment. Minisquats and single-leg balance can be performed once the athlete can tolerate full weight bearing with minimal pain. These exercises promote cocontraction around the joint and still keep the joint in midrange. The final phase involves higher-level exercises through the full ROM. Pain-free calf raises and proprioceptive exercises such as the wobble board should be introduced.

Once full ROM and good strength are achieved, it is important to make sure the athlete can meet the demands of the position he or she plays prior to returning to the field. This should include functional testing of the athlete. The player should demonstrate the ability the start and stop, break from a jog to a sprint, and change directions quickly. The athlete may or may not require taping or bracing to perform these activities. Make certain that the player is performing these activities on the same playing surface and in the same shoes that he or she intends to wear when training or competing. Allowing the player to perform these activities in running shoes, when they will be playing in cleats, may alter the results of the testing. Drills should include figure-eight runs and shuttle runs to test the player's ability to stop, start, and change directions (see Chap. 13 for illustrations of additional drills). Multidirectional running is also important to test for functional ability on the field. Soccer players often backpedal to position themselves for an air ball or to receive a pass. This is important for all soccer players, regardless of their position. Single-leg hops to simulate jumping for challenges on air balls also should be performed. Deficits on any of these tests need to be addressed in an on-going rehabilitation program.

Just because a player returns to the field does not necessarily mean that he or she has completed the rehabilitation process, especially if there is a history of chronic ankle sprains. Fifty-six percent of all ankle injuries in soccer involved players with a history of sprains.[10] Sending a player back to competition too soon can result in chronic problems for the athlete. The athlete should be reevaluated continually so that he or she is progressed appropriately and is well prepared for return to the playing field. Functional stability is one of the primary problems after an ankle injury, so emphasis must be placed on peroneal strengthening and proprioceptive training.[10] It is also necessary to provide the player with opportunities to strengthen the entire lower kinetic chain because of the compensatory reactions that may occur at other joints as a result of ankle instability.

Shin Splints *Shin splints* is a term often used as a "catch-all" for lower leg pain but normally refers to anterior tibialis or posterior tibialis tendinitis or stress fracture syndromes. Numerous problems of the lower leg can be attributed to overuse. Besides shin splints, compartment syndromes and stress fractures can occur as a result of repetitive use of the lower extremities. Mechanisms of injury include improper training, improper footwear, and biomechanical abnormalities of the foot and lower extremity. Inflammation of the posterior tibialis tendon is the primary cause for the pain along the medial tibia. Medial tibia pain is often referred to as *medial shin splints*. Inflammation of the anterior tibialis tendon or the extensor tendons of the digits is the primary cause for pain in the anterior compartment. This pain is often referred to as *lateral shin splints*. Factors that may cause shin splints to occur include the running surface, pes planus, genu varum/tibial varum, overuse, muscle fatigue, body chemical imbalance, and poor reciprocal muscle coordination between the anterior

and posterior aspects of the lower extremity. Usually with lateral shin splints there is a shock-absorption problem, and with medial shin splints there is overuse of the posterior tibialis from eccentrically controlling excessive pronation.

The symptoms of shin splints include a nondescript pain over the anteromedial or anterolateral aspect of the lower leg. Shin splints can be graded based on complaints of pain. Grade 1 cases exhibit pain after activity. A grade 2 case presents with pain before and after activity. Performance is usually not affected. Grade 3 cases present with pain before, during, and after activity. At this stage, performance is hindered. A grade 4 classification of shin splints is defined by pain so severe that competition at any level is impossible.[21]

Treatment for this condition must include determining the cause and removing the stimulus to allow healing. A thorough history will help the clinician ascertain the proper course of treatment. For instance, changing running shoes or running surfaces may provide relief to the athlete. Examination for biomechanical faults in the foot may result in an easy correction with orthotics. If pain persists after the stimulus has been removed and the athlete has rested, then examination by a doctor may be necessary to rule out stress fractures, muscle tears, or compartment syndrome.[21]

Rehabilitation for this injury includes modalities to decrease pain and inflammation along with a comprehensive stretching program. Ice massage may be one of the most effective modalities in reducing pain. Ice massage should be performed for 5 to 7 min until the area is numb. Orthotics or taping for arch support may benefit some athletes with this condition if there is a biomechanical problem of the foot. Stretching, towel gathering, and marble pickups should be initiated in the early stages. Stretching should include the muscles of both the posterior and anterior compartments. It is a good idea to have the athlete stretch before and after competition, as well as after the ice application.[21] If weakness is detected, strengthening should be initiated. Exercises can be started in a non-weight-bearing position but should progress to closed-chain exercises. Emphasis is then placed on endurance, using body weight and high repetitions to stimulate the demands of running. The athlete should progress back to jogging as symptoms resolve.

Compartment Syndrome Compartment syndrome is often seen in soccer players due to the amount of running they perform in both practice and games. The anterior compartment is most often affected, but sometimes the deep posterior compartment may be involved. The anterior compartment contains the tibialis anterior, deep peroneal nerve, extensor digitorum longus, and the anterior tibial artery and vein. The deep posterior compartment contains the posterior tibialis, tibial nerve, flexor muscles of the toes, and the peroneal and posterior tibial arteries and veins.[21]

Compartment syndrome occurs when the tissue fluid pressure has exceeded normal levels and thereby places pressure on the muscles, tendons, blood vessels, and nerves. With this increase in pressure, ischemia occurs. This can cause permanent damage to the athlete's extremity in severe cases. Compartment syndrome can be either acute or chronic. Acute compartment syndrome is a medical emergency and requires immediate care by a physician. The player with chronic compartment syndrome will report pain as there is a gradual rise of pressure during an activity, and the pain will decrease as the pressure falls when the activity is stopped. Neurologic signs are rarely present in this case. In serious cases, there is associated weakness of the dorsiflexors and toe extensors, as well as swelling on the dorsum of the foot. Often, because of the symptoms, com-

partment syndrome is confused with a stress fracture.[21]

Treatment for this includes rest, ice, and elevation. If this condition does not resolve with conservative treatment, a surgical release may be indicated. After surgery, the athlete may begin light exercises 7 to 10 days postoperatively.[21] Exercises following surgery will include ROM, strengthening, balance, and proprioceptive training. Progression back to sports activities is performed once the pain has subsided and ROM, strength, and balance are restored.

Knee Injuries

The second most commonly injured joint for soccer players is the knee.[18] Knee ligament injuries cause the longest absence from the sport, making them the number one major injury in soccer.[10] Nearly half of all knee injuries occur during tackling.[10,22] Knee sprains and strains caused the greatest amount of subjective complaints postinjury, with chronic pain and swelling being the primary complaints recorded.[10] Other injuries to the knee include meniscus injuries, osteoarthritis, patellofemoral pain, and patellar subluxations and dislocations.[24,26,27]

ACL Injuries Understanding the mechanism of an injury gives the health care provider an insight into rehabilitation of the athlete.[25] The primary mechanism of injury of the ACL is a noncontact moment.[20,23–25] Seventy-eight percent of all ACL injuries in soccer occurred as a result of landing from a jump or sudden deceleration accompanied by an abrupt change in direction on a planted foot.[20,23,25] Videotapes of these knee injuries revealed a valgus force at the knee along with tibial rotation.[23] Internal and external rotation of the tibia occurred equally during these injuries.[25] Videotapes also showed that deceleration prior to a change in direction was a more common cause of injury than was pivoting around a planted foot.

This deceleration force involves an eccentric contraction of the quadriceps. The quadriceps can exert enough force to displace the tibia anteriorly in relation to the femur. This displacement is greatest in males at 30 degrees of flexion and in females at 60 degrees or less of flexion. This increase in the knee angle could explain the increase in incidence of ACL injuries among females. A review of noncontact injuries showed that most injuries occur near heel strike with an average knee flexion angle of 21 degrees. At this point, the quadriceps are contracting eccentrically, generating maximum force in the muscle. Additionally, activities that involve rapid deceleration and landing produce eccentric contraction of the quadriceps. Maximum eccentric contraction of the quadriceps with the right amount of knee flexion may result in significant anterior translation of the tibia, producing a rupture of the ACL.[25]

The ACL can be ruptured during direct contact with another player. Usually there is a valgus force from the opponent striking the lateral side of the leg during a slide tackle. A slide tackle occurs when one player leaves his or her feet and slides to make contact with the ball in an attempt to force the player with the ball to lose possession or control of the ball. Occasionally, the sliding player may collide with the oncoming player as well as the ball, and an injury may occur.

This mechanism can injure multiple structures within the knee. O'Donoghue's unhappy triad often occurs during a contact injury and has been described as a tear of the ACL, medial collateral ligament (MCL), and medial meniscus.[25] Other studies have shown that the lateral meniscus also can be involved with an injury to the ACL and MCL. The most common mechanism of injury for the meniscus is rotation on the weight-bearing limb.[25]

Knowledge of the differences between male and female athletes can help tailor rehabilitation efforts more specifically to female athletes after an ACL injury. Females tend to have increased incidence of genu recurvatum and joint laxity. In rehabilitation, focus needs to be on controlling knee position for stability with closed-chain exercises that involve various knee angles. Females have been found to have a smaller intercondylar notch index than males.[20,23] This has been implicated as a reason for ACL failure.[20] Excessive pronation may need to be controlled more in female athletes. Females also have a wider pelvis than their male counterparts, which diminishes muscular force.[23] Sufficient quadriceps strength is important for knee stability and therefore is important to address in the rehabilitation process of females as well as males.

Understanding the extrinsic and intrinsic factors involved in ACL injuries provides us with the knowledge necessary to devise a rehabilitation program tailored to the individual soccer player's needs. The goal of an ACL program is to return an athlete back to competition as quickly and as safely as possible. A criterion-based approach requires the athlete to complete certain objectives before advancing to the next phase of rehabilitation. Most programs are divided into different phases based on the stage of the injury and time frames related to tissue healing.[23]

In the preoperative phase, goals include decreasing inflammation, swelling, and pain and restoring ROM, strength, and gait.[23] Exercises include quad sets; straight-leg raises for hip abduction, adduction, flexion, and extension; and closed-chain exercises such as minisquats, toe raises, step-ups, and standing resistive knee extension exercises with tubing. There must be excellent form with these exercises. Any exercises that increase anterior translation of the tibia must be avoided. Functional electrical stimulation may be used to elicit a contraction of the quadriceps if the athlete is having difficulty contracting the quadriceps on his or her own volition. For ROM, passive prone knee extension hangs and active assisted knee flexion in the supine and prone positions are used. Careful attention should be given to the end feel. Occasionally, a torn meniscus can be mechanically blocking the ROM. In this case, the ROM should not be forced. In this phase, modalities such as ice and electrical stimulation are used to control swelling. Providing the athlete with a postoperative home exercise program (HEP) is essential for early success after surgery.

Immediately after surgery, the goals are to restore full passive extension, decrease swelling and pain, gradually increase knee flexion to normal values, and initiate a good quadriceps contraction. Exercises include quad sets with electrical stimulation as needed, patellar mobilizations, and straight-leg raises for hip abduction, adduction, flexion, and extension. Based on the physician's approach, the leg raises may be performed with the brace locked at zero, especially if the patient has poor quadriceps control and cannot maintain 0 degrees of extension with the exercises. The quality of the exercise is extremely important at this time. The therapist should ensure that full knee extension can be maintained isometrically with these movements. Hamstring stretches are performed along with other ROM exercises for full extension. The knee flexion goal is at least 90 degrees in the first 5 to 7 days postoperatively. Heel slides or wall slides typically are used to increase ROM at this time. Progression after the first 2 weeks includes exercises such as multiangle isometrics, quarter-depth minisquats, weight shifting, and single-limb balance.[23] Modalities include ice and electrical stimulation for pain and edema control. A continuous passive motion machine often is used in the patient's home in this initial phase of therapy to gain ROM.

The early phase of rehabilitation lasts from 2 to 6 weeks and includes the aforementioned goals in addition to increased patellar mobility and independent ambulation. At this point, isotonic machines such as the leg press are added. Hamstring curls with and without cuff weights, bicycle training, step-ups, and proprioceptive training are integrated into the therapy program. The criteria to progress the patient to this phase of rehabilitation include full passive knee extension, knee flexion to 90 degrees, good patellar mobility, good quadriceps control, minimal joint effusion, and independent ambulation.[23]

The intermediate phase lasts from approximately week 4 through week 10. At this point, full active ROM should be the primary goal. The criteria to enter this phase include active ROM from 0 to 115 degrees, minimal to no joint effusion, and no joint-line pain. All exercises from phase 1 are continued. Additional closed-chain exercises such as the stairstepper and wobble board are added. Depending on the physician, isotonic knee machines in limited range for extension, isokinetics, plyometrics, and pool running are initiated in weeks 8 to 10.[23]

The advanced phase is when the athlete can begin sport-specific training. Criteria for this phase include full active ROM, no pain or effusion, quadriceps strength of at least 70 percent of contralateral side, and hamstring strength 100 percent of the contralateral side.[23] In this phase, single-leg volleying exercises with the soccer ball are initiated. Tubing for resistance around the player's waist while kicking, trapping, or heading the ball also can be used. Hopping drills are more difficult for the athlete. The athlete balances on one foot, performs a task such as volleying (kicking the ball while it is in the air) the ball back to the therapist, and then hops onto the opposite lower extremity and repeats the drill with the other extremity. This is a very good drill to help rebuild the athlete's confidence in the injured leg before returning to the playing field. A running program is initiated and, by week 12, cutting and pivoting are introduced. Depending on the progress of the athlete and the physician, it is 6 to 12 months before the athlete returns to competition.

Meniscal Tears As discussed earlier, meniscal tears often are associated with ligament injuries to the knee. However, they also can occur in isolation. Rehabilitation of a meniscal injury can be more aggressive than that of an ACL injury. A comprehensive strengthening program often helps the athlete avoid surgery. If surgery is indicated, then arthroscopy is usually performed. Since this procedure is less invasive than an open surgical procedure, healing occurs at a faster rate. The goals of rehabilitation are similar to those of the ACL protocol, focusing on increasing ROM, decreasing pain and swelling, and normalizing gait and strength. Exercises discussed earlier for ACL patients are similar for these patients, but progression occurs more rapidly. As long the partial meniscectomy is performed in isolation, there are no contraindications for aggressive rehabilitation. Once again, care should be taken to make sure that the athlete can perform the functional tasks necessary for soccer before releasing him or her back to the playing field. The average postoperative rehabilitation of a meniscectomy patient lasts 4 to 6 weeks.

Osteoarthritis Osteoarthritis (OA) is often found in athletes, especially after an ACL tear. The explanation for the fast progression of OA after an ACL injury is possibly the high forces that are involved in the initial injury. Blunt trauma that occurs along with the injury also may be a predisposing factor to the development of OA. Loss of proprioception and a change in gait pattern are additional causative factors in the progression of OA.[24] While OA cannot be prevented after an injury, additional trauma can be minimized through the restoration of strength, ROM, and proprioception and by teaching proper technique. Lack of knowledge about proper injury rehabilitation by soccer players can

lead to further complications. Many players attempt to treat themselves after an injury and often end up with complications.[10] It is the health care provider's responsibility to make certain that the athlete understands the injury and the importance of adequate rehabilitation.

Thigh Injuries

Contusions After ankle and knee injuries, contusions have the next highest incidence in soccer players.[2] The most commonly involved muscle is the quadriceps. Usually the deep vastus muscles adjacent to the bone are involved. Symptoms include pain with movement or muscle contraction, swelling, and stiffness. Muscle testing can reveal weakness on evaluation.[29] More acute care than actual long-term rehabilitation is required in the management of a contusion. Contusions usually result from a blunt impact to the muscle tissue.[29] An impact to a contracted, nonfatigued muscle is more resistant to injury and usually results in a less severe contusion. The advent of shin guards in soccer has reduced the number of lower leg contusions significantly, but nonetheless they still occur. Common treatment includes ice, pulsed ultrasound, electrical stimulation, and relative rest.

Myositis Ossificans Myositis ossificans is one complication of a muscle contusion. Ectopic bone forms in the quadriceps muscle belly. It is often caused by the lack of proper rest after a contusion.[21] Diagnosis is made by x-ray that is usually taken as a result of the athlete's continued complaints of pain, swelling, and the presence of a lump on palpation.[29]

Thigh Strains Muscle strains usually occur in two joint muscles during forceful eccentric contractions. The musculotendinous junction is most often the site of the lesion. The quadriceps, hamstrings, and hip adductors are the most common sites for strains in soccer players. Minor strains often occur before major ones. It is also more common to see strains occur during practice rather than during game situations. They are also more common in fatigued muscles because they absorb less energy and are therefore less resistant to a stretch. The athlete who has an increase in lumbar lordosis is also more likely to suffer from muscle strains.[29]

For these reasons, the health care team should educate soccer players on proper conditioning. This will allow the muscles to absorb more energy and avoid a fatigued state that will predispose them to injury.[29] As part of preseason conditioning, a focus on trunk strengthening can promote lumbar stability and decrease the risk of hamstring muscle strains. The athlete with a history of muscle strains needs to understand the importance of warming up and cooling down.

Symptoms of muscle strains include pain with activity or with an isometric muscle contraction. Usually the athlete will report feeling the muscle pull while he or she is running or playing. There is loss of function and the presentation of increased tone but little discoloration with muscle strains.[21]

Treatment for strains involves modalities, ice, and rest. Immediate compression also reduces swelling. Massage performed too deep may increase the risk of myositis ossificans, so caution should be used with this procedure.[29] Any athlete who does not improve with treatment in 1 to 2 days needs to be seen by a physician to rule out further injury.

Groin Injuries Groin injuries can encompass many different diagnoses. Because of the numerous structures in the area, differential diagnosis is often difficult. The injuries of the groin include inguinal hernias, adductor tendinitis, osteitis pubis, and muscle strains of the adductor longus and brevis as well as the gracilis.[30]

Hernias produce discomfort with prolonged standing or walking more so than with participation in sports. With an inguinal hernia, there is usually a palpable lump with coughing. There is little the rehabilitation specialist can do when a hernia is present. Often the athlete can participate in soccer without surgical intervention.[31] In more severe cases, the athlete will need surgery to repair the defect. The loss of time from soccer can be up to 6 weeks. The soccer player can still use an upper body bike to maintain some degree of fitness.

The adductor muscles are commonly injured when a quick change in direction occurs with an associated external rotation and/or abduction movement.[31] Adductor strains also can occur when an athlete fails to warm up properly.[32] The adductors are commonly injured because of the lack of focus placed on these muscles in conditioning programs. Symptoms include acute pain, usually at the adductor's insertion into the pelvis in more severe cases and distally in the muscle belly in less severe injuries.[31] Pain is exacerbated by resisted adduction and passive abduction.[32] Treatment includes ice, rest, gentle stretching, and isometrics. Once the pain decreases, strengthening exercises with ankle weights or therapeutic tubing with a progression to eccentric exercises will help to build the strength and endurance of the muscle so that it is more resistant to injury.[31,32]

Osteitis pubis used to be the most common diagnosis of groin pain in soccer players and is now more appropriately referred to as symphysis pubis instability. The incidence of injury is not as frequent as was once thought. It is actually inflammation at the symphysis pubis secondary to increased movement. Symptoms include pain over the midline of the symphysis pubis. Treatment involves prolonged rest. Injections and surgery occur only in severe cases that do not resolve with rest.[32]

The term *athletic pubalgia* has become popular in recent years. This term refers to weakness or a defect near the pubic insertion of the rectus abdominis and internal oblique aponeurosis in the inguinal area. The microtearing of the pelvic floor musculature near the inguinal ring may be a result of the repetitive stresses of sprinting and kicking. Nerve irritation also may contribute to this painful condition. Physical examination will reveal pain with resisted hip flexion, adduction, internal rotation, and abdominal muscle contractions. Palpation of the pubic tubercle typically elicits pain, but the hip flexors and adductors should not be tender. The presence of a hernia should be ruled out.[35]

Treatment for this condition begins with rest and nonsteroidal anti-inflammatory drugs (NSAIDs). Physical therapy is often beneficial to restore muscle balance around the pelvis. Trigger-point massage to the piriformis, hamstring, and gluteus medius can be beneficial. After a few days, light stretching to the adductors, abductors, hamstrings, hip flexors, hip rotators, and low back should be started. As pain decreases, abdominal strengthening including the rectus abdominis and the obliques should be initiated, followed by adductor strengthening. Combining abdominal exercises on a gym ball with isometric adduction can be a good challenge for the athlete. The stationary bike and other cardiovascular training techniques should be used until the athlete can return to painfree running. As with other injuries, the athlete should progress to higher-level exercises that simulate game situations such as sprinting, cutting, and tackling. If the athlete fails to respond to conservative treatment, surgery may be indicated. It can take up to 4 months after surgery for the athlete to return to play.[35]

Other injuries include stress fractures of the femoral neck or the inferior pubic ramus. These injuries are very rare in soccer players, however. Occasionally, a soccer player may develop trochanteric bursitis, iliopsoas bursitis, or adductor tendinitis. Diagnosis of these conditions is often difficult because of the nondescript pain the athlete reports. The treatment of these conditions is usually conservative. With NSAIDs and rest, the athlete usually can return to play in 4 to 6 weeks.[32]

LOWER EXTREMITY REHABILITATION

Once the clinician has determined what is indicated for full return to sport, he or she can begin to incorporate sport-specific activities during the recovery process. Many lower extremity injuries result in a decrease in balance and proprioception. These deficits need to be addressed prior to return to the playing field. Other sport-specific activities need to be included into the athlete's rehabilitation to ensure that he or she is ready to return to competition.

When dealing with lower extremity injuries, closed-chain exercises should be incorporated in the strengthening phase. Several basic closed-chain exercises can be modified to incorporate soccer skills that will not only progress the player toward his or her goals but also will help restore confidence. Players can begin with basic inside and outside passing.

Closed-chain activities such as the slide board can be modified to create sport-specific drills for goalkeepers. As the goalkeeper pushes off from the side, the therapist tosses the ball in the direction that the player is heading on the slide board. The athlete must catch the ball using proper technique for a goalkeeper. This exercise incorporates the side-to-side mobility necessary for the goalkeeper along with performance of a position-specific technique. This drill can be performed with the ball being tossed to both sides with varying rest periods between throws to simulate game demands.

Basic balance and proprioception exercises include activities that require a single-leg stance. The player can balance while stabilizing the ball in different positions (Fig. 14.3).

Balance activities also can include balancing on a minitrampoline, foam roll, or wob-

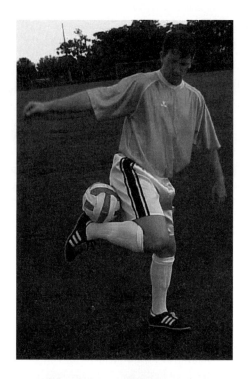

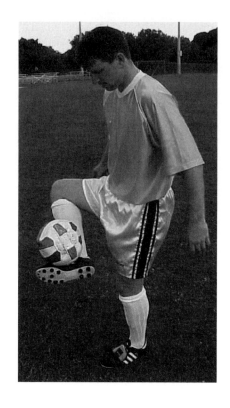

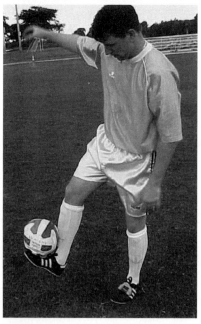

FIGURE 14.3

Single-leg balance with the ball in different positions.

ble board to work on balance and proprioception training. To challenge the soccer player, the therapist can involve skills such as heading or volleying while performing balance exercises. The therapist stands 5 to 10 ft away from the athlete and tosses the ball to the player's head. The athlete heads the ball back to the therapist. In addition, the uninvolved leg can be used for a series of half-volley drills while balancing. In this drill, the ball is tossed toward the athlete's foot, and the athlete kicks the ball back to the therapist or bounces it for repetitions. The athlete may be required to use the instep, dorsum of the foot, or thigh in these drills. These exercises also can be performed on a wobble board, foam roll, or minitrampoline to challenge the athlete's balance.

To progress activities, a sport cord can be placed around the athlete's waist while he or she steps forward, backward, or to the side, usually leading with the involved extremity. The angle of pull on the athlete can be altered to vary the muscular demands. After this has been mastered, the athlete can perform side lunges with the sport cord in place. Balance exercises can be performed with the athlete standing on the injured leg and the cord positioned around the uninvolved ankle. He or she then quickly kicks forward, backward, medially, and laterally while maintaining his or her balance on the injured extremity. Repetitions can vary based on the level of proficiency displayed by the athlete. Performing these exercises for set time intervals will further challenge the athlete. This gives the athlete the opportunity to perform activities as he or she is building up endurance.

The sport cord also can be placed behind an athlete's knee while standing with the involved lower extremity posterior to the uninvolved lower extremity. The athlete then flexes and extends the involved knee while keeping the foot flat on the floor. The opposite knee remains extended. This closed-chain terminal knee extension activity facilitates good control of knee extension that is necessary for gait, running, and kicking.

Once a dynamic component is appropriate for the athlete's rehabilitation, heading, half-volley, and trapping drills with movement can be performed. Volleying the ball requires the athlete to kick the ball in a controlled manner while it is still in the air. Trapping is slowing down the speed of the ball and bringing it under control. The athlete starts by hopping forward about 1 to 2 ft on the involved leg. Using a soccer ball, the therapist throws the ball to the player while he or she balances on the involved leg. The athlete then traps the ball and volleys it back to the therapist. Immediately after the ball leaves the player's body, the athlete hops forward on the involved leg without placing the uninvolved leg on the ground. The process is repeated as the player progresses forward in a straight line by hopping after each time the ball is returned to the therapist. Having the player hop backwards or diagonally can advance this drill.

By placing a row of cones 2 to 3 ft apart, the therapist can direct the athlete to hop over the cones, alternating one leg after the other. Next, the athlete remains balanced on the injured leg and hops through the row of cones. To advance the drill, the therapist can have the athlete hop from the inside of one cone to the outside of the next cone. When this is performed with some level of competence, rows of 8 to 10 cones are placed 2 to 3 ft apart. The athlete stands on the inside of the first cone in the row. The player balances on the injured extremity. The therapist stands 5 to 10 ft in front of the athlete and throws the ball for the athlete to head or volley back without placing the kicking leg or uninvolved leg on the ground. Immediately after the athlete returns the ball to the therapist, he or she hops forward on the involved leg to the opposite side of the next cone or, in this example, to the outside of the cone. The athlete continues to progress forward, hopping from one side of the cone to the opposite side of the next cone, until the end of the row is reached.

UPPER EXTREMITY INJURIES

Fractures

Upper extremity injuries are more common in goalkeepers than in field players. Fractures to the elbows, fingers, and wrists are the most common upper extremity injuries in soccer.[18] These injuries are usually the result of a fall or collision. Pain and deformity are usually present.[21] After the fracture is healed and the rehabilitation process begins, it is important to restore motion, strength, and function. The health care provider must take into consideration the position of the player during rehabilitation. A field player may be able to return to play with the injured area protected by a cast. This is not practical for goalkeepers because of the different demands of the position. With the rehabilitation of upper extremity injuries, functional training to include catching and throwing will be necessary to return the athlete to competition. If a goalkeeper is injured, more emphasis will be placed on throwing and catching than with a field player. Special consideration also should be given to the diving techniques of the goalkeeper. Coaches need to review proper landing techniques in order for the player to avoid excessive stress on the upper extremities due to poor mechanics. Plyometrics with weighted balls can be a valuable strengthening exercise when rehabilitating the upper extremities.

Occasionally, a soccer player fractures the clavicle when falling on an outstretched arm or hitting the shoulder on the ground. Treatment consists of a sling or clavicle strap until bony healing has occurred. The athlete can begin a throwing program usually after 6 to 8 weeks.[30] It is important to keep the field player from returning too soon following this injury. Although the player may feel that he or she can compete after 1 to 2 weeks, the bone may not be healed enough to absorb forces from routine contact with other players during the game.

Acromioclavicular Separations

Common shoulder injuries include acromioclavicular (AC) sprains. These can occur in field players as well as goalkeepers. The most common mechanism of injury to the goalkeeper's shoulder is usually landing on the ground or colliding with the goalpost. Field players also can experience shoulder injuries during collisions with other players, with the ground, and occasionally, with the goal posts. More specifically, AC sprains are usually the result of a direct blow to the lateral aspect of the shoulder girdle, forcing the acromion downward, or an upward force through the long axis of the humerus.[21]

AC sprains are graded according to severity. A grade 1 sprain is characterized by point tenderness over the AC joint and pain with shoulder flexion and abduction. No deformity is present. A grade 2 sprain presents with deformity at the AC joint and the lateral end of the clavicle prominent on inspection. The athlete has pain with motion and is unable to fully abduct or horizontally adduct the involved side. A grade 3 sprain involves complete disruption of the AC and coracoclavicular ligaments. Gross deformity is present. There is severe pain, loss of shoulder stability, and severe loss of motion.[21]

Treatment of AC separations includes immobilization with a sling to allow for healing for 2 to 10 days, followed by progressive rehabilitation. Taping of the AC joint should be used to decrease pain and speed up the restoration of function.[33] Rehabilitation of an AC sprain includes closed-chain exercises to promote stability as well as ROM exercises to prevent adhesive capsulitis. Periscapular and rotator cuff strengthening exercises are imperative to restore the correct firing of the muscles of the shoulder in order to restore full normal excursion of the involved extremity.

Shoulder Dislocations

Shoulder dislocations are not common but do occur in soccer. An athlete may be predisposed to subluxations or dislocations due to capsular laxity. If this is detected in a preseason screening, a comprehensive strengthening program that allows the dynamic stabilizers to aid in supporting the humerus in the glenoid fossa can reduce the risk of dislocations. In the event that a player dislocates the shoulder, he or she should be removed from competition immediately. The athlete should seek medical attention to reduce the upper extremity. Normally, the athlete will be immobilized in a sling, and depending on the physician, rehabilitation can be initiated immediately to reduce inflammation with modalities, and isometrics are begun to the wrist, elbow, and the shoulder. Rehabilitation consists of gentle ROM in all directions, with special caution to avoid humeral head translation in the direction of instability. Identifying tight structures and performing manual stretching of those structures, often the posterior capsule, will allow for better alignment of the humerus in the glenoid. For an anterior dislocation, the patient should be restricted from external rotation in an abducted position. Once the pain has decreased and ROM in flexion and internal rotation is restored, strengthening exercises should be started. Strengthening the surrounding muscles will contribute to support of the shoulder girdle. (See Chap. 10 for more discussion of rehabilitation for an anterior glenohumeral joint dislocation.)

UPPER EXTREMITY REHABILITATION

For upper extremity injuries, Theraband can be used to rehabilitate the shoulder, elbow, and wrists. Plyometric training also can be performed with tubing in functional positions such as 90 degrees of shoulder and elbow flexion, with an eccentric phase preceding a concentric phase to maximize strengthening for throwing.

Medicine ball exercises are also useful in the rehabilitation of upper extremity injuries. Although the goalkeeper is the only player allowed to use the hands, an injury to the upper extremity of any field player could limit his or her ability to play to potential. Medicine ball drills can be performed with the athlete lying supine. The therapist stands at the head of the athlete and lightly releases the ball. The starting position of the athlete is with the arms fully extended upward toward the ceiling. The athlete catches the ball and brings the ball into the chest. As the athlete begins the movement away from the body, the ball is released, throwing it back to the therapist. The focus is on a continuous movement back to the start position. The athlete should not pause while the ball is near the chest.

In addition, minitrampolines can be used for plyometric training. The athlete stands 5 to 10 ft away from the trampoline and throws the ball in a variety of patterns. Overhead throwing uses both upper extremities to simulate a soccer throw in from the sidelines. The athlete brings the ball back behind the head and then releases the ball toward the trampoline as the arms come forward over the head. Throwing also can be performed from a seated or kneeling position. A rotational component can be performed with the ball by introducing diagonal throwing patterns. These exercises are beneficial in rehabilitation of back injuries as well as upper extremity injuries.

Plyometric wall push-ups are performed with assistance of the therapist. The athlete places his or her hands shoulder width apart at shoulder height. The athlete's feet are 2 to 3 ft away from the wall. The individual performs a push-up. As the elbows are extended, the hands break contact with the wall. The therapist is positioned behind the individual, and as the athlete's body approaches the therapist, he or she exerts a force on the athlete's back strong enough to force the individual back in the opposite direction, or toward the wall. The force is not varied, but the timing of when the force is delivered can be altered.

The treadmill and stairstepper can be used in unconventional ways for closed-chain stabilization of the upper extremities. These exercises help to promote proximal stability of the involved limb. From a kneeling position, the athlete positions both hands on the belt of the treadmill. Once the treadmill is turned on at a slow speed, the athlete moves one hand in front of the other to mimic a walking motion. This closed-chain exercise requires minimal coordination. The stairstepper also can be used for similar results but has a higher degree of difficulty involved. From the same position, the individual places each hand on the step of the stairstepper and pushes the step up and down in the same manner as using the feet. Because this can be a very taxing exercise, shorter time increments or lower repetitions should be performed.

HEAD INJURIES

Head injuries are not overly common in soccer, but they can occur during collisions with other players and the goalpost. By definition, head injuries include dental, ophthalmologic, and closed head injury. Soccer players have about a 3 percent risk of head injury during a game or practice.[1] Symptoms of serious head injuries usually appear within 36 h. The symptoms include nausea, vomiting, dizziness, headaches, seizures, swelling, bruising, bleeding, and memory loss. Collisions with the goalposts can be very severe and are the number one cause of death in soccer.[17]

Concussions (Injury Rate)

Although concussion injuries are not addressed from a rehabilitative standpoint, it is important to manage them correctly. Trainers and coaches should remove an athlete from competition if there is any indication of ring-

ing in the ears, nausea, or headache. (See Chap. 12 for more information on concussions.)

Return to Sport

With the increase in participation in soccer comes an increase in soccer-related injuries. For rehabilitation specialists working with soccer players, it is important to have a good understanding of the demands of the sport on the athlete. This includes biomechanics of kicking and heading, rules of the game, demands of individual positions, and incidence and mechanism of injury. Rehabilitation specialists can then define the parameters for rehabilitation through their knowledge of injuries and the demands of soccer on the individual. With a basic understanding of soccer, many everyday rehabilitation techniques can be modified to simulate a sport-specific activity.

Creativity in the recovery process is a key element in keeping athletes motivated while preparing them for return to the playing field and is only limited by the rehabilitation specialist's imagination.

For players to return to game play, they should have 90 percent of their strength and good proprioception. Agility drills such as the single-leg hop test or the shuttle run can be helpful. The athlete should be able to start, stop, cut, jump, and run during any of these tests. Also, skill drills such as kicking, passing, and running through cones while controlling the ball can be helpful in planning the athlete's progression back to the competition.

References

1. Metzl JD, Micheli LJ: Youth soccer: An epidemologic perspective. *Clin Sports Med* 17: 664–674, 1998.

2. Hoy K, Lindblad BE, Terkelsen CJ, et al: European soccer injuries: A prospective epidemiologic and socioeconomic study. *Am J Sports Med* 20:318–322, 1992.

3. Garrett WE, Kirkendall DT, Contiguglia SR: *The US Soccer Sports Medicine Book.* Baltimore: Williams & Wilkins, 1996.

4. Bangsbo J: The physiology of soccer, with special reference to intense intermittent exercise. *Acta Physiol Scand Suppl* 619:1–155, 1994.

5. Barfield WR: The biomechanics of kicking in soccer. *Clin Sports Med* 17:712–728, 1998.

6. Safran MR, Garrett WE, Seaber AV, et al: The role of warm-up in muscular injury prevention. *Am J Sports Med* 16:123–128, 1988.

7. Ekstrand J, Gillquist J, Liljedahl S: Prevention of soccer injuries: Supervision by doctor and physiotherapist. *Am J Sports Med* 11:116–120, 1983.

8. Hergenroeder AC: Prevention of sports injuries. *Pediatrics* 101:1057–1063, 1998.

9. Ekstrand J, Gillquist J, Moller M, et al: Incidence of soccer injuries and their relation to training and team success. *Am J Sports Med* 11:63–67, 1983.

10. Nielsen AB, Yde J: Epidemiology and traumatology of injuries in soccer. *Am J Sports Med* 17:803–807, 1989.

11. Keller CS, Noyes FR, Buncher CR: The medical aspects of soccer injury epidemiology. *Am J Sports Med* 15:230–237, 1987.

12. Hedrick A: Soccer specific conditioning. *Strength Condit J* 21:17–21, 1999.

13. Baechle TR: *Essentials of Strength and Conditioning,* 2d ed. Champaign, IL: Human Kinetics, 2000.

14. Hewett TE, Stroupe AL, Nance TA, et al: Plyometric training in female athletes: Decreased impact forces and increased hamstring torques. *Am J Sports Med* 24:765–773, 1996.

15. Boden BP: Leg injuries and shin guards. *Clin Sports Med* 17(4):769–777, 1998.

16. Matser JT, Kessels AG, Jordan BD, et al: Chronic traumatic brain injury in professional soccer players. *Neurology* 51:791–796, 1998.

17. Janda DH, Bir C, Wild B, et al: Goal post injuries in soccer: A laboratory and field testing analysis of a preventive intervention. *Am J Sports Med* 23:340–344, 1995.

18. Lindenfeld TN, Schmitt DJ, Hendy MP, et al: Incidence of injury in indoor soccer. *Am J Sports Med* 22:364–371, 1994.

19. Engstron B, Johansson C, Tornkvist H: Soccer injuries among elite female players. *Am J Sports Med* 19:372–375, 1991.

20. Arendt E, Dick R: Knee injury patterns among men and women in collegiate basketball and soccer. *Am J Sports Med* 23:694–701, 1995.

21. Arnheim DD, Prentice WE: *Principles of Athletic Training.* St. Louis: Mosby–Year Book, 1993.

22. Bjordal JM, Arnoy F, Hannestad B, et al: Epidemiology of anterior cruciate ligament injuries in soccer. *Am J Sports Med* 25:341–346, 1997.

23. Wilk KE, Arrigo C, Andrews JR, et al: Rehabilitation after anterior cruciate ligament reconstruction in the female athlete. *J Athlet Train* 34:177–191, 1999.

24. Roos H: Are there long term sequelae from soccer? *Clin Sports Med* 17:819–830, 1998.

25. Delfico AJ, Garrett WE: Mechanisms of injury of the anterior cruciate ligament in soccer players. *Clin Sports Med* 17:780–785, 1998.

26. DeHaven KE, Lintner DM: Athletic injuries: Comparison by age, sport, and gender. *Am J Sports Med* 14:218–224, 1986.

27. Brynhildsen BJ, Ekstrand J, Jeppddon A, et al: Previous injuries and persisting symptoms in female soccer players. *Int J Sports Med* 11:489–492, 1990.

28. Alexander MJ: Peak torque values for antagonist muscle groups and concentric and eccentric contraction types for elite sprinters. *Arch Phys Med Rehabil* 71:334–339, 1990.

29. Saartok T: Muscle injuries associated with soccer. *Clin Sports Med* 17:811–817, 1998.

30. Moriarity JM: Injuries in football and soccer, in Sallis RE, Massimo F (eds): *Essentials of Sportsmedicine.* St. Louis: Mosby–Year Book, 1997, pp 592–601.

31. Garrick JG, Webb DR: *Sports Injuries: Diagnosis and Management,* 2d ed. Philadelphia: Saunders, 1999.

32. Gilmore J: Groin pain in the soccer athlete, fact, fiction, and treatment. *Clin Sports Med* 17:788–793, 1998.

33. Shamus J, Shamus E: A taping technique for the treatment of acromioclavicular joint sprains: A case study. *J Orthop Sports Phys Ther* 25:390–394, 1997.

34. Brewington P: Headers face scrutiny in soccer. *USA Today,* December 8, 1999.

35. Meyers WC, Foley DP, Garrett WE, et al: Management of severe lower abdominal or inguinal pain in high-performance athletes: PAIN (Performing Athletes with Abdominal or Inguinal Neuromuscular Pain Study Group). *Am J Sports Med* 28(1):2–8, 2000.

36. Bir CA, Cassatta SJ, Janda DH: An anaylsis and comparison of soccer shin guards. *Clin J Sport Med* 5:95–99, 1995.

37. Gainor BJ, Piotrowski G, Puhl JJ, et al: The kick, biomechanics and collision injury. *Am J Sports Med* 14:231–233, 1986.

38. Lohnes JH, Garrett WE, Monto RR: Soccer, in Fu F, Stone DA (eds): *Sports Injuries: Mechanisms, Prevention, Treatment.* Baltimore: Williams & Wilkins, 1994, pp 603–624.

Additional References

Anderson SJ: Soccer, a case-based approach to ankle and knee injuries. *Pediatr Ann* 29(3): 178–188, 2000.

Bishop NC, Blannin AK, Robson PJ, et al: The effects of carbohydrate supplementation on immune responses to a soccer-specific exercise protocol. *J Sports Sci* 17(10):787–796, 1999.

Boden BP, Lohnes JH, Nunley JA, Garrett WE Jr: Tibia and fibula fractures in soccer players. *Knee Surg Sports Traumatol Arthrosc* 7(4): 262–266, 1999.

Davids K, Lees A, Burwitz L: Understanding and measuring coordination and control in kicking skills in soccer: Implications for talent identification and skill acquisition. *J Sports Sci* 18(9):703–714, 2000.

DiFiori JP: Stress fracture of the proximal fibula in a young soccer player: A case report and a review of the literature. *Med Sci Sports Exerc* 31(7):925–928, 1999.

Dorge HC, Andersen TB, Sorensen H, et al: EMG activity of the iliopsoas muscle and leg kinetics during the soccer place kick. *Scand J Med Sci Sports* 9(4):195–200, 1999.

Drust B, Cable NT, Reilly T: Investigation of the effects of the pre-cooling on the physiological responses to soccer-specific intermittent exercise. *Eur J Appl Physiol* 81(1–2):11–17, 2000.

Francisco AC, Nightingale RW, Guilak F, et al: Comparison of soccer shin guards in preventing tibia fracture. *Am J Sports Med* 28(2): 227–233, 2000.

Grote C, Donders J: Brain injury in amateur soccer players. *JAMA* 283(7):882–883, 2000.

Hansen L, Bangsbo J, Twisk J, Klausen K: Development of muscle strength in relation to training level and testosterone in young male soccer players. *J Appl Physiol* 87(3):1141–1147, 1999.

Helsen WF, Hodges NJ, Van Winckel J, Starkes JL: The roles of talent, physical precocity and practice in the development of soccer expertise. *J Sports Sci* 18(9):727–736, 2000.

Heidt RS Jr, Sweeterman LM, Carlonas RL, et al: Avoidance of soccer injuries with preseason conditioning. *Am J Sports Med* 28(5):659–662, 2000.

Houshian S: Traumatic duodenal rupture in a soccer player. *Br J Sports Med* 34(3):218–219, 2000.

Karageanes SJ, Blackburn K, Vangelos ZA: The association of the menstrual cycle with the laxity of the anterior cruciate ligament in adolescent female athletes. *Clin J Sport Med* 10(3): 162–168, 2000.

Malina RM, Pena Reyes ME, Eisenmann JC, et al: Height, mass and skeletal maturity of elite Portuguese soccer players aged 11–16 years. *J Sports Sci* 18(9):685–693, 2000.

McCarroll JR, Meaney C, Sieber JM: Profile of youth soccer injuries. *Phys Sports Med* 12(2): 113–117,1984.

McGarry T, Franks IM: On winning the penalty shoot-out in soccer. *J Sports Sci* 18(6): 401–409, 2000.

McGregor SJ, Nicholas CW, Lakomy HK, Williams C: The influence of intermittent high-intensity shuttle running and fluid ingestion on the performance of a soccer skill. *J Sports Sci* 17(11):895–903, 1999.

Morris T: Psychological characteristics and talent identification in soccer. *J Sports Sci* 18(9): 715–726, 2000.

Nicholas CW, Nuttall FE, Williams C: The Loughborough intermittent shuttle test: A field test that simulates the activity pattern of soccer. *J Sports Sci* 18(2):97–104, 2000.

Putukian M, Echemendia RJ, Mackin S: The acute neuropsychological effects of heading in soccer: A pilot study. *Clin J Sport Med* 10(2):104–109, 2000.

Putukian M, Knowles WK, Swere S, et al: Injuries in indoor soccer, the lake placid dawn to dark soccer tournament. *Am J Sports Med* 14:317–322, 1996.

Reilly T, Bangsbo J, Franks A: Anthropometric and physiological predispositions for elite soccer. *J Sports Sci* 18(9):669–683, 2000.

Rienzi E, Drust B, Reilly T, et al: Investigation of anthropometric and work-rate profiles of elite South American international soccer players. *J Sports Med Phys Fitness* 40(2):162–169, 2000.

Shephard RJ: Biology and medicine of soccer: an update. *J Sports Sci* 17(10):757–786, 1999.

Sozen AB, Akkaya V, Demirel S, et al: Echocardiographic findings in professional league soccer players: Effect of the position of the players on the echocardiographic parameters. *J Sports Med Phys Fitness* 40(2):150–155, 2000.

Templeton PA, Farrar MJ, Williams HR, et al: Complications of tibial shaft soccer fractures. *Injury* 31(6):415–419, 2000.

Van-Yperen NW, Duda JL: Goal orientations, beliefs about success, and performance improvement among young elite Dutch soccer players. *Scand J Med Sci Sports* 9(6):358–364, 1999.

Williams LR: Coincidence timing of a soccer pass: Effects of stimulus velocity and movement distance. *Percept Motor Skills* 91(1):39–52, 2000.

Williams AM: Perceptual skill in soccer: Implications for talent identification and development. *J Sports Sci* 18(9):737–750, 2000.

CHAPTER 15

Martial Arts

George J. Davies
Chris Durall
Dennis Fater

The martial arts have evolved over millennia as a means to kill or disable. It is only in the last few decades that the martial arts have been marketed and sold as sport. It would appear that the transition to sport is incomplete.[81]

There has been a veritable explosion of interest and participation in the martial arts globally. Commercial entrepreneurism, media promotion, the health and fitness resurgence, and international diplomacy and goodwill have attracted at least 75 million participants worldwide.[8] The United States has been particularly infected with martial arts fever in the last few decades, with an estimated 8 million practitioners. In many countries, the annual growth rate is expected to be 20 to 25 percent.

The twentieth century brought rising popularity for the martial arts as sports forms and the attraction of a young and exuberant audience, likely due in part to the popular use of martial arts in films. Approximately 20 percent of martial arts participants are children.[44] Martial arts training has been advocated for individuals of all ages and abilities, including the elderly,[57,62,129–132] patients with rheumatoid arthritis,[48] and patients with spinal cord injuries[37,38,83] for conditioning and fitness, self-defense, health and recreation, self-confidence, self-discipline, social and environmental support, sports competition, artistic expression, and psychological, philosophical, and religious transformation.

Many styles of martial arts are practiced today, each with its own subtypes, schools, and individual philosophy of discipline. Training in all the martial arts is time-intensive and focuses on mental and physical endurance. Most martial arts incorporate a balance of body, mind, and spirit and emphasize focus, concentration, physical fitness, flexibility, strength, speed, power, agility, balance, reaction time, and coordination.[44] In several martial arts forms, seasoned practitioners have demonstrated an ability to accelerate their feet from 0 to 30 mi/h and kick an opponent with a force of 675 lb/in.[2,125] Recent medical reports provide evidence that this onslaught is probably harder on human bodies than most other sports.[123]

Research on the physical forces, morbidity, and mortality involved in martial arts practice is sparse compared with many other sports.[126] The study of karate, for instance, has been limited primarily to hand traumatology and conditioning.[18] This lack of information has spawned many false notions and perpetuated the aura of mystery surrounding the martial arts. While it is recognized that there are benefits to participation in the martial arts, like most sports, participation involves a risk of injury. However, some of the risks engendered by kickboxing and the martial arts as practiced are unwarranted and preventable.[81] The available evidence on martial arts practice can be used to provide valuable insights on the prevention and rehabilitation of injuries associated with the sport.

Therefore, the purposes of this chapter are to:

1. Present an overview of various martial arts forms.
2. Discuss the epidemiology, mechanisms, locations, and types of martial arts injuries.
3. Describe the kinetics and kinematics associated with selected martial arts activities.
4. Discuss techniques for injury prevention.
5. Provide recommendations regarding specific functional rehabilitation for martial arts participants.

In addition, references are provided to kinesiologic analyses of several karate kicks in this chapter.

History

Throughout much of history, the martial arts have been shrouded in mystery. The term *martial arts* refers to arts concerned with the waging of war and loosely refers to any of the offensive and/or defensive fighting styles or systems of fighting techniques derived in whole or part from the Far East and using one or more body parts.[8] Weapons use also may be incorporated. In the twentieth century, martial arts are no longer practiced entirely for military purposes. Instead, the martial arts have evolved into "the way" to develop character or higher moral standards.[126]

Thousands of different schools, systems, and styles of martial arts exist, and most are associated with a way of life based on Eastern philosophy. Most systems teach unarmed self-defense techniques as well as the use of weaponry and incorporate a spiritual and philosophical component designed to psychologically transform the practitioner. The term *martial ways* focuses primarily on the psychological aspects, with the combative components being secondary. *Martial disciplines* collectively refers to both the martial ways and the fighting arts. All forms have some system of achievement designation. Typically, belt or sash color is used to identify skill level (lighter colors denote less experience, and darker colors are reserved for advanced levels of proficiency). Only about 1 in 500 participants achieves the coveted black belt, which is the departure point for advanced studies.[8]

Martial arts may be divided into those with a strong sport or competitive element (karate, tae kwon do, judo, wrestling) and those with other foci, e.g., self-defense (akido, hapkido) or spiritual development (tai chi chuan). Martial arts also can be divided on the basis of techniques they employ. *Striking arts* are those which rely primarily on kicking or punching techniques and include karate, tae kwon do, kung fu/washa, kickboxing, and hapkido. *Grappling arts* are those which use techniques to throw the opponent to the ground and pin him or her there and include jujutsu, judo, akido, wrestling, and sumo. *Weaponry arts* involve techniques of attack and defense using the sword, staff, nunchaku, and bow and arrow.[9] Although there are many martial arts forms, research on martial arts practice has focused primarily on karate, tae kwon do, judo, and tai chi chuan.

Karate

Karate is both an art and a sport; it incorporates precise movement and body coordination with controlled fight situations.[13] The word *karate* was derived from the Japanese symbol meaning "empty hand" (*kara* = "empty," *te* = "hand"). Traditionally, karate has been a martial art without weapons or protective devices.[115] About 1600 A.D., the Okinawa government confiscated all weapons on the island and enforced a strict prohibition of combative activity or training in any form. For 400 years, though, Okinawans secretly developed and refined karate techniques, and karate flourished as a major martial art. In Korea, a similar martial art is called *tae kwon do*.

Judo

Judo is unique in its competitive element from the other grappling martial arts. Judo evolved from jujutsu after the more dangerous strikes, throws, and joint locks were removed to create a sport. The world headquarters for judo, the Kodokan, has a very active program of medical research. Since its creation in 1882, no fatalities have been reported in the sport as a result of shime-waza (choke holds).[52] Most interest has focused on the neurologic effects of syn-

cope induced by carotid sinus compression.[9] However, outside the sport, fatalities have occurred from tracheal, vertebral, and autonomic nervous system injury. Studies into the possibility of anoxic brain damage as a result of a single or multiple episodes of induced syncope are equivocal. This is discussed in more detail later in this chapter. Injuries from falls and joint locks in judo are similar to those in other grappling arts. Typically, falls onto an outstretched arm produce injury to the wrist, elbow, shoulder, and clavicle (as in tae kwon do).[9] Proper instruction must be provided with respect to falling safely without striking the head on the mat.

Tai Chi Chuan

Tai chi ("supreme ultimate") chuan ("fist") was devised more than 300 years ago in the late Ming and early Quin dynasties of China.[131] The 108 tai chi "forms" evolved from shadow boxing into a martial art used to ward off foreign invaders and to suppress peasant insurrections.

Present-day tai chi chuan practice is typically less combative and slower than other martial art forms, with an emphasis on improved vitality and health. Responses to prolonged tai chi practice include reduced blood pressures,[20,132,134] increased peak oxygen uptake,[10,20,56–58,102] greater flexibility,[58] lower percentage of body fat,[58] increases of T-lymphocytes in the bloodstream,[133] and greater postural/balance control in comparison with sedentary counterparts.[118,129,132,134] Of all the martial arts, tai chi chuan is perhaps the most accessible for the elderly and patients with rheumatoid arthritis.[62] Tai chi chuan exercises may be integrated into therapeutic exercise programs.[48] Ryan[96] presented an excellent descriptive article on the practice of tai chi chuan and some of the background and performance of the activity.

Biomechanics of the Martial Arts

FORCES/KINETICS

There are limited studies in the world's literature that actually describe the biomechanics of performing various martial arts activities. Therefore, this section will review the available studies and make appropriate recommendations throughout. Many researchers are fascinated by the ability of skilled practitioners from various disciplines to break bricks and boards with their hands and feet and consequently have studied such acts from the perspectives of anatomy, biomechanics, and physics.[11] There are relatively few data in the medical literature on the biomechanics of punching and kicking in the martial arts.[103] The speed and force generated by common upper and lower body techniques in the martial arts have been studied and recorded.[7,35,103,122] The forces generated by the kicks, punches, sweeps, and throws are typical of the martial arts.[8]

The incidence of injuries to the lower extremity is not surprising when one considers the power of a well-placed kick. A kick's peak acceleration rivals that of a boxer's punch[11]; thus kicks may fracture ribs and cause organ damage or even death.

The martial arts punch involves forces in excess of 600 ft·lb and speeds approaching 25 m/s.[35] A study by Feld et al.[35] demonstrated that the speed of a straight punch is around 7 m/s, whereas that of a roundhouse kick is about 10 m/s. These blows can exert a force of around 675 lb/in^2.

The sidekick has been shown to produce the most power under laboratory conditions and has caused at least one death.[7,103,122] In kinetic studies, tae kwon do kicks have been shown to have very high injury potential.[34]

To investigate the relative force of kicks and punches, Schwartz et al.[103] developed an instrumented dummy that was mounted to collect the force data. Fourteen karate experts kicked and punched the dummy. Accelerometer measurements in the 90 to 120 $\times$ g range indicated that hand protectors and foot padding did not reduce acceleration of the dummy. Ten-ounce boxing gloves mitigated peak acceleration to some extent. Kicks and punches produced accelerations in the same range. Violent acceleration of the head by any means can produce injury. The authors conclude that if full-contact karate is widely practiced, cases of kickboxer encephalopathy will soon be reported. Their study demonstrated the following points with karate punches and kicks: The peak acceleration is lower for kicks than for punches but continues for a greater length of time. Punches to the side of the head using the back of the fist (with or without safety gloves) produced greater peak acceleration on average than kicks to either the side or the front of the head. Punches to the side of the head produced greater peak accelerations than punches to the front. There was no significant difference between kicks to the side and kicks to the front of the head. Kicks to the side of the head produced greater maximum accelerations than punches to the front of the head. In summary, for bare or karate-style equipment-protected hand and foot blows, punches to the side of the head produced greater peak accelerations than did kicks to the front and to the side, which in turn produced greater acceleration than did punches to the front of the head.

Safety-chop karate-style protective handwear did not significantly alter the peak accelerations of the head, but 10-oz boxing gloves did significantly reduce the peak acceleration of punches. In contrast, safety-kick protective footwear resulted in increased peak acceleration values. It should be noted that there was a difference in the style of kicks to the side of the head, with and without the protective footwear, because barefoot blows were struck with the ball of the foot and padded kicks were struck with the instep.[103]

In general, the punching force of top-performance boxers correlates with body weight. Accelerometers have been bandaged to the heads of fighters, and accelerations up to $100 \times g$ have been measured when their opponents wore 6-oz boxing gloves. Sixteen-ounce boxing gloves reduced peak accelerations to $50 \times g$ or less. In the current study, accelerations of $90 \times g$ were recorded on several occasions, and one value of $120 \times g$ was recorded. This corresponds to the force to which the head of an unrestrained passenger in a low-speed automobile collision might be subjected to when striking the dashboard.[103]

Karate-style safety handgear and safety kick footgear failed to mitigate peak accelerations. With the caveat that kicks to the side of the head with and without padding differed slightly in style, it would appear that the karate-style protective hand- and footwear was perceived by the subjects in the study as protection for the wearer rather than for the opponent.[103]

In competition tae kwon do, points are scored when contact made to the torso or head is sufficient to produce a "trembling shock." Approximately 80 percent of the competitive techniques executed are kicks, as opposed to hand strikes. For these kicks to be effective, they must contain a large amount of force and energy and thus pose a high injury potential to the opponent. Serina and Lieu[104] measured velocities, and energy was calculated. Typical values for basic swing kicks (roundhouse and spin roundhouse kicks) were 15 m/s and 200 J. Basic thrust kicks (sidekicks and back kicks) possessed 45 percent less velocity but 28 percent more energy than swing kicks. Linkage models were developed to simulate the motion and kinetics of the kicking leg. Models were then developed, and these models predict a significant probability of serious injury with all kicks, with thoracic deflections from 3 to 5 cm and peak viscous tolerance values from 0.9 to 1.4 m/s, when no protective body equipment is used.

JOINT MOTIONS, KINEMATICS

Tae Kwon Do Kicks

Serina and Lieu[104] developed a linkage-based model of the tae kwon do kicks and determined that the kicking motion could be divided into three phases: windup, strike, and recovery.

Windup As the entire body accelerates, gaining momentum and energy, the kicking leg is extended toward the target. In swing kicks, the body rotates about the axis of the pivot leg. In thrust kicks, the upper body leans in a direction opposite the direction of the kicking leg motion. The supporting leg remains stationary and perpendicular to the floor for all kicks.

Strike In swing kicks, just prior to impact, the upper body and thigh stop completely, and a large percentage of their energy and momentum is transferred to the lower kicking leg. In thrust kicks, the motion of the foot follows a line extending straight from the hip marker to the target.

Recovery After striking the target, the remaining energy and momentum are transferred from the kicking leg back to the body as the kicking leg decelerates. In swing kicks, body movement continues in the same manner as prior to impact. For thrust kicks, the entire body, including the kicking leg, comes to a complete stop with the leg fully extended.

The observed velocity of the hip and knee markers relative to the foot showed that the hip remained relatively motionless during the strike for all the kicks performed. At impact, its velocity reached a maximum of 3 percent of the velocity of the ball of the foot for swing kicks and a maximum of 8 percent of the heel velocity for thrust kicks. In swing kicks, the knee also was relatively stationary, having a velocity of 7 percent of the foot velocity at impact. For swing kicks, a line approximated the short arc traversed by the foot prior to impact. For thrust kicks, the foot traveled in a straight line to the target.

For swing kicks, the mass is nearly constant. For thrust kicks, the effective mass increases dramatically as full leg extension is approached. Thus, as with many slider-crank mechanisms, greater mechanical advantage may be imparted to the target at these positions. This demonstrates mathematically a practice that martial artists have always emphasized. All the subjects struck their targets with the kicking leg approximately 15 cm from full extension, where the effective mass was relatively constant at 55 percent of the total leg mass for thrust kicks.

A comparison of the foot velocities of all kicks shows that swing kicks possess greater foot velocities than thrust kicks. The average foot velocity of swing kicks (15.9 m/s) is 80 percent greater than the average foot velocity of thrust kicks (8.8 m/s) (Fig. 15.1).

In addition, kicks having an initial spin are faster than those without. The apparent purpose of the initial spin is to generate a greater kick velocity. For thrust kicks, all back kicks had larger foot velocities than

sidekicks. It is interesting to note that the foot velocity difference between thrust kicks and swing kicks was not affected significantly by the initial spin.[104]

The leg energy content was greater for thrust kicks than for swing kicks. The greater effective leg mass of thrust kicks contributed to this difference. This resulted from the addition of a translational velocity of the lower leg and the added motion of the thigh, with nearly twice the mass of the lower leg and the foot combined. A more influential factor is the additional rotational and translational velocities of the thigh and translational velocity of the lower leg during thrust kicks. Thus using the entire leg instead of the lower leg and foot alone generated more energy.[104]

Based on the injury criteria models, Serina and Lieu[104] concluded that thrust kicks have the potential for greater chest compression than swing kicks. With the compression criterion, they are clearly predicted to be more dangerous than swing kicks. Using the viscous criterion, however, swing kicks appear to be more dangerous. Thus, on the basis on the injury criteria, the risk of internal organ and soft tissue damage, on which the viscous criterion is based, may be greater with swing kicks. Skeletal injury may be more likely with thrust kicks due to greater chest compression. Kicks having a spin prior to kick execution possessed greater potential for thoracic injury, according to both criteria.

Conclusions drawn by Sernia and Lieu[104] were:

1. Swing kicks are faster and have a greater potential for soft tissue damage.
2. Thrust kicks can generate larger chest compressions and thus may have more potential for skeletal injury than swing kicks.
3. The addition of a spin prior to kick execution results in greater foot velocities and thus increases the injury potential of a kick.

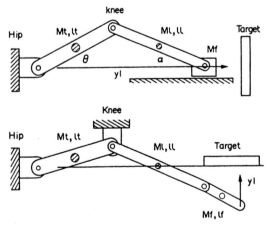

FIGURE 15.1

Linkage models comparing the thrust kick (top) and the swing kick.

4. Injury to an unprotected thorax by tae kwon do kicks is primarily through soft tissue or internal organ damage, seen by high peak viscous tolerance values.

5. Without the use of protective equipment, tae kwon do kicks exceed the proposed thoracic tolerance limit of 25 percent probability of serious injury. Therefore, current safety equipment can reduce the chance of thoracic injury and should be worn in all tae kwon do involvement when full contact is possible, whether it may be accidental or purposeful.

Karate Chop

Cavanagh and Landa[18] performed a biomechanical analysis of the karate chop. A kinematic analysis showed a sequential pattern of action at the shoulder and elbow joints, with shoulder extension normally 70 percent complete before elbow extension began. Angular velocities at the elbow joint reached 24.5 and 29.5 rad/s for two and three boards, respectively. Electromyography (EMG) supported the finding of the sequential pattern of action at the shoulder and elbow joints by revealing a sequential pattern of muscular action. Triceps brachii activity was only 200 ms in duration, and some activity in the biceps brachii was present immediately before impact, which would demonstrate the eccentric deceleration pattern of the musculature.

Treating the problem in a linear manner, hand velocities from 28 to 31 mi/h were found in experienced subjects, and forces at impact from 28 to 132 lbF were reported. These velocities in the extremity created a whiplike action of the upper limb.[18] This is a good illustration of the kinetic chain principle and the summation of forces through multiple joints.

When analyzing the karate chop, it was demonstrated that the movement was completed in 150 ms. The orientation of the trunk in space remained relatively fixed until the second half of the movement, when forward lean was initiated. It is clear from the kinematic analysis that a sequential rather than a simultaneous extension at the shoulder and elbow characterized upper limb movement during the karate chop. Typically, shoulder extension was at least 70 percent complete before joint extension began. The sequential pattern of movement occurs from the top of the backswing, at zero elbow angular velocity, and a peak velocity of 9 rad/s occurred during shoulder extension. At this time, the elbow joint had not begun to extend. The peak velocity of 25 rad/s at the elbow joint occurred 70 ms later, just prior to impact. This is a quantitative representation of the whiplike action, sometimes referred to as *summation.*[18]

The kinetic analysis of the karate chop demonstrated a peak linear acceleration in the region of $7 \times g$ (corrected for the effect of gravity) that occurred shortly before contact. Considerable differences were noted when an analysis was performed on a subject when he attempted to break boards with both the preferred and the nonpreferred hand, with the nondominant hand having a time interval 30 percent greater. This difference suggests the lack of coordination that would be expected from the nonpreferred arm. Using kinetic analysis may prove to be an extremely useful teaching device that provides immediate feedback in an important aspect of the skill.[18]

EMG analysis demonstrates a sequence of muscle activity that is seen clearly, with trunk, shoulder, and elbow muscles exhibiting consecutive phasic activity. It is interesting to note that activity in the biceps brachii was present 50 ms before contact. This activity, in anticipation, is a demonstration of the lag between electrical activity and the development of tension. The estimates of force at contact resulted in average forces of 540 and 270 lbF, respectively.[18]

Punching

Whiting et al.[124] performed three-dimensional analysis of four experienced boxers as they threw a series of punches at a practice bag. Three-dimensional coordinates of each boxer's shoulder, elbow, wrist, and glove were used to estimate linear and angular kinematics of the upper extremity. Average velocities at contact ranged from 5.9 to 8.2 m/s, whereas peak velocities of 6.6 to 12.5 m/s reached 8 to 21 m/s prior to hand/glove contact with the bag. Significant differences in shoulder and wrist velocities, elbow angle excursions, and elbow angular velocities were seen when comparing hooks and jabs. Few differences were evident when comparing the kinematics of gloved versus bare-handed punches.

Smith and Hamill[111] carried out a study to determine selected relative mechanical impact characteristics of the foam karate glove and the conventional boxing glove. The results revealed that high-skilled subjects generated greater bag momentum than both intermediate and low-skilled groups. No fist velocity differences were detected. Greater bag momentum was generated by the boxing glove than by either the karate glove or bare-fisted conditions, which did not differ from each other. Since subject masses and fist velocities among groups did not differ, it was concluded that high-skilled subjects transferred greater momentum under the boxing glove than the karate glove or bare-fisted conditions. Since the body momentum was highest for the skilled punchers with no difference in punching velocities among skill levels, evidence exists that the high-skilled subjects were better able to coordinate body momentum applied to the bag than intermediate- and low-skilled subjects. This particular finding supports the concepts of focus and force summation such that body momentum concentrated at the fist can be learned in order to generate larger forces.

The punch velocities in this study were higher than those reported previously. The present study[111] revealed an overall average of 11.5 m/s. It is likely the values reported here are representative of the general population of karate reverse punches due to the hip's contribution to the movement. The overall body momentum mean of 47.37 N/s was similar to previously reported data. With the fist velocity at 11.5 m/s immediately prior to impact and resulting body momentum at 47.37 N/s, the mass striking the bag would be 4.1 kg. The authors hypothesized that by using greater mass during the impact, subjects of lower skill levels delivered punches capable of surpassing concussion-level impacts for any of the glove conditions. In general, neither glove can be called "safe" for boxing or full-contact karate. With human punching capabilities, neither glove would prevent an opponent from being knocked out. However, the karate glove would have more effect in reducing breakage of bones and cartilage, especially after the first few impacts.

MUSCLE FUNCTION

Kinesiologic Analysis

The details of the karate roundhouse kick were described thoroughly in the sports performance series[41] (Fig. 15.2). A kinesiologic analysis with strength and conditioning principles of the tae kwon do sidekick was described thoroughly in the sports performance series[107] (Fig. 15.3).

Kinematics of Motor Learning

Zehr et al.[136] performed a study to determine differences in movement performance and the occurrence of agonist EMG premovement depression (agonist PMD) in highly trained karate practitioners and untrained control subjects. Karate-trained subjects produced significantly higher isometric and ballistic peak torques. Karate-trained subjects also had significantly higher peak rate of torque development under different loading conditions than did control subjects. Peak acceler-

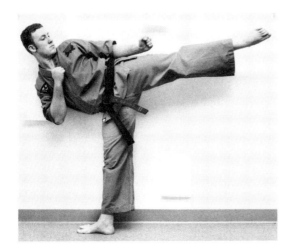

FIGURE 15.2

Correct biomechanics of executing the roundhouse kick. There is good eye focus on the target. The trunk is upright and in a "balanced" position. The hands are up for follow-up with hand techniques. The trunk, hips, knees, ankles, and feet are all in proper alignment with the open kinetic chain leg—left kicking leg in this figure. The ankle is plantarflexed so that the martial artist hits the target zone with the dorsum of the foot. The stance (closed kinetic chain—right leg in this figure) is in straight alignment, and there is a proper pivot of the entire lower extremity to generate the most power.

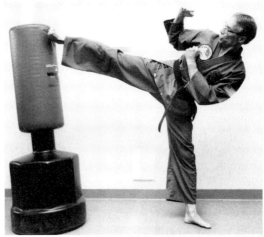

FIGURE 15.3

Correct biomechanics of executing the side kick. There is good eye focus on the target. The trunk is upright and in a "balanced" position. The hands are up for follow-up with hand techniques. The trunk, hips, knees, ankles, and feet are all in proper alignment with the open kinetic chain leg—right kicking leg in this figure. The ankle is dorsiflexed so that the martial artist hits the target zone with the plantar surface of the heel. The stance (closed kinetic chain—left leg in this figure) is in straight alignment, and there is a proper pivot of the entire lower extremity to generate the most power.

ation was significantly higher in the karate-trained as compared with control subjects. The superior movement performance of the karate-trained subjects could not be explained in terms of agonist PMD. It is concluded that agonist PMD should not be considered to be a naturally occurring training effect or learned motor response.

Zehr and Sale[135] evaluated ballistic elbow movements in moderately trained karate practitioners: peak torque, velocity, acceleration, and the agonist premovement silence. The data indicate no difference in ballistic performance between the left and right arms in karate practitioners who place equal em-phasis on both limbs during training. Premovement silence does not appear to be a consistent feature of ballistic movements, even in athletes who employ ballistic movements in training.

Injury Prevention

There is limited information in the medical or scientific literature regarding conditioning and training programs for martial artists preparing for belt promotions, black belt testing, and recreational to competitive sparring. Most of the conditioning and training programs have evolved as "hand-me-down programs" from instructors to students, with the philosophy that if it worked for me, then it should work for you. However, much of the conditioning and training has no scientific basis to it. In a recent study by Sanders and Antonio,[98] a strength and conditioning program for submission fighting was described. These authors performed an analysis of the sport based on the cardiovascular effects and the musculoskeletal systems used and developed recommendations. No specific outcomes or results of their recommended program are described, however.

This is an area where we think that involvement of sports-oriented clinicians could have a substantial impact on martial arts. Analyzing the demands of the sport from a systems approach (musculoskeletal, cardiorespiratory, neurophysiologic, etc.) and then developing scientifically based programs to enhance performance and to prevent injuries would make a substantial contribution to the martial arts. Injury prevention in all sporting activities begins by developing sufficient flexibility, strength, and balance/coordination to practice and compete safely. In addition, preparticipation screenings, protective equipment, and enforcement of rules/regulations are important factors in preventing injury.

Schmidt,[101] in describing the "sports traumatology syndrome," states that any lessening of physiologic conditioning, emotional stability, alertness, or morale increases the potential risk of sports injuries. However, the occurrences of these types of injuries in karate training are totally inexcusable. Only those students who have undergone a period of adequate physical conditioning and who have demonstrated competence in the basic free sparring techniques should engage in free sparring (Table 15.1).

WARM-UP

Ideally, each martial arts training or competitive session should begin with a physiologic warm-up. The intent of the warm-up is to raise the temperature in the exercising muscles to increase their elasticity[13] and decrease the risk of strain. Many instructors use outmoded methods of warm-up and push students past their limits of flexibility.[53] This is obviously an area where the clinician has a lot of experience and can educate teachers and students of martial arts about the proper principles and techniques of warm-ups and stretching. Often the prevailing philosophy in the martial arts dojo is that if my instructor made me do these warm-ups and I am as good as I am, then you are going to perform similar warm-ups.

STRETCHING

Flexibility of the musculotendinous unit is the primary objective of a stretching program and one of the most important aspects of conditioning that a martial artist can work on. This is important for preventing injury and for enhancing performance, e.g., increasing kick height. Martial artists should be instructed to perform stretching exercises following the warm-up for maximum benefit. Stretching exercises for the hamstrings, quadriceps, hip flexors, hip adductors, gastrocnemius-soleus complex, spinal extensors, spinal rotators, and pectorals should be included in the preparticipation stretching program.

The stretching program should consist of static stretching followed by dynamic/transitional/functional stretching. Static stretching should be performed to the point of tension in the muscles but not to the point of pain. Pain elicits the myotatic stretch reflex via the Golgi tendon organs that cause the muscle to contract in order to protect it from injury. This contraction prevents muscle lengthening

TABLE 15.1

Number and Severity of Injuries by Activity

Activity	Number	Percent	Severity
Fighting	30,417	74	2.1
Forms	2,047	5	1.3
Weapons	814	2	1.6
Basics	5,757	14	1.5
Miscellaneous	2,051	5	2.3
Total	41,086	100	
Average			1.88

Source: From Birrer RB: Trauma epidemiology in the marital arts. *Am J Sports Med* 24:S72–S79, 1996.

and improvements in flexibility. All static stretches should be held for 30 s and repeated three times for maximal benefit.

Following static stretching, there should be a phase involving dynamic/transitional/functional stretching that involves ballistic activity. Ideally, this should replicate some of the kicks and punches that will be used in classes or the workout. Furthermore, it is best to begin the dynamic flexibility exercises in a progressive manner by performing the movements in a progression from slower to faster and easier to harder. This will help prevent injury by preventing elicitation of the myotatic stretch reflex and allowing dynamic stretching to proceed.

Partner stretching may be implemented in combination with, or in lieu of, individual stretching. The martial arts instructor with a strong exercise background could instruct students to perform partner stretching using the principles of proprioceptive neuromuscular facilitation (PNF). For instance, PNF can be used to stretch the hamstrings when the leg is passively flexed to its limit. Once the leg is flexed, the hamstrings are briefly contracted isometrically by pushing into an im-

movable object, in this case a partner's shoulder. Following the isometric contraction, the hamstrings stretch reflex is depressed briefly, and the hip may be actively or passively flexed further. Partner stretching using PNF and/or static stretching techniques increase the variety of stretches possible and may improve the sense of cooperation and unity in the dojo.

The primary muscle groups and stretching exercises that we recommend include:

- Hamstrings—modified hurdler's stretch
- Quadriceps/hip flexors—front lunge, pull heel to butt
- ITB/TFL—long sitting, leg to be stretched crossed over the straight leg and stretch outside of hip
- Adductors—butterflies, side splits
- Lumbar spine—knees to chest
- Anterior chest and shoulders—arm circles, grab hands behind back
- Posterior chest and shoulders—arm circles, arm stretches crossing in front

Certainly, many different flexibility exercises can be used. These are the minimum that we recommend. Certainly the martial artist needs to be evaluated, and then specific muscle groups can be targeted with specific flexibility exercises designed for that area.

STRENGTHENING

Closed and Open Kinetic Chain Exercises

A martial artist must be capable of exerting tremendous forces to perform kicking, punching, and blocking maneuvers. Strengthening the trunk and extremities improves the capacity to safely exert (and absorb) such forces. Lower extremity strengthening should consist of both closed kinetic chain (e.g., squats) and open kinetic chain exercises (e.g., isolated knee extension) to prepare for closed kinetic chain (e.g., stance leg) and open kinetic chain (e.g., kicking) activities. The lower extremity resistance-training program should include exercises for the hip flexors, hip abductors, hip adductors, hip extensors, quadriceps, hamstrings, gluteus maximus, and gastrocnemius-soleus complex.

Examples of strengthening exercises for the following muscle groups have direct applications to the following activities in the martial arts:

- Plantarflexors—to improve height with jump kicks
- Quadriceps—used for front, round, and sidekicks
- Hamstrings—used for hook kick and to decelerate most other kicks
- Hip extensors—used for side and axe kicks
- Hip flexors—used primarily for front kicks
- Hip abductors—provide stability for round, side and outside crescent kicks
- Hip adductors—used primarily for inside crescent kicks

Like the lower extremities, upper extremity strengthening for the martial arts should involve both open kinetic chain exercises (e.g., lateral deltoid raises) and closed kinetic chain exercises (e.g., push-ups) to prepare for open kinetic chain activities such as punching or closed kinetic chain activities such as grappling. The lower extremity resistance-training program should include exercises for the pectorals, latissimus dorsi, deltoids, biceps, triceps, wrist extensors, and wrist flexors. Trunk strengthening should be included in a martial arts training program to improve the generation and transfer of forces between the legs and the arms and to increase the ability to absorb impact forces. An integrated series of strength, power, and endurance exercises should be performed to adequately prepare for the demands of the martial arts.

Examples of strengthening exercises for the following muscle groups have direct applications to the following activities in the martial arts:

- Scapulothoracic muscles—provide stabilization for the shoulder and arm; protraction is used for all punches
- Anterior deltoids—used in punches, particularly jab, hook, and rear-hand punches and uppercuts; also important in most blocking techniques
- Posterior deltoids—used for stabilization of punches
- Pectoralis major—used in hook and rear-hand punches
- Biceps—effective with the uppercut
- Triceps—used with the jab and back-fist punches
- Forearm and wrist muscles—used to stabilize the fist for punches and for blocking

Plyometrics

Plyometric exercise readily lends itself to martial arts training because it replicates the explosiveness needed for many martial arts movements, particularly in karate and tae kwon do. Plyometric (or stretch-shortening) exercise consists of three phases: (1) an eccentric prestretch that "loads" the muscle's connective tissue with potential energy, (2) the amortization phase, which is the time from cessation of the eccentric action to onset of the concentric action, and (3) the concentric (or power execution) phase. The amortization phase is the key to plyometrics; the shorter the amortization, the more forceful is the resulting concentric contraction. Plyometric training promotes the explosive ability required to perform many martial arts techniques.

Numerous plyometric drills can be used. Some examples include rope jumping, jumping with both feet in place and in different directions, hopping with one-foot drills, and shock drills of jumping from a mat, etc. Performing different types of power lifts also incorporates the use of plyometrics in performing, decelerating, and controlling the movements.

BALANCE/PROPRIOCEPTIVE/ KINESTHETIC TRAINING

The successful martial artist must be capable of highly coordinated movement. To facilitate this, balance, proprioceptive, or kinesthetic training should be incorporated into a training program for the martial arts. Single-leg stance drills with the eyes open or closed can be incorporated in a variety of ways to improve balance. Agility exercises (e.g., cariocas) can be incorporated to develop dynamic balance and coordination. Punching or striking exercises using a speed bag or punching bag can facilitate upper extremity kinesthesia.

CARDIORESPIRATORY TRAINING

Martial arts practice is typically both aerobic and anaerobic in nature. Stricevic et al.[114] performed a study to determine the cardiovascular response to the karate kata. The mean heart rate for the 50 subjects was 178 beats per minute during interval training consisting of 15 repetitions of the karate kata.

This represented 91 percent of the age-predicted maximal heart rate. The overall mean heart rate for the entire 21½-min exercise session was 163 beats per minute, which represents 84 percent of the age-predicted maximal heart rate. From the results of this study, it appears that the karate kata performed as interval training can stimulate heart rates that are greater than 80 percent of the age-predicted maximal heart rate. This suggests that with frequent training sessions (three to four times per week), cardiovascular fitness will improve.

Shaw and Deutsch[106] performed a study that evaluated heart rate and oxygen uptake response to performance of the karate kata. Data from this study indicate that only certain katas and protocols for training elicited heart rate responses that would be expected to bring about a cardiovascular training effect. Although it is possible that more experienced karateka perform their training routines at a greater intensity, in this study there was no significant correlation between experience and the mean exercise heart rate achieved with any of the protocols used in this study. The momentary static component of kata movements in combination with the repeated movements may have influenced the heart rate response to this otherwise moderately intense activity, as judged by $\dot{V}$ values. While these findings may suggest limitations of this activity in the development of cardiovascular fitness, they do not preclude kata training as an adjunct to physical activities designed to enhance general physical fitness. It is apparent that properly conducted karate training could in fact provide a minimal training stimulus for healthy individuals with a relatively low initial $\dot{V}O_2$ max. Schmidt and Royer[100] used a case study and recorded telemetered heart rates during karate katas to monitor heart rate responses with these exercises. The results demonstrated that the response patterns were essentially the same for all katas performed. The average time taken for each kata performance was 25.8 s. It is a generally accepted finding that vigorous exercise, the duration of which is less than 1 min, relies primarily on anaerobic pathways for its energy source. From the analysis of these data, it appears that karate kata performance for this study was primarily anaerobic in nature.

While strength training will enhance anaerobic capacity, the aerobic energy system must be trained with endurance activities. Running, cross-country skiing, swimming, and biking are examples of appropriate cardiovascular conditioning activities for the martial arts practitioner. If feasible, cross-training with a variety of aerobic activities should be used to improve endurance for martial arts exercise.

PREPARTICIPATION SCREENING

The preparticipation physical examination carried out by a physician, as recommended for youth sports in general, also should be required for every junior tae kwon do athlete who seeks enrollment in a tae kwon do club. Maturity assessment should be part of the preparticipation physical examination.[89] Jaffe and Minekoff[44] suggest that prophylaxis begins with a screening examination by both a pediatrician and an orthopedic surgeon to determine potential hazards of participation.

A prebout clearance system for all fighters should be implemented for all competitive martial arts contests.[8] A thorough prefight medical examination should be encouraged in all full-contact fighters, and this should be endorsed for subsequent contests as well.[72] In addition, standard suspensions from training and competition that are based on the number and severity of concussions should be developed for all contact sports.[90] We agree with the recommendations throughout

the literature that preparticipation screenings should be performed for the safety of participants.

MEDICAL STANDARDS

Certifiable medical standards should be established for instructors, referees, and physicians involved with the martial arts.[8] Since all three authors of this chapter have participated in some form of martial arts and are also professional clinicians, we strongly encourage more regulation and improvement in this area. As with many other things in the martial arts, much of what is done is because of tradition and is not necessarily the best thing for the martial artist. Similar to many coaching certification programs, it would be appropriate to require martial arts instructors to take courses on the basics of teaching motor skills, psychology of teaching, acute injury management, first aid, and basic principles of strengthening and conditioning.

MEDICAL COVERAGE

It is suggested that specific guidelines and plans be created for medical coverage at all competitive events, whether contact or non-contact.[8,70] Because of the high incidence of injuries that occur at competitions, it would certainly be appropriate to have adequate coverage available. It is recommended that minimum standards and certification should be established for medical practitioners who supervise these martial arts tournaments.[81] In view of the potential severity of karate injuries, a doctor should be present at all competitions. There seem to be fewer serious injuries in amateur boxing, and this has been attributed to the fact that there is usually a medical officer present at boxing competitions.[71]

Wilkerson[126] and McLatchie[73] developed several recommendations for medical officers attending karate competitions. It is important that adequate medical coverage be available for competitors. It has already been shown that there is a relatively high incidence of injury in competition and that this also can be mitigated to some degree. The physician's duties include examining competitors before the competition if requested by officials. The fighting areas should be inspected to ascertain that adequate flooring is in use. It is recommended that padded flooring be used because head injury is a common sequel to falls on hard floors. The physician also should treat any minor injuries sustained, such as lacerations and sprains, but should refer more serious injuries for hospital examination. Furthermore, the medical officer present should be able to advise the referees, where requested, as to the fitness of a competitor to continue in a competition and also as to the potential danger of various techniques when dubious points are under discussion.

Karate should be subject to the same stringent medical measures as boxing. All competitors are required to satisfy a strict medical examination, and the use of padded floors and padded footwear is encouraged. Serious injuries have resulted from spinning kicks, and it is believed that such techniques should be outlawed because they are uncontrollable once initiated.

We also think that appropriate medical coverage at competitive martial arts tournaments is appropriate. However, coverage does not always need to be provided by a physician because physicians are often not available and/or not familiar with acute injuries in competitive sporting events. The following practitioners would be appropriate for competitive martial arts coverage, including, but not limited to, sports physical therapists, physical therapists, certified athletic trainers, physicians, physician assistants, paramedics, emergency medical technicians, first responders, and registered nurses. Obviously, prac-

titioners with more experience in covering athletic events are preferred.

TECHNIQUE INSTRUCTION

Falling Techniques

Proper instruction must be provided with respect to falling safely without striking the head on the mat.[9] Regardless of the orientation of the martial art, the instructors should teach the basic mechanics of falling to prevent injuries. Even in a "hard martial art" such as karate, where little grabbing and minimal grappling are involved, occasionally falling will be part of the workout from either being knocked down or in a real situation where one were to grab or push the martial artist to the ground. Therefore, being aware of the distribution of forces when falling (trying to land on as large a surface area of the body as one can), preventing the typical reflexive response of putting the arm down directly toward the surface, striking the ground with the entire flat surface of the arm to distribute forces, rolling with the impact, and getting to a ready position as quickly as possible are all basic skills involved in teaching falling techniques.

Blocking Techniques

Kujala et al.[53] stated that in general a greater focus should be placed on diminishing rough and violent contact between athletes to help decrease the incidence of injuries in sports, particularly the martial arts.

Distal ulnar fractures can occur from using the forearm to block a blow. Most martial arts schools teach (in the opinion of Buschbacher et al.[12]) an incorrect blocking technique. They teach students to block overhead with a pronated forearm to cause impact with the distal ulna, which is the weakest in this position. Buschbacher et al.[12] recommend blocking with the radius and ulna together on the dorsum of the forearm.

Punching Techniques

Today's martial artist is usually taught to punch with a twist so that the fist moves from a supinated to a pronated position on impact. Buschbacker et al.[12] believe that this technique is improper. In the proximal forearm, the ulna is thicker and stronger than the radius, whereas distally the radius is stronger. When pressure is exerted on the fist, 80 percent of it is transmitted into the radius. A horizontal punch causes the radius and ulna to cross, which we believe causes a folding and weakening of the interosseous membrane. We investigated this relationship by dissecting a cadaver forearm and discovered that in a full-twist punch position the central interosseous membrane is slack. When the twist is continued only three-quarters of the way to horizontal (to 45 degrees), this slack disappears. Thus it would appear that the martial artist might be able to punch with greater power and less risk of injury if this alternate technique were practiced.[12] From an anatomic and biomechanical standpoint this concept makes sense; however, to teach this approach to martial artists who have "perfected" their punching abilities over years and years of practice would be difficult. Although it makes sense from the anatomic and biomechanical standpoints, more studies are needed to see if there really are differences in punching power and the incidence of injuries with the two positions.

Hand Techniques

Jaffe and Minkoff[44] suggest that the practice of toughening the knuckles probably should be discouraged to avoid fractures and unacceptable cosmesis in later years. Nieman and Swan[80] have reported a case of weakness and wasting of the hypothenar eminence due to traumatic neuropraxia in a karate student who "hardened" his hands by repeatedly striking them on firm objects. It is the opinion of McLatchie et al.[75] that the wood-break-

ing techniques are unnecessarily damaging to the hands. Larose and Kim[61] state that karate is the only martial art that attempts to build up callus formation on the hands, feet, and other potential striking areas. Two basic routines exist for hand conditioning. The "savage" technique consists of severely punishing the knuckles with multiple blows until the skin breaks and exposes the tendon of the extensor digitorum muscle and its expansion. The callus that develops from this technique is supposed to be more firmly anchored to the hand and cannot be moved passively across the knuckles, as can the skin on a normal hand. The milder routine for hand conditioning consists of striking a series of progressively firmer and coarser objects. The callus developed by this method will be attached to the skin and not to the extensor tendon. It is important to let the damaged soft tissues over the striking point partially repair themselves before another cycle of damage and repair is started. Various medications have been applied to stimulate callus formation and speed up the healing. Tannic acid and benzoin preparations are the most popular. Some decrease in manual dexterity will result from prolonged hand conditioning. Part of the effect would come about merely by increasing the amount of muscle in the hand. Larose and Kim presented a case report on a Korean-Japanese martial artist who holds an eighth-degree black belt and is probably most famous for killing bulls by a blow to the head with his fist. He began hand conditioning by the savage technique and continued the hand conditioning for 30 years.[61]

Serious hand conditioning is unnecessary in the present state of the art in the United States. Many students merely hand condition to the point where knuckle push-ups on a hardwood floor do not hurt. These students, who concentrate on execution, often can break as many boards as their heavily muscled and well-callused counterparts.

Fractures will occur when a punch is thrown with an improperly held fist.[60] It would not be unrealistic to expect degenerative arthritis at the second and third metacarpophalangeal joints in future case reports of hand conditioners. This would be true especially if the savage technique of hand conditioning were used.

Kelly et al.[47] indicate that most of the index metacarpal fractures could have been prevented if thrusts had been executed properly. Thrusts executed with equal axial compression of the index and long finger metacarpal heads, without torsional or angular stresses, could eliminate all the fracture patterns observed except for those occurring from blocked kicks or board breaking. The wood-breaking techniques, although impressive for spectators and also satisfying for the competitors, produce grotesque deformities of the hands and possible subsequent osteoarthritis of the metacarpophalangeal joints.

Kicking Techniques

McLatchie[76] recommends the outlawing of certain uncontrollable methods of attack. He particularly recommends that the spinning back kick should be outlawed, since once initiated, it cannot be controlled. Furthermore, he recommends that strict control regarding contact with roundhouse kicks should be exercised.

DEVELOP, STANDARDIZE, AND ENFORCE RULES

In order to maximize safety, standardization and enforcement of rules across organizations and styles for all forms of competition (i.e., forms, weapons, breakage, and fighting, both noncontact and contact), especially multiple sequential bouts, must be done.[8] Oler et al.[81] recommend that no head contact be allowed for children and only light head contact for certain experienced adults. Rules should be changed to restrain contact while allowing a good cardiovascular workout.[81]

Weight Classes

McLatchie[76] recommends the introduction of weight classes as one method of helping to decrease injuries in karate. Similar to other sports (Pop Warner football, wrestling, etc.), matching opponents by size does have merits, particularly for younger and less experienced martial artists. It does appear that most competitive karate tournaments do have "general weight categories" as well as belt ranks.

Maturity Assessment and Matching

Maturity assessments also could be used to match junior tae kwon do athletes for competition. Matching young athletes based on their maturity rather than on chronological age has been recommended for participation in other sports as well.[89]

DISQUALIFICATIONS

When participation in the martial arts includes competitive sparring, Wilkerson[127] would disqualify persons with the following medical disorders: carditis, severe uncontrolled hypertension, severe congenital heart disease, absence or loss of one eye, absence of one kidney, heptomegaly, splenomegaly, poorly controlled seizure disorder, pulmonary insufficiency, and atlantoaxial instability. When individuals with any of these conditions wish to participate in the martial arts for self-defense, fitness, or flexibility, without ever participating in full-contact sparring, he recommends individual assessment. Based on such assessment, some may be allowed to train, but only in a noncontact environment.[127]

Guidelines regarding disqualification to participation in collision or contact sports also should be applied for competitive sparring in the martial arts. Several sources are available for recommendations as to what conditions constitute contraindications for participating in collision or contact sports.

Regulations

If preventive efforts through regulation are to be implemented, both competitors and administrators must see change as desirable. From the perspective of competitors and coaches, it is more likely that regulation would be accepted if it could be shown clearly that prior injury had a deleterious effect on performance. However, this was not the case in Feehan and Waller's study.[34] None of the injury-related variables were significantly associated with fight success or failure. These findings were unexpected and warrant replication. It is also possible that those who had received the most severe injuries during the lead-up to the competition did not enter or may even have dropped out of the sport altogether.

Certifications

Judo instructors and officials should be certified and registered by the national governing body to be qualified to teach, and they should be familiar with the latest contest rules. The rules should be changed to severely penalize contestants who perform hazardous moves.[51]

As with many professional societies, there are national certifications and standardization of competencies for performing various activities. Because of so much diversity in the martial arts, it would be difficult to create a unifying national body to perform national certification for standardization of the basics of teaching, first aid, and acute injury management and basics principles of conditioning. However, it probably would be beneficial as a means of quality assurance that the client is getting the best instruction for his or her dollar to determine if an instructor is certified or not.

Rules

There are several potential ways to decrease injuries in the martial arts. The most likely way to reduce serious injuries is to exclude the head as a target area.[70,81] Oler et al.[81] reported a fatality from a spinning hook kick to the face. A back-spinning kick or back hook kick cannot necessarily be thrown with control. If it is thrown too slowly, the opponent will kick the aggressor (possibly in the back). If it is thrown with proper speed, it cannot be controlled to decrease the impact. Wilkerson,[127] as the team physician for several martial arts tournaments, convinced the masters putting on the tournaments to disallow the back kick and back-spinning kicks to the head because of potential injury. Furthermore, only front leg kicks to the head, such as a round kick, could be performed in a controlled fashion. This change markedly decreased the chance of serious injury. No head contact for children in tae kwon do competition also should be considered.[89]

Another factor in the reduction of injuries is stricter control of the contests by the referee and judges. Disqualification, instead of a warning, for uncontrolled techniques should be more common. Participants therefore are more aware of the importance of good, well-controlled techniques for scoring.[72] Standard suspensions from training and competition that are based on the number and severity of concussions should be developed for all contact sports.[90]

Incentives for good control should be developed. Since much of the purpose of point-competitive sparring is based on the concept of speed and quickness, demonstrating good control should be valued as much as good solid contact, particularly with some of the forceful kicking techniques. The awarding of points for good control, however, must be recognized by the judges and probably would decrease the incidence of injury. After all, it probably takes more skill to "pull" a punch or kick inches from the contact areas as it does to follow through with a solid "shot" to the opponent.

Choke Out

In judo, the participants are taught to "choke" properly and in turn have been "choked." They have the ability to realize its effects before unconsciousness ensues. The officials, referees, judges, and coaches can recognize the competitor when he or she is "choked out" (becomes unconscious).[52] However, they need to recognize when the athlete is almost out, because to "choke out" repetitively over time may be detrimental, as discussed previously in this chapter.

EQUIPMENT

Martial arts pads absorb and rebound with each contact, but their role is questionable. The essence of the martial arts is learning control over the body, and in a well-run school, there should be only light contact. Several schools of karate do not encourage protective clothing and devices because the practice of karate is based on the discipline of accurate focusing. Protective wear causes punches and kicks to stop short of the target, and violence is substituted for discipline.[115] Furthermore, pads alter reach, especially of the arms, and may interfere with learning proper control. They also may encourage overly vigorous technique because they give the martial artists a false sense of security. Nevertheless, they are probably here to stay. In some settings they have been found to decrease injury rate and severity.[13]

There is also some evidence to suggest that some martial arts equipment serves to protect the attacker rather than the defender, allowing for greater force than would otherwise be applied.[34] On the other hand, use of more padding and protective helmets may increase the confidence of the competitors, which may increase the number of minor injuries. An increase in the occurrence of minor injuries and a decrease in the occurrence of more severe injuries were found to be associated with the use of hand padding. Competitors may punch and kick harder and faster when their opponents are better protected. Thus, use of more protective padding should be combined with further modification of the rules to avoid such unfavorable developments.[119]

There is some evidence that the increased use of padding has decreased the number of sprains in the extremities and contusions in the trunk and limbs.[46,71,72] To decrease the number of injuries to the head, safety precautions should be taken further. Mouth guards protect the teeth but not the surrounding soft tissue. McLatchie et al.[75] state that it would seem reasonable to require padding for the fists, forearms, shins, and feet and to make the use of gum shields compulsory. Mouth guards are most likely advisable, and shin pads can help protect fighters from painful but otherwise benign blows to the lower leg usually from blocking kicks.[13]

An earlier study by McLatchie and Morris[72] states that there is a significant reduction in the number of injuries when padding is used. Kurland[54] indicated that 72 percent of injuries could have been prevented by using hand, foot, and chest protectors.

Shoes

The majority of injuries both for defenders (81 percent) and attackers (84 percent) occurred in settings where no protective equipment was used.[8,70] It appears that in the absence of protective shoes, the digits constitute that area most vulnerable to injury in the practice of the martial arts. Burks and Satterfield[11] suggest that a lightweight, protective shoe be worn during participation in the martial arts to reduce the incidence of digital injuries, even in noncontact settings.

Footgear

Some of the most popular martial arts safety equipment has been found to be inadequate. In a study by Schwartz et al.,[103] the effect of hand and foot protection on the peak accelerations imparted to dummies was assessed. They determined that 10-oz boxing gloves decreased peak accelerations but that a popular brand of martial arts hand protection did not. The same popular brand of foot protection actually increased accelerations imparted to the dummies. Consequently, such equipment protects the wearer primarily and facilitates the use of greater force in attacking.

Pieter et al.[87] suggested using padding for the instep of the foot during tae kwon do competition to help decrease the occurrence of injuries to that body part. However, it also was found that wearing safety equipment would protect the attacker more than the one being attacked. In other words, although foot padding may help in decreasing injuries to the foot in tae kwon do, it also may give the attacker the possibility to kick harder and therefore could cause brain damage when hitting the head/face area.

Agnew[1] indicated that practitioners of martial arts develop their feet and hands through repeated minor trauma to deaden pain and hypertrophy certain muscles, bones, and areas of skin. Some modern martial artists strike rigid objects with their hands and feet for this purpose. Because powerful strikes with the foot can sprain, dislocate, or even fracture bones and joints, Agnew proposed a method of taping the most vulnerable joints to help prevent these injuries.

Hand Pads/Gloves

Hand pads primarily protect the attacker. They also increase the shear force imparted to the brain by a blow to the head. Head gear protects from lacerations, abrasions, and contusions but not necessarily against brain injury.[13] Johannsen and Noerregaard[46] did not find any statistically significant difference between those wearing fist padding and those who did not in terms of cerebral concussions. Although fist padding may decrease the severity of head injuries, it may contribute to an increased incidence.

Johannsen and Noerregaard[46] conducted a study to analyze the effects of knuckle protection on the type and incidence of injuries in traditional karate contests. The results of their study demonstrated that fist pads offer some protection against injuries, especially to the hands, but additional measures are needed. Head injuries were more common in tournaments where fist pads were used, but the difference was not statistically significant. A possible explanation for the increased incidence of head injuries where fist pads were used could be that competitors delivered harder or less controlled blows, trusting in the ability of the fist pads to prevent obvious outer signs of trauma in cases of accidental excessive contact, thereby reducing their risk of disqualification. The use of knuckle protection did not influence the frequency of knocked-out or groggy contestants. The pattern of head injuries, however, was clearly different when knuckle protection was used. There were considerably more minor injuries, primarily contusions. Injuries to the extremities decreased dramatically per match when knuckle protection was used. This was due mainly to a reduction in the number of injuries to the fingers or hands, which were almost nonexistent when knuckle protection was used. Most injuries to the fingers or hands were self-inflicted, caused by punching into the opponent's blocks or bony prominences.

Smith and Hamill[111] found that after only the fifth impact during punching, the karate glove would no longer give adequate protection. Furthermore, the impact forces resulting from a punch after the fifth impact would be within the zone of concussion.

Groin Protective Cups

All males should wear specially designed martial arts protective groin cups.[13]

Headgear

Siana et al.[108] evaluated the injuries that occurred at the tae kwon do World Championships and reported that more than 4 percent of the competitors were admitted to the hospital. The majority of the severe injuries were to the head and neck. Encouraging the use of protective padding, mouth guards, and a face shield would seem reasonable in view of the severity of tae kwon do injuries.

It is recommended that more substantial headgear should be developed and that there should be mandatory use of headgear, mouth guards, torso protection, groin protection, and padded floors or canvas rings.[81] Protective padding of the arms, legs, feet, and hands and the use of gum shields and protective boxes appeared to reduce the incidence and severity of injury. Protective padding should be encouraged, especially among lower-grade fighters.[71]

Unfortunately, higher accelerations are not mitigated by safety padding,[103] such as the helmet worn in tae kwon do competitions. The neurosurgical literature indicates that wearing headgear increases the shearing injury to nerve fibers and neurons in the brain in proportion to the degree of acceleration to the head. However, the helmet will dissipate the force of a kick and also will provide some protection if the head hits the mat after the blow and therefore should still be worn. Schmid et al.[99] performed laboratory testing of the effects on wearing headgear. They found that the use of the headgear reduced the acceleration amplitude from a frontal blow to 70 percent of the original value. The acceleration from a side blow dropped to about 60 percent of the original value. For jaw blows, the changes are hardly perceptible, which could be explained mainly by the little layer of padding under the jaw. One also can ascertain that the time of acceleration is less than 0.1 s almost in all measured cases. It is evident from all the quotations that the decisive effect of a blow on a fighter's head is in the direction of the blow. The protective effect of the headgear after blows with boxing gloves is apparent. Nevertheless, all results show that the protective effect of the headgear depends in a great part on the fighter's individual ability to catch the blow. On average, one can say, due to the headgear, that the fall in acceleration and therefore also of the inertial forces acting on the boxer's head after a blow is about 15 to 25 percent.

Another advantage of introducing headgear is that injury of the eyebrow (cut eye), so often seen in boxing, has practically vanished. Summing up the results of laboratory experiments and observations at contests, we can say that the introduction of headgear does not limit knockouts but nevertheless means a substantial reduction of the hazard of this sport and another step in cutting down injuries and chronic damage in this sport.

Estwanik and Boitano[31] evaluated boxing injuries at the national championships. The most frequent injuries were head blows, soft-tissue hand injuries, and facial lacerations. Forty-eight matches were stopped because of head blows, which occurred at the rate of 4.38 percent. All other injuries occurred at a rate of 4.75 percent. Amateur boxing injuries could be reduced if the sport were included in the scholastic milieu and if the headgear, mats, and gloves were better designed.

Tuominen[119] analyzed data from personal interviews with participants in six national karate competitions in Finland. Injuries occurred to 16 percent of the competitors and were greatest among adult males in the final bouts. Of all injuries diagnosed by physicians for the competitions, more than 95 percent were localized to the head. The majority of the injuries were minor injuries. Experienced competitors were more injury prone than beginners. Most injuries and penalties, as well as full scores, were caused by direct punches to the head more than any other technique. From these findings it was concluded that a protective guard for the head together with modification of competition rules could significantly reduce injuries.

Training and Competition Environments

Coaches and referees need to create and maintain safe training and competition environments.[8] The use of protective equipment, including mouth guards, headgear, and adequate floor padding should be mandatory for sparring practice. Such measures have been shown to reduce the number (from 42 to 16 percent) and severity (from 66 to 44 percent) of injuries.[9] Floor padding also has been recommended to prevent injury to a contestant when hitting the floor.[76]

One of the recurrent themes from the literature is the importance of adequate floor padding to help decrease injuries. This is particularly important from the standpoint of preventing head injuries when a competitor falls to the mat. Therefore, if just having adequate floor padding is recommended and could help prevent a potentially catastrophic injury, then adequate floor coverings also should be included as part of the rules and regulations.

TEACHING/COACHING/SUPERVISION

Teaching

It has been suggested that three-quarters of martial arts injuries could be prevented if instructors and students learn to recognize potentially hazardous situations.[9] Proper instruction must be provided with respect to falling safely without striking the head on the mat. This training must come before instruc-

tion on throwing techniques. The teachings should conform to the safety standards emphasized in proper throwing, falling, and holding techniques.[51]

Backward-spinning hook kicks can cause injury to the head (or elsewhere) because the person kicking has poor visibility through much of the kick and because once initiated, the kick is hard to control. Therefore, its use should be discouraged.[13]

Coaching

Inadequate training techniques include sparring while excessively fatigued, gross mismatches in skill levels, premature entry of youth and inexperienced persons into sparring, inadequate sparring time, inadequate coaching before competition, and unrestrained full-contact fighting. Many fighters do not practice adequate head protection techniques. As an example, competitors frequently drop their hands in order to maintain balance, especially while kicking. With these inadequacies in mind, it is recommended that minimum standards and certification should be established for martial arts instructors.

Hirano and Seto[40] have recommended mandatory supervision of those providing karate instruction in an effort to prevent the occurrence of serious injuries. Coaches are advised to work on the blocking skills of their junior tae kwon do athletes.[89]

For those providing instruction in karate, preventive intervention in the form of modification of potentially hazardous training procedures is recommended in an effort to eliminate unnecessary, fatal, or traumatic injuries. It is further recommended that instructors initiate emergency first aid protocols in their schools in an effort to effectively assist with life-threatening situations.

Supervision

Kurland[54] contends that 72 percent of the injuries reported were preventable. This may relate not only to inadequacies in physical preparation but also to improper supervision of events.

Proper instruction of students is a vital factor in reducing injuries. The instructor must be able to teach not only proper technique but also proper attitude. A karate student whose techniques are inappropriate will sustain or cause unnecessary injuries. Contact should be kept to a minimum even with the use of protective gear, which sometimes provides a false sense of security.

RECORD KEEPING

Injuries should be tracked through a standardized registry.[8] This would be an excellent opportunity to more accurately track injuries. Consequently, an analysis could be performed regarding the mechanisms of injuries. Then specific prevention and performance-enhancement programs could be developed.

PSYCHOLOGICAL ASPECTS

Enjoying great popularity today, both within and outside the scope of sports proper, is the field of martial arts. Martial arts have been loosely defined as styles of combat originating in the Orient that offer a way of life based on the Eastern philosophy.

There exist thousands of different types of martial arts. While techniques and principles will vary from one style to another, most share a common heritage in teaching unarmed self-defense techniques as well as the use of weaponry. Further, many (though not all) traditions have philosophical and spiritual teachings that seek to effect a psychological transformation of the practitioner. Maliszewski's paper[67] proposes to review the evidence supporting this claim and assesses the pros and cons of engaging in this combat-oriented activity from a psychological perspective.

Writings that have explored the psychological effects of participation in martial arts

present mixed findings. Some reveal positive psychological effects, whereas others are more negative in their findings. Exposure to the psychological and philosophical aspects of a martial art may play a significant role in determining the type of impact it has on practitioners. One study demonstrated that those who participated in the traditional martial arts showed decreased aggressiveness, lowered anxiety, increased self-esteem, increased social adroitness, and an increase in value orthodoxy. Students who participated in a "modern" version of martial arts that did not emphasize the psychological/philosophical aspects of the sport showed a large increase in aggressiveness and an even greater tendency toward delinquency. The control group showed no changes.[67] These data suggest that training in the traditional martial art of tae kwon do is effective in reducing juvenile delinquent tendencies.

In another study, both the akido and traditional psychotherapeutic treatment groups significantly improved their scores as opposed to the control group. The results of the akido group were significantly better than the psychotherapy group.[67] In conclusion, while a variety of medical injuries have been reported, the concerns voiced about injuries inflicted by martial arts weapons appear to be exaggerated. Positive psychological changes have been noted through participation in martial arts, and preliminary findings suggest that the "appropriate" psychological stance may weigh considerably in effecting such gains.

From the psychological aspect, McLatchie[76] stated that he wonders frequently if participation in combat sports creates an overall increase in aggressiveness. In sports such as karate, motivation may prompt an injured student to continue to practice, which does not allow for proper healing and rehabilitation. Instructors who teach students to work through the pain encourage this. This attitude may have been a good attribute on the battlefield, but we do not consider it an enlightened viewpoint for this era of sports medicine.[54] Developing a good self-concept at a young age can help children develop throughout the remainder of their lives.

MEDIA PROMOTION

McLatchie[76] suggests that the media hype may influence individuals' responses to participation in the martial arts. Combat-oriented sports and activities have come under increasing scrutiny by the media and professional groups. While injuries stemming from boxing have been a primary topic of concern, the martial arts also have received public attention. To date, no medical or professional groups have provided any policy statement regarding involvement in such activity. However, it is important to determine at this stage what is known regarding the extent and type of injuries reported as well as the psychological effects of participation in the martial arts. Therefore, Maliszewski[67] provides a review of various studies that have appeared on these subjects.

Etiology of Injuries

EPIDEMIOLOGY

Epidemiologic data on martial arts injuries are sparse. Martial arts injuries occur most commonly to the face and head, digits, legs, and abdominal organs, with more severe injuries typically occurring to the face and head (approximately 8 percent).[4,13] The overwhelming majority of injuries (86 percent) in the martial arts, i.e., contusions, sprains/strains, abrasions, and lacerations, are mild to moderate.[13]

The Consumer Products Safety Commission (CAPS) estimates that between the years 1994 and 1999 over 100,000 martial arts–re-lated injuries were treated in hospital emergency rooms.[13] Over 60 percent of the victims were between the ages of 5 and 24 years. Interestingly, the number of weapon-related injuries was too small to derive a national estimate. The incidence of injury from martial arts practice in the 5- to 14-year-old age group was found to be significantly lower than for many other sports. In this age group, approximately 10 per 100,000 injuries were attributed to martial arts practice compared with wrestling (55.2), basketball (289.3), and football (437.1) (Neiss data highlights based on CPSC data). A separate investigation across all age groups, however, found that karate and judo have higher injury rates than ice hockey, soccer, basketball, and volleyball.[53]

An extensive survey of injuries to martial arts athletes of all ages revealed that the number of injuries[24,112] was four times the number of participants.[4] Injuries from martial arts practice appear to be evenly divided between genders.[34] Approximately 74 percent of martial arts injuries occur during sparring in practice or during competitions.[8,13] Most serious injuries, especially head injuries, occur during sparring in practice or during competitions. The incidence of injury appears to be inversely proportional to the level of expertise and training; therefore, most injuries occur in less experienced practitioners. A study of 41,086 injuries in 15,017 participants demonstrated that younger participants (12- to 19-year-olds) and less-experienced participants (particularly those with less than 1 year of training) had the highest rates and severity of injury[8] (Table 15.2).

Approximately 50 to 84 percent of martial arts injuries are unreported.[5,8,13,34] This may be due to athletes dismissing minor injuries, failing to report injuries, or fear of an instructor's disapproval. Practitioners of several martial arts, particularly advanced students, develop higher pain thresholds and historically have been trained to feel invulnerable. This may result in a tendency to withhold injury informa-

TABLE 15.2

Number and Severity of Generic Injuries

Injury	Number	Percent	Severity
Contusions	17,676	43	1.30
Sprains/strains	11,083	27	1.60
Abrasions/lacerations	5,335	13	2.20
Fractures	2,467	6	3.70
Dislocations	2,063	5	3.80
Miscellaneous	2,462	6	3.90
Total	41,086	100	
Average			1.88

Source: From Birrer RB: Trauma epidemiology in the marital arts. *Am J Sports Med* 24:S72–S79, 1996.

tion, particularly during competition, a phenomenon known as *tournament psychology*.[5] In one investigation, 35 percent of tae kwon do competitors reported that on the day of competition they had a current injury that was affecting their ability to perform.[34]

Several studies have demonstrated that injuries tend to be more severe under tournament conditions.[5,71] An analysis of 295 karate contests found that injuries occurred in 25 percent of the contests; 10 percent of the injuries were severe enough to cause the participant to withdraw, and 75 percent of injuries occurred in grades below the brown belt level. Injuries were more prevalent in the first hour of each day's competition, suggesting that inadequate warm-up or participation anxiety may be contributory factors.

The medical literature contains references to other horrific injuries resulting from misapplied or ignorantly directed attacks. Injuries of this magnitude fortunately are uncommon, comprising 0.2 percent of all martial arts injuries.[9] Birrer and Birrer[4] reported similar results in that only 1 in 500 injuries was serious (0.2 percent). In addition, the severity of injuries proportionately increased with the amount of contact permitted and the inexperience of the athlete. A number of severe injuries did occur. Cerebral concussions represented 63 percent of these injuries—over five times as frequent as long bone fractures (11 percent), the next most common form of severe trauma. Even though the incidence of severe injuries was low (0.033 injuries per participant per year), some of these injuries (69 of 41,086, or 0.17 percent)) were life-threatening. There were six fatalities recorded that occurred after trauma to the head (one strike, one kick, two falls), the neck (one, a single-handed blow to the carotid region), and the chest (one, a single punch).[8]

Certain martial arts styles have been associated with particular injury patterns: increased lower extremity trauma in tae kwon do, predominance of left-side injuries in kendo, increase incidence of head trauma due to kicks in tae kwon do, and increased frequency of trauma related to karate styles.[8] Feehan[34] described the various types of injuries. In an analysis of karate injuries, an injury occurred once in every four fights, and a disabling injury occurred once in every ten fights.[71]

A number of unusual acute and chronic injuries have been reported in the literature.[7,26,36,40,47,61,80,81,94,95,113,121] Some have been life-threatening, and many have been associated with prolonged disability.[16,59,75,76,79] Fatalities from head, neck, and chest trauma have been reported.[81,101]

Approximately 20 percent of judo injuries have been found to be serious.[43] The rates and distribution of injuries are the same for male and female participants in judo.[51] Deaths have been reported in judo as a result of the use of choke holds,[52,82,93] the majority involving brain and cervical cord trauma. Koiwai[51] presented case reports of 19 judo fatalities. Judo is a contact sport, and deaths can be expected in any contact sport. This brings up the question of the use of accepted methods of choking in judo. Unless the choked participant submits (taps out), the opponent can choke until the other loses consciousness. This will be discussed in more detail later in this chapter.

INTRINSIC FACTORS

Like all athletes, the martial artist with deficits in strength, flexibility, and/or proprioception may be predisposed to injury. Poor flexibility of the hamstrings, for instance, may increase the propensity toward hamstring strains while performing front kicks. Weakness of the hamstrings also may lead to strains during the eccentric activity of a front kick. Deficits in proprioception also may increase the risk of injury. If proprioceptive deficits are present in the ankle, for example, the martial artist's balance will be affected, and the likelihood of sustaining an ankle sprain is increased.

Experience Level of Participants (Belt Rank)

As the level of experience increases, the number of reports of osseous injuries increases. Burks and Satterfield[11] propose that as martial artists become more advanced, their incidence of severe injuries increases, but their incidence of minor injuries remains the same. One explanation for this finding is that in all martial arts, as the rank increases, so does the level of difficulty. For example, in karate and tae kwon do, jumping and spinning maneuvers are performed only at the higher ranks. Judo uses more technically difficult maneuvers at the higher ranks and not necessarily kicking maneuvers. In many styles of martial arts, board and brick breaking are required for advancement through the ranks. Moreover, the greater demands placed on the experienced student certainly provide more opportunities for more severe injuries to occur.[11]

It has been shown that serious head injuries occur most frequently in the inexperienced color belts[9] and that injuries decrease as expertise increases. Birrer and Birrer[4] pointed out that the majority of the serious head injuries caused by martial arts occur most frequently in the inexperienced color belts (lower ranks) because participants lack coordination and control.

A higher level of risk is present for those who are male, of a younger age group, and lack experience. McLatchie,[71] in an analysis of karate injuries, reported an injury to occur once in every four fights and a disabling injury once in every ten fights (Table 15.3).

EXTRINSIC FACTORS

Failure to use protective equipment, improper use of equipment, or faulty equipment is directly associated with increased numbers and severity of injuries.[8] Unsupervised activity or inadequate medical and coaching supervision that condones poor training habits or inappropriate aggression (e.g., excessive head contact) is directly correlated with increased injury rates and severity. Poor training environments and lack of attention to basic first aid are directly associated with an increased number and severity of injuries.

TABLE 15.3

Number and Severity of Injuries by Training Level

Training Level	Number	Percent	Severity
Beginner			
10	2,060	5.0	1.2
9	3,291	8.0	1.4
Advanced beginner			
8	5,019	12.2	1.9
7	5,344	13.0	2.4
Intermediate			
6	5,768	14.0	2.2
5	4,925	12.0	2.3
4	4,517	11.0	2.0
Advanced intermediate			
3	3,701	9.0	1.9
2	2,872	7.0	1.8
Advanced			
1	1,649	4.0	1.8
2	1,223	2.1	1.6
3	618	1.2	1.5
4	362	0.9	1.4
5	169	0.4	1.2
>5	76	0.2	1.1
Total	41,086	100.0	
Average			1.88

Source: From Birrer RB: Trauma epidemiology in the marital arts. *Am J Sports Med* 24:S72–S79, 1996.

Styles and schools of martial arts that incorporate close supervision with a sense of self-discipline, particularly through traditional teaching methods, philosophy, and meditation, are associated with fewer numbers and severity of injuries.[8]

Like any sport, the martial arts carry a risk of injury. The injuries sustained are often indicative of the nature of the maneuvers performed.[11] In karate, kung fu, and tae kwon do, injuries can occur in any of the four stages of training: (1) noncontact solo exercises, (2) striking implements and objects, (3) noncontact prearranged sparring, and (4) free sparring with full contact (wearing protective gear or minimal protective gear), light to medium contact, and noncontact. Using bare feet to strike, as well as sitting in exercise positions with severe knee flexion, may cause previous injuries to flare up.[54]

In many of the martial arts, contact is either nonexistent or minimal. The reasoning behind this is that a skilled martial artist should be able to aim a punch or kick with enough control to be able to stop short of actual contact.[11]

Blocking

Unblocked attacks are the major cause of injury in both boys and girls.[89] Despite the physical control developed through practice, injuries still occur from mistakes in blocking.[3] Because the martial arts are practiced in bare feet, they are more conducive to many lower extremity injuries compared with other sports. Digital fractures and digital jamming are good examples. In a survey, digital injuries accounted for 37 percent of the total number of reports of injuries.[11]

Most fractures of the metatarsals are due to incorrectly blocked kicks or, less frequently, direct trauma (Fig. 15.4). Hand fractures occur most frequently as a result of an accidental direct blow from the heel in a kick or from poor blocking by novices.[3]

Foot Sweeping

McLatchie[71] reported incidences of ankle sprains and digital sprains and dislocations that all resulted from foot-sweeping maneuvers.

Striking

In the case of a strong crescent kick striking the opponent's extended front kick, it can cause a contusion and possible fracture of the proximal fibula, damage to the peroneal nerve, and some degree of tearing of the lateral collateral ligament and perhaps the lateral meniscus. The mechanism of injury is the important factor.[3] Although Birrer et al.[3] indicate that a strong crescent kick to the outside of the leg can cause injuries to the structures indicated, often a blow to the outside of the leg will create a valgus force and actually injure the medial collateral ligament of the knee.

Punching

Most experienced martial artists know that the punching motion primarily should direct the forces along the longitudinal axis of the second and third metacarpals. This is the most stable part of the hand from an osseous standpoint. Overenthusiastic novices commonly injure the fifth metacarpal in the typical Western boxing fashion, creating the "boxer's fracture" (Fig. 15.5).

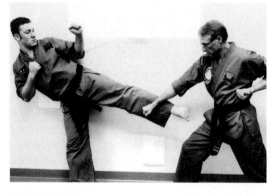 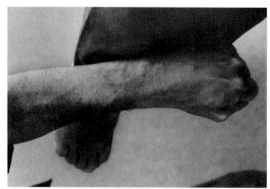

FIGURE 15.4

Example of an injury that could occur from blocking. A downblock performed in the manner illustrated here is a commonly used blocking technique. However, the distal end of the weaker of the forearm bones is used for the block, which predisposed the ulna to a fracture.

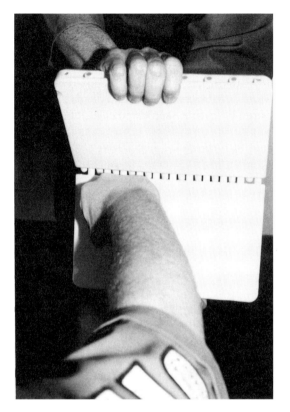

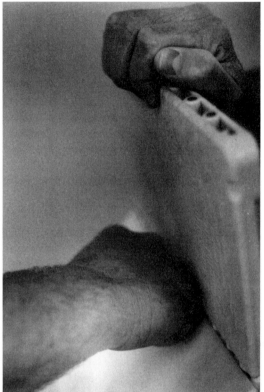

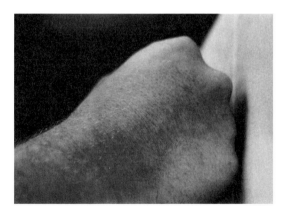

FIGURE 15.5

Example of an injury that could occur from striking. This is one of the most common injuries that occurs with striking called the "boxer's fracture." The martial artist hits with the fourth and fifth metacarpals, which are the unstable part of the hand, rather than striking with the second and third metacarpals, which are the stable parts of the hand.

Stricevic et al.[115] noted that punches accounted for a higher injury ratio than did kicks. Such injuries result from repetitive action, direct impact, or ballistic and torsional maneuvers (Fig. 15.6).

Receiving Direct Blows

Direct blows to several areas in the body can result in fractures. A blow to the medial proximal tibia from a violent crescent kick can damage the medial collateral ligament and meniscus.[3] Although Birrer et al.[3] state that a blow to the proximal medial tibia would injure the medial collateral ligament, more often the varus forces created from the location of the kick actually would injure the lateral collateral ligament. Patellar trauma is frequently due not only to direct blows but also to missed falls in certain styles. The damage to the patella is usually to the articular cartilage and rarely an obvious fracture.[3] Since only 2 to 5 lb is required to fracture the

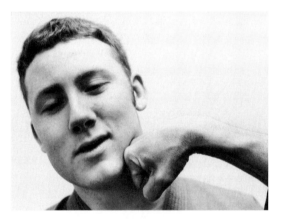

FIGURE 15.6

Example of an injury that could occur from punching. Punching with the wrist flexed places the carpals into a precarious position and can lead to a wrist sprain, strain, or fracture. The wrist should be in a straight line so that the carpals are supported by the radius and ulna and in a more stable position to transmit the force to the punching area. Of course, the recipient of the punch also can sustain an injury.

clavicle, moderate direct blows or indirect ones such as from missed falls can cause a fracture.[3]

According to the CPSC, between 1985 and 1994 there was one death directly related to a blow sustained during a karate competition.[11] Schmidt[101] discussed three cases of death following anterior chest trauma resulting from martial arts kicks. Aspiration and asphyxia, cardiac arrest, and traumatic rupture of the spleen caused the three cases of fatal anterior chest trauma. Failure to "pull" delivered techniques just short of anatomic impact was the primary mechanism responsible for death in all cases (Fig. 15.7).

The specific aspect of karate that the three martial artists were participating in when they were fatally injured is referred to as *kumite,* a Japanese word meaning "free sparring." Kumite consists of two unarmed opponents engaged in combat. They use four principles—*kiai* (yelling), *waza* (technique), *maai* (distance), and *ma* (timing)—in an attempt to strike a "disabling" or "killing" blow against their respective opponents. Both combatants attempt to deliver each technique with maximum force and velocity and "pull" (stop) the blows just short of actual anatomic impact. Unfortunately, however, injuries sometimes do occur as a result of improper technique or misjudgment in distance and/or timing. These fatalities all resulted from anterior chest trauma complicated by associated injuries and terminal sequelae. Although a pattern of injury hardly can be suggested by only three cases, perhaps the state of physiologic conditioning may have had some bearing on the severity of the injuries inflicted.[101]

Pieter and Pieter[88] presented a study to assess the exact conditions under which cerebral concussions occur in full-contact tae kwon do competition. The predominant injury mechanism in both males and females was receiving a blow. Although it has been suggested that the more experienced karate athletes sustain fewer total injuries, it is possible that if they do incur an injury, it may be

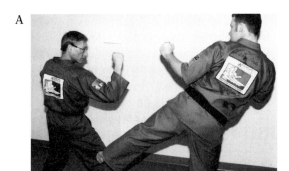

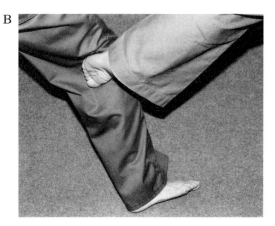

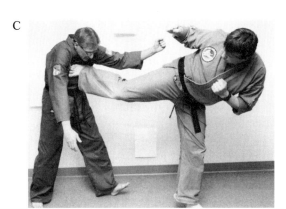

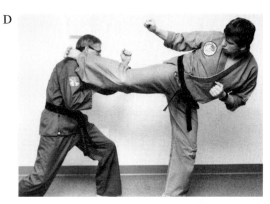

FIGURE 15.7

A,B. Example of an injury that could occur from receiving a blow. A "round kick" to the lateral aspect of the knee of the opponent can cause a potential injury to the medial side of the knee (MCL and ACL sprain, medial meniscus) or the lateral side of the knee (contusion). *C.* Example of an injury that could occur from receiving a blow. The side kick is one of the most powerful kicks and has been reported to cause deaths as well as other injuries in martial artists when received in the chest area. *D.* Example of an injury that could occur from receiving a blow. A spinning hook kick delivered to the opponent at the head/neck area has been reported to cause death or a variety of other injuries in martial artists.

of a more serious nature compared with their lesser-skilled counterparts. The dominant injury situation is an unblocked attack, and the dominant injury mechanism is receiving a blow for both male and female tae kwon do athletes. It is hypothesized that the un- blocked attack, as well as the blow received, involved a round kick. This rotational technique is believed to lead to higher accelerations to the head and a larger chance of sustaining a cerebral concussion. This is not to imply that translational techniques will not lead to cerebral concussion in tae kwon do, as was found elsewhere.[86]

Fighting/Sparring

The activity most commonly associated with injury, regardless of setting, is fighting (74 percent). The incidence and severity of injury are highest for free fighting and lowest for controlled sparring. The head, face, and neck are frequently injured during free-fighting situations, whereas the trunk and extremities are predominantly injured during controlled fighting. The distribution of injuries by activity is as follows: attacker (23 percent), defender (69 percent), and both (8 percent). Breakage (e.g., breaking boards or bricks) and weapons use (e.g., nunchaku, arnis, cutlery, tonfu, manrikigusari, and shuriken, or "throwing stars") are associated with the fewest injuries. Injuries from weapons are typically mild, whereas more serious injuries are associated with breakage (e.g., puncture wound from splinters, fractures, and concussions).[11]

Sparring in tournaments produces significantly higher injury rates and degrees of severity, particularly of the head and neck, presumably due to increased levels of aggression and unfamiliar settings associated with competition.[8] The magnitude of increase has been estimated to be 3 to 20 times. A number of studies have suggested that the risk for significant head injury in the competitive situation may approach or exceed the rate for other sports including football.[8,19,28,53,115,120] Phalangeal injuries are common in tae kwon do and often occur during sparring.[3]

Tournaments

The incidence of injury is higher in the tournament situation. There was some form of injury in one of four contests and an incapacitating injury in one of ten contests[5,71] (Table 15.4).

Karate injuries sustained in several national and international tournaments were reviewed by Stricevic et al.[114] They found that most injuries occurred during the second minute of the contest. Possibly the late occurrence of the afternoon injuries may be related to the fatigue factor. The significance of the competition was supported by this study finding that those final bouts in particular offered increased risk for injury. This finding contradicts McLatchie's[71] impression that injuries occur more commonly in the opening hour of the day. The competitors in this study probably were more tired in the final bouts than in the eliminations, which may have reduced their sensitivity and ability to control various techniques. In addition, the average rank of the injured athlete was always lower than the average rank of the opponent. This indicates that as the athletes become more experienced, they sustained fewer injuries. There were four times more injuries caused by punches than by kicks.

Two previous studies[8,115] also have shown that more experienced competitors are less injury prone than those with less experience. In some studies, lower-grade competitors have been reported to suffer more injuries than those of a higher grade. However, the belt grade is not necessarily a good indicator of experience. A person may have a black belt and very limited contest experience, whereas another person may have, for instance, only a green belt and much more contest experience.

Spin Kicks

McLatchie[76] states that the spinning back kick should be outlawed because once it is initiated, it cannot be controlled. The emphasis placed by competitors, judges, and spectators on "head shots" invites serious injuries. Spinning kicks to the head are especially dangerous. It is noteworthy that spinning hook kicks were developed by unarmed serfs to forcibly unseat sword-wielding horsemen.[81]

TABLE 15.4

Injury Data by Setting*

Location	No. of injuries (%)	Prevalence			Incidence			Severity
		Men	Women	Total	Men	Women	Total	
Competitive	12,176 (29.6)	3.83	2.18	3.4	2.42	1.36	2.22	2.4
Noncompetitive	28,910 (70.4)							1.7
Formal	19,678 (47.9)	2.83	2.19	2.52	1.79	1.26	1.54	1.6
Informal	9,232 (22.5)	3.37	2.26	3.08	1.84	1.22	1.68	2.1
Total	41,086 (100)							
Average		3.43	1.8	2.99	1.98	1.07	1.71	1.88

*Prevalence, injuries per participant; incidence, injuries per participant per year.
Source: From Birrer RB: Trauma epidemiology in the marital arts. *Am J Sports Med* 24:S72–S79, 1996.

Roundhouse Kick

The roundhouse kick has been reported to cause severe injuries.[76,115] As with any technique, learning proper execution and control is important. Control is particularly important when using advanced techniques that have significant forces and can be potentially injurious.

Choking

Experiments with human subjects and animals show the following effects from choking[52]:

1. Unconsciousness is due to the lack of oxygen and by the metabolites created in the brain as a result of acute cerebral anemia from pressure on the arteries and veins and shock, which is a reflex action initiated on the receptor organ in the carotid sinus
2. The appearance of flushing of the face is because of the disturbances in pressure in the carotid arteries and jugular veins
3. Tachycardia, hypertension, and mydriasis (dilated pupils) are caused by stimulation of the sympathetic nervous system (vagus nerve)
4. In some cases bradycardia and hypotension, whereas in others tachycardia and hypertension depending on the hypersensitivity of the carotid sinus and where the pressure was applied
5. Cardiac volume decreases but recovers 10 s after awakening
6. Vasoconstriction of the peripheral blood vessels in the muscle and skin
7. Stress on the circulatory and hypophysioadrenocortical system
8. With electroencephalographic (EEG) examination, convulsions during unconsciousness that are very similar to those of petit mal epilepsy, but no deleterious effects afterwards (It is considerably less dangerous than a knockout in boxing.)

Although not from participation in the martial arts per se, Reay and Eisle[92] reported two deaths that resulted from the use of "choke holds" by law enforcement officers. The hazards of choke holds are emphasized, and the authors reviewed those conditions where there is an increased risk for a fatal outcome when the choke hold is used. In addition to the circumstances where a choke hold is justifiable, it is imperative that the officer who would use such a hold has proper training in its use. Admittedly, there may be persons so skilled in the martial arts and judo techniques that they can act with quickness of movement and effectively squeeze the vessels in the neck in the classic carotid sleeper. The success of the maneuver depends on surprise as well as skill. No officer should be lulled into the false confidence that squeezing an arm about a neck is a safe and innocuous technique of subduing a suspect. It must be viewed as a potentially fatal tactic and reserved for situations that merit its risk.

Breaking

Many martial arts tournaments include breaking techniques (tameshiwari), which are known to be self-destructive forms of competition.[75,80] Once again, although the preceding statement is included in the literature, we feel that proper instruction and focus are critical to having martial artists break objects correctly and safely.

Throws

Jackson et al.[43] described blunt head injuries incurred by Marine recruits in hand-to-hand combat (judo training). The modus operandi of each of the cases of blunt head injuries was exactly the same; namely, the patient was thrown to the deck (floor), striking his shoulders. An accelerated secondary impact occurred when the occiput struck the floor. It is apparent that primary acceleration of the body and shoulders to the mat followed by the secondary acceleration of the occiput to the deck resulted in blunt injury to the brain with secondary cerebral edema and hemorrhage. Specific recommendations for the prevention of such injuries have been suggested. These include a definite program of neck strengthening exercises, periodic review of training techniques by judo experts, and an increased in the "density of recruit participa-

tion and physical training" to further improve participation in physical training per unit of time instruction.

Weapons Usage

There are limited studies on the injury rates associated with the use of weaponry in the martial arts, but in the epidemiologic study by Birrer[8] the infrequency and mild nature of injuries from weapon use were noted.

Common Injuries (Table 15.5)

In the grappling arts, injuries occur when (1) a breakfall (ukemi waza) is poorly executed, (2) a joint lock is overapplied or the opponent fails to submit, or (3) a choke or stranglehold (shime-waza) is applied incorrectly or held in place for too long.[9] Minor injuries (abrasions from mat friction burns) occur more commonly in these styles, with more serious injuries involving the head, neck (airway), and joints (wrist, elbow, shoulder, and knee).[9] Most attention has centered on judo/jujutsu, especially with respect to choking tactics.

JUDO

The rules of judo provide for strangulation techniques in which the blood supply to the brain is blocked by pressure on the carotid arteries; such techniques produce anoxia and possibly unconsciousness if the victim fails to submit. Anoxic brain damage is not a common form of sports injury, but the unique characteristics of judo suggest that under certain circumstances, an individual may develop signs of anoxic brain damage. The rules specify that one of the ways to win a judo contest is by means of "strangulation" techniques. Loss of consciousness follows rapidly with no pain or discomfort to the victim. Victory is achieved if the opponent either (1) in-

TABLE 15.5

Number and Severity of Injuries by Anatomic Site

Location	Number	Percent	Severity
Head	1,238	3	3.5
Face	3,272	8	3.8
Neck	406	1	2.8
Shoulder	2,067	5	2.0
Elbow	2,041	5	1.7
Arm/forearm	2,473	6	1.3
Wrist	2,451	6	1.5
Fingers/hand	4,518	11	1.9
Trunk	2,874	7	1.4
Groin	3,293	8	2.6
Hip	1,245	3	1.2
Knee	1,639	4	1.8
Thigh/leg	6,990	17	1.5
Ankle	825	2	1.6
Foot/toes	5,754	14	1.7
Total	41,086	100	
Average			1.88

Source: From Birrer RB: Trauma epidemiology in the martial arts. *Am J Sports Med* 24:S72–S79, 1996.

dicates submission as a result of the technique or (2) loses consciousness, having had the opportunity to submit, as a result of failing to do so. In both cases it is accepted practice that the hold is maintained until the referee has announced the awarding of the point. In addition, it should be noted that judo competitors are commonly strangled into unconsciousness during teaching either as an illustration of the technique or in order to demonstrate the judo resuscitation procedures (kuatsu). Such circumstances do not occur in any other sport. Consequently, years of participating in these types of activities may make one more susceptible to anoxic brain damage.[82]

Rodriguez et al.[93] examined 10 judoka at rest, and then in 7 of them as syncope was in-duced by judo choke holds. An EEG was recorded during the loss of consciousness while the regional cerebral blood flow (rCBF) was measured immediately after recovery. In all cases, the choking procedure was applied on the lateral side of the neck (katajuji-jime), and it was carried out until the subject had lost consciousness. It was immediately interrupted when, after a muscular contraction, the postural tone failed. The syncope obtained by choking was preceded by a "clouding" of the state of consciousness and by a general muscular contraction, and it was accompanied by muscular flaccidity followed by tonic-clonic contractions and irregular breathing. The subject's consciousness was restored after 10 to 15 s, and the awakening often was characterized by pleasant oneiric contents. Indeed, judo, despite the violent characteristics of some of its attack techniques, does not seem to be accompanied by the decline of cerebral function noted with other systems. It is interesting to underline that in other sports, such as boxing, both structural[16] and functional[93] pathologic modifications were seen. The findings suggest that there is no evidence of permanent central nervous system (CNS) functional changes due to judo practice and choking. The variable rCBF features soon after choking-induced syncope may reflect a different timing of recovery from cerebral ischemia for each subject.

Koiwai[52] evaluated deaths allegedly caused by the use of choke holds (shime-waza). He found that the shime-waza, when properly applied, should not cause death. Therefore, its primary purpose should be to subdue violent individuals. When properly applied, the choke hold causes unconsciousness in 10 to 20 s. No fatalities as a result of shime-waza have been reported in the sport of judo since its inception in 1882. Among the methods of "control holds" taught to law enforcement officers is a choke hold similar or identical to shime-waza. Using the choke hold, officers may afford themselves maximum safety while subjecting the suspect to a minimum possibility of injury. Koiwai[51] reviewed 14 fatalities with autopsy findings where death was allegedly caused by the use of choke holds. Based on this survey and the number of judo participants throughout the world, the number of fatalities associated with judo is minimal.

Judoists are taught to apply shime-waza using the principle "maximum efficiency with minimum effort." The maximum pressure is applied directly on the "carotid triangle" without applying pressure to other parts of the neck, causing unnecessary damage. If the carotid hold is applied properly, unconsciousness occurs in approximately 10 s

(8–14 s). The state of unconsciousness, according to investigators of the Society for Scientific Study in Judo, Kodokan, is caused by a temporary hypoxic condition of the cerebral cortex. After release, the subject regains consciousness spontaneously in 10 to 20 s. Neck pressure of 250 mmHg or 5 kg of rope tension is required to occlude carotid arteries. The amount of pressure to collapse the airway is six times greater.[52]

In judo, the player holds the opponent's neck by his or her hands or forearm, and the blood flow of the common carotid artery is obstructed. However, the vertebral artery is not obstructed. It has been confirmed that complete obstruction of blood flow to the brain or asphyxia by complete closure of the trachea will result in irreversible damage to the body that often results in death. While unconsciousness (ochi) caused by choking (shime) in judo is a temporary reaction that incapacitates the opponent for a short while, its execution is quite harmless.[52]

In the striking arts, targets of attack generally are limited to the chest and head.[9] Injuries occur from:

1. Noncontact practice on one's own (kata)
2. Striking objects (punching bag, wood, cement, etc.)
3. Sparring (kumite): noncontact, light contact, full contact

KARATE

A recent survey of karate practitioners found that older participants had a higher injury rate than younger participants, men had more injuries than women, and advanced students had more serious injuries than beginners. The injury rate was 2.7 per 1000 hours of karate practice.[13] Only 47 serious injuries were recorded at a rate of 1 in 500 injuries. Injuries from karate occur to three main areas: the head/neck, the abdominal organs, and the limbs.[76] It is not surprising that karate injuries can be severe, considering that karate was developed as a means to kill or maim an opponent.

TAE KWON DO

During the 1988 U.S. Olympic Tae Kwon Do Team trials, the injury rate for men was 40 percent higher than the rate for women.[138] Contusions were the predominant injury, with the foot and the head the most frequently injured areas. Concussions were recorded for both men and women. A large proportion (41 percent) of injuries in male participants was the result of direct blows from an unblocked attack, whereas women were more commonly injured (40 percent) while attacking with a kick. For both men and women, 15 percent of the reported injuries resulted in time lost to tae kwon do practice. The high velocities and momentum levels generated during tae kwon do kicking and the lack of proper blocking raise serious concerns about the safety of full-contact tae kwon do. Although protective equipment may be effective initially, it may be insufficient to withstand repeated violent impacts.

Injuries during tae kwon do practice occur in 7 of 10 competitors, and approximately 1 in 20 injuries are closed head injuries.[34] Because of careful training and control, most injuries are mild to moderate, and most are contusions—only 1 in 500 injuries is serious.[3] Boxing is the competitive sport to which karate may be most closely compared. Karate bouts are shorter, and there is no repeated trauma such as recurrent head injury; seasoned fighters, therefore, do not become "punch drunk," nor do they suffer from gross facial disfigurements.[71]

Most injuries in the striking martial arts occur to either the target of an attack (e.g., head, torso) or to the attacking weapon (e.g., hand, foot).[9] Injuries occur most frequently in the inexperienced color belts and decrease as expertise increases, although the severity of the injuries increases with the higher-level skills.

Pieter and Zemper[89] performed a prospective study evaluating injury rates in children participating in tae kwon do competitions. No differences were found between boys and girls.

LOWER EXTREMITIES

The CPSC reported that in 1984 that there were 2913 foot, 681 ankle, and 1381 toe injuries involving the martial arts.[11]

Foot

The foot receives about 18 percent of the injuries in tae kwon do, usually during sparring. The toes are easily jammed, resulting in contusion, dislocation, or fracture. More serious foot injuries can occur in sparring, particularly fracture of the metatarsals. Metatarsalgia and fractures also occur secondary to the stresses placed on the foot during kicks and jumps.[3]

In tae kwon do the primary weapon is the foot, and emphasis is often placed on jumping and/or spinning attacks to the upper chest and head. As with karate, the attacking part is frequently injured, and since the foot cannot be rolled up like a fist, fractures involve the phalanges, metatarsals, and less commonly, the tarsals.[9]

Ankle

Injuries to the ankle are relatively uncommon in tae kwon do and usually involve contusion to the malleoli, especially the lateral malleoli.[3]

Achilles Tendon

Novice martial arts practitioners (especially women) are often afflicted with Achilles tendinitis secondary to overenthusiastic application of the various stances in end range of dorsiflexion.[3]

Knee

In tae kwon do, the knee is prone to both accidental and intentional trauma. A classic injury caused by a kick to the lateral aspect of the knee is a fracture of the proximal fibula, a contusion of the peroneal nerve, and a sprain of variable degree to the medial collateral ligament with possible tearing of the medial meniscus.[3]

Thigh

In styles permitting contact, the thigh is in the legal striking zone in sparring and is often struck with great force, causing thigh contusions. This can cause not only a painful contusion but also a large hematoma.[3]

Muscle strains of the thigh (quadriceps and hamstrings) can occur frequently from excessive stretching or overly vigorous kicking and exercise.

UPPER EXTREMITY

In a longitudinal (7-year) epidemiologic study, Tenvergert et al.[117] found that the majority of injuries reported occurred to the upper extremities.

Hand

In karate, the hand is the primary striking tool. Most injuries involve the carpals and metacarpals, especially of the dominant hand. Injuries usually result from attempts to break wood, stone, ice, or concrete. The second and third metacarpals are injured more commonly in senior students, whereas junior students tend to suffer the "boxer's fracture" (fifth metacarpal).[9] Phalangeal injuries are common, including dislocations and fractures in association with tendon ruptures.[3]

Kelly et al.[47] contacted 18 karate schools and evaluated the incidence of index metacarpal fractures in karate. Most injuries occurred in the dominant hand and resulted from missed blows. Nine of the 11 metacarpal fractures showed elements of axial compression. Characteristic fractures of the hand have been associated with particular athletic activities. The punch fracture ("boxer's fracture") resulting from roundhouse blows usually involves the surgical neck of the little finger or ring metacarpal. The biomechanical stresses of karate explain the higher incidence of index metacarpal fractures in the sport. Karate training emphasizes use of the fists and arms. The correctly executed thrust (tsuki) and hand strike places axial compression forces on the index and long finger metacarpal heads. Inaccurate thrusts, roundhouse blows, and other opponent contact (such as blocking kicks) transmit angular and torsional forces to the metacarpals. When these forces are combined with axial loading, oblique diaphyseal fractures may result. Epiphyseal plate fractures also occurred in some individuals. A review of metacarpal fractures related to karate disclosed an unusually high incidence of index finger metacarpal fractures.

Larose and Kim[60] reviewed 50 consecutive cases of metacarpal fractures. The high incidence of knuckle fractures in the fourth and fifth metacarpals can be explained by the weaker structures of these metacarpals, by their lack of support in a bare-knuckle fist, and by the number of roundhouse punches that are thrown. A fracture of the fourth or fifth metacarpal head is often referred to as a *knuckle fracture, punch fracture,* or *boxer's fracture.* The fourth metacarpal is the most slender of the metacarpals. The cortex of the fifth metacarpal is eggshell thin. The thenar eminence only supports the second and third metacarpals in a bare-knuckle fist. Students of karate are taught to make a fist by first flexing the interphalangeal joints maximally and then flexing the metacarpophalangeal joints so that the thenar eminence supports the second and third metacarpals. The thumb is tucked out of the way in order to avoid a fracture of the first metacarpal base or possibly a Bennett's fracture-dislocation. Karate students also are taught to strike with the second and third knuckles and only with a maximally tightened fist. Twisting the wrist to the pronated position at impact has the double effect of reminding the striker to tighten the fist maximally and to also tear the opponent's skin.

Soft tissue injuries also occur in karate. Hypertrophy of the skin and the bones at the index and long metacarpal head regions is often found in association with karate. Vayssairat et al.[121] reported a case of arterial aneurysms of the hand. The only causal factor appeared to be repeated trauma to both hands. Therefore, it is tempting to link intensive karate practice with the occurrence of ulnar artery aneurysms. However, systematic investigation of hand arteries in the karateka population is required to confirm this hypothesis.

Danek[27] reviewed x-ray studies and physical examinations of the hands of karate experts, and the results were unexpected. There was no evidence of soft tissue calcification in the study group. He concludes that the three Cs of karate—*concentration*, *control*, and *contact*—make it possible for experts to smash through bricks and boards without a high incidence of hand and foot injuries.

Crosby[26] reviewed radiographic evidence of 22 karate instructors who had practiced the sport for a minimum of 5 years. Four activities seem to have the greatest potential for damage: doing push-ups on the knuckles, repeated punching of a firm target, sparring, and breaking objects. In conclusion, the long-term and routine practice of karate does not appear to predispose to the early onset of osteoarthritis or tendinitis in the hands and wrists.

Streeton and Melb[113] described a case of traumatic hemoglobinuria after karate exercises involving considerable trauma to the hands. Hemoglobinuria often has been described after marching, running, or walking and has been termed *march hemoglobinuria*. The area of the body surface exposed to trauma also may be an important factor be-

cause it would seem that the smaller the exposed body surface area and the greater the traumatizing force, the more likely it is that hemoglobinuria will ensue. Muscular exertion can be excluded as a causative factor in this case. There was no evidence of muscle cell damage during the exercises, and myoglobinuria was not demonstrated at any stage. Posture is also not related to the cause of march hemoglobinuria. In view of the findings in this case, it would seem that the term *march hemoglobinuria* is a misnomer, and the condition more properly should be referred to as *traumatic hemoglobinuria*.

Wrist/Forearm

Wrist injuries are infrequent in tae kwon do (4 percent) and usually consist of contusions from missed blocks and kicks.[3] In styles that use weapons, an occasional "nightstick" fracture can result. Even a violent crescent kick blocked by an outside-inside block can fracture the ulna. The elbow rarely receives injuries besides contusions. Distal ulnar fractures can occur from using the forearm to block a blow.[13]

Shoulder

Shoulder trauma includes dislocation, fracture, and brachial plexus damage. The most frequent fracture involves the clavicle. Rarely, shoulder separations (acromioclavicular sprains) result from a violent blow or a missed fall.[3] Cottalorda et al.[24] described the fracture of the coracoid process caused by a direct fall onto the shoulder while engaging in judo.

Nonmusculoskeletal Injuries

Nonmusculoskeletal injuries that have been reported in the martial arts include[3]:

- Eye injuries—corneal abrasion, subconjunctival hemorrhage, hyphema, globe contusions, and retinal tears and detachments

- Abdominal trauma—relatively common because the abdomen is in the designated striking zone (Often the wind is knocked out of the athlete, and no serious trauma results. However, a well-focused moderate blow in either upper quadrant has been known to produce liver and spleen contusions and lacerations. A forceful midepigastric punch can lacerate the left lobe of the liver, rupture the diaphragm, and contuse the pericardium and myocardium after fracturing the xiphoid.)
- Bladder rupture and spontaneous abortion in an undiagnosed pregnant woman due to a blow to the suprapubic area
- Kidney contusion or laceration from a well-placed kick or strike to the costovertebral region

Nielsen and Jensen[79] described a case report of total transection of the pancreas occurring during karate training. The mechanism of injury was a blow to the upper abdomen. This is a rather rare injury, and only a few cases due to sports accidents have been described. Mars and Pimendes[70] presented a case study where a karate participant was punched in the eye, was knocked unconscious, and fell to the floor. As a result of the injury, there was a blinding choroidal rupture in the karateka participant. A wide range of trauma has been recorded, and though rare, life-threatening injuries to the head, thorax, and abdomen have occurred[5,16,54] (Table 15.6).

HEAD INJURIES

Feehan and Waller[34] demonstrated the body sites of tae kwon do–related injuries. One in 20 injuries was a closed head injury. Of all registered injuries, more than 95 percent were localized to the head. However, the use of protective guards and padding was not significantly associated with the occurrence of injuries. Among adult males, competitors with more than 5 years of competitive experience had 4.9 times the odds of sustaining injury as compared with those with less than 2 years of experience.[119]

Studies reported in the neurosurgical literature[69,103] have compared peak acceleration of blows to the head, with and without headgear, using punches to the front and the side of the head. These punches were with bare hands, "safety-chuck hand protectors," and 10-oz boxing gloves. Kicks also were delivered to the head, with and without headgear, using bare feet and "safety kick" padding. These studies showed that bare karate-style equipment punches to the side of the head produced greater peak accelerations than kicks to the front and side. Kicks produced greater acceleration than did punches to the front of the head. Safety equipment failed to soften or lessen peak accelerations with or without headgear. The subjects in the study perceived that safety equipment for hands and feet was protection for the wearer rather than for the opponent.[126]

Unequivocal evidence exists that repeated brain injury of concussive or even subconcussive force results in characteristic patterns of brain damage and a steady decline in the ability to process information efficiently. Furthermore, the effects of repeated blows to the head from a punch or kick are cumulative. Although some blows may be more severe than others, none is trivial, and each has the potential to be lethal. Blunt head blows cause shearing injury to the nerve fibers and neurons in proportion to the degree that the head is accelerated, and these acceleration forces are transmitted to the brain. Blows to the side of the head tend to produce greater acceleration forces than those to the face, whereas blows to the chin (which acts as a lever) produce maximal forces. (Headgear and protective padding to the hands and feet may lessen the force of brain acceleration. Thus extra padding may reduce the chances

TABLE 15.6

Severe Injuries

Injury	No.
Pneumothorax	8
Contusion	
Lung	2
Brain	7
Heart	2
Spinal cord	3
Renal	4
Laceration	
Spleen	5
Liver	3
Kidney	3
Pancreas	2
Rupture	
Diaphragm	1
Bladder	3
Hematoma	
Brain	4
Spinal cord	1
Pericardium	1
Retroperitoneum	1
Fractures	
Cricothyroid/larynx	3
Long bone	79
Epiphysis	14
Skull	42
Spine	9
Cerebral concussion	433
Testicular torsion	9
Eye	
Hyphema	17
Retinal detachment	7
Globe contusion	19
Lens dislocation	4
Miscarriage	6
Total	692 (1.7%)

Source: From Birrer RB: Trauma epidemiology in the martial arts. *Am J Sports Med* 24:S72–S79, 1996.

of death, but it will not prevent brain damage due to tearing of brain substance.[103])

"Punch-drunk syndrome," or dementia pugilistic, is a traumatic encephalopathy that may occur in anyone subjected to repeated blows to the head from any cause. Fight fans recognize the syndrome as "cuckoo," "goofy," "slug-nutty," or "cutting paper dolls."

Butler et al.[14] performed a prospective, controlled investigation of the cognitive effects of amateur boxing. No evidence of neuropsychological dysfunction due to boxing was found either following a bout or after a series of bouts at follow-up. None of the range of parameters, including number of previous contests, recovery from an earlier bout, number of head blows received during a bout, and number of bouts between initial assessment and follows-up, was found to be related to changes in cognitive functioning.

Critchley[25] discussed the medical aspects of boxing, particularly from a neurologic standpoint. Critchley concludes that there is much in boxing of concern to neurologists, and special attention should be focused on (1) the phenomenon of groggy states as occurring during or after a contest and (2) the condition known as *traumatic progressive encephalopathy* (or punch-drunkenness). Owing to the extreme paucity of pathologic data, it is highly desirable that the opportunity should be afforded to neuropathologists to study the appearance and structures of the brain of punch-drunk individuals. There is a scope for further study of boxers by EEG as well as clinical techniques at all stages, i.e., early as well as late in their careers and before and immediately after a contest, especially if a knockout has occurred.

Casson et al.[17] studied 18 former and active boxers who underwent neurologic examination, EEG, computed tomographic scan of the brain, and neuropsychological testing. Eighty-seven percent of the professional boxers had definite evidence of brain damage. All the boxers had abnormal results on at least one of the neuropsychological tests. Brain damage is a frequent result of a career in professional boxing.

Many authorities actually separate boxing from the more traditional martial arts. However, because there is so much more research on head injuries in the boxing literature, we decided to include a few comments here regarding the effects of repetitive contact to the head and the residual sequelae. Some authors[103] think that it is just a matter of time before some of the effects that have occurred from boxing also will start to show up in martial artists who do a lot of full-contact fighting.

Return to Sport

FUNCTIONAL SPORT-SPECIFIC REHABILITATION TECHNIQUES

Clinical protocols for return to play need to be established (consider a passbook system).[8] Jaffe and Minkoff[44] recommend stretching and strengthening exercises be performed as needed. Loose or unstable joints, particularly the knees and ankles, may require braces to permit participation. Jaffe and Minkoff[44] state that injury begets injury. Once injured, an individual often develops weakness and contracture of the injured area and escalates the likelihood of additional injury or reinjury.

Musculoskeletal injuries occur in karate practice due to an emphasis on solo practice. Most chronic problems result from karate techniques that cause inadequately rehabilitated previous injuries to flare up.[54]

GENERAL REHABILITATION PRINCIPLES

We recommend that as with the development of a rehabilitation program for a patient in any sport, an understanding of the biomechanics of the sport, the mechanisms of injuries involved, and the pathomechanics that result is necessary. The traditional methodologies performed (physical therapy modalities, etc.) in developing a rehabilitation program still need to be applied to the patient as the foundation. Then specific martial arts rehabilitation or performance-enhancement programs can be developed based on the aforementioned criteria. At this time, the rehabilitation program diverges from traditional rehabilitation because of the specific requirements of the particular martial art in which the patient participates.

Range of Motion/Flexibility

Increasing joint range of motion (ROM) and the flexibility of the musculotendinous unit are important aspects of rehabilitating any injury.

Closed Kinetic Chain/Open Kinetic Chain Exercises

Examples of activities for the lower extremities that would be included would be a variety of closed kinetic chain activities replicating the stance or support leg when kicks are being thrown. Likewise, open kinetic chain exercises need to be performed because most of the kicking techniques are open kinetic chain movement patterns. Therefore, an integrated approach to the rehabilitation must be performed. Working on muscular strength, power, and endurance is important as part of the total rehabilitation program.

Depending on the martial art, upper extremity rehabilitation may involve either primarily open kinetic chain activities, i.e., punching in karate, or primarily closed kinetic chain patterns, i.e., with some of the grappling sports like judo. Consequently, an integrated approach using both open and closed kinetic chain activities is warranted with rehabilitation of the upper extremities in the martial artist, with attention being paid to the particular activity and the amount of emphasis on the details of the rehabilitation program. Once again, emphasis must be placed on muscular strength, power, and endurance.

Core (Trunk) Stabilization

Because of the kinetic chain link between the legs and the arms for most martial arts activities, the trunk also must be included in the rehabilitation program for core stabilization. Using basic calisthenics is an effective means of core stability by performing sit-ups, rotations, and trunk extensions. However, almost all activities involved in martial arts training and conditioning incorporate the need for trunk musculature strengthening and stabilization.

Cardiorespiratory Training

In addition, various energy systems must be trained for both the cardiorespiratory and musculoskeletal systems. Research has shown that performing katas (participating in sparring workouts or competitive matches) creates an aerobic training response, whereas practicing individual skills or techniques puts more emphasis on the anaerobic system. Once again, there needs to be an integrated approach to training the energy systems as part of the total comprehensive training program.

Balance/Proprioceptive/ Kinesthetic Training

Balance, proprioceptive, and kinesthetic training plays an integral part in the total training program for the martial artist. One of the main reasons for this is the "focus" necessary when "pulling" a punch or a kick. The martial artist must have the ability to accelerate the punch or the kick from being still to striking or almost striking ("pulling") the object within milliseconds. This is one of the most critical factors that would need to be redeveloped in returning the martial artist back to successful participation.

Specificity Training
Exercises: Plyometrics

Some exercises that readily lend themselves to martial arts training are plyometrics. Plyometrics involves the concept of a stretch-shortening cycle. There are three phases to a plyometric exercise: (1) the eccentric prestretch motion that "loads" the connective tissue with potential energy to facilitate phase 3, (2) the amortization phase (which is the key to plyometrics in that the shorter the phase, the more effective is the plyometric motion), which involves the time from the cessation of the eccentric action to onset of the concentric action, and (3) the concentric or power execution phase. The primary reason is that the plyometric motion replicates the explosiveness needed for many of the jumps required in several of the martial arts such as karate and tae kwon do. Plyometric training helps promote the explosive ability to correctly perform the specific techniques in martial arts.

Use of medicine ball techniques can be included in the training program to replicate specific movements to enhance performance. For example, medicine ball throws from the chest are effective in increasing the power of several punching techniques. Using the jump rope is an example of in-place response-speed plyometrics that can help improve the speed and footwork of the martial artist.

Neuromuscular Control/Agility Training

Other types of training, such as coordination training and agility training, become critical as well. Neuromuscular control and agility training are key to the patient's ability to perceive and control his or her body in space. This is the essence of many of the jumping and twisting techniques used in the martial arts. Consequently, rehabilitation and performance-enhancement programs require specificity training in a controlled reactive training situation to prepare the martial artist to return to the reactive, realistic training environment.

Sport-specific drills, which are broken down into component parts and practiced, are the foundation. The component parts are molded back into the total functional motion. Along with integration of the basics into more advanced techniques, the principles of progression and overload are also used as part of specificity training programs. An example of a drill to improve the round kick might be as follows: Have the martial artist lift the leg to the chamber position as quickly as possible with the proper pivoting motion. Next, from the chamber position, have the martial artist work on just the kicking motion. Then perform the kicking motion, but focus on rechambering as quickly as possible. After the rechamber, have the martial artist return to the ready position as quickly as possible. Finally, of course, the entire sequence needs to be performed. This can begin with slower movements and progress to faster speeds. The principle of progression also can be applied by starting with submaximal efforts and progressing to maximal intensity and power.

DETERMINING READINESS TO RETURN TO MARTIAL ARTS ACTIVITY

Assessing readiness to return to full activity is challenging. To assist in the decision-making process, Davies created a functional testing algorithm (FTA) that consists of a series of progressively challenging tests. Test scores must meet the minimal clinician-established criteria before the athlete is progressed to a more challenging test. The FTA can be referred to during serial reassessments to determine readiness to return to activity. Based on the results of testing within the algorithm, the clinician can update and customize the clinical rehabilitation program.

Davies' Functional Testing Algorithm (FTA)

- Basic measurements (visual analog pain scales, anthropometric measurements, goniometric measurements, etc.)

- KT 1000 testing for ACL/PCL ligament injuries
- Kinesthetic/proprioceptive/balance testing
- Closed kinetic chain (CKC) supine isokinetic testing
- Open kinetic chain (OKC) isokinetic testing
- CKC squat isokinetic testing
- Functional jump test
- Functional hop test
- Lower extremity functional test
- Sport-specific testing
- Discharge and return to activity

Research

Additional research on (1) the pathogenesis of injuries, (2) equipment design, safety, and testing by a recognized certification organization, and (3) long-term effects of macro- and microtrauma, particularly to the CNS, is needed. Furthermore, a better research base is needed to evaluate injury pathogenesis, promote better training techniques, design better safety equipment, and establish better rules for competition.[81]

Observations made during the course of investigation of the injuries in national and international karate tournaments support this need for more research.[115] For tae kwon do competitions specifically, future research is needed to confirm the association between the force of kicks and the occurrence of cerebral concussions and the incidence of injury for participants differing in skill level.[90]

Summary

This chapter has provided an introduction to martial arts and the myriad types of activities involved, the epidemiology of injuries, the mechanisms of injuries, the types and locations of injuries, and the kinetics and kine-matics of some of the activities in the martial arts. This chapter also has described various injury prevention techniques and finally specific recommendations for rehabilitation and/or performance enhancement for the martial artist.

References

1. Agnew PS: Taping of foot and ankle for Korean karate. *J Am Podiatr Med Assoc* 83(9): 534–536, 1993.
2. Birrer RB, Birrer CD: *Medical Injuries in the Martial Arts*. Springfield, IL: Charles C Thomas, 1981.
3. Birrer RB, Birrer CD, Son DS, Stone D: Injuries in tae kwon do. *Phys Sports Med* 9(2): 97–103, 1981.
4. Birrer RB, Birrer CD: Martial arts injuries. *Phys Sports Med* 10(6):103–108, 1982.
5. Birrer RB, Birrer CD: Unreported injuries in the martial arts. *Br J Sports Med* 17(2): 131–134, 1983.
6. Birrer RB, Halbrock SP: Martial arts injuries: The results of a five-year national survey. *Am J Sports Med* 16:408–410, 1988.
7. Birrer RB, Robinson T: Pelvic fracture following karate kick. *NY State Med J* 91:503, 1991.
8. Birrer RB: Trauma epidemiology in the martial arts: The results of an eighteen-year international survey. *Am J Sports Med* 24(6): S72–79, 1996.
9. Bonneville S: Martial arts injuries: A review. *Sports Med: http://publish.uwo.ca/~ahpandya/spmarti.html*; accessed June 25, 1999.
10. Brown DD, Mucci WG, Hetzler RK, Knowlton RG: Cardiovascular and ventilatory responses during formalized t'ai chi chuan exercise. *Res Qt* 60(3):246–250, 1989.
11. Burks JB, Satterfield K: Foot and ankle injuries among martial artists: Results of a survey. *J Am Podiatr Med Assoc* 88(6):268–278, 1998.
12. Buschbacher RM, Coplin B, Buschbacher L: Proper punching technique in the martial arts (abstract). *Arch Phys Med Rehabil* 73:1019, 1992.

13. Buschbacher RM, Shay T: Martial arts. *Phys Med Rehab Clin North Am* 10(1):35–47, 1999.

14. Butler RJ, Forsythe WI, Beverly DW, Adams LA: A prospective controlled investigation of the cognitive effects of amateur boxing. *J Neurol Neurosurg Psychol* 56:1055–1061, 1993.

15. Cantu C, Voy R: Second impact syndrome: A risk in any contact sport. *Phys Sports Med* 23:27–34, 1995.

16. Cantwell JD, King JT: Karate chops and liver lacerations. *JAMA* 224(10):1424, 1973.

17. Casson IR, Siegel O, Sham R, et al: Brain damage in modern boxers. *JAMA* 251(20):2663–2667, 1983.

18. Cavanagh PR, Landa J: A biomechanical analysis of the karate chop. *Res Q* 47(4):610–618, 1976.

19. Chambers RB: Orthopedic injuries in athletes (ages 6 to 17): Comparison of injuries occurring in six sports. *Am J Sports Med* 7:195–197, 1979.

20. Channer KS, Barrow D, Barrow R, et al: Changes in hemodynamic parameters following tai chi chuan and aerobic exercise in patients recovering from acute myocardial infarction. *Postgrad Med J* 72:349–351, 1996.

21. Chui DT: Karate kid finger. *Plast Reconstr Surg* 91(2):362–364, 1993.

22. Columbus PJ, Rice DL: Psychological research on the martial arts: An addendum to Fuller's review. *Br J Med Psychol* 61:317–328, 1988.

23. Conkel BS, Braucht J, Wilson W, et al: Isokinetic torque, kick velocity and force in tae kwon do. *Med Sci Sports Exerc* 20(2S):S5, 1988.

24. Cottalorda J, Allard D, Dutour N, Chavrier Y: Fracture of the coracoid process in an adolescent. *Injury* 27(6):436–437, 1996.

25. Critchley M: Medical aspects of boxing, particularly from a neurological standpoint. *Br Med J* 1:357–362, 1957.

26. Crosby AC: The hands of karate experts: Clinical and radiological findings. *Br J Sports Med* 19:41–42, 1985.

27. Danek E: Martial arts: The sound of one hand clapping. *Phys Sports Med* 7:3, 1979.

28. de Loes M, Goldi I: Incidence rate of injuries during sport activity and physical exercise in a rural Swedish municipality: Incidence rates in 17 sports. *Int J Sports Med* 9(6):416–467, 1988.

29. DeMeersman RE, Wilkerson JE: Judo nephropathy, trauma versus nontrauma. *J Trauma* 22(2):150–152, 1982.

30. Dvorine W: Kendo: A safer martial art. *Phys Sports Med* 7(12):87–89, 1979.

31. Estwanik JJ, Boitano M, Ari N: Amateur boxing injuries at the 1981 and 1982 USA/ABF National Championships. *Phys Sports Med* 12(10):123–128, 1984.

32. Fabian RL: Sports injury to the larynx and trachea. *Physician Sports Med* 17(2):111–118, 1989.

33. Fahrer M: Anatomy of the karate chop. *Bull Hosp Joint Dis Orthop Inst* 44(2):189–198, 1984.

34. Feehan M, Waller AE: Precompetition injury and subsequent tournament performance in full-contact tae kwon do. *Br J Sports Med* 29(4):258–262, 1995.

35. Feld MS, McNair RE, Wilk SR: The physics of karate. *Sci Am* 240:150–158, 1979.

36. Gardner RC: Hypertrophic infiltrative tendinitis (HIT syndrome) of the long extensor: The abused karate hand. *JAMA* 211:1009–1010, 1970.

37. Goodman G, Satterfield MJ, Yasumura K: Combining traditional physical therapy and karate in the treatment of a patient with quadriplegia. *Int J Rehabil Res* 3(2):236–239, 1980.

38. Gordon SK, Scalise A, Felton RM, et al: Ueichi-Ryu karate in spinal cord injury rehabilitation: The Sepulveda experience. *Am Correct Ther J* 34:166–168, 1980.

39. Greene L, Kravitz L, Wongsgathikun J, Kemmerly T: Metabolic effect of punching tempo. *Med Sci Sports Exerc* 31(suppl 5):157, 1999.

40. Hirano K, Seto M: Dangers of karate. *JAMA* 226:1118–1119, 1973.

41. Hobusch FL, McClellan T: The karate roundhouse kick. *NSCA J* 12(6):6–89, 1990.

42. Imamura H, Yoshimura Y, Nishimura S, et al: Oxygen uptake, heart rate, and blood lactate responses during and following karate training. *Med Sci Sports Exerc* 31:342–347, 1999.

43. Jackson F, Earle KM, Beamer Y, Clark R: Blunt head injuries incurred by Marine recruits in hand-to-hand combat (judo training). *Milit Med* 132:803–808, 1967.

44. Jaffe L, Minkoff J: Martial arts: A perspective on their evolution, injuries and training formats. *Orthop Rev* 17(2):208–221, 1988.

45. Johannsen HV, Noerregaard FOH: Karate injuries in relation to the qualifications of participants and competition success. *Ugeskr Laeger* 148:1786–1790, 1986.

46. Johannsen HV, Noerregaard FOH: Prevention of injuries in karate. *Br J Sports Med* 22(3): 113–115, 1988.

47. Kelley DW, Pitt MJ, Mayer DM: Index metacarpal fractures in karate. *Phys Sports Med* 8(3):103–106, 1980.

48. Kersteins AE, Dietz F, Hwang S-M: Evaluating the safety and potential use of a weight-bearing exercise, tai chi chuan, for rheumatoid arthritis patients. *Am J Phys Med Rehabil* 70(3):136–140, 1991.

49. Klein KK: The martial arts and the Caucasian knee: "A tiger by the tail." *J Sports Med* 3(1): 44–47, 1975.

50. Klein KK: Why Caucasian martial artists have greater knee problems. *J Am Correct Ther Assoc* 7(1):51–56, 1976.

51. Koiwai EK: Fatalities associated with judo. *Phys Sports Med* 9(4):61–66, 1981.

52. Koiwai EK: Deaths allegedly caused by the use of "choke holds" (shime-waza). *J Forens Sci* 32:419–432, 1987.

53. Kujala UM, Taimela S, Antti-Poika I, et al: Acute injuries in soccer, ice hockey, volleyball, basketball, judo, and karate: Analysis of national registry data. *Br Med J* 311: 1465–1468, 1995.

54. Kurland H: Injuries in karate. *Phys Sports Med* 8(10):80–85, 1980.

55. Kurosawa H, Nakasita K, Nakasita H, et al: Complete avulsion of the hamstring tendons from the ischial tuberosity: A report of two cases sustained in judo. *Br J Sports Med* 30: 72–74, 1996.

56. Lai J-S, Lan C, Wong M-K, Teng S-H: Two-year trends in cardiorespiratory function among older tai chi chuan practitioners and sedentary subjects. *J Am Geriatr Soc* 43:1222-1227, 1995.

57. Lan C, Lai J-S, Chen S-Y, et al: 12-month tai chi training in the elderly: Its effect on health fitness. *Med Sci Sports Exerc* 30(3):345–351, 1998.

58. Lan C, Lai J-S, Wong MK, Yu ML: Cardiorespiratory function, flexibility, and body composition among geriatric tai chi chuan practitioners. *Arch Phys Med Rehab* 77:612–616, 1996.

59. Lannuzel A, Moulin T, Amsallem D, et al: Vertebral-artery dissection following a judo session: A case report. *Neuropediatrics* 25: 106–108, 1994.

60. Larose JH, Kim DS: Knuckle fracture-a mechanism injury. *JAMA* 206(4):893–894, 1968.

61. Larose JH, Kim DS: Karate hand-conditioning. *Med Sci Sports* 1(2):95–98, 1969.

62. Levandoski LJ, Leyshon GA: Tai chi exercise and the elderly. *Clin Kinesiol* 44(2):39–44, 1990.

63. Liebert PL, Buckley T: Providing medical coverage at karate tournaments. *J Musculoskel Med* 1992.

64. Lindsay KW, McLatchie GR, Jennett B: Serious head injury in sport. *Br Med J* 281(6243): 789–791, 1980.

65. Liu SH, Henry M, Bowen R: Complications of type 1 coronoid fractures in competitive athletes: Report of two cases and review of the literature. *J Shoulder Elbow Surg* 5(3): 223–227, 1996.

66. Maffuli N, So WS, Ahuja A, et al: Iliopsoas hematoma in an adolescent tae kwon do player. *Knee Surg Sports Traumatol Arthrosc* 3: 230–233, 1996.

67. Maliszewski M: Injuries and effects of martial arts. *J Asian Martial Arts* 1(2):16–23, 1992.

68. Maliszewski M: Meditative-religious traditions of fighting arts and martial ways. *J Asian Martial Arts* 1(2):1–15, 1992.

69. Martland HS: Punch-drunk. *JAMA* 91(15): 1103–1107, 1928.

70. Mars JS, Pimendes D: Blinding choroidal rupture in a karateka. *Br J Sports Med* 29(4): 273–274, 1995.

71. McLatchie GR: Analysis of karate injuries in 295 contests. *Injury* 8:132–134, 1976.

72. McLatchie GR, Morris EW: Prevention of karate injuries: A progress report. *Br J Sports Med* 11:78–82, 1977.

73. McLatchie GR: Recommendations for medical officers attending karate competitions. *Br J Sports Med* 13:36–37, 1979.

74. McLatchie GR: Surgical and orthopaedic problems in sport karate: A case for medical control. *Medisport* 1(1):41–44, 1979.

75. McLatchie GR, Davies JE, Caulley JH: Injuries in karate: A case for medical control. *J Trauma* 20(11):956–958, 1980.

76. McLatchie GR: Karate and karate injuries. *Br J Sports Med* 15(1):84–86, 1981.

77. Nakata M, Shirahata N: Statistical observation on injuries resulting from judo. *Jpn J Orthop Assoc* 18:1146–1154, 1943.

78. Naylor AR, Walsh ME: Aikido foot: A traction injury to the common peroneal nerve. *Br J Sports Med* 21(4):182, 1987.

79. Nielsen TH, Jensen LS: Pancreatic transection during karate training. *Br J Sports Med* 20(2): 82–83, 1986.

80. Nieman EA, Swan PG: Karate injuries. *Br Med J* 1(742):233, 1971.

81. Oler M, Tomson W, Pepe H, et al: Morbidity and mortality in the martial arts: A warning. *J Trauma* 21(2):251–253, 1991.

82. Owens RG, Ghadiali EJ: Judo as a possible cause of anoxic brain damage: A case report. *J Sports Med Phys Fitness* 31:627–628, 1991.

83. Pandavela J, Gordon S, Gordon G, et al: Martial arts for the quadriplegic. *Am J Phys Med* 65(1):17–29, 1986.

84. Paup DC, Finley PL: A comparison of male and female injury incidence in martial arts training. *Med Sci Sports Exerc* 26(5):S14, 1994.

85. Perez HR, O'Driscoll E, Steele J, et al: Physiological responses to two forms of boxing aerobics exercise. *Med Sci Sports Exerc* 31(suppl 5):157, 1999.

86. Pieter W, Lufting R: Injuries at the 1991 tae kwon do World Championships. *J Sports Traumatol Rel Res* 16:49, 1994.

87. Pieter W, Van Ryssegem G, Lufting R, Heijmans J: Injury situation and injury mechanism at the 1993 European tae kwon do Cup. *J Hum Mov Stud* 28:1, 1995.

88. Pieter W, Pieter F: Speed and force of selected tae kwon do techniques. *Biol Sport* 12(4): 257–266, 1995.

89. Pieter W, Zemper ED: Injury rates in children participating in tae kwon do competition. *J Trauma* 43(1):89–96, 1997.

90. Pieter W, Zemper ED: Incidence of reported cerebral concussion in adult tae kwon do athletes. *J R Soc Health* 118(5):272–279, 1998.

91. Plancher KD, Minnich JM: Sport-specific injuries. *Clin Sports Med* 15(2):207–218, 1996.

92. Reay DT, Eisle JW: Death from law enforcement neck holds. *Am J Forens Med Pathol* 3(3):253–258, 1982.

93. Rodriguez G, Francione S, Barth JT, et al: Judo and choking, EEG and regional cerebral blood flow findings. *J Sports Med Phys Fitness* 31:605–610, 1991.

94. Russel SM, Lewis A: Karate myoglobinuria. *N Engl J Med* 293(18):941, 1975.

95. Russo MT, Maffulli N: Dorsal dislocation of the distal end of the ulna in a judo player. *Acta Orthop Belg* 57(4):442–446, 1991.

96. Ryan AJ: T'ai chi chuan for mind and body. *Phys Sports Med* 2:58–61, 1974.

97. Saal JS: Flexibility training. *Phys Med Rehabil State of the Art Revs* 1:537–554, 1987.

98. Sanders MS, Antonio J: Strength and conditioning for submission fighting. *Strength Cond J* 21(5):42–45, 1999.

99. Schmid L, Hajik E, Votipka F, et al: Experience with headgear in boxing. *J Sports Med Phys Fitness* 8:171–176, 1968.

100. Schmidt RJ, Royer FM: Telemetered heart rates recorded during karate katas: A case study. *Res Q Exerc Sport* 44(4):501–505, 1973.

101. Schmidt RJ: Fatal anterior chest trauma in karate trainers. *Med Sci Sports* 7(1):59–61, 1975.

102. Schneider D, Leung R: Metabolic and cardiorespiratory responses to the performance of wing chun and t'ai chi chuan exercise. *Int J Sports Med* 12:319–323, 1991.

103. Schwartz ML, Hudson AR, Fernie GR, et al: Biomechanical study of full contact karate contrasted with boxing. *J Neurosurg* 64: 248–252, 1986.

104. Serina ER, Lieu DK: Thoracic injury potential of basic competition tae kwon do kicks. *J Biomech* 24(10):951–960, 1991.

105. Shapiro DH: Another cause of tennis elbow. *New Engl J Med* 323(20):1428, 1990.

106. Shaw DW, Deutsch DT: Heart rate and oxygen uptake response to performance of karate kata. *J Sports Med Phys Fitness* 22:461–468, 1982.

107. Shirley ME: The tae kwon do side kick: A kinesiological analysis with strength and conditioning principles. *NSCA J* 14(5):7–78, 1992.

108. Siana JE, Borum P, Kryger H: Injuries in tae kwon do. *Br J Sports Med* 20(4):165–166, 1986.

109. Smith PK: Transmission of force through the karate, boxing, and the thumbless boxing glove as a function of velocity, in Terauds J, Gwolitzke BE, and Holt LE (eds): *Biomechanics in Sports,* Vols III and IV. Del Mar, CA: Academic Press, 1987.

110. Smith PK, Hamill J: Karate and boxing glove impact characteristics as functions of velocity and repeated impact, in Terauds J, Barham JN (eds): *Biomechanics in Sports,* Vol II. Del Mar, CA: Academic Press, 1985.

111. Smith PK, Hamill J: The effect of punching glove type and skill level on momentum transfer. *J Hum Mov Stud* 12:153–161, 1986.

112. Srensen H: Dynamics of the martial arts high front kick. *J Sports Sci* 14(6):483–495, 1996.

113. Streeton JA, Melb MB: Traumatic hemoglobinuria caused by karate exercise. *Lancet* 2: 191–192, 1967.

114. Stricevic MV, Okazaki T, Tanner A, et al: Cardiovascular responses to the karate kata. *Phys Sports Med* 8(3):57–67, 1980.

115. Stricevic MV, Patel MR, Okazaki T, Swim BK: Karate: Historical perspective and injuries sustained in national and international tournament competitions. *Am J Sports Med* 11(5): 320–342, 1983.

116. Sun XS, Wang YG, Xia YJ: Determination of E-rosette-forming lymphocyte in aged subjects with tai ji quan exercise. *Int J Sports Med* 10:217–219, 1989.

117. Tenvergert EM, Ten Duis HJ, Klasen HJ: Trends in sports injuries, 1982–1988: An in-depth study on four types of sport. *J Sports Med Phys Fitness* 32(2):214–220, 1992.

118. Tse S-K, Bailey DM: T'ai chi and postural control in the well elderly. *Am J Occup Ther* 46: 295–300, 1992.

119. Tuominen R: Injuries in national karate competitions in Finland. *Scand J Med Sci Sports* 5:44–48, 1995.

120. Van Mechelen W, Hlobil H, Kemper HCG: Incidence, severity, etiology, and prevention of sport injuries. *Sports Med* 14(2):82–99, 1992.

121. Vayssairat M, Priollet P, Capron L, et al: Does karate injure blood vessels of the hand? *Lancet* 2(8401):529, 1984.

122. Vos JA, Binkhorst RA: Velocity and force of some karate arm-movements. *Nature* 211: 89–90, 1966.

123. Walker J: Karate strikes. *Am J Phys* 43: 845–849, 1975.

124. Whiting WC, Grogor RJ, Finerman GA: Kinematic analysis of human upper extremity movements in boxing. *Am J Sports Med* 16(2): 130–136, 1988.

125. Williams G: Karate creates patients one kick at a time. *Podiatry Today.com: http://www. podiatrytoday.com/march1.html/1999;* accessed June 25, 1999.

126. Wilkerson LA: Martial arts, in Mellion MB (ed): *Sports Medicine Secrets.* Philadelphia: Hanley & Belfus, 1994, pp 422–430.

127. Wilkerson LA: Martial arts injuries. *J Am Osteopath Assoc* 97(4):221–226, 1997.

128. Wirtz PD, Vito GR, Long DH: Calcaneal apophysitis (Sever's disease) associated with tae kwon do injuries. *J Am Podiatr Med Assoc* 78(9):474–475, 1988.

129. Wolf SL, Barnhart HX, Kutner NG, et al: Reducing frailty and falls in older persons: An investigation of tai chi and computerized balance training. *J Am Geriatr Soc* 44(5):489–499, 1996.

130. Wolf SL, Barnhart HX, Ellison GL, et al: The effect of tai chi quan and computerized balance training on postural stability in older subjects. *Phys Ther* 77:371–381, 1997.

131. Wolf SL, Coogler C, Tingsen X: Exploring the basis for tai chi chuan as a therapeutic exercise approach. *Arch Phys Med Rehabil* 8: 886–892, 1997.

132. Wolfson L, Whipple R, Derby C, et al: Balance and strength training in older adults: Intervention gains and tai chi maintenance. *J Am Geriatr Soc* 44(5):498–509, 1996.

133. Xusheng S, Yugi X, Yunijan X: Determination of E-rosette-forming lymphocytes in aged subjects with tai chi quan exercise. *J Sports Med* 10(3):217–219, 1989.

134. Young DR, Appel LJ, Jee S, et al: The effects of aerobic exercise and t'ai chi on blood pressure in older people: Results of a randomized trial. *J Am Geriatr Soc* 47(3):277–286, 1999.

135. Zehr EP, Sale DG: Ballistic elbow extension movements in moderately trained karate practitioners: peak torque, velocity, acceleration, and the agonist pre-movement silence. *Med Sci Sports Exerc* 25(4):S131, 1993.

136. Zehr EP, Sale DG, Dowling JJ: Agonist pre-movement depressions not a naturally acquired

learned motor response in karate-trained subjects. *Med Sci Sports Exerc* 26(5): S101, 1994.

137. Zehr EP, Sale DG, Dowling JJ: Ballistic movement performance in karate athletes. *Med Sci Sports Exerc* 29(10):1366–1373, 1997.

138. Zemper ED, Pieter W: Injury rates during the 1988 US Olympic team trials for tae kwon do. *Br J Sports Med* 23(3):161–164, 1989.

139. Zigun JR, Schneider SM: "Effort" thrombosis (Paget-Schroetter's syndrome) secondary to martial arts training. *Am J Sports Med* 16(2): 189–190, 1988.

Additional Reading

Aging in Medical Science Research Group: *Behavior of Tai Chi and Non-Tai Chi Participants* (People's Sports and Exercise Publication). Canton: People's Republic of China, 1983.

Ahn BH: Kinematic and kinetic analysis of tae kwon do kicking motions. Unpublished master's thesis, Purdue University, 1985.

Almer S, Westerberg CE: Discussion of the panorama of injuries associated with karate blows: Potential risks need new attention. *Lakartidningen* 82:2886–2888, 1985.

Almer S, Westerberg CE: Cerebral infarction following a karate fight. *Presse Med* 14:29, 1985.

American Council on Exercise: ACE helps exercisers kick their way to fitness with cardio kickboxing. Available at *http://www.acefitness.org/newsreleases/1999;* accessed May 20, 1999.

American Council on Exercise: ACE helps exercisers kick their way to fitness with cardio kickboxing. Available at *http://www.acefitness.org/newsreleases/1999;* accessed June 25, 1999.

American Council on Exercise: Cardio kickboxing packs a punch; ACE study confirms benefits of popular workout. *ACE Fitness Matters,* July–August:4–5, 1999.

Aotsuka A, Kojima S, Furumoto H, et al: Punch drunk syndrome due to repeated karate kicks and punches. *Rinsho Shinkeigaku* 30: 1243–1246, 1990.

Bentley A: Self-defense from a wheelchair. *Midnight* 23(40):7–10, 1977.

Birrer RB: Karate kids. *Sports Care Fit* 2(1):14–19, 1989.

Bjerrum L: Scapula lata induced by karate. *Ugeskr Laeger* 146:2022, 1984.

Blonstein JL: Medical aspects of amateur boxing. *Proc R Soc Med* 59:649, 1966.

Brettel VFH: Injuries by karate blows. *Gerichtlichen Med* 39:87–90, 1981.

Casson IR, Sham R, Campbell EA, et al: Neurological and CT evaluation of knocked-out boxers. *J Neurol Neurosurg Psychiatry* 45:170–174, 1982.

Corsellis JA, Brunton CJ, Freeman-Browne D: The aftermath of boxing. *Psychol Med* 3:270–303, 1973.

Council on Scientific Affairs: Brain injury in boxing. *JAMA* 249:254–257, 1983.

Courville CB: The mechanism of boxing fatalities. Report of an usual case with severe brain lesions incident to impact of boxer's head against the ropes. *Bull Los Angeles Neurol Soc* 29:59–69, 1964.

Creighton BW: Forum: Carotid restraint: Useful tool or deadly weapon? Trial. *The National Legal Newsmagazine* 19(5):102–106, 1983.

Dawson A: Personal best: A kick for mental health. *Womens Sports Fitness* 8:41–42, 1986.

Demos MA, Gitin EL, Kagen LJ: Exercise myoglobinemia and acute exertional rhabdomyolysis. *Arch Intern Med* 134:669–673, 1974.

Duke K: FitVids: FIT rates the latest exercise tapes: Advanced tae bo with Bill Blank. *Fit* January–February:86, 1999.

Fisher S: Golden gloves: Rules for injury prevention. *Phys Sports Med* 7:135–136, 1979.

Francescato MP, Talon T, diPramero PE: Energy cost and energy sources in karate. *Eur J Appl Physiol* 71:355–361, 1995.

Frey A, Muller W: Heberden-Arthrsen bei Judo-Sportlern. *Schweiz Med Wochenschr* 114: 40–47, 1984.

Funakoshi G: *Karate Do Kyohan: The Master Text.* Kodansha International, 1973.

Gong L, Jianan Q, Jisheng Z, Yang Q, Tao Q, et al: Changes in heart rate and electrocardiogram during tai ji quan exercise. *Chinese Med J* 94: 589–592, 1981.

Halbrook SP: Martial arts weapons injuries: They aren't what Congress cracks them up to be. *Black Belt* 6:3–11, 1986.

Hirata K: Injuries of karate in all Japan. *Jpn J Educ Med* 3:1213–124, 1967.

Hunter: Karate: Kardio kickboxing. Available at *http://www.hunterkarate.com/1999;* accessed April 8, 1999.

Hwang IS: Analysis of the kicking leg in tae kwon do, in Terauds J, Gowitzke B, Holt L (eds): *Biomechanics in Sports,* Vols III and IV. Del Mar, CA: Academic Press, 1987, pp 39–47.

Hwang IS: Biomechanical analysis of dwihuryo-chagi in tae kwon do, in *A Collection of Research Papers in the 1st World tae kwon do Seminar.* Seoul: Kukkiwon, 1985, pp 67–79.

Ikai M, Ishiko T, Ueda G: Physiological studies in choking in judo. *Bull Assoc Sci Stud Judo* 1: 1–12, 1958.

Ikai M, Ishiko T, Ueda G: Physiological studies in choking in judo: II. X-ray observations on the heart. *Bull Assoc Sci Stud Judo* 1:13–22, 1958.

Ishida Y, Kato Y: Observation of karatedo, in Larson L, Hermann D (eds): *Encyclopedia of Sport Sciences and Medicine.* New York: American College of Sports Medicine, 1971.

Jin PT: Changes in heart rate, noradrenaline, cortisol and mood during tai chi. *J Psychosomat Res* 33:192–206, 1989.

Jin PT: Efficacy of tai chi, brisk walking, meditation, and reading in reducing mental and emotional stress. *J Psychosom Res* 36:361–370, 1992.

Joch W, Krause I, Fritsche P: Punching power and motor speed in boxing. *Leistungssport* 12: 40–46, 1982.

Joon SN: An analysis of the dynamics of the basic tae kwon do kicks. *US tae kwon do J* 4:10–15, 1987.

Johnson J, Skorecki J, Wells RP: Peak acceleration of the head in boxing. *Med Biol Engrg* 13: 396–404, 1975.

Jorga I, Sarovic D, Jorga V, et al: Specific bone deformity of the fist of karate athletes caused by nonfunctional regular third-time practice. Presented at the Third Balkan Congress of Sports Medicine, Nis, Yugoslavia, October 1976.

Kaste M, Vikki J, Sainio K, et al: Is chronic brain damage in boxing a hazard of the past? *Lancet* 2:1186–1188, 1982.

Koh TC: Tai chi chuan. *Am J Chin Med* 9:15–22, 1981.

Koh TC: Tai chi and ankylosing spondylitis: A personal experience. *Am J Chin Med* 10:59–61, 1982.

Koiwai EK: Major accidents and injuries in judo. *Ariz Med* 22:957–962, 1965.

Kurland HL: Minimizing the accident complex. *Black Belt Magazine,* February–March, 1979.

Kurland HL: A short study of tournament injuries. *Karate Illus* 3:32–36, 1981.

Lai JS, Wong MK, Lan W, et al: Cardiorespiratory responses of tai chi chuan practitioners and sedentary subjects during cycle ergometry. *J Formos Med Assoc* 92:894–899, 1993.

Lampert PW, Hardman JM: Morphological changes in brains of boxers. *JAMA* 251: 2676–2679, 1984.

Lissner HR, Gurdjian ES: A study of the mechanical behavior of the skull and its contents when subjected to injury blows. *Proc Soc Exp Stress Analysis* 3:40, 1946.

Lucas J: Tae kwon do, pelote basque/jai-alai, and roller hockey-three unusual Olympic demonstration sports. *J Phys Educ Recreation Dance* April:80–82, 1992.

McGown IA: Boxing safety and injuries. *Phys Sports Med* 7:75–82, 1979.

Mawdsley C, Ferguson F: Neurological disease in boxers. *Lancet* 2:799–801, 1963.

Moore M: The challenge of boxing-bringing safety into the ring. *Phys Sports Med* 8:101–105, 1980.

Moore M: Apall over boxing. *Phys Sports Med* 11(1):21, 1983.

Nakayama N: *Dynamic Karate.* Palo Alto, CA: Kodansha International, 1966.

Nakayama N: *Official Manual of the Japan Karate Association.* Palo Alto, CA: Kodansha International, 1974.

Ng RKT: Cardiopulmonary exercise: A recently discovered secret of tai chi. *Hawaii Med J* 51: 216–217, 1992.

Nishiyama H, Brown RC: *Karate: The Art of Empty-Hand Fighting.* Rutland, VT: Charles E. Tuttle, 1965.

Nistico VP: *A Kinematic Investigation of Two Performance Conditions of the Karate Counterpunch Technique.* Eugene, OR: Microform Publications, 1982.

Noerragaard FO, Johannsen HV: Pattern of injuries in the Danish karate championships. *Ugeskr Laeger* 148:1785–1786, 1986.

Norton ML, Safrin M, Cutler P: Medical aspects of judo. *NY State J Med* 67:1750–1752, 1967.

Nyst M, Laundly P: Injuries incurred in the practice of karate. *Sport Health* 5:7–10, 1987.

O'Driscoll E, Steele J, Perez HR, et al: The metabolic cost of two trials of boxing exercise utilizing a heavy bag. *Med Sci Sports Exerc* 31(suppl 5):158, 1999.

Ogawa S, et al: Physiological studies on choking in judo-studies on choking with reference to the hypophysio-adreno-cortical system. *Bull Assoc Sci Stud Judo* 2:107–114, 1963.

Parker Academy of Martial Arts: Cardio karate for fun and fitness. Available at *http://www.kick-srus.com/1999;* accessed April 8, 1999.

Pieter W: Martial arts, in Caine D, Caine C, Lindner K (eds): *Epidemiology of Sport Injuries.* Champaign, IL: Human Kinetics, 1996.

Qu M: Tai ji quan: A medical assessment. *Chin Sports* 1:26–27, 1980.

Ratamess N: Weight training for ju jitsu. *Strength Cond J* 20(5):8–15, 1998.

Reay DT, Mathers RL: Physiological effects from use of neck holds. *FBI Law Enforc Bull* 52(7):12–15, 1983.

Reeder S: And in this corner: Boxercise. *Womens Sports Fitness,* August:52, 1986.

Roback MD: The injury debate. *Black Belt Magazine,* January 1979, pp 38–40.

Roberts AH: *Brain Damage in Boxers.* London: Pitman, 1969.

Ross RJ, Cole M, Thompson JS, et al: Boxers: Computed tomography, EEG, and neurological evaluation. *JAMA* 249:211–213, 1983.

Ryan AJ: Eliminate boxing gloves. *Phys Sports Med* 11:49, 1983.

Schanche DA: Common sense rules you'd better follow if you're into karate. *Today's Health,* July 1974, pp 28–33.

Serres P, Calas J, Guilbert F: Karate et fracture du malaire. *Rev Stomatol Chir Maxillofac* 74:177–178, 1973.

Shaik F: Physician challenges safety of youth boxing. *Phys Sports Med* 9:27, 1981.

Smith PK: Punching impact effect of the karate, boxing, and the thumbless boxing glove, in Terauds J, Gwolitzke BE, Holt LE (eds): *Biomechanics in Sports,* Vols III and IV. Del Mar, CA: Academic Press, 1987.

Spillane J: Five boxers. *Br Med J* 2:1205–1210, 1962.

Stull RA, Barham JN: An analysis of movement patterns utilized by different styles in the karate reverse punch in front stance, in Kreighbaum E, McNeil A (eds): *Biomechanics of Sports,* Vol VI: *Proceedings of the 6th International Symposium on Biomechanics.* International Society of Biomechanics in Sports and Department of Health and Human Development, Montana State University, Bozeman, 1990, pp 225–243.

Sung NJ, Lee SG, Park HJ, Joo SK: An analysis of the dynamics of the basic tae kwon do kicks. *US tae kwon do J* 6:10–15, 1987.

Suzuki K: Medical studies on choking in judo with special reference to electroencephalographic investigation. *Bull Assoc Sci Stud Judo* 1:23–48, 1958.

Tezuka M: Physiological studies on the ochi (unconsciousness) resulting from shime-waza (strangle hold) in judo. *Bull Assoc Sci Stud Judo* 5:71–73, 1978.

Thomaassen A, Juul-Jensen P, Olivarious B, et al: Neurological, electroencephalographic and neuropsychological examination of 53 former amateur boxers. *Acta Neurol Scand* 60:352–362, 1979.

Unterharnscheidt FJ: About boxing: A review of historical and medical aspects. *Texas Rep Biol Med* 28:421–495, 1970.

Van Gheluwe A, Van Schandevjil H: A kinematic study of the trunk rotation during gyaku-zuki using tilted-plane cinematography, in Matsui H, Kobayashi K (eds): *Biomechanics,* Vol VIII-B. Champaign, IL: Human Kinetics, 1999, pp 876–881.

Webb R: Unique new program teaches self defense for wheelers. *Paraplegia News,* January 1976.

Wohlin S: A biomechanical description of the tae kwon do turning hook kick. Unpublished master's thesis, Montana State University, 1989.

Wongsgathikun J, Kravitz L, Greene L: Metabolic response of trained and untrained boxers. *Med Sci Sports Exerc* 31(Suppl 5):158, 1999.

Wos W, Puzio J, Opala G: Traumatic internal carotid artery thrombosis following karate blow. *Pol Przegl Chir* 49(12):1271–1273, 1977.

Xu SW, Fan ZH: Physiological studies of tai ji quan in China. *Med Sports Sci* 28:70–80, 1988.

Yang JW: *Shaolin Chin Na-The Seizing Art of Kung Fu.* Hollywood, CA: Unique Publications, 1980, pp 115–117.

Zemper ED: Incidence of reported cerebral concussion in adult tae kwon do athletes. *J R Soc Health* 118(5):272–279, 1998.

Zhuo D, Shepard FJ, Plyley MJ, Davis GM: Cardiorespiratory and metabolic responses during tai chi chuan exercises. *Can J Appl Sport Sci* 9:7–10, 1984.

CHAPTER 16

Cycling

Susan Lefever-Button

Cycling is a many-faceted, popular activity. It is thought that there are as many as 100 million bicyclists in the United States currently, with adults making up one-third of this number. Membership in the U.S. Cycling Federation (USCF) has been stable at 35,000 for the last several years. A steady increase has been seen in the membership in the National Off-Road Bicycle Association (NORBA).[1] Cycling can be performed on a variety of terrains with different types of bicycles for different purposes. The goal of getting from one place to another requires some amount of energy expenditure. On land, cycling is an efficient means to accomplish this.[2] In addition, the use of stationary cycling has been advocated by numerous physicians to rehabilitate patients following surgeries or injuries to their lower extremities.[3-5]

To fully understand the sport and treat recreational or competitive cyclists effectively, it is necessary to have a working knowledge of the cyclist, the bicycle, and the interaction of the two. By integrating knowledge of both the bicycle and the rider, opti-

mal care can be given to cyclists. This chapter is designed to help clinicians understand basic bicycle function, elements of proper fit, basic muscle function used when cycling, injury prevention, common cycling injuries and their etiologies and treatment, and return-to-sport guidelines.

Participation in cycling can be done as either a sport or an exercise modality in the rehabilitation process. Cycling as a sport encompasses different types of riding as well as different types of bicycles. Four different types of bicycles can be identified: sport/touring, racing, mountain, and hybrid. The differences between these bicycles and their common uses will be explored. The geometry of the frame of the bicycle, i.e., the angle the seat tube makes with the ground, dictates how the bicycle will handle (Fig. 16.1). The typical range for most bicycles is from 70 to 74 degrees. The more shallow the seat tube angle, the less responsive the bicycle is to turning. Deciding what type of riding the cyclist is going to do with the bicycle will aid in selection of the proper type of bicycle.[6]

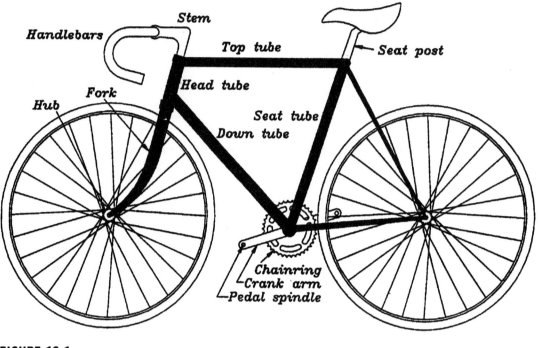

FIGURE 16.1

Anatomy of the bicycle.

Sport/Touring Bicycles

The sport/touring bicycle has a moderately steep angle. It is the best choice for riders who want a moderately comfortable but responsive bicycle. Fitness riding, touring 20 mi or longer, commuting, and organized club rides are activities best suited for sport/touring bicycles.[6]

Racing Bicycles

Racing bicycles are lightweight and very responsive. Cyclists involved in group riding, racing, fitness riding, and competing in triathlons probably would enjoy the quick handling of a racing bicycle. Racing bicycles differ from sport/touring bicycles in the geometry of the frame (steeper frame angle), narrower tires, and a stiffer ride.[6]

Mountain Bicycles

Mountain bicycles are characteristically easier to ride. The upright riding position, shallower frame angle, wide tires, and easy access to the brake and shift levers afford the rider more control. Riding off-road is the best venue for a mountain bicycle, although short road trips of less than 10 mi can be ridden comfortably on a mountain bicycle.[6]

Hybrid Bicycles

A hybrid bicycle takes the control and comfort of a mountain bicycle and adds the lighter frame design and speed of a sport bicycle. These bicycles have semiwide tires and either drop or flat handlebars and can be ridden either on- or off-road.[6] Many commuters find that this type of bicycle fits their needs in the urban setting.

By understanding and using the elements of forces, cadence, and symmetry and by establishing and maintaining proper position while riding, both competitive and recreational cyclists can improve their performance and reduce their chances of injury.

Biomechanics of Cycling

FORCES

Accelerating the bicycle and rider forward requires that the amount of force applied to the pedals by the cyclist exceeds the external physical forces of wind resistance, rolling resistance, gravity, and weight imparted to both the cyclist and the bicycle.[2] Modifying either side of this equation, i.e., either applying a more effective force to the bicycle or reducing the resistance, can improve the cyclist's performance. This section will discuss the effect these forces have on efficient cycling.

The first group of forces includes those imposed on the bicycle by the rider. As the cyclist pushes on the pedal, a force is transferred from the crank to the chain ring to the gears and finally to the back tire, resulting in movement of the bicycle.[2] The applied pedal force from the cyclist has two components: a perpendicular component and a parallel component[7] (Fig. 16.2). The perpendicular

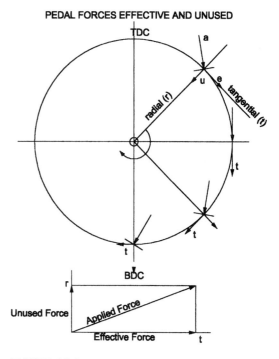

PEDAL FORCES EFFECTIVE AND UNUSED

FIGURE 16.2

Pedal forces and unused forces.

component of the applied force is perpendicular to the crank arm of the bicycle and is considered the effective force. The effective force is the only force that propels the bicycle. This can be seen in Fig. 16.2. As force is applied to the pedal (*a*), the perpendicular component (*t*) changes. It increases as the crank angle approaches 90 degrees. This occurs during the middle of the propulsive phase, as the knee is getting closer to 90 degrees. Correspondingly, peak activity of the quadriceps muscle is achieved (Fig. 16.3). During the last part of the propulsive phase, a higher tangential force can be applied perpendicular to the pedal if a technique called *ankling* is employed. Ankling involves plantarflexion of the ankle joint throughout a small circle to maintain a perpendicular force through the pedal. This is best illustrated at the bottom of the circle. In cycling terms, the bottom of the circle is called *bottom dead center* (BDC). A larger perpendicular force can be continued on the pedal by plantarflexing the ankle.[7]

Unused forces are all other forces that are not perpendicular to the crank arm. Included as unused forces are the parallel component of the applied force and any rotational or shearing forces applied by the foot to the pedal. Shearing forces are created when the foot is permitted to move or slide on top of

the pedal. Toe clips and cleated shoes improve efficiency by decreasing this sliding motion. Ultimately, a decrease in the shear force increases the driving force used to propel the bicycle. Using plantarflexion earlier in the cycle stroke applies a force that is more tangential to the circle. This also aids in improving the performance by limiting the unused forces[7] (see Fig. 16.2).

Improving cycling performance can be accomplished by either increasing the input or decreasing the resistance. In order to de-

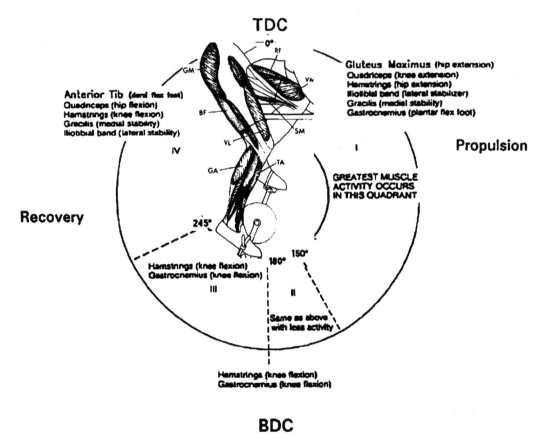

FIGURE 16.3

Muscular action during the cycle stroke.

crease the resistance, the cyclist must be aware of and understand how to overcome the physical forces acting on the bicycle. For example, wind resistance is an external force that must be overcome by the cyclist. At speeds above 40 km/h (25 mi/h), wind resistance is responsible for over 90 percent of the retarding force. The air drag of an object depends on the shape and roughness of its surface.[2] Cylindrical shapes have a high aerodynamic drag because of the air turbulence created in their wake. As the air separates from the object's trailing edge, a large low-pressure area is created. Streamlined objects, on the other hand, have a smooth flow of air over the trailing edge, resulting in decreased drag. About two-thirds of the aerodynamic drag during road racing is created by the wind resistance of the human body. The bicycle contributes to the other third of the aerodynamic drag. Methods used to decrease drag include altering the shape of the bicycle as well as the rider. Four methods can be employed to reduce wind resistance: learning to draft behind other riders, decreasing the frontal area of the cyclist, smoothing the rough surfaces, and streamlining the bicycle.[2]

The practice of *drafting* among racing cyclists is the oldest method for decreasing wind resistance, which in turn decreases energy consumption. Drafting involves following closely behind a fellow cyclist. Racing cyclists may draft as closely as 12 in. A wheel gap of approximately 5 ft. between cyclists can allow the drafting cyclist a 30 percent reduction in energy consumption secondary to the decrease in wind resistance. However, a decrease in wind resistance also decreases the effect that the wind has on cooling the drafting cyclist. The drafting cyclist should be reminded to drink more fluids when drafting to combat the thermal effect.[2]

The second method to reduce wind resistance involves *decreasing the frontal area of the rider.* The crouched racing position as well as elbow-rest handlebars are attempts to

do this. By forming a more streamlined shape, there is less area to resist the wind. The crouched racing position has been estimated to reduce the aerodynamic drag by 20 percent over the upright position.[2]

The third method to reduce wind resistance is to *minimize the rough surfaces.* As air flows in a parallel direction over rough surfaces, the resulting shear forces create a friction drag. By hiding exposed cables, wearing a rounded helmet and tight-fitting clothes and using aerodynamically shaped parts, air resistance can be further reduced.[2]

Another external force opposing power output is that of *rolling resistance.* This is the friction force created by the tires. As the tires move along the pavement, the tread and sidewalls deform, resulting in a loss of energy. Both the diameter of the tire and the amount of air pressure the tire carries affect this rolling resistance. Thinner tires and higher pressures lead to less resistance. This is secondary to a decrease in surface area. On the other hand, riding over rougher surfaces increases the amount of rolling resistance.[2,8]

An additional external force is *gravity.* The effect of gravity on the bicycle is most noticeable when a cyclist begins up an incline. There is a component of the cyclist's body mass that opposes the uphill motion. Increased weight increases inertia, thus requiring a greater amount of pedal force to move the bicycle forward. The final result is a slower rate of acceleration as the cyclist overcomes this increase in inertia.[8]

In summary, the physical retarding forces of wind resistance, tire rolling resistance, and gravitational forces must be overcome by the amount of force applied to the pedal by the cyclist. The more efficient the applied pedal forces, the higher is the power output. Likewise, the more streamlined the bicycle and the rider and the narrower the width of the tires, the smaller is the resistance to overcome. Limiting the resistance also increases power output. Additionally, power output can be increased by using optimal pedaling rate and symmetry.

CADENCE AND SYMMETRY

Pedal cadence is measured in revolutions per minute. Cadence × load = power output. Power output and pedaling rate generate the application of force. *Symmetry* refers to correspondence of the opposite sides of the body. There are two types of symmetry: force and work. *Force symmetry* applies to the amount of muscular effort applied by each leg. *Work symmetry* is the portion of the applied force that propels the bicycle forward. Ideally, there is both work and force symmetry between the two legs. In order to achieve this symmetry, smooth spinning should be practiced. Theoretically, sharing the load equally between the legs results in better performance.[7]

There are some conflicting reports in the literature concerning the optimal pedaling rate. Maximum metabolic efficiency requires a cadence of 60 to 80 rpm, whereas maximum power occurs between 120 and 130 rpm. Competitive cyclists competing in road races perform at 90 to 110 rpm. Track athletes may cycle at much faster speeds. On the other hand, the recreational cyclist spins at a slower, inefficient speed. Optimal pedaling rate depends on the power output.[7] There is a positive correlation between power output and pedaling rate. This would explain why well-trained competitive cyclists maintain higher optimal pedaling rates than recreational cyclists. The faster a cyclist spins above the optimal rate, the more he or she works against himself or herself during the recovery phase.[7] In order to achieve an optimal pedaling rate, proper position on the bicycle must be maintained.

PROPER POSITIONING OF THE CYCLIST ON THE BICYCLE

Proper positioning on the bicycle is essential both for optimal performance and injury prevention. The areas of the bicycle that can be adjusted to fit the cyclist include seat or saddle height, saddle fore/aft, saddle tilt, upper body position, handlebar position, crank arm length, and foot position. The following descriptions are approximate recommendations for an initial cyclist-bicycle fit. Some additional adjustments may be necessary once the cyclist is riding on a regular basis. When necessary, small adjustments of 0.25 in. should be made. Following any adjustment, the cyclist should ride numerous miles before readjusting.[6] A general rule of thumb in sizing a bicycle frame to a person involves measuring the distance from the top tube of the bicycle to the rider's pubic symphysis. When straddling the frame of a sport/touring or racing bicycle with the cycling shoes on, a 1- to 2-in. distance between the rider's pubic symphysis and the top tube should be present.[6]

Usually a mountain bicycle frame is sized a few inches shorter than a sport/touring bicycle. For a mountain bicycle, a 3- to 6-in. distance between the rider's pubic symphysis and the bicycle's top tube is recommended.[6] This shorter frame permits the rider to shift his or her center of mass more easily fore and aft to adapt for the different terrains. Most important, function should dictate selection of frame size. A bicycle that will be ridden on the road should have a slightly smaller pubic symphysis to top tube clearance than an off-road bicycle. Saddle height is the first and most important position to set.[6]

SADDLE HEIGHT

Numerous formulas have been developed to estimate optimal seat height based on power output and caloric uptake studies. These metabolic studies place the optimal seat height at 106 to 109 percent of the pubic symphysis height. Pubic symphysis height is measured standing on the ground bare-footed with a measurement taken from the pubic symphysis to the floor.[6]

Yet another formula uses the inseam-to-floor height. With the cycling shoes on, a measurement is taken from the pubic symphysis to the floor and multiplied by 1.09. A modification of this inseam formula, recommended by Greg Lamond, multiplies the inseam measurement by 0.883.[6] This lowers the first inseam formula by 0.5 to 2.5 cm but takes into consideration the height of the bottom bracket. Additionally, Lamond subtracts 3 mm from this total when using clipless pedals.[6]

Another formula recommends a knee flexion angle of 25 to 30 degrees at BDC. This allows for decompression of the knee joint, resulting in a decrease in anterior knee pain.[9]

A more practical method is to have the cyclist sitting on the bicycle supported on a wind trainer and pedaling comfortably wearing cycling shoes. Next, the cyclist places his or her heels on the bottom of the pedals and pedals backward. The knee should have a slight bend with the crank arm parallel to the seat tube, which usually occurs just after BDC (Fig. 16.4). This position of the crank arm places the knee in the longest position, preventing an overextension of the knee joint

while riding. (Remember, the cyclist will be riding with the ball of the foot on the pedal.) The cyclist should be able to pedal backward without the hips rocking from side to side and maintain a slight (10 degrees) bend in the knee at the limb's most lengthened position.[6,10]

On a mountain bicycle, the seat height is usually set slightly lower than on a road bicycle. This is to accommodate the higher bottom bracket and to keep the rider's center of mass lower, thus providing greater stability and maneuverability.[6]

SADDLE FORE/AFT

A couple of different methods can be used to align the forward and backward position of the seat. With the crank arms parallel to the floor, placing them in the three and nine o'-clock positions, the axis of rotation of the knee should be over the pedal spindle. A plumb line dropped from the lateral femoral condyle (knee joint axis) can be used to test

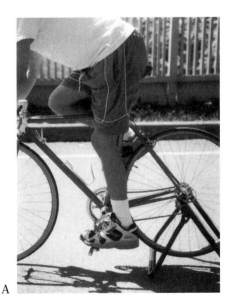

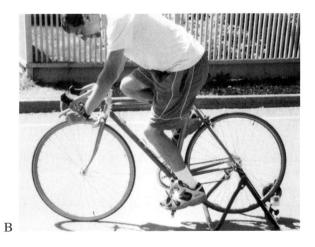

A B

FIGURE 16.4

A. Correct seat height. *B.* Incorrect seat height.

this position.[10] This fore/aft position places the knee in a safe position throughout the propulsive phase. As the highest effective pedal forces are applied through the lower limb, the knee remains perpendicular to the ground. By using the landmark of the patella, an additional method to measure seat fore/aft can be used. Keeping the crank arms in the same position, a straight edge is placed on the front of the patella, extended to the end of the crank arm, and aligned perpendicular to the floor. This keeps the patellofemoral joint from being placed in too much flexion during the propulsive phase.[6]

The seat fore/aft position for mountain bicycles differs slightly. More traction is required over the rear tire for climbing from a seated position. Consequently, the seat is set back slightly further. In this case, the front edge of the patella is about 1 cm behind the end of the crank arm when a straightedge is used. Some professional cyclists prefer to ride in a similar position so that they can remain seated and use a higher gear ratio while climbing.[6]

SADDLE TILT

The saddle should be level or tilted slightly higher in the front. A level may be placed along the length of the saddle to evaluate the amount of tilt. Saddle tilt can be used to maintain a specific position of the pelvis. If a flattened lumbar spine and a posterior pelvic tilt are desired, the saddle can be tilted higher in the front. In contrast, if an increased lumbar lordosis and an anterior position of the pelvis are desired, the front of the saddle may be tilted slightly downward. Some women prefer this slightly downward position to relieve pressure on the perineal area.[6]

UPPER BODY POSITION

Once the saddle adjustments are set, the length of the bicycle can be adjusted to fit the cyclist's "reach." From the "in the drops" position, the hands on the curved part of the handlebars, a plumb line dropped from the nose should bisect the handlebars in the center at the stem.[6] In this position, the back should be slightly lower than a 45-degree angle and should have no sharp bends. An overextended position places more stress on the lower back and hamstrings. A cramped position inhibits breathing.[10]

The position of the upper body is the most variable measurement of the bicycle fit positions. Lower back and hamstring flexibility will help determine the amount of trunk extension the cyclist can maintain.

The upper body position of the cyclist on a mountain bicycle is usually more upright. This is to accommodate the change in position necessary to traverse different terrains.[6]

When using aerodynamic handlebars, the cyclist must change his or her upper body position. Aerodynamic handlebars are used to reduce the amount of aerodynamic drag of the cyclist. By decreasing the frontal area of the rider, the air is directed around the cyclist. The cyclist begins by bringing the armrests closer together until he or she can ride comfortably with the forearms almost touching.[6] Next, a flattened back posture must be maintained. This is accomplished by rotating the pelvis forward in the saddle. Third, the chin must be dropped slightly to fill in the gap created between the forearms and the chest. Finally, the cyclist must not alter the movement of the knees. In order to miss hitting the elbows, there is a tendency to throw the knees outward. If this occurs, the handlebars should be raised until the knees can be held in while pedaling and the upper body maintains this aerodynamic posture.[6]

HANDLEBAR POSITION

The height of the handlebars should be at least 1 to 2 in. lower than the seat for a short cyclist and up to 4 in. lower than the seat for a tall cyclist. Handlebars that are too low may cause hand numbness and tingling.[6]

The width of the handlebars should match the width of the rider's shoulders. The distance between the acromion processes is the desired measurement. Handlebars that are too narrow may restrict breathing.[6]

The bottom of the handlebars on a road bicycle should be level or tilted slightly backward toward the middle of the rear wheel. On aerodynamic handlebars, most athletes keep the tilt between 15 and 30 degrees to enhance both comfort and performance.[6]

On a mountain bicycle, the height of the handlebars should be about 1 to 2 in. lower than the seat. A wide handlebar is used for slow speed control. Narrow handlebars are used for quicker maneuvering through wooded trails.[6]

CRANK ARM LENGTH

The crank arm length should be paired to the length of the leg. The standard crank length is 170 mm and is usually used by cyclists who are between 5 ft. 5 in. and 6 ft. tall. The length of the crank arm determines the size of the pedal circle. The *pedal circle* is the vertical distance the foot rises from the bottom to the top of the circle.[6]

Crank arm length affects both range of motion (ROM) of the lower leg and foot speed. For a given revolution per minute, a longer crank arm will result in an increase in ROM of the limb and an increase in foot speed. To maintain a comfortable range of hip and knee flexion at the top of the circle, a cyclist shorter than 5 ft. 5 in. should consider a shorter, more proportional crank arm.[6]

FOOT POSITION

The widest portion of the foot should be placed over the pedal spindle. When using cleated shoes, a natural or neutral angle of the foot should be used. Do not force the toes in or toes out. Instead, think of the foot as a rigid lever that needs only to flex and extend. Any sideways motion (pronation) will

rotate the knee, wasting energy and increasing stress on the knee.[6]

The primary goal of a properly fitted bicycle is that of comfort and consequently injury prevention. In order to accomplish this, proper adjustments in saddle height, saddle fore/aft, saddle tilt, upper body position, handlebar position, crank arm length, and foot position have been presented. Adjusting the bicycle to fit the person so that there is minimal rider adaptation is the aim of a properly fitted bicycle.

Now that the proper riding position has been established, the mechanics of the cycling stroke will be examined. This includes the phases of propulsion and recovery and the basic muscle and joint functions throughout these phases.

Biomechanics of the Cycling Stroke

The basic unit of bicycling is the *cycle stroke.* The cycle stroke is one revolution of the pedal from the top of the circle, or top dead center (TDC), to TDC of the same limb. It encompasses two phases: the propulsive phase and the recovery phase. The *propulsive phase* occurs just after TDC to just before BDC. Peak muscular activity occurs during this phase as the bicycle is driven forward. During the recovery phase, just after BDC to just before TDC, the muscles are preparing to work (see Fig. 16.3).

PROPULSIVE PHASE

Compilations of numerous studies approximate the ROM and muscle activity during seated steady-state cycling.[11–14] In general, the joints of the lower extremities begin the cycle stroke in a more flexed posture and extend throughout the range to end in a less flexed posture midway through the cycling stroke. In the forthcoming paragraphs a specific analysis of hip, knee, and ankle joint function throughout the cycling stroke will be given.

During the propulsive phase, the trunk is fixed in 20 to 35 degrees of flexion. The erector spinae and abdominal muscles are working to hold this posture. The hip joint is in 71 degrees of flexion at TDC and moves to 28 degrees of flexion just before BDC, for a total of 43 degrees of hip extension. The gluteus maximus and hamstrings account for approximately 27 percent of the total work in this phase[11–14] (see Fig. 16.3).

The knee joint has a total of 74 degrees of knee extension. At TDC, the knee is in 111 degrees of flexion and moves to 37 degrees of flexion before BDC. Maximal internal rotation of approximately 13 degrees occurs when the knee is flexed at 87 degrees. The amount of knee flexion depends on seat height. The higher the seat height is, the less is the knee flexion that takes place. Muscle activity includes the quadriceps, tensor fasciae latae (lateral stabilizers), and gracilis (medial stabilizer), which accomplish approximately 39 percent of the total work[11–14] (see Fig. 16.3).

Ankle joint motion depends on cycling style but usually involves 15 degrees of dorsiflexion to 20 degrees of plantarflexion. Peak dorsiflexion occurs at a 50- to 70-degree crank angle for a total of 35 degrees of motion. Muscular activity is seen in the anterior tibialis, gastrocnemius, soleus, and deep posterior calf muscles, which account for approximately 20 percent of the total work. Thirty-eight percent of this work has been attributed to the posterior tibialis, flexor digitorum longus, and flexor hallucis longus[11–14] (see Fig. 16.3). It is hypothesized that subtalar joint motion follows the movement of the lower limb. That is, as the knee extends and externally rotates and the ankle joint plantarflexes, subtalar joint supination occurs. This foot posture results in a rigid lever to apply force to the pedal.[14]

RECOVERY PHASE

The joints of the lower extremities begin the recovery phase in a more extended position and flex throughout the recovery phase to end at TDC in a more flexed posture. The biggest difference between the two phases is in muscle function. The primary focus of muscle function during the recovery phase is to unload the pedal. A specific analysis of hip, knee, and ankle joint function throughout the recovery phase follows.

The hip joint begins the recovery phase in 28 degrees of flexion before BDC and ends further flexed to 71 degrees at TDC for a total range of 43 degrees. The muscle action of the quadriceps produces 4 percent of the total work[11–14] (see Fig. 16.3).

The motion of the knee joint shows a total of 74 degrees of flexion. The knee joint begins the recovery phase at 37 degrees of flexion and further flexes to 111 degrees at TDC. Muscle action is that of the hamstrings and gastrocnemius as they work to decelerate knee joint extension and accelerate knee joint flexion. These muscles account for approximately 10 percent of the total work[11–14] (see Fig. 16.3).

During the recovery phase, the motion of the ankle joint begins in approximately 20 degrees of plantarflexion and reaches its peak of 15 degrees of dorsiflexion at 50 to 70 degrees of crank angle. The total amount of motion is 35 degrees at the ankle. The amount of ankle joint motion varies greatly and depends mostly on individual cycling style. The more a cyclist ankles, the greater is the amount of plantarflexion he or she demonstrates. The muscle activity is that of the gastrocnemius, soleus, deep posterior calf group, and tibialis anterior[11–14] (see Fig. 16.3).

Motion of the subtalar joint is hypothesized to follow knee joint motion and tibial rotation. As the knee joint flexes and internally rotates, the ankle joint dorsiflexes, and the subtalar joint pronates.[14]

Understanding the biomechanics of the cycle stroke as it relates to proper positioning, environmental forces, and muscle and joint function is important in developing an effective injury prevention program. This includes identifying the musculoskeletal demands and possible areas of muscle imbalance as well as recognizing biomechanical malalignments and correcting improper training programs performed by cyclists.

Injury Prevention

Injury prevention for cyclists should include an adequate warm-up, strengthening exercises, appropriate stretching, and balance and agility activities to efficiently control and propel the bicycle. Additionally, proper bicycle fit, appropriate training, and bicycle safety education to prevent impact injuries will be discussed.

WARM-UP

Cycling is predominately an aerobic activity. Therefore, an aerobic warm-up period of 5 to 10 min. at a low intensity should be performed before beginning cycling. Warming up the muscles prior to stretching can improve flexibility by increasing muscle temperature.[15] Brisk walking and riding a stationary cycle while spinning with low resistance are good aerobic warm-up activities for cycling. These warm-up activities can be performed prior to stretching. Once on the road, begin spinning with a low resistance, gradually increasing the workload while maintaining the same cadence.

STRETCHING EXERCISES

Stretching plays a major role in preventing overuse injuries. Stretching may be performed before, during, and after a ride and should incorporate the entire spine, shoulders, and lower extremity musculature.[16] Two methods of stretching will be discussed. Passive stretching uses a sustained position,

which should be held for 15 to 30 s, until muscle tightness begins to lessen. This passive stretch should be repeated two to five times.[17] A slow sustained stretch will inhibit an overactive stretch reflex, permitting improved flexibility.[18,19]

Another method to improve flexibility is active stretching. Active stretching works more on the dynamic flexibility of muscle and joint forces. One type of active stretching is the paired-muscle stretch. The paired-muscle stretch uses the relationship of the muscle agonist-antagonist. For example, to actively stretch the hamstring muscle in a seated position, the cyclist actively extends the knee, activating the quadriceps muscle to enhance a relaxation of the hamstring muscle. Active stretching can be held momentarily at the end of the contraction and should be performed five to ten times.[17]

Specific upper extremity flexibility exercises for cyclists should include the wrist extensors, pectoralis major and minor, posterior shoulder girdle, and levator scapulae muscles. Lower extremity stretches should include the hamstrings, quadriceps, hip flexors, iliotibial band, hip rotators, and the gastrocnemius and soleus muscle groups. The cat/camel stretch for the lumbar and thoracic spine and an upper trapezius stretch for the cervical spine complete the stretching routine.[16,20,21]

To prevent either overuse or impact injuries, a cyclist must have adequate strength. Strengthening exercises should be performed in addition to a proper warm-up and stretching activities. Included in a strengthening routine are exercises for the trunk, cervical musculature, upper body, and lower extremity musculature.

STRENGTHENING EXERCISES
Lumbar Spine

Spinal stabilization via lower back and abdominal muscle strength is necessary to maintain a prolonged flexed posture and balance the bicycle. In cycling, the upper extremity muscles must perform both pulling and pushing motions. The upper body pulls on the handlebars during hill climbing or sprinting. Pushing activities aid with supporting the cyclist on the handlebars, shock absorption, controlling the bicycle, and balance. Lower extremity muscle strength is necessary to balance and propel the bicycle efficiently.[16,20,21]

Spinal stabilization exercises can be performed beginning in a supine position and progressing through pelvic bracing, bridging progressions, and quadruped and kneeling stabilization routines.[16] The spine can be challenged and balance reactions improved by performing these exercises on a physioball. Specific lower-back strengthening exercises include prone bilateral leg lifts and prone back extensions. Care should be taken to avoid extreme hyperextension of the lumbar spine. Seated rowing activities are useful to strengthen the lower and midback musculature. One-arm rows and middle and lower trapezius exercises complete the upper back strengthening program.[16,21]

Abdominal Muscles

Abdominal strengthening activities should focus on a balance between all four abdominal muscles. Frequently, the transversus abdominis and external obliques are relatively weak. In addition, there is a shortening of the upper fibers of the rectus abdominis and upper front fibers of the internal obliques. Performing a crunch-type exercise would only serve to enhance this muscle imbalance. A program of controlled leg lifting with a neutral spine at an appropriate strength level is recommended. Once mastery of supine leg-lifting exercises has occurred, sitting positions then should be mastered.[22]

Cervical Spine

Isometric cervical spine strengthening, as well as gravity-resisted lateral bending, extension, and flexion, should be performed to prevent neck trauma. Once a basic level of strength is established, a bicycle helmet can be used to add additional weight for strengthening.[16]

Upper Extremities

Upper extremity strength in cycling is important for maintaining balance and control of the bicycle, shock absorption, and maintaining posture. Exercises to improve upper body pushing function include the chest press, push-ups with a plus, dips, triceps extensions, wrist curls, and triceps push-downs. Additionally, upper body strength is necessary when climbing hills or sprinting. Exercises to enhance upper body pulling on the bicycle include lat pull-downs, biceps curls, upright rowing, and low rowing.[20,21] The muscle groups to target include the biceps, pectoralis, posterior shoulder girdle, middle and lower trapezius, and latissimus dorsi.

Lower Extremities

Lower extremity muscle strengthening activities should focus on the quadriceps, hip flexors, hamstrings, gluteals, and calf musculature. These are the muscle groups most responsible for propulsion of the bicycle. Squats, lunges, hamstring curls, dead lifts, step-ups, and calf raises are basic strengthening activities for these areas. The hamstrings should be strengthened to four-fifths the level of the quadriceps to prevent premature leg fatigue.[20]

Plyometric Exercises

Plyometric exercises can be used to enhance strength and power of the lower extremity musculature. The use of plyometric exercises can result in improved performance and bicycle handling.[19,21] Plyometric exercises should be performed only after a sound conditioning base and regular stretching program have been achieved. Proper landing on a shock-absorbing surface should be mastered before any jumping is initiated. Four types of jumps are recommended for beginners to plyometric training. These include jumping up, bouncing, single-leg hops, and combination jumps. Jumping up should be performed on a stable 6-in. box, progressing to 8 to 12 in.. Jumping up teaches the takeoff action and uses the lower extremity musculature to contract concentrically to accomplish this. A controlled step-down is used instead of jumping down. Once jumping up has been accomplished, bouncing can be performed. Bouncing is basically rope jumping without the rope and can help teach quick reaction off the ground. Hops are next in the progression and are performed initially with both legs and progress to a single leg. The standing long jump is an example of an activity included in the single-leg hop. Horizontal displacement of the center of gravity is learned through single-leg hops. The final type of jump is the combination jump. The purpose of combination jumps is to add more velocity. Skipping would be an example of combination jumps.[19,21]

Cycling-Specific Activities

Cycling-specific activities to enhance injury prevention include balance and agility exercises. These exercises include the balance-ready position, the ability to maintain a straight line, and slalom activities designed specifically for road cyclists. Lifting the front wheel, lifting the back wheel, and finally, the "bunny hop" are good agility drills for mountain bike riders.[20] Proficiency in balance and agility activities can help prevent falls and other impact injuries.

Furthermore, prevention of impact-related injuries should involve bicycle safety education, correct bicycle fit, a properly maintained bicycle, practice of the "rules of the road," and use of bicycle safety equipment.[23,24] Bicycle safety education should target safe riding behavior, including the use of hand signals, riding single file, and using lights for night riding. Practicing the rules of the road includes obeying all traffic laws, including wearing a helmet in some states.[23] The chance of head injury can be reduced by 85 percent with the use of a helmet.[25] Wearing protective headgear and face protection will reduce the incidence of head and face injuries.[23,26]

Improper fit of the bicycle to the rider and improper training techniques are the two important factors to consider when discussing the prevention of cycling injuries.

As with many aerobic activities, improper training techniques contribute to injury. It is important to remind cyclists to progress gradually with their training programs.

Etiology of Injuries

Understanding the cause of an injury can help in prevention or when returning a cyclist to the sport. Two general classifications of factors are those which are intrinsic or inherent to the interplay between the cyclist and the bicycle and those which are extrinsic to the sport or can be seen in many aerobic sports. Improper fit of the bicycle to the rider and the cyclist's biomechanical alignment are two intrinsic factors to consider when discussing the etiology of cycling injuries.

INTRINSIC FACTORS

Biomechanical Factors

There are alignments within the lower extremity that cause the limb to move through excessive motions. These motions can result in excessive stress placed on soft tissues, resulting in overuse syndromes. Additionally, stationary cycling is frequently included in the rehabilitation process following surgery or injury to the lower extremity.[3-5] Specifically, cycling has been advocated following anterior cruciate ligament (ACL) reconstruction. It is important to remember to evaluate the biomechanical alignment of the lower limb prior to using the bicycle on all postoperative lower extremity patients. To keep adverse stresses from inhibiting the healing tissue, the foot must be maintained parallel to the ground.

Forefoot Varus   Forefoot varus is an inverted position of the forefoot on the rear foot. In order for the foot to function like a rigid lever, it must function around neutral. Compensation for a forefoot varus results in excessive subtalar joint pronation with internal rotation of the lower leg, an increased valgus stress across the knee, and adduction of the thigh in the frontal plane. This stretches the medial structures and compresses the lateral structures. Types of injuries include extensor mechanism or "lateral tracking" problems, a medial collateral ligament sprain, quadriceps tendinitis, patellar tendinitis, and medial plica syndrome.[27]

Forefoot Valgus   Forefoot valgus is an everted position of the forefoot on the rear foot. Compensation for a forefoot valgus results in excessive subtalar joint supination with external rotation of the lower leg, an increased varus stress across the knee, and abduction of the thigh in the frontal plane. This stretches structures on the lateral aspect of the knee, compresses medial structures, and forces the patella more medially. Some of the common injuries are a lateral hamstring strain and lateral plica and extensor mechanism syndrome.[27]

Knock Knees   "Knock knees" (genu valgum) are a frontal plane deformity where the knees are close together in a valgus position. As the knee flexes, there is increased internal rotation of the tibia, resulting in stretching of the medial structures and compression of the lateral structures.[27]

Abnormal Angle of Gait   An abnormal angle of gait results in an excessive toe-in or toe-out position of the foot. In this case, the cleat should be adjusted so that the ankle,

knee, and thigh remain parallel. If excessive malleolar torsion is present, caution should be taken to limit the amount of toeing in.[28] Excessive toeing in of a naturally toed-out limb may place undue stress on the anterior cruciate ligament by excessively rotating the tibia anterolaterally.

Leg-Length Discrepancies   Leg-length discrepancies can involve a lengthened femoral or tibial component. A long leg usually will try to shorten its length through excessive compensatory movements. This excessive motion can take place at the foot, knee, or hip. At the foot, a long leg may pronate excessively. If this occurs, increased internal rotation of the lower leg can cause an increased stress at the knee. Injuries from this increased stress can simulate a forefoot varus malalignment. The short leg may supinate, resulting in injuries similar to a forefoot valgus malalignment. At the knee, in the frontal plane, the long leg may assume either a bowlegged or knock-kneed position to shorten. The bowlegged position will stretch the lateral knee structures and compress the medial structures. Conversely, the knock-kneed position will stretch the medial structures and compress the lateral knee structures. At the knee in the sagittal plane, the long leg typically stays more flexed than the shorter limb. At the pelvis, the short leg may try to lengthen by tilting to the same side. This will cause trunk rotation to the opposite side, placing abnormal stress on the lower back. Treatment for a leg-length discrepancy depends on which segment is short. It is recommended to use a shorter crank if the thigh is short and to lift the shoe if the tibial component is short.[29]

EXTRINSIC FACTORS

Extrinsic factors contributing to cycling injuries include improper training practices and improper riding technique. As with many aerobic activities, cyclists do not allow enough time to progress to their goal. Enough preparation time prior to an event must be scheduled to permit a safe progression of frequency, duration, and intensity of miles on the bicycle. A heart rate monitor is one method to apprise a cyclist if he or she is progressing at a reasonable rate or overtraining.

Improper Training

As with many aerobic activities, improper training techniques contribute to injury. It is important to remind cyclists to limit distance and intensity when starting out. This will allow the soft tissues time to adapt to the increased demands of cycling. A general rule of thumb is to limit weekly mileage increases to 10 percent divided throughout the entire week's training schedule.[16] Additionally, early-season rides should focus on low-resistance, high-cadence workouts with an emphasis on proper riding technique. Some cycling specialists recommend that serious cyclists begin each season with 1000 mi of spinning at a high cadence with the handlebars in a slightly higher position, gradually lowering the handlebars and assuming a more aerodynamic position. Excessive climbing or using low gears for an extended time should be limited during the early season.[16] As mentioned in Chap. 9, the body *responds* to small increments in change but *reacts* to large increments in change. This is the philosophy a cyclist should follow in the early season.

Heart rate should be a guiding factor for evaluating the level of intensity of an aerobic activity and as a measure of nonadaptive responses of the body to training demands. A heart rate monitor may be helpful in quantifying the physiologic demands placed on the body during exercise. The continuous feedback enables a quick adjustment of intensity to stay within a desired range. Different heart rate zones can be identified based on a percentage of maximum heart rate. A basic starting percentage of 50 to 60 percent maximum heart rate should be set when just beginning a fitness program. As aerobic fitness increases, 60 to 70 percent maximum heart

rate should be attained. Once a basic level of fitness is achieved, most workouts should be done in the 70 to 80 percent maximum heart rate zone. Higher levels of heart rate training in the 80 to 90 percent and 90 to 100 percent zones are used when anaerobic power training is desired for small amounts of time. As training is performed at an increasingly higher percentage of maximum heart rate, there is a proportionately higher risk of musculoskeletal and cardiovascular injury. Heart rate also can be used as a measure of overtraining. Once a baseline for morning resting heart rate is established, the cyclist can evaluate his or her body's response to training. A morning resting heart rate that is elevated by 5 to 10 beats per minute can be a sign of overtraining.[30]

Improper Cyclist-Bicycle Fit

Generally speaking, an improperly fitted bicycle can contribute to many overuse injuries. The most common site of overuse injuries in the lower extremity is the knee joint. Saddle height, saddle fore/aft, and crank arm length should be evaluated when treating patients with knee joint injuries.

Riding Technique

A rigid riding posture with the elbows locked or in an extended position for prolonged periods of time can lead to overuse syndromes of the upper extremities, neck, and back. Frequent changing of hand position to at least three different positions while on the bicycle, stretching, and changing the neck position can help to eliminate injuries to the upper extremities, back, and neck.[16,31]

Common Injuries and Their Rehabilitation

Understanding the biomechanics of the cycle stroke can help explain the origin of injuries associated with cycling. There are basically two broad categories of injuries: (1) those due to an impact with an external object and (2) those created by overuse.[32] Numerous studies have cited crashing as the major factor in impact cycling injuries.[32–34] For road bicycles, falling by losing control of the bicycle accounts for approximately 50 percent of the impact injuries. Only 17 percent were a result of collisions with automobiles.[23] In contrast, 81.2 percent of acute injuries due to falling downhill was recorded in off-road bicycle racing.[33] Of all impact injuries, abrasions constitute the majority of injuries, followed by contusions, lacerations, and fractures.[32,33]

Overuse injuries make up the second category of cycling injuries. They include injuries secondary to repetitive microtrauma and poor training techniques as well as those due to improper bicycle fit and poor biomechanical alignment.[9,16,28,32] This section will discuss common cycling injuries and their treatment and will focus on both impact and overuse injuries for the upper extremities, lower extremities, and trunk.

UPPER EXTREMITIES

Impact injuries for the upper extremities usually occur when trying to break a fall. In recreational cyclists over 35 years of age, the upper extremities remain the most frequent site of fractures at 41.9 percent.[35] The scaphoid, distal radius, radial head, and radial neck are the most common upper extremity fracture sites. Additionally, clavicle fractures and acromioclavicular (AC) separations are common shoulder injuries.[33] The incidence of clavicular fractures in racers is high.[26,32]

Ulnar Nerve Neuropathy

Ulnar nerve neuropathy is characterized by loss of sensation or muscular weakness along the area supplied by the ulnar nerve. It is most commonly the result of prolonged compression. During passage through the ulnar tunnel, the nerve splits into a deep and superficial branch. The superficial branch supplies sensation to the hypothenar eminence, the volar ring, and the little fingers. The deep branch supplies motor function to the interosseous muscles, the abductor digiti quinti and flexor digiti quinti, and the flexor pollicis brevis musculature. Three syndromes have been identified and are associated with compression ranging from sensory loss to motor loss to a combination of both sensory and motor loss. Typically, the type of syndrome corresponds to the site of the compression. When only sensory changes are evident, the superficial sensory branch of the nerve has been affected. Motor loss indicates compression of the deep motor branch only. Both sensory and motor loss indicates that the compression has occurred prior to the division of the nerve. The mechanism of injury is prolonged pressure to the wrist or repetitive stress. It is usually brought on by poor bicycle-rider fit and poor riding technique. A bicycle that has too long of a "reach" (the distance from the toe of the saddle to the handlebars) will result in increased pressure on the cyclist's wrists. Changing the stem length and raising the handlebars will decrease this stress. Proper adjustment should result in keeping less than one-third of the cyclist's weight on his or her hands. Additionally, changing the hand position frequently to at least three different postures helps to decrease stress to the ulnar nerve. The addition of padded gloves and padded handlebars is recommended to decrease the stress as well.[36]

Median Nerve Neuropathy

Median nerve neuropathy in cyclists is less common and is characterized by numbness along the median nerve distribution usually as a result of compression. The mechanism of injury is prolonged pressure over the carpal tunnel. The roof of the carpal tunnel is heavier and stiffer than the ulnar tunnel and is thus more resistant to prolonged pressures. The biomechanical factors and treatment are the same as for ulnar nerve compression.[31,36]

DeQuervain's Tenosynovitis

Tenosynovitis of the extensor pollicis brevis and abductor pollicis longus tendons is characterized by pain on abduction and extension of the thumb. Pain also may occur with flexion of the thumb and ulnar deviation of the wrist. This is usually seen in off-road cyclists secondary to the increased gripping and continuous shifting necessary in this type of cycling. The mechanism of injury may be direct trauma, overuse, repetitive stress, excessive vibration, or movements creating a sharp bend of the tendons. Changing the type or position of the gearshift levers may be helpful in decreasing the stress on the tendons. Using a good suspension system on the front of the bicycle may decrease the stress from vibration.[36]

Treatment for upper extremity overuse injuries in cycling usually involves rest and repositioning of the forces through the upper extremity. Forearm flexion and extension exercises in a limited range using the Body Blade may assist with improved muscle function necessary to manage the increased stress of excessive vibration.

LOWER EXTREMITIES

Impact injuries in the form of fractures are relatively uncommon. Occasionally, spoke injuries occur when the foot is caught between the wheel and the frame. Of greater importance is the incidence of lower extremity overuse injuries.

In cyclists, pain in and around the knee is the most common lower extremity overuse injury.[9] It has been reported that knee injuries account for 25 percent of the reported cycling injuries.[14] Management of all nontraumatic cycling injuries should include an evaluation of the rider-bicycle fit, a biome-

chanical alignment evaluation, and an assessment of the cyclist's training practices.[9,16] The following discussion on overuse injuries will take into consideration these topics.

Chondromalacia Patella

Chondromalacia patella is characterized by a wearing of the articular cartilage of the posterior aspect of the patella or chronic synovial inflammation.[9,31] The pain may be brought on by hilly rides, too slow a cadence, or "pushing" large gears. The mechanism of injury is excessive patellofemoral loading throughout the pedal stroke. This might be due to a saddle height that is too low and/or too far forward.[9,31]

Biomechanical alignment may show either dynamic or static malalignment of the patellofemoral joint. The patella may exhibit poor tracking. Treatment should include correction of the seat position, a thorough quadriceps and hip external rotator strengthening program, and visual feedback to ensure that the patella traces an elliptical line through space that is centered over the middle of the pedal. Hamstring and tensor fasciae latae–iliotibial band stretching exercises and McConnell taping should be performed to help decrease the lateral tracking. Training practices should include easy spinning with low resistance on flat surfaces.[9,31]

Patellar Tendinitis

Patellar tendinitis is characterized by complaints of patellar pain at the insertion of the tendon on the inferior patellar pole. The pain is usually brought on by an increase in hill work or mileage. The mechanism of injury during cycling is usually excessive angular traction. This might be due to a saddle that is either too low or too far forward.[9,31]

Biomechanical alignment reveals internal malleolar torsion or excessive subtalar joint pronation. Treatment is centered on proper positioning, participation in only painfree cycling, cycling orthoses (which are more rigid and longer than running orthoses), and/or floating-cleat systems. When floating-cleat systems are used, the float is limited to 5 degrees.[1,9] Treatment emphasizes a decrease in stress across the patellar tendon until the pain subsides.

Quadriceps Tendinitis

Quadriceps tendinitis is characterized by pain at the suprapatellar area. The pain may be either medial or lateral and may have been brought on by an increase in mileage, hill work, or riding into a head wind. The mechanism of injury is repetitive overload of the quadriceps tendon. The saddle position may be too low and/or too far forward. In addition, the cleats may be too far forward or excessively rotated. Poor training techniques early in the season are frequently to blame.[1,9,31]

Biomechanical alignment reveals an excessive varus or valgus angle within the lower extremity. An excessive varus angle stretches the lateral structures of the knee. Spacers placed between the pedal and crank arm can be used to improve the stance width and thus the alignment. An excessive valgus angle stretches the medial structures of the knee. Cants placed between the pedal and the shoe on the medial side of the pedal can help to reduce the valgus angle. Cycling orthoses also may improve the valgus malalignment. Floating-pedal systems should be used to limit the floatation to 5 degrees. Regaining an adequate training base is one of the goals of treatment. Only painfree weight training and high-cadence miles are recommended in the treatment of quadriceps tendinitis.[9,31]

Medial Plica/Medial Patellofemoral Ligament

Medial knee pain is seen commonly in cyclists and usually is the result of irritation of either the medial plica or the medial patellofemoral ligament. The function of the medial patellofemoral ligament is to passively restrict patellar excursion. The cyclist may describe the medial knee pain as disabling, with a popping sensation occurring with each pedal stroke. The mechanism of injury is excessive traction on the medial patellofemoral ligament as the patella is pulled away laterally from the midline. Internal tibial rotation, excessively externally rotated cleats, or improper saddle position may be the reason the patella is pulled laterally. In this case, the saddle may be either too high or set too far back.[9]

Biomechanical alignment may reveal internal tibial rotation, valgus knees, or active pronation. Cleat position should be corrected to mirror the position of the tibial rotation. Cants placed between the shoe and the pedal on the medial side of the pedal can help to reduce the valgus angle. Cycling orthoses may improve the valgus alignment. Floating-pedal systems should be used to limit flotation to 5 degrees. Painfree cycling, easy spinning, and no hills are recommended in the treatment of medial knee pain. Surgical intervention may be necessary to remove a thickened plica.[9]

Iliotibial Band Syndrome

Iliotibial band (ITB) syndrome is characterized by pain on the lateral aspect of the knee. This irritation is the result of repetitive friction force across the lateral femoral condyle.[9,31] During the cycling stroke, the ITB is pulled anteriorly on the downstroke and posteriorly on the upstroke. The mechanism of injury may include excessive pronation with internal tibial rotation, excessively internally rotated cleats, or improper saddle height. In this case, the saddle might be too high or set too far back.[1,9]

Biomechanical alignment may reveal a varus knee or forefoot position. Saddle height and cleat position should be corrected. Spacers can be placed between the pedal and the crank arm to decrease the stress. Excessive pronation should be corrected with foot orthoses. Floating pedals may be of some benefit in limiting the amount of internal tibial rotation. Regaining an adequate training base is one of the goals of treatment. Only pain-free weight training and high-cadence miles are recommended in the treatment of ITB syndrome.[9]

Biceps Femoris Tendinitis

Biceps femoris tendinitis is characterized by posterolateral knee pain. There is point tenderness of the insertion of the tendon into the fibular head. Saddles that are too high or too far forward may stress the biceps tendon, as may excessively toed-in cleats.[9]

Biomechanical alignment reveals a knee varus or a long leg. Saddle position and cleat position should be corrected. This is performed by lowering the seat and reducing the toe-in position of the cleats. Spacers between the pedal and crank arm may improve the varus alignment. Correction of the short leg for a tibial length difference can be accomplished by placing a lift between the shoe and the cleat. For a short femoral length, a shorter crank may be necessary or repositioning of the foot on the pedal.[1] The short leg should be moved back about a third of the leg-length difference, and the long leg should be moved forward the same amount.[9] Only painfree riding and a restriction in weight training exercises are recommended.

Achilles Tendinitis

Foot and ankle injuries to cyclists are rare due to the decreased joint compressive forces that cycling affords. Achilles tendinitis is characterized by pain on the heel at the insertion of the Achilles tendon. The mechanism of injury usually involves excessive ankling, improper shoe wear, improper foot placement, or excessive pronation.[9]

Biomechanical alignment reveals an excessive pes planus foot and/or a leg-length discrepancy. Foot placement over the pedal spindle and without excessive toeing in should be corrected. Evaluation of the stiff-

ness of the cycling shoe should be performed. A stiff-soled cycling shoe is desired. Cycling orthoses may be helpful in treating athletes with a pes planus foot type. If the short leg has not been treated, excessive plantar flexion is necessary to reach the pedal. Appropriate treatment of a leg-length discrepancy is necessary. Only painfree riding on flat terrain should be permitted until the symptoms subside. A change in riding technique by decreasing ankling may be necessary to improve the cyclist's condition. Taping the ankle to assist with plantarflexion may be helpful in reducing symptoms.[9]

Once changes in the rider-bicycle fit and an evaluation of the rider's biomechanical alignment have been completed, specific therapeutic exercises should be incorporated into the cyclist's rehabilitation program. For patellar and quadriceps tendinitis, isometric quadriceps strengthening activities followed by isotonic strengthening exercises should be emphasized. The sport of cycling uses the muscles of the lower extremities in a predominately concentric fashion with a limited joint load. Therefore, either open or closed kinetic chain concentric quadriceps and hamstring strengthening activities would be appropriate in rehabilitation. For the treatment of chondromalacia patella, limiting the amount of knee flexion in closed kinetic chain activities while conversely limiting the amount of extension in open kinetic chain activities would be appropriate. All these conditions also would benefit from quadriceps and hamstring stretching activities as well as hip extensor and external rotator strengthening exercises. Incorporating hip strengthening will assist with excessive femoral internal rotation. ITB tendinitis treatment should include strengthening of the gluteus medius and hip rotator musculature and an aggressive tensor fasciae latae (TFL) stretching program. Bicycle stretches for the hamstrings and Achilles musculature can be performed while riding to help with treatment of biceps femoris and

Achilles tendinitis and improve the flexibility of these muscles.[9,16]

HEAD AND FACE INJURIES

Head and face injuries are common.[33] Off-road cyclists have about 20.5 percent more facial fractures than road cyclists. Fatalities due to cycling are approximately 0.1 percent, usually involve head injuries, and are most common in the riders between 5 and 15 years of age.[35]

SPINE

Impact injuries to the trunk are uncommon and usually are seen only in children. Overuse injuries to the spine are very common and incorporate all regions of the spine. These overuse injuries are associated with an increased load on the upper extremities to support the rider and hyperextension of the neck.[16,31] Because of the cycling posture and the position of the handlebars, injuries to the cervical spine are more common than injuries to the thoracic and lumbar areas. Two specific neck problems have been identified: myofascial trigger points caused by overuse and poor riding posture and multiple microwhiplash injury.[16]

Trigger Points

Trigger points are irritable portions in the muscle or fascia that send pain signals to the central nervous system, resulting in a spasm-pain-spasm cycle. Common sites for trigger points in cyclists include the levator scapulae, splenius capitis, trapezius, sternocleidomastoid, infraspinatus, supraspinatus, and rhomboid muscles.[16] The most common sites for trigger points in cyclists are the left levator scapula and trapezius muscles. This is presumably due to riding on the right side of the road while rotating left to look for overtaking traffic. In addition to a left levator scapula injury, prolonged hyperextension may result in bilateral levator scapulae injuries as these muscles work to hold the head in that position.[16]

Microwhiplash Injury

The second specific neck injury, multiple microwhiplash injury, occurs in endurance riders riding in the "drops" (hands in the curved portion of the handlebars). Cumulative microtrauma is imparted to the neck if it is held in a hyperextended position or when using overinflated tires. Multiple jarring motions are absorbed by the cervical tissues, resulting in severe pain and an inability to hold the neck in an extended position.[16]

Treatment for neck pain involves adjusting the position of the rider on the bike as well as encouraging specific strengthening and stretching exercises. On the bicycle, stretches for the levator scapulae and upper trapezius can help alleviate trigger point problems. Cervical stabilization activities and gentle cervical isotonic strengthening and a general postural strengthening program to decrease cervical hyperextension should be incorporated in the treatment of cervical overuse injuries.[16]

Decreasing the amount of hyperextension of the neck by altering the bicycle should be considered when treating cyclists with either of the neck syndromes mentioned. Methods to change the neck position include raising the handlebars, using handlebars with a smaller drop, using a shorter stem, or moving the seat forward.[16,31] Care must be taken so that altering the seat fore/aft position does not result in knee pain. Additional equipment changes may include padded handlebars, padded gloves, wider and minimally inflated tires to reduce the amount of road shock, use of a lighter helmet, addition of a mirror for rear viewing of traffic, and finally, changing to upright handlebars to allow a more upright position.[16]

Improving the rider's technique is equally important in treating neck pain. A static, rigid posture with locked elbows increases the amount of road shock, thus increasing the amount of stress transferred to the rider's shoulders and neck. A recommended cycling position is with the arms, upper back, and elbows relaxed. In addition, the frequent changing of hand positions and performing stretches while cycling can result in reduced shoulder and neck pain.[16,31]

Injuries to the thoracic spine have been reported in the French and Belgium medical literature. Signs of Scheuermann's disease have been reported in as many as 40 percent of the bicycle racers less than 20 years of age.[16] Scheuermann's disease encompasses a narrowing or wedging of the anterior portion of the vertebral body. It is theorized that in the adolescent athlete, the extreme kyphotic posture places increased pressure on the vertebral end plates, remodeling the anterior aspect of the vertebral body into a wedge shape. Pulling too hard with the upper body while pedaling a large gear encourages the development of Scheuermann's disease.[16]

Treatment for thoracic spine injuries should include a good off-season cross-training and postural program to reduce the kyphotic position. Physioball or foam roller extension exercises as well as middle and lower trapezius strengthening exercises should be incorporated in programs for the young cyclist. Additionally, stretching of the pectoralis and anterior chest musculature should be employed. A stretch for the thoracic spine can be performed while riding the bicycle to reduce the tension in the muscles of the thoracic spine.[16]

As stated previously, the incidence of low-back pain is less than cervical pain and is usually associated with a poor rider-cycle fit. The pelvis and lower back constitute a platform that is responsible for powering the bicycle. The stability of this platform will decide the effectiveness of the cyclist. Therefore, the fore/aft and side-to-side position of the lumbar spine must be evaluated. The fore/aft position of the pelvis is controlled by a balance between the quadriceps and hamstring musculature. Tight iliopsoas and quadriceps muscle groups tend to pull the pelvis into an anterior pelvic tilt. Conversely, if the hamstrings are tight, anterior pelvic motion is restricted, resulting in increased flexion from the lumbar spine.[16]

For maximum power output and injury prevention, the rider should maintain the pelvis in a neutral position. An increase in the lordotic curve can be the result of poor rider-cycle fit. Possible reasons for this poor fit include a bicycle that is too long (either the stem or the top tube), handlebars that are too low, and too much downward tilt of the saddle. The result of an excessive lordotic curve is painful pressure on the posterior spinal elements. Conversely, too short of a top tube can result in extreme flexion of the lumbar spine causing intervertebral disk pain.[16]

Side-to-side balance of the pelvis is determined by the seat height. A rider who rocks from side to side in order to pedal is fit with a seat that is too high. A leg-length discrepancy also will create the same side-to-side movement. The side bending and rotation that occurs with this motion will stress the facet joints.

Treatment for low-back pain should include hamstring and lower-back stretching and many of the spinal stabilization activities discussed in the injury prevention section. The "on the bicycle stretches" for the hamstrings and calf musculature (Fig. 16.5) as well as lower and thoracic spine musculature previously presented should be incorporated into the rehabilitation program. Additionally, three cycling-specific functional abdominal exercises—the kneeling ball roll (Fig. 16.6), single-leg-stance trunk sidebending, and beachball oscillations while leaning forward in high kneeling—can facilitate a return to the sport.[20]

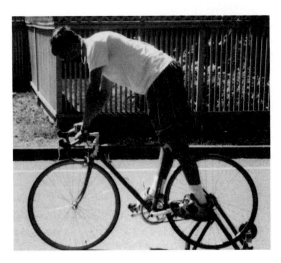

FIGURE 16.5

On-bike gastrocnemius stretch.

Return to Sport

Returning the cyclist to the sport of cycling following an injury can be a challenge for the health care professional. Recreational and competitive cyclists should begin with an amount of easy spinning at 80 to 90 rpm that can be accomplished without the return of symptoms. This may be as little as 5 to 10 min every other day.[29] Gradually, the cyclist increases the workout. To increase the time on the bicycle safely, an endurance training

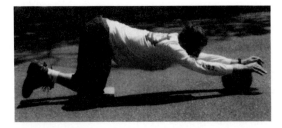

FIGURE 16.6

Kneeling ball rolling for flexibility and strength.

or aerobic base is established first. This is followed by fast interval training and finally by slow interval or anaerobic training. The variables of frequency, duration, and intensity are manipulated to accomplish these goals. Frequency of the activity is increased first, followed by duration and finally intensity.[29] Two programs will be presented for a safe return to cycling.

A program of progressing athletes through various levels of endurance, speed, and anaerobic training has been set forth by Garrick.[29] Level 1, the endurance training segment, begins with 5 to 10 min of easy spinning every other day and progressing to 30 min four times weekly. Garrick recommends that competitive cyclists expand this level to 90 min. At the end of level 1, short sprint training, or level 2, begins. This includes 5- to 15-s intervals of fast spinning with 30-s to 2-min rest intervals of easy spinning. If five or six cycling workouts are completed in a week, two or three of them are level 2. Progressing to level 3 can be accomplished once the cyclist can perform 20 min or more of 5-s sprints on the half-minute.[29]

Level 3 training comprises 30- to 60-s or more work intervals and shorter rest periods. The variable of intensity is increased as the cyclist maintains the same cadence and increases the workload while performing the work interval. An example would be to increase the workload every 5 min for 30 s by increasing the resistance. During the week, two level 1 workouts, two level 2 workouts, and two level 3 workouts should be completed before resuming event-specific cycling training.[29]

Training for a specific cycling event must take into consideration both the length of the event and the amount of preparation time available prior to the event. The second program addresses recommendations for adequate preparation times for selected cycling events. For example, riding 100 mi on the road or off-road cycling 5 h would require 9 weeks of preparation time. The preparation time is divided into three training phases, and weekly training plans are provided.[20]

The first phase includes basic cycling mileage. The second phase enhances strength and improves the cyclist's aerobic capacity. Finally, the third phase is training for a specific event. Once the event mileage is set, a program of weekly goal mileage is devised. It is necessary to count backward from the event date to determine these goals. A sample template proposed by Moren's return-to-cycling schedule[20] would be helpful in understanding this process. If the mileage of a selected event is 150 mi, 12 weeks are necessary to train safely for this event. Phase 1 is designed to allow for endurance training and is 5 weeks in length. The peak mileage goal (PMG) should equal the distance of the event (150 mi). Weekly mileage goals (WMG) are a percentage of the PMG. During phase 1, the WMG should be no more than 60 percent of the PMG. An 8 percent increase in miles per week will guarantee a slow progression toward the PMG. The general equation would be WMG = PMG × phase percent PMG – (percent increase/week × PMG × week number). For week 1 in phase 1, the equation would be as follows: WMG = 150 × 0.6 – (0.08 × 150 × 5). The WMG for week 1 in phase 1 would be 30 mi. A translation into road mileage would be a long ride of 30 mi for that week.[20]

Phase 2 is designed to enhance the cyclist's cycling aerobic capacity and is 4 weeks in length. WMG should be no more than 70 percent of the PMG. A 5 percent increase in miles per week should be realized to reach the PMG. The specific equation for week 4 in phase 2 would be as follows WMG = 150 × 0.7 – (0.05 × 150 × 1). Thus, 97.5 mi would be the WMG for week 4 during phase 2.[20]

Phase 3 is the specific preparation phase for the selected event. This phase is 3 weeks in length. The WMG during this week is 100 percent of the race distance. A 10 percent in-

crease in miles per week is included in this phase. The mileage equation for week 2 of phase 3 would be as follows: WMG = 150 – (0.10 × 150 × 2).

Once the WMG is fixed, a weekly training program can be established. This consists of 4 days of training. A percentage of the WMG is performed throughout the week. During phase 1, one workout of 45 percent, two workouts of 20 percent, and one workout of 100 percent WMG are performed. The duration of the workouts increases in phase 2 with an increase in the percentage of WMG. Phase 2 uses two workouts of 30 percent, one workout of 100 percent, and one workout of 25 percent WMG. Remember the weekly mileage increases as the week progresses. In addition to a percentage increase of the WMG in phase 2, Moren recommends interval training similar to Garrick. Phase 3 uses the same percentages of WMG as phase 2. Remember that the WMG during phase 3 is 100 percent of the race distance.[20]

Two return-to-sport scenarios have been presented to help the clinician return the cyclist to the sport in a painfree and systematic fashion. It should be noted that proper equipment, particularly cycling shoes, should be worn during all phases of these programs.

Summary

Bicycling remains a popular recreational, competitive, and rehabilitative activity for the general population, serious athletes, and recovering patients. Over the past decade, cycling has risen in popularity and stature, and bikes are no longer considered a toy for amusement. With a sound knowledge of the biomechanics of cycling, rider fit, and strengthening and conditioning principles, the majority of cycling injuries can be prevented or rehabilitated successfully.

References

1. Kronish R: Bicycling injuries, in Sallis RE, Massimino F (eds): *ACSM's Essentials of Sports Medicine*, St. Louis: Mosby–Year Book, 1996, p 571.

2. Kyle CR: Energy and aerodynamics in bicycling. *Clin Sports Med Bicycling Injuries* 13(1): 39–73, 1994.

3. Fleming BC, Beynnon BD, Renstrom PA, et al: The strain behavior of the anterior cruciate ligament during bicycling: an in vivo study. *Am J Sports Med* 26(1):109–118, 1998.

4. Henning CE, Lynch MA, Glick KR: An in vivo strain gage study of elongation of the anterior cruciate ligament. *Am J Sports Med* 13(1): 22–26, 1985.

5. McLeod WD, Blackburn TA: Biomechanics of knee rehabilitation with cycling. *Am J Sports Med* 8(3):175–180, 1980.

6. Burke ER: Proper fit of the bicycle. *Clin Sports Med* 13(1):1–14, 1994.

7. Cavanagh PR, Sanderson DJ: The biomechanics of cycling: Studies of the pedaling mechanics of elite pursuit riders, in Burke ER (ed): *Science of Cycling*. Champaign, IL: Human Kinetics, 1986, p 91.

8. Ryschon TW: Physiologic aspects of bicycling. *Clin Sports Med* 13(1):15–38, 1994.

9. Holmes JC, Pruitt AL, Whalen NJ: Lower extremity overuse in bicycling. *Clin Sports Med* 13(1):187–205, 1994.

10. Kolin MJ, de la Rosa DM: *The Custom Bicycle*. Rodale Press, 1979.

11. Ericson MO, Nisell R, Nemeth G: Joint motions of the lower limb during ergometer cycling. *J Orthop Sports Phys Ther* 9:273, 1988.

12. Jorge M, Hull ML: Analysis of EMG measurements during bicycle pedalling. *J Biomech* 19(9):683–694, 1986.

13. Ericson MO: Muscular function during ergometer cycling. *Scand J Rehabil Med* 20(1): 35–41, 1988.

14. O'Brien T: Lower extremity cycling biomechanics: A review and theoretical discussion. *J Am Podiatr Med Assoc* 81(11):585–592, 1991.

15. Musnick D: Exercise physiology, in Musnick D, Pierce M, Elliott SK (eds): *Conditioning for Outdoor Fitness*, 1st ed. Seattle: Mountaineers, 1999, p 16.

16. Mellion MB: Neck and back pain in bicycling. *Clin Sports Med* 13(1):137–164, 1994.

17. Zanoni M, Musnick D: Warm-up and stretching, in Musnick D, Pierce M, Elliott SK (eds): *Conditioning for Outdoor Fitness*, 1st ed. Seattle: Mountaineers, 1999, p 52.

18. Feingold ML: Flexibility standards of the US cycling team, in Burke ER (ed): *Science of Cycling*. Champaign, IL: Human Kinetics, 1986, p 3.

19. Burke ER: *Cycling Health and Physiology: Using Sports Science to Improve Your Riding and Racing*. College Park, MD: Vitesse Press, 1998.

20. Moren E: Conditioning for road and mountain bicycling, in Musnick D, Pierce M, Elliott SK (eds): *Conditioning for Outdoor Fitness*, 1st ed. Seattle: Mountaineers, 1999, p 271.

21. Burke ER: *Off-Season Training for Cyclists*. Boulder, CO: Velo Press, 1997.

22. Hall C, Pierce M: The abdominal region, in Musnick D, Pierce M, Elliott SK (eds): *Conditioning for Outdoor Fitness*, 1st ed. Seattle: Mountaineers, 1999, p 146.

23. Weiss BD: Bicycle-related head injuries. *Clin Sports Med* 13(1):99–112, 1994.

24. Ellis TH, Streight D, Mellion MB: Bicycle safety equipment. *Clin Sports Med* 13(1): 75–98, 1994.

25. Thompson RS, Rivara FP, Thompson DC: A case control study of the effectiveness of bicycle safety helmets. *New Engl J Med* 321(17): 1194–1196, 1989.

26. Gassner RJ, Hackl W, Tuli T, et al: Differential profile of facial injuries among mountain bikers compared with bicyclists. *J Trauma* 47(1): 50–54, 1999.

27. Francis PR: Injury prevention for cyclists: A biomechanical approach, in Burke ER (ed): *Science of Cycling*. Champaign, IL: Human Kinetics, 1986, p 185.

28. Markolf KL, Burchfield DM, Shapiro MM, et al: Combined knee loading states that generate high anterior cruciate ligament forces. *J Orthop Res* 13(6):930–955, 1995.

29. Garrick JG, Webb DR: Overuse injuries relative rest/alternative training, in Garrick JG, Webb DR (eds): *Sports Injuries: Diagnosis and Management*, 2d ed. Philadelphia: Saunders, 1999, p 40.

30. Sager-Dolan D, Musnick D: Aerobic conditioning and interval training, in Musnick D, Pierce M, Elliott SK (eds): *Conditioning for Outdoor Fitness,* 1st ed. Seattle: Mountaineers, 1999, p 22.

31. Conti-Wyneken AR: Bicycling injuries. *Phys Med Rehabil Clin N Am* 10(1):67–76, 1999.

32. Powell B: Medical aspects of racing, in Burke ER (ed): *Science of Cycling.* Champaign, IL: Human Kinetics, 1986, p 185.

33. Kronisch RL, Chow TK, Simon LM, et al: Acute injuries in off-road bicycle racing. *Am J Sports Med* 24(1):88–93 , 1996.

34. Dannenberg AL, Needle S, Mullady D, et al: Predictors of injury among 1638 riders in recreational long-distance bicycle tour: Cycle across Maryland. *Am J Sports Med* 24(6): 747–753, 1996.

35. Lofthouse GA: Traumatic injuries to the extremities and thorax. *Clin Sports Med* 13(1): 113–135, 1994.

36. Richmond DR: Handlebar problems in bicycling. *Clin Sports Med* 13(1):165–173, 1994.

Additional References

Ericson MO, Bratt A, Nisell R, et al: Load moments about the hip and knee joints during ergometer cycling. *Scand J Rehabil Med* 18(4): 165–172, 1986.

Ericson MO, Bratt A, Nisell R, et al: Power output and work in different muscle groups during ergometer cycling. *Eur J Appl Physiol* 55(3): 229–235, 1986.

Ericson MO, Ekholm J, Svensson O, Nisell R: The forces of ankle joint structures during ergometer cycling. *Foot Ankle* 6(3):135–142, 1985.

Ericson MO, Nisell R: Efficiency of pedal forces during ergometer cycling. *Int J Sports Med* 9(2):188–122, 1988.

Ericson MO, Nisell R: Patellofemoral joint forces during ergometer cycling. *Phys Ther* 67(9): 1365–1369, 1987.

Ericson MO, Nisell R: Tibiofemoral joint forces during ergometer cycling. *Am J Sports Med* 14(4):285–290, 1986.

Ericson MO, Nisell R, Arborelius UP, Ekholm J: Muscular activity during ergometer cycling. *Scand J Rehabil Med* 17(2):53–61, 1985.

Hull ML, Jorge M: A method for biomechanical analysis of bicycle pedalling. *J Biomech* 18(9): 631–644, 1985.

Mellion MB: Common cycling injuries, management and prevention. *Sports Med* 11(1): 52–70, 1991.

Rivara FP, Thompson DC, Thompson RS: Epidemiology of bicycle injuries and risk factors for serious injury. *Inj Prev* 3(2):110–114, 1997.

Weiss BD: Clinical syndromes associated with bicycle seats. *Clin Sports Med* 13(1):175–186, 1994.

Index

Page numbers followed by f indicates figures; page numbers followed by t indicates tables.

A